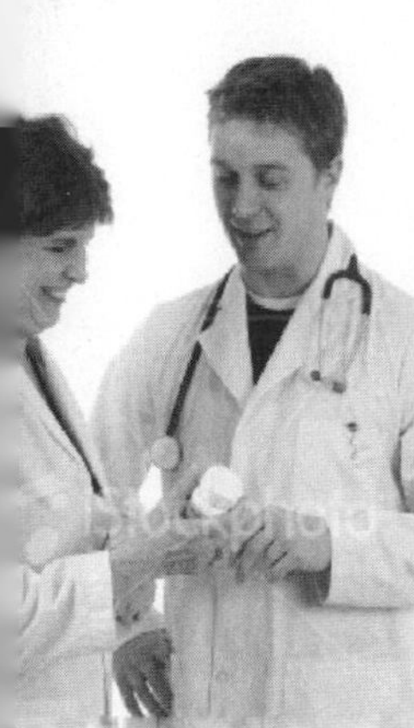

PHARMACY MANAGEMENT

ESSENTIALS FOR ALL PRACTICE SETTINGS

Notice

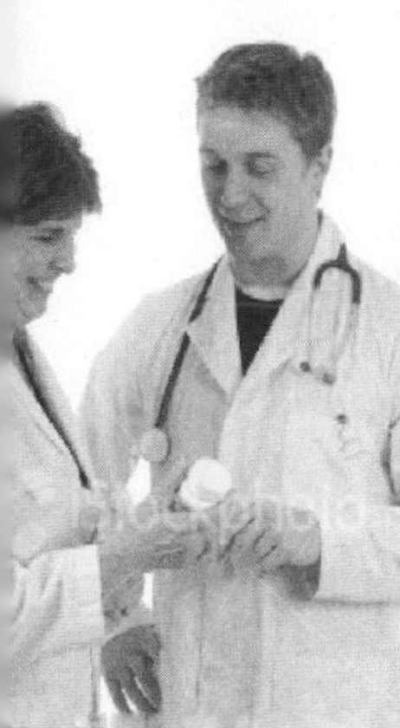

PHARMACY MANAGEMENT

ESSENTIALS FOR ALL PRACTICE SETTINGS

THIRD EDITION

Shane P. Desselle, RPh, PhD, FAPhA
Dean and Professor
College of Pharmacy
California Northstate University
Rancho Cordova, California

David P. Zgarrick, PhD
Professor and Chair
Department of Pharmacy Practice
School of Pharmacy
Bouvé College of Health Sciences
Northeastern University
Boston, Massachusetts

Greg L. Alston, PharmD
Associate Professor and Assistant Dean
for Assessment
Wingate University School of Pharmacy
Wingate, North Carolina

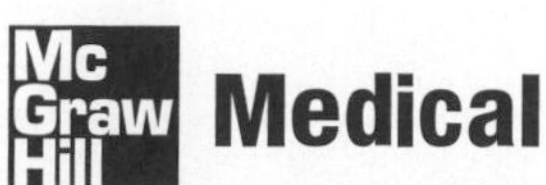

New York Chicago San Francisco Lisbon London Madrid Mexico City
Milan New Delhi San Juan Seoul Singapore Sydney Toronto

Pharmacy Management: Essentials for All Practice Settings, Third Edition

1 2 3 4 5 6 7 8 9 0 DOC/DOC 17 16 15 14 13 12

ISBN 978-0-07-177431-4
MHID 0-07-177431-9

This book was set in Adobe Garamond by Aptara®, Inc.
The editors were Michael Weitz and Christina M. Thomas.
The production supervisor was Sherri Souffrance.
Project management was provided by Sandhya Joshi of Aptara®, Inc.
The cover designer was LaShae V. Ortiz; the cover image is by George Doyle, the left inset is by moodboard, the center inset is by Bruce Ayres, and the right inset is by Fuse, all from Getty Images.
RR Donnelley was printer and binder.

This book is printed on acid-free paper.

Library of Congress Cataloging-in-Publication Data

Pharmacy management: essentials for all practice settings/[edited by] Shane P. Desselle,
David P. Zgarrick, Greg L. Alston. — 3rd ed.
p. ; cm.
Includes bibliographical references and index.
ISBN 978-0-07-177431-4 (soft cover : alk. paper) – ISBN 0-07-177431-9 (soft cover : alk. paper)
I. Desselle, Shane P. II. Zgarrick, David P. III. Alston, Greg L.
[DNLM: 1. Pharmacies—organization & administration. QV 737]
615′.1068—dc23

2011046287

DEDICATION

To Deborah and Brittney (S.P.D.)
To Michelle, Elle, Seamus and Zoe (D.P.Z.)
and
To June (G.L.A.)

CONTENTS

CONTRIBUTORS

Greg L. Alston, PharmD
Associate Professor and Assistant Dean for Assessment, Wingate University School of Pharmacy, Wingate, North Carolina

Melvin F. Baron, PharmD, MPA
Associate Professor, University of Southern California School of Pharmacy, Los Angeles, California

Michele A. Belsey, RPh
Vice President for College Relations and Professional Recruitment, Rite-Aid Corporation, Enola, Pennsylvania

John Bentley, PhD
Associate Professor, Department of Pharmacy Administration, School of Pharmacy, University of Mississippi, University, Mississippi

Dr. Joseph C Blizzard B.S. Pharm, PhD Pharmacoeconomics
Director of Operations for Beam Pharmacies Inc. Saint Matthews, South Carolina

Joseph K. Bonnarens, PhD
Associate Dean for Student Affairs, Associate Professor School of Pharmacy, Manchester College, Fort Wayne, Indiana

Leigh Ann Bynum, PharmD, MS
Graduate Student, University of Mississippi School of Pharmacy, University, Mississippi

Steven Chen, PharmD
Associate Professor, Department of Clinical Pharmacy and Pharmaceutical Economics and Policy, Hygeia Centennial Chair in Clinical Pharmacy, Director, Pharmacy Practice Residency in Primary Care, University of Southern California, Los Angeles, California

Michelle Chui, PhD
Assistant Professor, Social and Administrative Sciences, University of Wisconsin School of Pharmacy, Madison, Wisconsin

Bartholomew Clark, PhD
Associate Professor, Creighton University School of Pharmacy and Allied Health Professions, Omaha, Nebraska

Ed Cohen, PharmD
Senior Manager, Product Development, Walgreens Corporate Innovation Group, Deerfield, Illinois

Michael R. Cohen
President, Institute for Safe Medication Practices, Huntington Valley, Pennsylvania

Shane P. Desselle, PhD
Dean and Professor, College of Pharmacy, California Northstate University, Rancho Cordova, California

Kevin C. Farmer, PhD
Professor of Clinical and Administrative Sciences, University of Oklahoma, College of Pharmacy, Oklahoma City, Oklahoma

Laura L. Feeney, PharmD
Clinical Pharmacist, Clinicas Del Camino Real, Inc., Ventura, California

Brent I. Fox, PhD, PharmD
Assistant Professor, Department of Pharmacy Care Systems, Harrison School of Pharmacy, Auburn University, Auburn, Alabama

Caroline M. Gaither, PhD
Professor, Department of Pharmaceutical Care and Health Systems, Assistant Dean, Professional Education Division, College of Pharmacy, University of Minnesota, Minneapolis, Minnesota

David Gettman, PhD
Professor and Chair, D'Youville College School of Pharmacy, Buffalo, New York

William A. Gouveia, MS, FASHP, DHL
Director of Pharmacy (Retired), Tufts-New England Medical Center; Associate Professor of Medicine, Tufts University School of Medicine, Boston, Massachusetts

Matthew Grissinger, RPh, FISMP, FASCP
Director, Error Reporting Programs, Institute for Safe Medication Practices, Huntington Valley, Pennsylvania

Wesley R. Haltom, PharmD
Assistant Professor and Director of IPPE, Wingate University School of Pharmacy, Wingate, North Carolina

Dana Hammer, RPh, MS, PhD
Director, Bracken Pharmaceutical Care Learning Center, University of Washington School of Pharmacy, Seattle, Washington

Donald Harrison, PhD
Associate Professor University of Oklahoma College of Pharmacy, Oklahoma City, Oklahoma

David Holdford, RPh, MS, PhD
Associate Professor, Department of Pharmacotherapy and Outcome Science, School of Pharmacy, Virginia Commonwealth University School of Pharmacy, Richmond, Virginia

Erin R. Holmes, PhD, PharmD
Assistant Professor, University of Mississippi School of Pharmacy, University, Mississippi

Stephanie Iniguez, PharmD
Pharmacy Manager, Ventura Pharmacy, Ventura, California

Frank Massaro, PharmD
Pharmacy Practice Manager, Tufts-New England Medical Center, Boston, Massachusetts

Randal McDonough, PharmD
Co-owner, Towncrest and Medical Plaza Pharmacies, Adjunct Professor, College of Pharmacy, The University of Iowa, Iowa City, Iowa

Rashid Mosavin, PhD
Associate Professor and Chair, Loma Linda University School of Pharmacy, Loma Linda, California

Gretchen L. Peirce, PharmD, MS
Graduate Assistant, College of Pharmacy, University of Oklahoma Health Sciences Center, Tulsa, Oklahoma

Jason Perepelkin, BA, Bcomm, MSc, PhD
Assistant Professor of Social and Administrative Pharmacy, Director, Centre for the Study of Social and Administrative Pharmacy, University of Saskatchewan College of Pharmacy and Nutrition, Saskatoon, Saskatchewan, Canada

Glen Schumock, PharmD, MBA
Professor, Department of Pharmacy Practice, Director, Center for Pharmacoeconomic Research, University of Illinois at Chicago College of Pharmacy, Chicago, Illinois

Virginia G. Scott, PhD, MS, RPh
Professor and Director of Continuing Education, Department of Pharmaceutical Systems and Policy, West Virginia University School of Pharmacy, Morgantown, West Virginia

Mark Siracuse, PharmD, PhD
Associate Professor and Vice Chair, Department of Pharmacy Sciences, Center for Health Services Research and Patient Safety, Creighton University School of Pharmacy and Allied Health Professions, Omaha, Nebraska

Mark H. Siska, BS Pharm, MBA/TM
Assistant Director, Informatics and Technology, Pharmacy Services, Mayo Clinic, Rochester, Minnesota

Alan R. Spies, RPh, SD, MBA, PhD
Director of Professional Development and Associate Professor, University of Oklahoma College of Pharmacy, Oklahoma City, Oklahoma

JoAnn Stubbings, BS Pharm, MHCA
Clinical Associate Professor, University of Illinois at Chicago, College of Pharmacy, Ambulatory Care Pharmacy Department, Department of Pharmacy Practice, Chicago, Illinois

Benjamin S. Teeter, BS
Graduate Student, Department of Pharmacy Care Systems, Auburn University Harrison School of Pharmacy, Auburn, Alabama

Brad Tice, PharmD, PMP, FAPhA
Chief Clinical Officer, PharmMD Solutions, LLC, Brentwood, Tennessee

Julie Urmie, PhD
Associate Professor, University of Iowa College of Pharmacy, Iowa City, Iowa

Terri L. Warholak, PhD, RPH
Assistant Professor, University of Arizona College of Pharmacy, Tucson, Arizona

Donna West-Strum, RPh, PhD
Chair and Associate Professor, Department of Pharmacy Administration, University of Mississippi School of Pharmacy, University, Mississippi

Salisa Westrick, PhD
Associate Professor of Pharmacy Care Systems, Auburn University Harrison School of Pharmacy, Auburn, Alabama

Godwin Wong, PhD
Visiting Associate Professor, Haas School of Business, University of California Berkeley, President, US Management Center, San Francisco, California

David P. Zgarrick, PhD
Professor and Chair, Department of Pharmacy Practice, School of Pharmacy, Bouvé College of Health Sciences Northeastern University, Boston, Massachusetts

PREFACE

WHY DID WE CREATE THIS TEXTBOOK?

Pharmacy remains a very exciting profession; in fact, more opportunities are available for pharmacists, pharmacy students, and educators than ever before. The roles of pharmacists in interdisciplinary health care teams continue to evolve, as does their recognition by payers and policy makers. Pharmacists are in the midst of a transformation in the delivery of services to accentuate the critical nature of public health and proactive health care. But with new opportunities also come challenges, including the challenge of how to manage the personal and professional resources necessary to succeed in today's ever-changing environment.

Educators must not only keep up with changes in pharmacy practice, but also anticipate and prepare our students for opportunities and contingencies that will arise throughout their professional careers. In our efforts to best prepare students, pharmacy management educators have increasingly had to gather teaching materials from a variety of textbooks, journals, and other educational resources. This is due to the fact that many resources only focus on a specific management function (marketing, personnel, accounting, and finance) or a specific practice setting (independent pharmacies, hospital pharmacies). We believed that there would be value in a comprehensive pharmacy management textbook that covered many content areas and gathered a variety of resources into one text. We also aimed to develop a text that uses "evidence-based management"; that is, material derived from the best and most contemporary primary literature, but that which at the same time focuses on the application of knowledge into skills that pharmacists will use everyday.

NEW CONTENT IN THIS EDITION!!

In planning for a third edition of this text, we sought input from faculty who pharmacy management, as well as from pharmacy students and pharmacists who apply management principles in their daily practice. We listened carefully to users also while scanning the latest advances in teaching strategies to produce the third edition. Of course, we also considered the many changes in pharmacy practice, management, and health systems reform that have occurred during the past few years.

- Every chapter has been updated to reflect the fluid nature of their respective management topic.
- New trends in the management literature are reflected in each of the chapters, including management trends within and beyond pharmacy.
- Some chapters have been revised substantially and with new authors to provide users of the text with the most relevant information. Examples include the following:
    - The establishment and management of medication therapy management services
    - Evaluating outcomes of medication therapy management services as a component of operations
    - Training employees to provide customer service and engender loyalty among patrons
    - New technology to assist with managing inventory, and for value-added services
    - Financial position analyses most commonly undertaken by pharmacists in several key settings

    - Impact of state and federal legislation, including Affordable Care Act, accountable care organizations, contextualizing pharmacy within medicine's transformation into medical home models of care
    - Exploring the roles of pharmacists in the provision of population-based public health services
    - Focusing on intrapreneurship, in addition to entrepreneurship, to help readers connect with all the possibilities of innovation within their own organization, not just opportunities that exist outside of that context
- We have added several new chapters to promote a more global understanding of pharmacy management in the spirit of its growth, evolution, and penetration into new settings.
    - We added a chapter on to help users sell themselves, their services, and all key stakeholders.
    - We added a chapter on Applications in Managed and Specialty Environments to better describe pharmacy managers play in storing, handling, and distributing specialty drug products, such as biologics and impending pharmacogenomic goods and services.
    - There is a new chapter on Management of Comprehensive Pharmacy Services in Safety Net Clinics to illustrate the challenges and opportunities for pharmacists in a widening array of programs aimed at to economically disadvantaged populations.
    - A new chapter on Pharmacy Management Applications in Varied Health Care Systems appeals not only to users outside the United States, but also helps users in the United States further apply the principles of management espoused throughout the text.

NEW FEATURES IN THIS EDITION!!

Teaching (and learning) management within a pharmacy curriculum presents. This edition's new features will help promote learning and application, while increasing the fun factor! On McGraw-Hill's Online Resource Center, 3rd edition instructors will have access to [sample syllabi], active learning exercises, slide presentations to accompany each chapter, and a bank of test questions created using The National Board of Medical Examiners Item Writing Guide (http://www.nbme.org/PDF/ItemWriting_2003/2003IWGwhole.pdf) for authoring reliable and valid multiple choice test items guidelines for test question development. The active learning exercises help to underscore what this edition is all about; that is, application of the knowledge gained directly into skills useful for practice.

WHAT WILL THE READER FIND IN THIS TEXTBOOK?

This textbook is organized to reflect all of the major management functions performed by pharmacists in any practice setting. The book is divided into sections representing each function, and is further divided into chapters that detail the various components of each function.

Our experience as educators has taught us that students are the most effective learners when they are "ready" to learn. Many students selected pharmacy as a major in part from the desire to help people, but also due to their fascination and intrigue with how such small amounts of various medicinal substances have such profound effects on the body. Many of these students also believe that they only need to learn about management after they graduate, and then only if they take on a managerial or administrative position at their pharmacy. The first section of this book makes the case that management skills are important for all people and pharmacists, regardless of their position or practice setting. In an environment of increasingly scarce resources and higher accountability, we also help the reader to understand and create the value proposition for themselves, their services, and their organization. After establishing the need for management in both our personal and professional lives, the next four sections describe the management functions and resources that are common to all pharmacy practice settings (operations, people, money, traditional pharmacy goods, and services). Chapters within each section focus on important aspects of each function or resource.

As pharmacy practice moves from a product orientation to a patient orientation, there are unique challenges that arise in managing the value-added services that pharmacists are developing to meet patient needs in medication therapy management. A section of this book is dedicated to the planning, implementation, and reimbursement of these new patient care services offered by pharmacists.

Several chapters are dedicated to describing the risks inherent in pharmacy practice, and the impact that laws, regulations, and medication errors have on pharmacy management. The final section describes how management functions are applied in specific pharmacy practice settings (independent, chain, health systems, managed environments, safety net operations), and settings in unique health systems.

HOW EACH CHAPTER IS ORGANIZED

Each chapter is divided into several sections to facilitate the reader's understanding and application of the material. Chapters begin with a list of learning objectives that outline the major topics to be addressed. A brief scenario is used to describe how a pharmacy student or pharmacist may need or apply the information described this chapter in their daily lives or practice. Questions at the start of each chapter provide direction and assist the reader in understanding what they can expect to learn.

The text of each chapter provides comprehensive coverage of the content and theory underlying the major concepts. References to the management and pharmacy literature are commonly used to provide readers with links to additional background information. Explanations and applications are also used to help readers better understand the need to master and apply each concept. Questions at the end of each chapter encourage readers to think about what they have just learned and apply these concepts in new ways.

WHAT WE HOPE YOU WILL GAIN FROM THIS BOOK

If you are a pharmacy student, we hope that using this book will help you gain an appreciation for the roles of management in pharmacy practice, regardless of your future position or practice setting. This book will also provide you with a variety of management theories and tools that you can apply in your daily life.

We realize that many pharmacists have not had much management coursework in their formal education or professional training. We hope that this book serves as a valuable guide to pharmacists who may require some assistance in dealing with matters they did not anticipate when embarking on their careers. For those pharmacists with formal management education and experience, we hope that this book serves as a valuable reference or as a source of new ideas that can be applied in daily practice.

For educators, this book has been designed as a comprehensive pharmacy management textbook. As a whole, it is meant to be used in survey courses that cover many areas of pharmacy management. The section format also allows the book to be used in courses that focus on specific pharmacy management functions or topics. The sections and content of each chapter are meant not only to provide valuable information that is easy for students to understand, but also to stimulate further discussion and motivate students to learn more on their own.

WE WOULD LIKE TO HEAR FROM YOU!

Textbooks today have a great deal in common with. The creators of each have put a great deal of time and effort into getting their final outputs ready for consumers, but it rarely can be considered a "finished product." Textbooks, like, are "works in progress" that can always be improved. The best way to improve these products is to seek input from their users. As you use this book, we would like to learn what you like about it, what could be improved, and what topics or features you would like to see included in the future. Please feel free to share your thoughts at any time by contacting us through *pharmacy@mcgraw-hill.com.* We plan to improve this book over future editions by listening to your feedback and continuing to reflect changes in the management sciences and pharmacy practice.

ACKNOWLEDGMENTS

We would like to thank the colleagues who have played an important role in our development throughout our undergraduate and graduate studies, as well as at our institutions. In addition, as our careers have advanced, we also have come to know many great academicians in other disciplines, and other leaders in pharmacy who have greatly influenced our careers and provided keen guidance. We have learned so much from all these people, and feel fortunate that they have been willing to share their knowledge and experience with us.

Thanks must also go to all the faculty, staff, and administrators at the University of Oklahoma, California Northstate University, Northeastern University, and Wingate University, who have provided an environment that makes this type of endeavor possible. We would also like to thank all of the students we have taught who have inspired us to continue to strive to become better educators.

We would like to thank everyone at McGraw-Hill, and in particular our editor, Michael Weitz, for working with us to improve this comprehensive pharmacy management textbook.

Finally, we would like to acknowledge the efforts of each of our chapter authors. We chose our authors not only because of their expertise, but also because of their dedication to teaching and the professional development of pharmacy students and pharmacists. There is no way in which we could have completed this textbook without their efforts.

SECTION I

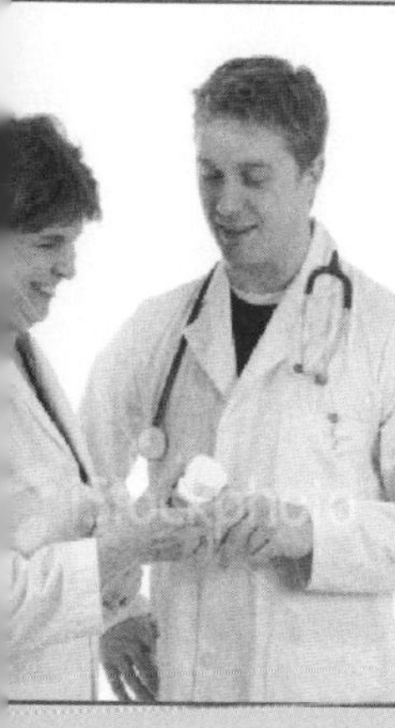

WHY STUDY MANAGEMENT IN PHARMACY SCHOOL?

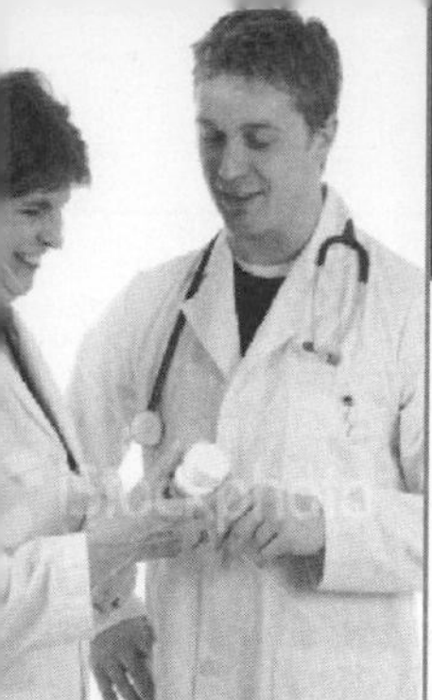

1

THE "MANAGEMENT" IN MEDICATION THERAPY MANAGEMENT

Shane P. Desselle

About the Author: Dr. Desselle is Dean and professor at the California Northstate University, College of Pharmacy. He received a B.S. degree in pharmacy and a Ph.D. in pharmacy administration from the University of Louisiana at Monroe. He has practice experience in both community and hospital pharmacy settings. He teaches courses in American health care systems, health care economics, social and behavioral aspects of pharmacy practice, and research methods. His research interests include performance appraisal systems in pharmacy, quality of work life among pharmacy technicians, direct-to-consumer prescription drug advertising, Web-based pharmacy services, and pharmacy benefit design. Dr. Desselle won the Duquesne University School of Pharmacy's President's Award for Teaching and President's Award for Scholarship and was recognized for his contributions to pharmacy by being named a Fellow of the American Pharmacists Association in 2006.

LEARNING OBJECTIVES

After completing this chapter, readers should be able to

1. Identify changes in the roles of pharmacists since the early 1900s.
2. Describe how pharmacy practitioners and educators viewed the need for management skills as the roles of pharmacists evolved.
3. Identify principal domains of pharmacy care. Describe how management skills and functions fit within the context of providing medication therapy management services.
4. Identify myths surrounding the practice of pharmacy and health care as a business.
5. Evaluate the need for a management perspective to better serve patients and improve outcomes to drug therapy.
6. List the managerial sciences and describe their use as tools to assist pharmacists in practice.

SCENARIO

Mary Quint has just completed the first 2 years of a doctor of pharmacy curriculum. Despite many long hours of hard work and a few anxious moments preparing for examinations, she has been pleased with her educational experience. She perceives that as she continues progressing through the curriculum, the upcoming courses will be more integrated and directly applicable to pharmacy practice. She is especially excited about taking courses in pharmacology and therapeutics so that she can "really learn about how to be a pharmacist." As she glances down at her schedule and sees that she is enrolled in a required course in pharmacy management, her enthusiasm becomes somewhat tempered. She immediately consults with fellow students on what they have heard about the course, and they tell her that the course is about "finance, accounting, personnel management, and marketing." Despite some positive comments provided by students having already completed the course, she is concerned. "What do I have to take this course for? I did not come to pharmacy school for this. I'm very good at science. If I liked this kind of stuff, I would have majored in business. How is this going to help me to become a better pharmacist?" she asks herself.

After some thought she comes to realize that, at worst, taking this course will not be the end of the world, and even better, it simply might be a moderate intrusion in her Monday–Wednesday–Friday routine. She begins to focus on other issues, such as her part-time job at Middletown South Pharmacy. Lately, she has been dreading each day that she goes to work. The staff consistently seems rushed and impatient. There always seems to be conflict among the employees, and as soon as one fire has been put out, another larger one begins to burn. She regrets her decision to quit her job at Middletown North Pharmacy 3 months ago, even though it took 20 minutes longer to get there. Things always seemed to run smoothly at Middletown North. Mary even noticed that the patients at Middletown North seemed happier and healthier than those at Middletown South.

CHAPTER QUESTIONS

1. How have pharmacists' roles in delivering goods and services evolved over the past few decades? What roles and functions do pharmacists perform today?
2. What is the significance of management within the context of the profession's movement toward the provision of medication therapy management services? Why has its significance typically been over looked by pharmacists and pharmacy students?
3. What are some of the myths surrounding the confluence of business practices and the provision of patient care by pharmacists?
4. What evidence exists that a business perspective is critical to providing effective pharmacy services to patients?
5. What are the managerial sciences, and how can pharmacy practitioners use them effectively?

INTRODUCTION

The preceding scenario, though perhaps overly simplistic, captures the feelings of many students who select pharmacy as a major. They generally are interested in science, have a desire to help people in need, and prefer a career offering long-term financial security. Given that the pharmacy curriculum consists of courses that apply knowledge from physics, chemistry, anatomy, physiology, and therapeutics, most pharmacy students achieved success in science and math courses throughout their prepharmacy studies (Keshishian et al., 2010). Second, students selecting pharmacy as a major typically are attracted to health care fields and may have contemplated nursing, medicine, or other health professions. Research has demonstrated that people in health care are caring and empathic and seek personal reward and self-actualization through the helping of others (Carmel and Glick, 2001; Fjortoft and Zgarrick, 2003; Keshishian, 2010; Kunyk and Olsen, 2001). Finally, many pharmacy students also consider the relatively high salaries of their chosen profession prior to choosing a college major and a career pathway. While few fields guarantee graduates a job, and certainly not one with entry-level salaries in the six figures, pharmacy students take comfort in knowing that employment in their profession will provide them with a generous and steady stream of income. It comes as no surprise that pharmacists and pharmacy students have been shown to be risk-averse individuals who do not deal with uncertainties particularly well (Gaither, 1998a; Latif, 2000). This further explains their gravitation toward science-oriented courses that offer straightforward solutions to problems.

Unbeknown to many pharmacy students is that the actual practice of pharmacy does not present a succession of problems that can be resolved in such a linear manner. While the sequential processes involved in community pharmacy practice have remained the same—patients present with prescriptions, pharmacy personnel fill them, and the necessary counseling is offered or provided by the pharmacist—a careful introspection reveals that the profession has undergone a rapid, head-turning transformation over just the past few decades. Pharmacists now are increasingly involved with providing services in addition to medications, and are taking greater responsibility for patients' outcomes arising from drug therapy. Pharmacists have become more integrated into health care delivery teams that coordinate patient care through the implementation of guidelines and treatment algorithms. This has been even further accelerated by recent changes in states' pharmacist scope of practice regulations, reimbursement incentives from payers, and the reorganization of health care delivery into medical home models (Johnson et al., 2010; Lee et al., 2006).

For students to better understand the way that pharmacy is practiced today, time should be devoted to understanding the major forces that have shaped the profession. This chapter begins with a brief history of the evolution of pharmacy practice in the twentieth century. This history, coupled with a snapshot of contemporary pharmacy practice, will make it clear that the past and current pharmacy practice models are as much about management as they are about clinical pharmacy practice. The chapter proceeds by pointing out myths about the exclusivity of the pharmacy business and patient outcomes and by providing evidence that what is best for the operation of a pharmacy business is often also best for the patients that it serves. The chapter concludes with a brief discussion of the managerial sciences—tools that every practitioner will find useful at one point or another regardless of the practice setting. This chapter and all other succeeding chapters use an *evidence-based approach* to discuss pharmacy management, relying on recent literature and research findings to describe and explain what is happening in practice today. Students are encouraged to explore readings of interest among the references cited throughout the text.

A BRIEF HISTORICAL OVERVIEW OF PHARMACY PRACTICE

Pharmacy Practice Prior to the 1940s

There have been several noteworthy efforts to describe the evolution of pharmacy practice. Some have described the process within the context of "waves," or shifts, in educational and industrial forces (Hepler, 1987), another through identifying stages of professional identity (Hepler and Strand, 1990), and still another through describing momentous occurrences in the health care delivery system whose effects rippled throughout the pharmacy profession (Broeseker and Janke, 1998). While these approaches appear quite different, their descriptions of the principal drivers of change closely mirror one another.

Pharmacy in the Early Twentieth Century

Pharmacy in the United States began the twentieth century much like it existed in the latter 1800s. Pharmacy was, at best, a "marginal" profession. Most practitioners entered the occupation through apprenticeships rather than formal education. The pharmacist's principal job function was described as the "daily handling and preparing of remedies in common use" (Sonnedecker, 1963, p. 204). Pharmacists, or "apothecaries," often were engaged in the wholesale manufacture and distribution of medicinal products. Pharmacists' roles during this time were considerably different than they are today. In the early twentieth century, pharmacists' primary roles were to procure raw ingredients and extemporaneously compound them into drug products for consumer use. While pharmacists had yet to achieve recognition as health care professionals, they often had considerable autonomy in their practice. There was no clear distinction between "prescription" and "nonprescription" drugs. Although physicians were engaged in the process of writing prescriptions, pharmacists were not precluded from dispensing preparations without a physician's order. Consumers commonly relied on their pharmacists' advice on minor ailments, and often entrusted the nickname of "doc" to their neighborhood pharmacist (Hepler, 1987).

Pharmacists had little choice but to have sharp business acumen to survive. Since few of the products they dispensed were prefabricated by manufacturers, pharmacists had to be adept at managing inventories of bulk chemicals and supplies used in compounding the preparations they dispensed. They also had to have a keen sense of how to manage time and people to accomplish a series of complex tasks throughout the workday.

A series of studies commissioned by the US government in the early 1900s produced what became known as the "Flexner Reports" in 1915. These reports were critical of health care professionals and their education, including pharmacists. The reports questioned the validity and necessity of pharmacists as health care professionals. Shortly thereafter, the American Association of Colleges of Pharmacy (AACP) commissioned a study directed by W. W. Charters that ultimately served as the basis for requiring a 4-year baccalaureate degree program for all colleges of pharmacy (Hepler, 1987). These and other forces led to dramatic changes in pharmacy in the coming years.

Pharmacy in the Middle of the Twentieth Century

The 1940s through the 1960s often have been referred to as the "era of expansion" in health care (Relman, 1988). The Flexner Reports paved the way for a more scientifically sound, empirically based allopathic branch of medicine to become the basis by which health care was practiced and organized. The federal government invested significant funds to expand the quantity and quality of health care services. The Hospital Survey and Construction (Hill-Burton) Act of 1946 provided considerable funding for the renovation and expansion of existing hospitals and the construction of new ones, primarily in underserved inner city and rural areas (Torrens, 1993).

Ironically, pharmacists began to see their roles diminish during this era of expansion in health care. Among the factors responsible for this decline were advances in technology and in the pharmaceutical sciences, coupled with societal demands that drug products become uniform in their composition. These brought about the mass production of prefabricated drug products in tablet, capsule, syrup, and elixir dosage forms, thus significantly reducing the need for pharmacists to compound prescription orders. The passage of the Durham-Humphrey amendment to the Food, Drug, and Cosmetic Act in 1951 created a prescription, or "legend," category of drugs. Pharmacists did not have the ability to dispense these drugs without an order from a licensed prescriber. Finally, pharmacy's own "Code of Ethics" promulgated by the American Pharmaceutical Association (APhA) stated that pharmacists were not to discuss the therapeutic effects or composition of a prescription with a patient (Buerki and Vottero, 1994, p. 93). This combination of forces relegated the role of the pharmacist largely to a dispenser of pre-prepared drug products.

The response of schools and colleges of pharmacy to these diminishing professional roles was the creation of curricula that were more technical, scientific, and content driven. A fifth year of education was added to the 4-year baccalaureate degree by colleges and schools of pharmacy during the late 1940s and early 1950s following the AACP Committee on Curriculum report entitled, "The Pharmaceutical Curriculum" (Hepler, 1987). It was during this time that pharmacology, pharmaceutics, and medicinal chemistry matured as disciplines and became the fabric of pharmacy education. Pharmacy students were required to memorize an abundance of information about the physical and chemical nature of drug products and dosage forms. Courses in the business aspects of pharmacy took a secondary role, whereas education in patient care (e.g., communications, therapeutics) was for all intents and purposes nonexistent.

With the APhA Code of Ethics suggesting that pharmacists not discuss drug therapies with patients, the profession lost sight of the need for pharmacists to communicate effectively with patients and other health care professionals. As the number of hospital and chain pharmacies expanded, resulting in pharmacists being more likely to be an employee than a business owner, the importance of practice management skills was not stressed in schools of pharmacy. Ironically, studies such as the "Dichter Report" commissioned by the APhA revealed that consumers regarded pharmacists more as merchants than as health care professionals (Maine and Penna, 1996).

Pharmacy in the Latter Part of the Twentieth Century

The era of expansion slowed in the 1970s when society began to question the value obtained from the larger amount of resources being allocated toward health care. Congress passed the Health Maintenance Act of 1973, which helped to pave the way for health maintenance organizations (HMOs) to become an integral player in the delivery of health care services. Governments, rather than the private sector, took the lead in attempting to curb costs when they implemented a prospective payment system of reimbursement for Medicare hospitalizations based on categories of diagnosis-related groups (Pink, 1991).

In 1975 The Millis Commission's report, *Pharmacists for the Future: The Report of the Study Commission on Pharmacy* (Millis, 1975), suggested that pharmacists were inadequately prepared in systems analysis and management skills and had particular deficiencies in communicating with patients, physicians, and other health care professionals. A subsequent report suggested incorporating more of the behavioral and social sciences into pharmacy curricula and encouraged faculty participation and research into real problems inherent in pharmacy practice (Millis, 1976).

Prior to these reports, the American Society of Hospital Pharmacists had published *Mirror to Hospital Pharmacy* stating that pharmacy had lost its purpose, falling short of producing health care professionals capable of engendering change and noting that frustration and dissatisfaction among practitioners was beginning to affect students (Hepler, 1987, p. 371). The clinical pharmacy movement evolved in the 1970s to capture the essence of the drug use control concept forwarded by Brodie (1967) and promoted the pharmacist's role as therapeutic advisor. The clinical pharmacy movement brought about changes in pharmacy education and practice. After being introduced in 1948, the 6-year Doctor of Pharmacy (Pharm.D.) degree became the only entry-level degree offered by a small number of colleges of pharmacy as early as the late 1960s and early 1970s. The additional year of study was devoted mostly to therapeutics or "disease-oriented courses" and experiential education. The Doctor of Pharmacy degree became the entry-level degree into the profession in the late 1990s, with colleges of pharmacy phasing out their baccalaureate programs (American Association of Colleges of Pharmacy, 1996).

These trends toward a more clinical practice approach may at first glance appear to be an ill-conceived response given recent changes in health care delivery. These changes placed a heightened concern over spiraling costs and have resulted in the deinstitutionalization of patients and the standardization of care using tools such as protocols, treatment algorithms, and critical pathways. Adoption of a clinical practice approach may also appear to fly in the face of changes in the organization of the pharmacy workforce and current market for pharmaceuticals. With the proportion of independently owned community pharmacies at an all-time low in the year 2000, chain, supermarket, and mass-merchandiser pharmacies had garnered nearly 64 percent of the outpatient prescription drug market (National Association of Chain Drug Stores, 2010). Studies have long suggested that pharmacists willing and knowledgeable enough to provide patient-oriented clinical services face significant barriers when practicing in a chain environment (Miller and Ortmeier, 1995). In addition, two relatively new venues for outpatient pharmacy services virtually exclude face-to-face consultation with patients. Mail order pharmacy has become a formidable venue for the distribution of pharmaceuticals and is used by the Veterans Administration system and many pharmacy benefits managers. Traditional brick-and-mortar pharmacy operations have even gotten into the mail order business themselves. The new millennium also saw the implementation of Internet pharmacy sites, many of which are owned and operated by traditional "brick and mortar" chain pharmacy corporations. While providing consumers with a convenient way to obtain drug products, this form of commerce may further remove the pharmacist from patients who could benefit from their clinical services.

PHARMACEUTICAL CARE AND MEDICATION THERAPY MANAGEMENT AS MANAGEMENT MOVEMENTS?

With these changes in mind, adopting pharmaceutical care as a practice philosophy in the 1990s would have appeared "a day late and a dollar short" for both the profession and the patients it serves. And indeed, that might have been the case if the concept of pharmaceutical care were entirely clinical in nature. The originators of the concept fervently stressed that pharmaceutical care was not simply a list of clinically oriented activities to perform for each and every patient but was, in fact, a new mission and way of thinking that takes advantage of pharmacists' accessibility and the frequency to which they are engaged by patients—a way of thinking that engenders the pharmacist to take responsibility for managing a patient's pharmacotherapy to resolve current and prevent future problems related to their medications.

It has been argued that the focus on preventing and resolving medication-related problems is simply an extension of *risk management* (Wiederholt and Wiederholt, 1997, see also Chapter 27). Risks are an inherent part of any business activity, including the provision of pharmacy services. Common risks to business practice include fire, natural disasters, theft, economic downturns, and employee turnover, as well as the fact that there is no guarantee that consumers will accept or adopt any good or service that is offered to them. The practice of pharmacy involves additional risks, specifically the risk that patients will suffer untoward events as a result of their drug therapy.

These events are significant because they may result in significant harm and even death to a patient and also can pose serious detriments to pharmacists, such as feelings of guilt and stress, the potential for litigation from patients and their families, the threat of punitive action by state boards of pharmacy, and the loss of social esteem enjoyed by the profession as a whole. Risk management suggests that risk cannot be avoided entirely, but rather that it should be assessed, measured, and reduced to the extent feasible (Flyvbjerg, 2006).

The idea that pharmaceutical care should be viewed strictly as a clinical movement was called into question (Wilkin, 1999). Evidence that pharmaceutical care existed in part as a management movement was provided in a study that sought to identify standards of practice for providing pharmaceutical care (Desselle and Rappaport, 1996). A nationwide panel of experts identified 52 standards of pharmacy practice, only to have a statewide sample of pharmacists judge many of them as unfeasible to implement in everyday practice (Desselle, 1997). Of the practice standards that were judged to be feasible, further research yielded a system of "factors" or "domains" in which these standards could be classified (Desselle and Rappaport, 1995). These practice domains can be found in Table 1-1. Figuring very prominently into this classification was the "risk management" domain, which included activities related to documentation, drug review, triage, and dosage calculations. However, the contributions of the managerial sciences do not stop there. The remaining four domains connote significant involvement by pharmacists into managerial processes. Two of the domains ("services marketing" and "business management") are named specifically after managerial functions.

Table 1-1. Pharmacy Care Practice Domains

I. *Risk management*
- Devise system of data collection
- Perform prospective drug utilization review
- Document therapeutic interventions and activities
- Obtain over-the-counter medication history
- Calculate dosages for drugs with a narrow therapeutic index
- Report adverse drug events to FDA
- Triage patients' needs for proper referral
- Remain abreast of newly uncovered adverse effects and drug–drug interactions

II. *Patient advocacy*
- Serve as patient advocate with respect to social, economic, and psychological barriers to drug therapy
- Attempting to change patients' medication orders when barriers to compliance exist
- Counsel patients on new and refill medications as necessary
- Promote patient wellness
- Maintain caring, friendly relationship with patients
- Telephone patients to obtain medication orders called in and not picked up

III. *Disease management*
- Provide information to patients on how to manage their disease state/condition
- Monitor patients' progress resulting from pharmacotherapy
- Carry inventory of products necessary for patients to execute a therapeutic plan (e.g., inhalers, nebulizers, glucose monitors, etc.)
- Supply patients with information on support and educational groups (e.g., American Diabetes Association, Multiple Sclerosis Society)

IV. *Pharmacy care services marketing*
- Meet prominent prescribers in the local area of practice
- Be an active member of professional associations that support the concept of pharmaceutical care
- Make available an area for private consultation services for patients as necessary
- Identify software that facilitates pharmacists' patient care–related activities

V. *Business management*
- Utilize technicians and other staff to free up the pharmacist's time

From Pharmaceutical Care to Medication Therapy Management

While the pharmaceutical care movement made an indelible mark on the profession, its use in the modern lexicon describing pharmacists' services is fading. It is being replaced with terminology that more accurately reflects pharmacists' growing roles in the provision of public health services and reorganization of care into medical homes. In recognizing the morbidity and mortality resulting from medication errors as a public health problem, the profession has begun to embrace the concept of medication therapy management (MTM). MTM represents a comprehensive and proactive approach to help patients maximize the benefits from drug therapy and includes services aimed to facilitate or improve patient compliance to drug therapy, educate entire populations of persons, conduct wellness programs, and become more intimately involved in disease management and monitoring. The MTM movement has been especially strengthened by language in the Medicare Prescription Drug, Improvement and Modernization Act (MMA) of 2003 (Public Law Number 108–173, 2010), which mandates payment for MTM services and proffers pharmacists as viable health professionals that may offer such services. The place of MTM in health care delivery was advanced even further in the Patient Protection and Affordable Care Act, which established pilots for integrated care delivery, comprehensive medication review for Medicare beneficiaries, and grants specifically for medication therapy management programs (Public Law Number 111–148, 2010). As such, MTM is now considered a key component in the provision of pharmacy care services.

MYTHS CONCERNING THE CONFLUENCE OF BUSINESS PRACTICE AND PHARMACY

Despite evidence that would suggest otherwise, the need for a management perspective in pharmacy is often overlooked and even shunned by some pharmacy students and practitioners. Common misconceptions about the need for a management perspective have been documented (Tootelian and Gaedeke, 1993, p. 23):

- *The practice of pharmacy is ethically inconsistent with good business.* The origin of this myth probably evolved from the unethical business practices of some organizations. Scandals involving abuses by corporate executives at large international firms in the early 2000s have done little to mitigate these perceptions. Physicians, pharmacists and other professionals who commit insurance fraud or knowingly bill for goods and services they did not provide demonstrate that health care professions are not without unscrupulous members (Stafford, 2002). Furthermore, some people believe that companies involved in the sale of health care goods and services should be philanthropic in nature and are upset that companies profit from consumers' medical needs. Despite occasional examples of misconduct, most companies and persons involved in business operations conduct themselves in an appropriate manner.
- *Business is not a profession guided by ethical standards.* Pharmacists and pharmacy students generally are cognizant of the vast number of rules and regulations that govern pharmacy, but are less aware of the standards governing practice in advertising, accounting, and interstate commerce. Many of the rules and regulations governing pharmacy practice were borrowed from legislation existing in sectors other than health care.
- *In business, quality of care is secondary to generating profits.* This misconception likely results from the efforts by payers of health care and by managers to control costs. In light of the fact that in 2009 health care accounted for over 18 percent of the United States' gross national product and cost over $7,000 per person (OECD, 2010), health care consumers have little choice but to become more discerning shoppers of health care goods and services. Because resources are limited, the number of goods and services provided to consumers cannot be boundless. Conscientiousness in the allocation of resources helps to ensure that more of the right people receive the right goods and services at the right time and place. Many people do not stop to think that if a company in the health care business is not able to pay its own workforce and cover its other costs of doing business, it will have little choice but to close its doors, leaving a void in the array of goods and services previously afforded to consumers. Even nonprofit entities have to pay the bills, because if they cannot break even, they too have to shut down operations. Students may be surprised to learn that most nonprofit companies in health care both depend on and compete with companies that are structured on a for-profit basis.
- *The good pharmacist is one who is a "clinical purist."* This is perhaps a manifestation of the other misconceptions, in addition to a false pretense that the complexities of modern drug therapy do not allow time for concern with other matters. On the contrary, a lack of knowledge on how to manage resources and a lack of understanding on how to work within the current system of health care delivery will only impede the pharmacist's goal to provide medication therapy management services. Pharmacists

who "don't want to be bothered with management" face the same logistical constraints, such as formularies, generic substitution, prior authorizations, limited networks, employee conflict and lack of productivity, breakdowns in computer hardware and software, budgetary limitations, and changes in policy, that all other pharmacists face. The problem with the "don't want to be bothered with management" pharmacists is that they will be less likely to operate efficiently within the system, becoming frustrated and ultimately less clinically effective than the pharmacists who accept these challenges as part of their practice.

The profession has come under more intense pressure to reduce the incidence of medication errors in both institutional and ambulatory settings (Institute of Medicine, 2006). This is placing a burden on pharmacists to be especially productive, efficient, and error free. Productivity is a function of a pharmacist's ability to manage workflow, technology, the quality and efficiency of support personnel, phone calls, and other problems that arise in day-to-day practice.

Moreover, pharmacy administrators reward pharmacists who can manage a pharmacy practice. New Doctor of Pharmacy graduates may obtain entry-level administrative positions (e.g., pharmacy department manager, area manager, clinical coordinator) within their first few years of practice. It is not uncommon to see pharmacy graduates move up into even higher-level administrative positions (e.g., district or regional manager of a chain, associate director or director of a hospital pharmacy department) within 5 to 10 years of graduation. Pharmacists who can manage a practice successfully (i.e., increase volume, reduce errors, engender customer satisfaction, improve profitability, reduce employee turnover) are in the best position for promotions.

A final point to consider is that even if a pharmacist does not ascend to an administrative position, that person inherently "manages" a practice the instant he or she takes a position as a pharmacist. Staff pharmacists in every practice setting manage technicians and clerks every hour of every day. They also manage the flow of work through their sites and the use of medications by patients. Closely tied to this issue is the issue of personal job satisfaction. The pressures on the modern pharmacist are unmistakable. Satisfaction with one's job and career are important because they are closely related to one's satisfaction with life (Gaither et al., 2008). Pharmacists' ability to manage their work environment can have a significant impact on their ability to cope with the daily stressors of practice, increasing job satisfaction, and diminishing the likelihood of career burnout or impairment through the abuse of alcohol and drugs.

GOOD MANAGEMENT PRACTICE AND MEDICATION THERAPY MANAGEMENT—A WINNING COMBINATION

Evidence of the success of a management perspective in pharmacy practice abounds. A series of studies examined the use of strategic planning by pharmacists in both community and hospital settings (Harrison and Ortmeier, 1995, 1996; Harrison and Bootman, 1994). These studies showed that among community pharmacy owners, those who fully incorporated strategic planning saw higher sales volume and profitability than did those who did not or who did so just partially. Pharmacies owned by "strategic planners" also were significantly more likely to offer clinical or value-added services than pharmacies run by owners who were not. Likewise, better administrative, distributive, and clinical performance among hospital pharmacies also was associated with their respective directors' involvement in the strategic planning process.

Another study pointed out that support from supervisors and colleagues had a positive impact on the commitment that pharmacists display toward their respective organizations, thus enhancing the likelihood that these pharmacists would not quit their jobs (Gaither, 1998b). Other studies suggest that pharmacists' perceived ability to adhere to standards of pharmacy practice hinged considerably on the effectiveness of supervisors to provide them with feedback and facilitate their satisfaction on the job (Desselle and Tipton, 2001). The same study also demonstrated that pharmacists designating themselves as "managers" were less satisfied with their own jobs, likely as a result of their lack of training in such areas.

Surveys of pharmacists commonly indicate that, looking at their practices today, they wish they had more training in management during their professional education. One study suggested that a business/work orientation was the skill most critical in implementing a successful clinical practice (Speedie et al., 1974). It was suggested in another survey that lack of time and poor communication were primary obstacles to delivering pharmacy care services (Ciancanglini et al., 1994). Still another study concluded that it would benefit practicing pharmacists to seek continuing education in management, health care systems and policy, and pharmacotherapeutics (Desselle and Alafris, 1999). It has been argued that to achieve excellence in the implementation of medication therapy management services, pharmacists must obtain and properly allocate resources, design efficient distribution systems, select and train adequate support staff, develop systems for disseminating knowledge on new drugs and technology, and document and evaluate the cost-effectiveness of the services provided—all of which are tasks that require management skills (Smith, 1988). The author of this chapter once visited a noted community pharmacist and observed his practice of giving away small gifts to patients who had been on time for several months in a row to acquire their refill medications. This concept—incentivize patients to be adherent to a medication regiment and also secure their patronage as a pharmacy customer—is a perfect example that clinical acumen and business skills often form a winning combination.

Table 1-2 summarizes many of the principal factors that affect the delivery of pharmacy goods and services and is used to further illustrate the existing synergy between patient care and good business practice. First, the demographic composition of the patient population has changed dramatically. The mean age of Americans continues to increase, as does their life expectancy. This results in a greater proportion of patients presenting with multiple disease states and complex therapeutic regimens. Although many of our nation's seniors lead normal, productive lives, their visual acuity, sense of hearing, mobility, and ability to use and/or obtain viable transportation may be compromised. Pharmacists must take on additional responsibilities in managing these patients' care and coordinating their services. Also, the population of patients that pharmacists serve is becoming more diverse in age/generational beliefs, race/ethnicity, socioeconomic status, and in other ways. Good pharmacy managers will benefit from a heightened sensitivity toward the needs of all patients and efforts to provide goods and services that appeal to specific populations.

Table 1-2. Factors Affecting the Delivery of Pharmacy Goods and Services

Patient demographics
Aging population
Females as decision makers
Ethnic composition of patients
Attitudes and belief systems
Beliefs about disease, sick role, and medication taking
Trust in the health care delivery system
Direct-to-consumer advertising of prescription drugs
Third-party payers and coverage issues
Complexity/differences among payers' policies
Formularies
Limited networks
Limited access for some patients
Lack of knowledge by patients
Competitive markets
Diminished margins
Diversity in the types of providers offering products and services
Technology
Software
Automated dispensing technology

The shift in the demographic composition of patients also brings to bear the varying beliefs people have about treating their disease states, taking medications, and their trust in the health care delivery system. All the clinical and scientific knowledge in the world is rendered useless if pharmacists lack basic knowledge about the patients whom they serve. Even the most carefully devised and therapeutically correct pharmaceutical care plan will not work if the patient does not put faith in the pharmacist's recommendations. Good pharmacists are able to relate to patients of all persuasions and convince them to put faith in the consultation they provide. This requires cultural competence by pharmacists and other pharmacy personnel. An additional consideration is the increased marketing of health care products directly to consumers. This has resulted inevitably in an increase in the frequency of medication-specific queries from patients. Good pharmacists do not bias their answers but are able to triage the patient's request with appropriate information and recommendations.

A management perspective is indispensable when it comes to issues dealing with third-party payers (e.g., private insurers, government-sponsored programs—see Chapters 19 and 20). Unlike other countries, whose health care systems are founded on single-payer reimbursement structures, practitioners in the United States face a mix of payers, including individual patients, private insurers, employers, and government health plans. Each payer differs in its formularies (list of approved drugs), rules for reimbursement, and the network of pharmacists qualified to accept its coverage. The management-minded pharmacist is able to identify payers that afford the pharmacy the opportunity to provide quality patient care while maintaining an appropriate level of profit. Pharmacists must provide appropriate information about coverage to patients, who often do not know about the intricacies of their plans and the health care system (Fronstin, 2000). In addition, pharmacists must coordinate therapeutic plans for cash-paying patients whose financial situation may preclude them from receiving certain therapies and services.

An additional challenge facing pharmacies and pharmacists is that of shrinking profit margins. A pharmacy's net profit margin is the excess of revenues after covering expenses that it secures as a percentage of its total revenues. As the percentage of prescriptions paid for by sources other than patients has increased, pharmacy profit margins have decreased. In addition to selecting the right mix of plans in which to participate, the management-minded pharmacist looks for other opportunities to bring in additional revenues and decrease expenses, such as implementing patient care services, selling ancillary products, effectively purchasing and maintaining proper levels of inventory, effective marketing, and having the appropriate amount and type of personnel needed to do the job. This is especially important in light of the fact that consumers have more choices than ever in seeking health care solutions, ranging from nontraditional sources (complementary and alternative medicine) to more traditional sources (grocery stores, convenience stores, gift shops, the Internet).

The management-minded pharmacist also maintains software and automated dispensing technologies that free up time formerly spent in the dispensing process. This gives pharmacists more time to provide patient care and perform other practice and management functions.

Changes in the legal and regulatory environments, which have impacted both the types of goods and services pharmacists may provide as well as their levels of reimbursement, further underscore the need for practice management skills among pharmacists. In addition to knowledge required to help patients navigate the health care system, pharmacists must be able to maximize efficiency in human, capital, technological resources to serve patients, provide services, and take advantage of the unique opportunities arising to gain reimbursement for their goods and services.

THE MANAGERIAL SCIENCES

Although mentioned throughout this chapter, a more formal examination of the managerial sciences should put into perspective their use as tools to implement pharmacy services effectively. The managerial sciences are summarized in Table 1-3. The reason they are

Table 1-3. The Managerial Sciences

Accounting
- Keep the books
- Record financial transactions
- Prepare financial statements
- Manage cash flows
- Analysis of profitability
- Determine business strengths and weaknesses
- Compute taxes owed to federal, state, and local governments

Finance
- Determine financial needs
- Identify sources of capital
- Develop operating budgets
- Invest profits
- Manage assets

Economics
- Determine optimal mix of labor and capital
- Determine optimal output
- Determine optimal hours of business operation
- Determine levels of investment into risk management

Human resources management
- Conduct job analyses
- Hire personnel
- Orient and train personnel
- Motivate personnel for performance
- Appraise personnel performance
- Allocate organizational rewards
- Terminate employment

Marketing
- Identify competitive advantages
- Implement competitive advantages
- Identify target markets
- Evaluate promotional strategies
- Implement promotional strategies
- Evaluate promotional strategies
- Select proper mix of merchandise
- Properly arrange and merchandise products
- Price goods and services

Operations management
- Design workflow
- Control purchasing and inventory
- Perform quality assurance initiatives

Value creation
- Sell yourself and/or your ideas to stakeholders
- Leverage knowledge and skill sets to enhance success
- Develop or enhance a process or good that enhances a stakeholder's position
- Leverage existing knowledge, skills, and abilities to develop a product or service offering for stakeholders:
  - At the correct price
  - With the proper amount of additional service
  - To be freely chosen as a viable alternative in the marketplace

referred to as *sciences* is that their proper application stems from the scientific process of inquiry, much the same as with other pharmaceutical sciences. The science of *accounting* (see Chapter 17) involves "keeping the books," or adequately keeping track of the business' transactions, such as sales revenues, wages paid to employees, prescription product purchases from suppliers, rent, and utility bills. This must be done to ensure that the company is meeting its debts and achieving its financial goals. Accounting is also used to determine the amount of taxes owed, make reports to external agencies and/or auditors, and identify areas where the company's assets could be managed more efficiently. While accounting is used to evaluate a company's financial position, *finance* is more concerned with the sources and uses of funds (e.g., Where will the money come from to pay for new and existing goods and services? Which goods and services are most likely to enhance profitability for a pharmacy?).

The other managerial science commonly associated with managing money is *economics*. However, the use of economics transcends financial considerations.

Economics is a tool to evaluate the inputs and outcomes of any number of processes. It can be used to determine the right mix of personnel and automated dispensing technologies, the optimal number of prescriptions dispensed given current staffing levels, whether or not a pharmacy should remain open for additional hours of business, and how much to invest in theft deterrence. It is also used to determine the most appropriate drugs to place on a formulary or to include in a critical pathway.

Human resources management (see Chapter 12) is used to optimize the productivity of any pharmacy's most critical asset—its people. It involves determining the jobs that need to be done, recruiting people for those jobs, hiring the right persons for those jobs, training them appropriately, appraising their performance, motivating them, and seeing that they are justly rewarded for their efforts. It also involves issues such as determining the right mix of fringe benefits and retirement, setting vacation and absentee policies, assistance with career planning, ensuring employees' on-the-job safety, and complying with laws and rules established by regulatory bodies.

It may be easy to assume that *marketing* is simply another word for *advertising* (see Chapters 21–24). However, while promotional activities are a significant component of marketing, its activities include identifying the company's strengths over its competitors, properly identifying consumer bases to which marketing strategies will be directed, carrying the right mix of goods and services, arranging these products for optimal "visual selling," and establishing the right prices for goods and services. Price setting is critical not only for goods but also especially for services. It is here that pharmacists often make mistakes when trying to establish patient care services. Services priced too low are unprofitable, perhaps even a money-losing proposition, whereas services priced too high will fail to attract customers.

Operations management (see Chapter 6) involves establishing policies delineating the activities of each employee on a day-to-day basis, what tools they will use to accomplish the tasks, and where those tasks will be performed (i.e., workflow design). It also entails maintaining the proper inventory of prescription and nonprescription products so that, on the one hand, the pharmacy is not consistently running out of drug products that patients need, and on the other hand, there are not excess amounts of products reaching their expiration date prior to sale or otherwise taking up valuable space that could be used for other purposes.

Knowledge and skill sets in each of these areas assist and inform yet another very important component of management, which is *value creation*, which can be defined as the art of utilizing foundational assets (e.g., knowledge, skills, and experiences) to generate the ability to create value for other stakeholders in the healthcare marketplace. This employs some aspect of personal selling, but also requires a firm grasp of internal and external environments to help you and/or your employing organization gain the most from current resources, and/or acquire needed resources to improve a business or create a new niche. In that way, it is an application of all the other managerial sciences and will be elaborated upon in Chapter 3.

"SMOOTH OPERATIONS"—REVISITING THE SCENARIO

The preceding discussion of the managerial sciences, especially the issue of workflow design in operations management, brings us back to the scenario involving Mary Quint. Pharmacy students questioning the significance of management and the importance of having a management perspective need not look much further than this case. Mary is faced with a dilemma probably all too common to pharmacy students and practitioners. Students who have worked in numerous environments probably can recall that in some of these places things just seemed to be "going well." Both the customers and the employers were happy, and it was not completely unpleasant to have to show up at work. At other places, there always appears to be a crisis. Immediately on waking up in the morning, the first thoughts are of dread at having to go to work that day. While this may be somewhat of an oversimplification, the latter places are not being managed well, whereas the former ones probably are. The tremendous variability that exists from one workplace to another is indicative of how critical management is for both the employees working there and the patients they serve. Now ask yourself, Where do you think that you would rather work, and where do you think that patients are receiving the best care, Middletown North Pharmacy or Middletown South Pharmacy?

CONCLUSION

Contrary to popular belief, good business practice and good patient care are not mutually exclusive. In fact, they are almost entirely mutually dependent. Superior patient care and the implementation of clinical services are made possible by pharmacists who are skilled in management. Pharmacists must be attuned to the internal and external forces that shape the practice of pharmacy. The managerial sciences of accounting, finance, economics, human resources management, marketing, and operations management are indispensable tools for today's practitioner.

QUESTIONS FOR FURTHER DISCUSSION

1. Would you be willing to extend your commute or make other similar sacrifices to work at a place where you enjoyed your job? Why or why not?
2. How do you feel about the role that management plays in the practice of pharmacy?
3. Can you identify someone in a managerial position who is very good at what he or she does? What is it that makes him or her effective?
4. Do you believe that you are going to be an effective pharmacist? What makes you think so?
5. Do you think that you are going to ascend eventually to a managerial position? Why or why not?

REFERENCES

American Association of Colleges of Pharmacy. 1996. Paper from the Commission to implement change in pharmaceutical education: Maintaining our commitment to change. *Am J Pharm Educ* 60:378.

Brodie DC. 1967. Drug-use control: Keystone to pharmaceutical service. *Drug Intell* 1:63.

Broeseker A, Janke KK. 1998. The evolution and revolution of pharmaceutical care. In McCarthy RL (ed.) *Introduction to Health Care Delivery: A Primer for Pharmacists.* Gaithersburg, MD: Aspen, p. 393.

Buerki RA, Vottero LD. 1994. *Ethical Responsibility in Pharmacy Practice.* Madison, WI: American Institute of the History of Pharmacy.

Carmel S, Glick SM. 2001. Compassionate-empathic physicians: Personality traits and social-organizational factors that enhance or inhibit this behavior pattern. *Soc Sci Med* 43:1253.

Desselle SP. 1997. Pharmacists' perceptions of pharmaceutical care practice standards. *J Am Pharm Assoc* NS37: 529.

Desselle SP, Alafris A. 1999. Changes in pharmacy education sharpen counseling skills. *US Pharmacist* 24:78.

Desselle SP, Rappaport HM. 1995. Feasibility and relevance of identified pharmaceutical care practice standards for community pharmacists. Paper presented at the American Association of Pharmaceutical Scientists Annual Meeting, Miami, FL, November 7.

Desselle SP, Rappaport HM. 1996. Establishing standards of care in the community setting. *J Pharm Care* 1:1.

Desselle SP, Tipton DJ. 2001. Factors contributing to the satisfaction and performance ability of community pharmacists: A path model analysis. *J Soc Admin Pharm* 18:15.

Fjortoft N, Zgarrick D. 2003. An assessment of pharmacists' caring ability. *J Am Pharm Assoc* 43:483.

Flyvbjerg B. 2006. From Nobel Prize to project management: Getting risks right. *Proj Manage J* 37:5.

Fronstin P. 2000. Confidence and confusion: The health care system in the United States. *Stat Bull* 81:18.

Gaither CA. 1998a. Investigation of pharmacists' role stress and the work/non-work interface. *J Soc Admin Pharm* 15:92.

Gaither CA. 1998b. Predictive validity of work/career-related attitudes and intentions on pharmacists' turnover behavior. *J Pharm Market Manage* 12:3.

Gaither CA, Ou HT, Doucette W, et al. 2008. Pharmacist and practice characteristics related to pharmacists' commitment, stress, satisfaction, and perceptions of health. Paper presented at the American Association of Colleges of Pharmacy Annual Meeting, Chicago, IL, July 19.

Harrison DL, Bootman JL. 1994. Strategic planning by institutional pharmacy administrators. *J Pharm Market Manage* 8:73.

Harrison DL, Ortmeier BG. 1995. Levels of independent community pharmacy strategic planning. *J Pharm Market Manage* 10:38–52.

Harrison DL, Ortmeier BG. 1996. Predictors of community pharmacy strategic planning. *J Pharm Market Manage* 11:21–34.

Hepler CD. 1987. The third wave in pharmaceutical education: The clinical movement. *Am J Pharm Educ* 51:369.

Hepler CD, Strand LM. 1990. Opportunities and responsibilities in pharmaceutical care. *Am J Hosp Pharm* 47:533.

Johnson KA, Chen S, Cheng IN, et al. 2010. The impact of clinical pharmacy services integrated into medical homes on diabetes-related clinical outcomes. *Ann Pharmaco* 44:612.

Institute of Medicine. 2006. *Preventing Medication Errors: Quality Chasm Series.* Washington, DC: National Academy of Sciences.

Keshishian F. 2010. Factors influencing pharmacy students' choice of major and its relationship to anticipatory socialization. *Am J Pharm Educ* 74:75.

Keshishian F, Brocavich JM, Boone RT, Pal S. 2010. Motivating factors influencing college students' choice of academic major. *Am J Pharm Educ* 74:46.

Kunyk D, Olson JK. 2001. Clarification of conceptualizations of empathy. *J Adv Nurs* 35:317.

Latif DA. 2000. Relationship between pharmacy students' locus of control, Machiavellianism, and moral reasoning. *Am J Pharm Educ* 64:33.

Lee JK, Grace KA, Taylor AJ. 2006. Effect of pharmacy care program on medication adherence and persistence, blood pressure, and low-density lipoprotein cholesterol: A randomized controlled trial. *JAMA* 296:2563.

Maine LL, Penna RP. 1996. Pharmaceutical care: An overview. In Knowlton C, Penna R (eds.) *Pharmaceutical Care.* New York: Chapman & Hall, p. 133.

Miller MJ, Ortmeier BG. 1995. Factors influencing the delivery of pharmacy services. *Am Pharm* NS35:39.

Millis JS. 1975. *Pharmacists for the Future: The Report of the Study Commission on Pharmacy.* Ann Arbor, MI: Health Administration Press.

Millis JS. 1976. Looking ahead: The Report of the Study Commission on Pharmacy. *Am J Hosp Pharm* 33: 134.

National Association of Chain Drug Stores (NACDS). 2010. The Chain Pharmacy Industry Profile: 2003. Alexandria, VA: National Association of Chain Drug Stores.

OECD (Organization for Economic Co-operation and Development). OECD Health Data 2010—Frequently Requested Data. Available at http://www.oecd.org/document/30/0,3343,en_2649_34631_12968734_1_1_1_1,00.html; accessed on December 6, 2010.

Pink LA. 1991. Hospitals. In Fincham JE, Wertheimer AI (eds.) *Pharmacists and the U.S. Healthcare System.* Binghamton, NY: Pharmaceutical Products Press, p. 158.

Public Law 108–173. 2010. Available at http://www.medicare.gov/medicarereform/108s1013.htm; accessed on December 6, 2010.

Public Law 111–148. 2010. Available at http://www.gpo.gov/fdsys/pkg/PLAW-111publ148/pdf/PLAW-111publ148.pdf; accessed on December 6, 2010.

Relman AS. 1988. Assessment and accountability: The third revolution in medical care. *New Engl J Med* 319:1220.

Smith WE. 1988. Excellence in the management of clinical pharmacy services. *Am J Hosp Pharm* 45:319.

Sonnedecker G. 1963. *Kremers and Urdang's History of Pharmacy.* Philadelphia, PA: Lippincott.

Speedie SM, Palumbo FB, Leavitt DE. 1974. Pharmacists' perceptions of the antecedents of success in pharmacy. *Contemp Pharm Pract* 3:189.

Stafford M. 2002. *Ex-Pharmacist Gets 30 years for Diluting Cancer Drugs.* Associated Press, December 5.

Tootelian DH, Gaedeke RM. 1993. *Essentials of Pharmacy Management.* St. Louis: Mosby.

Torrens PR. 1993. Historical evolution and overview of health service in the United States. In Williams JS, Torrens PR (eds.) *Introduction to Health Services,* 4th edn. Albany, NY: Delmar, p. 3.

Wiederholt JB, Wiederholt PA. 1997. The patient: Our teacher and friend. *Am J Pharm Educ* 61:415.

Wilkin NE. 1999. Pharmaceutical care: A clinical movement? *Mississippi Pharm* 26:13.

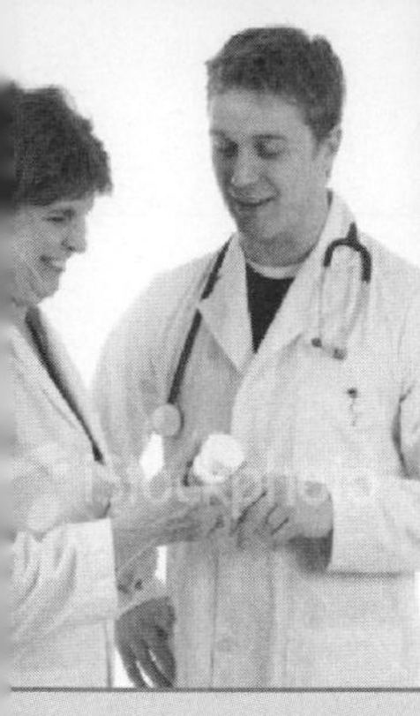

2

MANAGEMENT FUNCTIONS

David P. Zgarrick

About the Author: Dr. Zgarrick is professor and chair of the Department of Pharmacy Practice in the School of Pharmacy at Northeastern University's Bouvé College of Health Sciences. He received a B.S. degree in pharmacy from the University of Wisconsin and an M.S. and Ph.D. in pharmaceutical administration from The Ohio State University. He has practice experience in both independent and chain community pharmacy settings. He teaches courses in pharmacy management, business planning for professional services, and drug literature evaluation. His research interests are in pharmacist workforce issues, professional service development, and the use of evidence-based medicine by pharmacists.

LEARNING OBJECTIVES

After completing this chapter, readers should be able to

1. Define the terms *management* and *manager.* Describe how concepts in management figure into our everyday lives.
2. Compare and contrast *management* and *leadership.*
3. Compare and contrast classical views of management with modern views.
4. Describe the management process within the contexts of what managers do, resources they manage, and levels at which managers perform their roles.
5. Integrate modern views of management with the management process.
6. Apply the management process to all personal and professional activities.

SCENARIO

Krista Connelly is a second-year pharmacy student. Like most second-year students, she describes her life as "incredibly stressed out." A typical day consists of getting up at 6 a.m., getting dressed and running out the door by 7 a.m., and driving to school to get to her first class by 8 a.m. (making sure to avoid the accident on the expressway that she heard about on her way out the door). While at school, she finds time to squeeze in cups of coffee and snack bars between the lectures, labs, and workshops that usually last until at least 4 p.m. She also makes a point to go to the library to prepare upcoming assignments, as well as to meet with her professors to review how she did on her exams.

After class today, Krista has an Academy of Students of Pharmacy (ASP) meeting. Krista is the president of her chapter and works with committee chairs to accomplish the goals of the organization. In the past few weeks, she has helped the new professional service chairperson develop a brown bag seminar, talked her fund-raising chairperson out of quitting, and wrote a report on each committee's activities for the chapter Web site. While Krista enjoys her leadership role in ASP, she finds some of the people she works with to be frustrating and wonders how she can motivate them to do a better job.

After her meeting, Krista drives to a fast-food restaurant to grab a quick dinner on her way to her part-time pharmacy intern job. If she is not working, she will head to a friend's house to study for an upcoming exam. She usually gets back to her apartment by 10 p.m. and mentally prepares for what she needs to do in the next few days. She might catch a little bit of TV before heading to bed by midnight.

On weekends, Krista catches up on what one might call "activities of daily living." She does her laundry, pays her bills, surfs the Internet, calls her parents and friends back home, and gets together with her friends on Saturday nights. When Krista and her friends (most of whom are also pharmacy students) go out, they often talk about their plans after they graduate from pharmacy school. They talk about how exciting it will be to counsel patients, work with other health care professionals, and finally start making those high salaries they have heard so much about. None of them says that they want to be pharmacy managers. "The pharmacy manager at my store is always on my case about coming in late or having to arrange my hours around my exam schedule," said Krista. "I don't see how being a manager can help me do the things I want to as a pharmacist."

CHAPTER QUESTIONS

1. Why is it that all pharmacists should be considered managers regardless of their titles or positions?
2. Why should pharmacy students study management?
3. What is the difference between management and leadership?
4. How does management affect every aspect of our daily lives?
5. Will the same approach to management be effective for all types of situations encountered by pharmacists?

WHAT IS MANAGEMENT?

For many people, a distinct set of images comes to mind when they hear the word *management.* First and foremost, they think of a person (or possibly a group of people) who is "the boss" to whom they report at work. While some people view their relationships with management as positive, many of us have had experiences where this has not been the case. This is why when you ask people what they think of management, they often provide negative views and experiences. Ask pharmacy students what they think about entering careers in pharmacy management, and you likely will get answers similar to those provided by Krista Connelly and her friends in the scenario.

Perhaps it may be better to start by looking a bit more closely at the term *management.* The stem of the word is *manage,* which according to *Webster's Dictionary* is a verb meaning "to control the movement or behavior of, to lead or direct, or to succeed in accomplishing" (Allee, 1990). Think about how this definition applies to your daily life. Have you ever controlled the movement or behavior of someone or something (even if it was just yourself)? Have you ever succeeded in accomplishing a task (even if it was just getting to an examination on time)?

According to Tootelian and Gaedeke (1993), *management* is "a process which brings together resources and unites them in such a way that, collectively, they achieve goals or objectives in the most efficient manner possible." Contrary to what many people believe, management is a *process,* which is simply a method of doing something. Processes are used to perform simple everyday tasks (e.g., swinging a golf club or driving to school) as well as more complex activities (e.g., hiring a pharmacy technician or dosing an aminoglycoside drug). People perform processes because they want to achieve a goal or objective. Goals and objectives can be personal (e.g., a low golf score or getting to school on time) or professional (e.g., a smoothly operating pharmacy or high-quality patient care). Because processes require resources, and because resources are scarce (they are not present in unlimited supply), it is important that resources be used in such a way as to achieve goals and objectives in the most efficient manner possible. While one could achieve one's goal of getting to school on time by driving 90 miles an hour, one also could argue that this would not be the most efficient use of the driver's resources, especially if there is a sharp turn ahead or a police officer waiting around the corner.

Managers are simply people who perform management activities. While people whom we think of as "the boss" and those with administrative appointments within an organization certainly are managers, the fact is that anyone who has a task to accomplish or a goal to achieve is also a manager. Pharmacy students and pharmacists who say that they do not want to be managers may not desire the authority and responsibilities of having an administrative position, but there is no getting around their need to use resources efficiently to perform the tasks related to their jobs. Thus all pharmacists, regardless of their job responsibilities or position, should view themselves as managers.

Another term that is often used in concert with management is *leadership.* While some people use the terms interchangeably to describe characteristics that are expected of people who are "in charge" of organizations, leadership is a distinctly different skill from *management.* Leadership involves the ability to inspire or direct others. While it certainly is desirable that all managers also have leadership skills, they do not necessarily go hand in hand.

CLASSICAL AND MODERN VIEWS OF MANAGEMENT

While management and managers have been with us since humans have had tasks to perform and goals to accomplish (e.g., gathering food or finding shelter), the study of management as a scientific and academic curriculum is relatively new. Before the industrial revolution of the eighteenth and nineteenth centuries, most people lived and worked alone or in small groups. While people at that time still had goals and objectives that needed to be accomplished efficiently, there was little formal study of the best ways to do so. The advent of the industrial revolution brought together groups of hundreds and thousands of people who shared a common objective. To get large groups of people to work together effectively, industrialists and academics established hierarchies and systems that allowed large industrial organizations to accomplish their goals (especially those related to growth and profitability).

Around the turn of the twentieth century, an American industrialist and a French engineer began to publish observations in what would become known as the *classical,* or *administrative,* school of management thought. F. W. Taylor, an executive with Bethlehem Steel, published *The Principles of Scientific Management* in 1911. He was among the first to espouse applying scientific principles to management of the workplace. Henri Fayol, a French mining engineer and corporate executive, published *Administration Industrielle et Generale* in 1916. Both Taylor and Fayol argued that all organizations, regardless of size or objective, had to perform a standard set of functions to operate efficiently. Fayol's five management functions (i.e., forecasting and planning, organizing, commanding, coordinating, and controlling) became widely accepted throughout the industrialized world. Both Fayol's five management functions and 14 principles for organizational design (Table 2-1) are still used by managers

Table 2-1. Classical Management Theory (Fayol)

Fayol's five management functions
1. Forecast and plan
2. Organize
3. Command
4. Coordinate
5. Control

Fayol's 14 principles for organizational design and effective administration
- *Specialization/division of labor.* People should perform tasks specific to their skills. No one should be expected to perform all the skills needed to run an organization.
- *Authority with corresponding responsibility.* People with responsibility also have sufficient authority within an organization to ensure that a task is performed.
- *Discipline.* People should follow rules, with consequences for not following rules.
- *Unity of command.* The organization has an administrator who is recognized as having the ultimate authority (e.g., CEO or president).
- *Unity of direction.* The organization has a sense of direction or vision that is recognized by all members (e.g., mission statement).
- *Subordination of individual interest to general interest.* The goals of the organization supercede the goals of any individuals within the organization.
- *Remuneration of staff.* Employees should be paid appropriately given the market for their skills and their level of responsibility.
- *Centralization.* Performing similar tasks at a single location is more effective than performing these tasks at multiple locations.
- *Scalar chain/line of authority.* Each employee has one, and only one, direct supervisor.
- *Order.* Tasks should be performed in a systematic fashion.
- *Equity.* Supervisors should treat employees with a sense of fairness.
- *Stability of tenure.* Benefits should go to employees who have stayed with an organization longer.
- *Initiative.* Organizations and employees are more effective when they are proactive, not reactive.
- *Esprit de corps.* Teamwork, harmony.

today. For example, while in the scenario Krista Connelly has the responsibility for working with her ASP chapter's committee chairs, she cannot be effective in her ability to carry out her responsibilities unless her position provides her with authority that is recognized by the committee chairs. Chapter 11 provides more information on Fayol's principles of organizational design.

Much of Taylor's and Fayol's work was developed based on the workplace conditions of the nineteenth and early twentieth centuries. The great industries of those times focused primarily on the mass production of tangible goods. Very few people were educated beyond grammar school. The few people with higher levels of education (almost always men) generally were given administrative positions. They were expected to supervise large numbers of less educated production-line employees. In this hierarchy, the role of administrators generally was to command and control their employees, and the role of workers was to carry out the tasks at hand without question.

On the other hand, the workforce and workplace of the late twentieth and early twenty-first centuries have evolved into something quite different. According to the US Bureau of Labor Statistics (2011), more than three times the number of people are involved in the provision of services than in the production of tangible goods. Today's workforce is better educated and more highly skilled than workers had been in the past. In many cases, today's administrators have less formal education and fewer technical skills than the people they are supervising.

These trends have led many to question the relevance of classical management theories in today's rapidly changing world. Walk down the "Business" aisle of practically any bookstore and you'll find literally hundreds of books written by management "gurus" such as Covey, Drucker, Peters, and many others espousing modern management techniques and offering "hands on" advice about how to deal with day-to-day workplace issues. Researchers apply scientific methods to the study of management and publish their results in scholarly journals, similar to what we see in pharmacy and medicine. These books and research studies make important contributions to management science, given the continued need to use scarce resources to achieve goals and objectives in an ever-changing business climate. However, classical management theory still has a place in today's pharmacies, as well as in our personal lives.

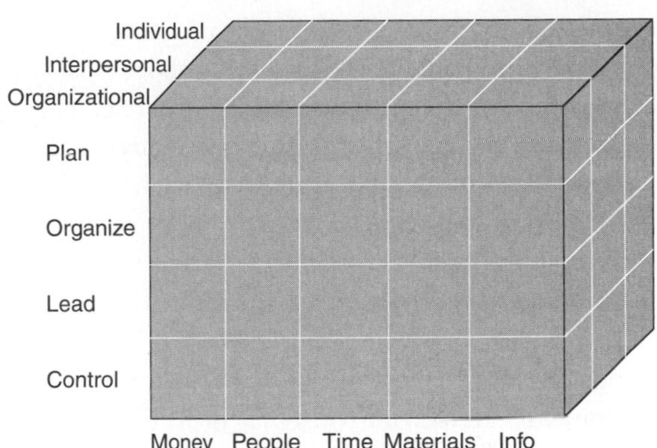

Figure 2-1. The management process.

THE MANAGEMENT PROCESS

Figure 2-1 describes one way in which Fayol's management functions can be adapted to describe what managers do in today's world. There are three dimensions of management: (1) activities that managers perform, (2) resources that managers need, and (3) levels at which managers make decisions. Every action taken by a manager involves at least one aspect of each of the three dimensions.

Management Activities

Fayol's five management functions have been adapted to describe four activities that all managers perform. While managers who hold administrative positions in their organizations may have formal ways of performing these activities (and are evaluated on their ability to get them done), all managers (which means all of us!) perform each of these activities every day, whether we are thinking of them or not.

The first of these four activities is planning. *Planning* is predetermining a course of action based on one's goals and objectives. Managers must consider many factors when planning, including their internal and external environments. The chief pharmacist at a community pharmacy or the director of a hospital pharmacy will develop plans to predetermine which drug products she wishes to carry or what professional services she might offer. Some pharmacists will even go so far as to develop formal strategic and business plans for their pharmacies (see Chapters 4, 5, 25, and 26). On the other hand, planning can also be very informal. Anyone who goes to work or school in the morning develops a plan for how he will get there (i.e., What time do I need to arrive? What form of transportation should I take? What route should I follow?).

The next management activity is organizing. *Organizing* is the arrangement and relationship of activities and resources necessary for the effective accomplishment of a goal or objective. Once a pharmacist has decided which drug products or services she should offer, she needs to ask herself *what* resources she needs to provide them, *how* she will go about obtaining these resources, and then determine *when* she will need to obtain them. Once the person going to work or school has a plan, he needs to think about what else he may need to do to accomplish his goal (e.g., check the weather and traffic reports, get gas in his car, drop his kids off with a child care provider, etc.).

The next step is the leading or directing step. This step combines Fayol's command and coordinate steps to provide a better description of what managers actually do in today's world. *Leading* or *directing* involves bringing about purposeful action toward some desired outcome. It can take the form of actually doing something yourself (the person going to work or school just needs to get up and go) or working with others to lead them to where you want your organization to be. A pharmacist eventually may offer the goods and services described in her plans, but almost certainly will need to work with a number of other people within her organization to accomplish this task. In the scenario, Krista Connelly, in her role as president of her ASP chapter, is responsible for seeing that the chapter's committees work effectively to accomplish their objectives. Working with others often requires leadership skills, which will be discussed in Chapter 16.

The fourth step is the control or evaluation step. *Control* or *evaluation* involves reviewing the progress that has been made toward the objectives that were set out in the plan. This step involves not only determining *what* actually happened but also *why* it happened. Performing quality-control checks to help ensure that patients are receiving the desired medication in the appropriate manner is a very important function of a pharmacy practice. Pharmacists also can ask themselves if the goods and services they offered met their goals. These goals can be from the perspective of their patients (e.g., Did the goods and services result in high-quality patient care or improved clinical outcomes?), as well as from other perspectives (e.g., Did the service improve the pharmacist's job satisfaction? Did it improve the profitability of the pharmacy or organization?). The person going to work or school not only should ask himself if he arrived on time, but also should know why he did or did not (e.g., the traffic accident on the expressway, hitting the snooze button that third time before getting up, etc.). Chapters 8, 9, and 29 review methods that pharmacists use to evaluate the outcomes of their services, ensure the quality of their operations, and reduce the occurrence of medication errors.

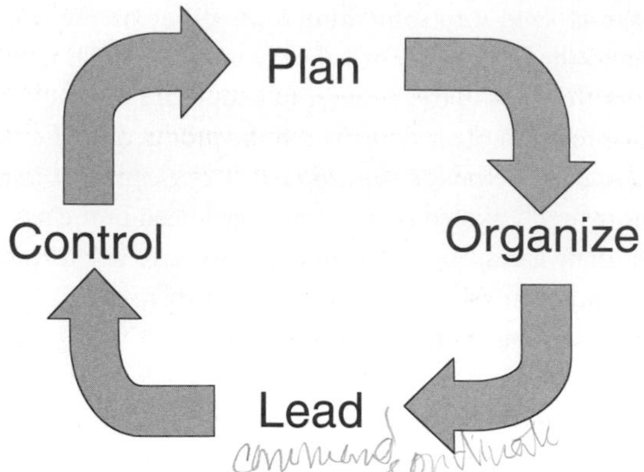

Figure 2-2. Management activities cycle.

Management activities should be performed in order, starting with the planning step. They are also meant to be cyclic, meaning that what a manager learns in the control and evaluation step should be incorporated back into the planning step the next time she needs to accomplish that objective (Fig. 2-2). For example, if a pharmacy student receives a score on an examination that did not meet his goal, he should use what he learned in the evaluation step (e.g., what questions he got wrong, time spent studying, etc.) to help him plan for the next examination.

Resources That are Managed

Regardless of their level or position within an organization, managers must use resources to achieve their goals and objectives. Keep in mind that resources are scarce, meaning that they are not available in unlimited supply. Both organizations and individuals must use resources efficiently to achieve their goals and objectives.

The first resource that many managers think of is money. Customers generally provide money to pharmacies and pharmacists in exchange for goods and services. Employers generally pay their employees money in exchange for the services they provide to the organization. Managing money is important to any organization or individual, and several chapters of this book are dedicated to explaining how pharmacies and pharmacists manage money and use economic information to make decisions (see Chapters 17 to 20). Money in and of itself can be an important yardstick for measuring the success of an organization or an individual. However, most managers value money for its ability to allow them to obtain additional resources that are necessary to achieve other goals and objectives.

Another resource that is very important to managers is people. In pharmacy practice, there is very little that any one person can accomplish on his or her own, regardless of the practice setting. Pharmacists must work with other employees in their pharmacies, other health care professionals, and especially the patients and customers they serve. Given the importance of this topic, an entire section of this book (Chapters 11 through 15) is dedicated to the management of people.

How many times have you heard someone say, "I'd have got that done if I'd have had more time"? Of all the resources managers have at their disposal, time can be the most limiting. After all, there are only 24 hours in a day! Time management is essential for today's busy pharmacist, as well as for most other people. In the scenario, Krista Connelly is a great example of a pharmacy student who could benefit from time and stress management. Chapter 10 is dedicated to time management, stress management, and organizational skills that can help you to get the most out of this precious resource.

When many people think of pharmacy, they still think of a pharmacist standing behind a counter compounding drug products and dispensing prescriptions. While pharmacy practice continues to evolve from a product to a patient orientation, managing material resources is still an important function in any pharmacy. Community pharmacies filled 3.6 billion prescriptions in 2009, an increase of over 30 percent over the past decade (NACDS, 2010). The costs of these drug products, as well as the costs of the equipment and supplies necessary to dispense them safely and efficiently to patients, continues to rise in all practice settings. Just as people need to assess their needs and supplies of material goods (e.g., food, clothing, household supplies, etc.) before going on a shopping trip, pharmacies need to make the same assessments before purchasing drug products, equipment, and supplies. Chapters 6, 23, and 24 are all designed to help readers learn more about managing material resources.

While the eighteenth and nineteenth centuries were known as the time of the industrial revolution, the twenty-first century certainly will be known as the information age. The advent of the computer and the Internet in the late twentieth century has resulted in an explosion of information that is literally at most people's fingertips. This already has had a tremendous impact on pharmacy practice, providing pharmacists with information about drugs and patients that they did not have only a few years ago. While it is not certain what implications this will have for pharmacy practice in the future, it is certain that information management is becoming an important job for pharmacists. Chapter 7 provides an overview of technologies that pharmacists use to manage information, as well as insights into what role information management may have in the future of pharmacy practice.

Levels of Management

When managers perform management activities, they can do so at a number of levels within an organization, and with a variety of different purposes in mind. While some people think of management activities occurring only in corporations and other complex organizations, management activities take place in all types of organizations, involving all levels of interactions among their members.

There is not a person reading this book who has not performed self-management activities. Just the fact that you are a pharmacy student or pharmacist attests to the fact that you have performed a number of activities on your own just to get to this point. Self-management is the most frequently occurring level of management, if for no other reason than that practically every decision we make every day (both professional and personal) requires self-management. For example, pharmacists must prioritize and manage their time efficiently so that they can accomplish the wide variety of tasks, from ensuring that every prescription is dispensed accurately to making sure that they have time to counsel their patients.

Next to self-management, the most frequent level on which managers find themselves performing is the interpersonal level. Interpersonal management occurs between the manager and one other person. In a pharmacy, this might involve a pharmacist counseling a patient about a medication or training a technician on how to submit a claim for a medication therapy management service with a third-party payer. Our personal lives are full of interpersonal relationships, including those with our parents, siblings, spouse, children, friends, and significant others.

The level of management that occurs the least often is organizational management. This involves actions that affect groups of people. We frequently think of this occurring at work, especially when a pharmacist needs to develop a policy or make a decision that may affect many people at the pharmacy. High-level administrators in large organizations (e.g., pharmacy chains, hospitals, etc.) often make decisions that affect everyone within the organization. Keep in mind that people who hold administrative positions are not the only ones who perform organizational management. Anyone who has ever had to make an "executive decision" among a group of classmates who are studying for an examination or deciding where to go for lunch can relate to the kinds of organizational-level decisions that business leaders make every day.

INTEGRATING MODERN AND CLASSICAL VIEWS OF MANAGEMENT

Much of what was first described by Taylor and Fayol at the beginning of the twentieth century is still applied today by managers at all levels of administration in all types of organizations. However, much has changed in both pharmacy practice and the workplace over that time, and management science has exploded to keep up with those changes.

In the past, the relationship between an administrator and a worker was often hierarchical. The authority of the administrator generally went unquestioned, and workers simply did what they were told. In today's workplace, there is often more of a partnership between administrators and workers. While administrators are still responsible for achieving organizational goals and objectives, workers generally expect to have input as to how goals and objectives will be developed, and expect to share in the rewards when those goals are accomplished.

Health care organizations such as hospitals and pharmacies present a number of managerial challenges to administrators. Unlike the workers of Taylor's and Fayol's day, most health care workers are highly educated and skilled professionals. Trends toward specialization among health care professionals often create situations where staff-level health care workers have more knowledge and expertise of their particular area than their administrators. As you can imagine, administrators of health care professionals who attempt to use their authority to command and control these employees may find this not to be an effective way to achieve organizational goals and objectives. According to Drucker, "knowledge workers" in today's information age need to ask "what *should*" they be doing in light of their own values, in accordance with the objectives and values of the organization (Drucker, 1999).

Modern views of management suggest that managers must adapt their management activities to their workers. These functions generally occur in addition to the classical management functions. According to Nelson and Economy (2003), today's manager also needs to

- *Energize.* Today's managers need to have a vision of what they want to create and the energy to make it happen. When you think of good managers with whom you have worked with, they are probably not the kind of people who just want to keep doing the same thing every day for the rest of their lives. They have ideas about what they would like to see their organizations become in the future, and the energy and enthusiasm to attract others to want to join them in achieving their goals. They are always trying to make the best stressful situations, especially when the level of resources available may be less than they desire. In pharmacy today, good managers are often pharmacists who want to see the profession move forward by developing new goods and services, especially those that improve patient care. Their energy and enthusiasm attract motivated pharmacists and other personnel who share their vision and want to work with them. These managers also seem to find the resources they need to carry out their vision or make the most of what they already have. Not only does the power of energy and enthusiasm work for pharmacists, but it also benefits pharmacy students. Do you think that Krista Connelly would be as an effective leader if she did not have a high level of energy and enthusiasm for ASP's goals and objectives?

- *Empower.* If you are a highly educated and skilled health professional, the last thing you want is to have an administrator questioning your decisions and telling you how you should do your job. In today's environment, managers should empower their employees to do what needs to be done. In many ways, today's manager is very much like the coach of a team. Coaches develop a game plan; select players; provide them with training, resources, and advice; and then step back and let the players execute the game plan. Good coaches empower their players to carry out the game plan. Managers who empower their employees provide them with training, resources, and advice and then let the employees get the job done. Krista Connelly can empower her ASP committee chairpersons by providing them with goals, resources, and advice and then letting them get to work.

  This is not to say that managers do not need to supervise their employees. Managers are still responsible for seeing that organizational goals are met, which may mean having to intervene with workers. Just as coaches need to provide resources and advice to their players during a game, and occasionally replace a player who is not executing the game plan, managers need to provide resources, advice, and occasionally discipline to see that organizational goals are met.

- *Support.* After a manager has empowered her employees to do their jobs, she should not just leave them on their own, especially when things start to go wrong. Today, good managers need to be coaches, collaborators, and sometimes even cheerleaders for their employees. Providing support for employees does not mean that managers should be willing to do their employees' work or always agree with the decisions employees make on the job. It does mean that managers need to provide employees with the training, resources, and authority needed to do their jobs. Managers also need to be good coaches, letting employees know when they have done a good job, as well as helping them learn when things are not going so well. Even pharmacy students like Krista Connelly know that a few kind words to her committee chairpersons will help the ASP chapter in the long run.

  In providing support, managers must also be mindful to balance the needs and resources of their organizations with what employees need. As much as a manager may wish to give a valued employee a big raise, the manager must also consider how much money is available for a raise amongst other potential uses of his organization's financial resources.

- *Communicate.* In today's information-laden environment, communication between managers and employees is more important than ever. While managers can energize, empower, and support their employees, if they cannot communicate their messages, they will not be effective and their organizations will suffer. The cornerstone of communications in any environment is trust. If employees feel that they can bring up any question or concern to a manager, they will likely be more receptive to what the manager has to say.

  One major challenge for managers and employees today is the vast number of ways in which they can communicate. Communication that once took place between managers and employees in person now can take place over the telephone, via voice mail or e-mail, in a text message, or even through a social network such as Facebook or Twitter. While these additional methods can make it easier for managers and employees to communicate with each other, care must be taken in using these methods. As you can imagine, not every method of communication is appropriate for every type of message (e.g., disciplining or firing an employee in a text message is *not* a good idea).

WHY SHOULD I STUDY MANAGEMENT?

After reading the first two chapters of this book, you still may be asking yourself, "Why should I study management?" You may think that being a good manager just involves using your common sense and applying the Golden Rule (act toward others as you would have others act toward you). After all, you probably have done a good job managing yourself up to this point without taking a management course or reading a management textbook. Can managing a pharmacy practice be that much different?

While there is certainly a role for applying self-management skills, most pharmacy managers agree that managing a pharmacy practice successfully requires a unique set of skills. Some of these skills can be quite technical [e.g., financial management (see Chapters 17 through 19) and marketing (see Chapters 21 through 24)], requiring a knowledge base that goes beyond what many pharmacists bring to their practices. These skills should be learned just as one would learn medicinal chemistry, pharmacology, or therapeutics.

Something else to keep in mind is that in today's workplace, what might be common sense to you may not make sense at all to the other people you encounter. Pharmacists today work with employees, other health professionals, and especially patients who come from a wide variety of racial, ethnic, cultural, and educational backgrounds. People from diverse backgrounds bring with them an incredible amount of insight and experience. Pharmacists who do not take this diversity into account when working with people may find themselves frustrated and not able to achieve their goals and objectives effectively.

This book presents material that is relevant to both pharmacy students and pharmacists. Pharmacy students who use this book will find that many of the scenarios that start each chapter are directed toward experiences to which they can relate. There may be some of you right now who think that your life has a lot in common with Krista Connelly's. We anticipate that this is the case. The information provided in each chapter not only will help students to better deal with management issues they are currently experiencing but will also help to prepare them for what to expect in the future as pharmacists.

Pharmacists who use this book often have a good idea of why they need to have management skills. After all, they are living pharmacy practice management on a daily basis! The information provided in this book should help provide pharmacists with the skills they will need to better meet the challenges they face every day. In addition, the last six chapters of this book (Chapters 31 through 36) describe how pharmacists in a variety of practice settings apply management skills on a daily basis.

QUESTIONS FOR FURTHER DISCUSSION

Listed below are three scenarios that represent how pharmacists use the management process on a daily basis. For each scenario, please describe (1) the level of management being performed, (2) the type of management activity being performed, and (3) the resources that the pharmacist needs to perform this activity.

Scenario 1: Sabin Patel, R.Ph., is trying to decide what form of education (nontraditional Pharm.D., certificate program, continuing education) would best allow her to maintain her practice skills.

Scenario 2: Doug Danforth, Pharm.D., is training a technician regarding information that needs to be collected during an initial patient interview.

Scenario 3: Casey Kulpinski, Pharm.D., is reviewing her pharmacy's financial statements to determine if her diabetes care center met her chain's financial goals.

REFERENCES

Allee JG (ed.). 1990. *Webster's Dictionary.* Baltimore, MD: Ottenheimer Publishers.

Drucker PF. 1999. *Management Challenges for the 21st Century.* New York: Harper Collins.

National Association of Chain Drug Stores (NACDS). 2010. *The Chain Pharmacy Industry Profile: 2010.* Alexandria, VA: National Association of Chain Drug Stores.

Nelson B, Economy P. 2003. *Managing for Dummies,* 2nd edn. New York: Wiley.

Tootelian DH, Gaedeke RM. 1993. *Essentials of Pharmacy Management.* St. Louis, MO: Mosby.

U.S. Bureau of Labor Statistics. 2011. http://www.bls.gov/webapps/legacy/cpsatab13.htm; accessed on August 5, 2011.

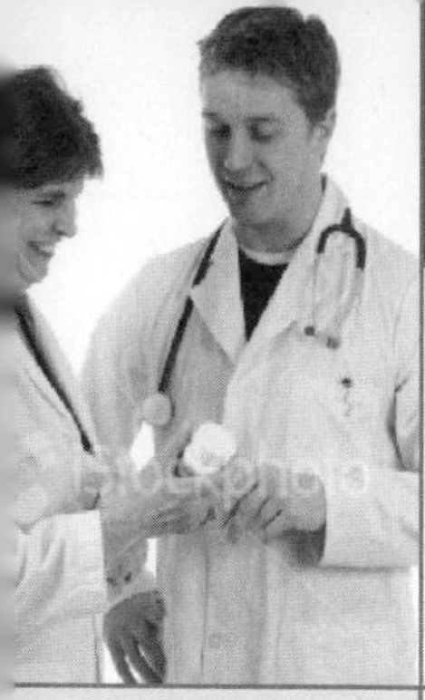

3

CREATING AND MANAGING VALUE

Greg L. Alston and Joseph C. Blizzard

About the Authors: Greg L. Alston is an associate professor of pharmacy management and assistant dean for assessment at Wingate University School of Pharmacy in North Carolina. Before coming to academia he had over 15 years of experience in chain drug and food/drug store management, as well as an additional 15 years of experience owning and operating multiple independent drug stores and other businesses. He earned a Doctor of Pharmacy degree from the University of the Pacific while simultaneously becoming a credentialed K-12 teacher through the School of Education. He teaches pharmacy management, community health outreach and pharmacy communications skills courses. His main research interest is in quantifying and qualifying the processes required to create viable professional niche business models.

Dr. Blizzard is director of operations for Beam Pharmacies, which operates approximately 30 independent pharmacies in North and South Carolina. After receiving a B.S. in Pharmacy from the University of Oklahoma and practicing independent pharmacy, he attended the University of South Carolina to earn his Ph.D. in Pharmacoeconomics. Dr. Blizzard taught courses in pharmacy management, leadership, and psychosocial and behavioral aspects of health care at Wingate University School of Pharmacy before returning to independent pharmacy management.

LEARNING OBJECTIVES

After completing this chapter, readers should be able to

1. Describe how value is created.
2. Describe the relative value theorem.
3. Describe the stakeholders in the health care marketplace.
4. Apply the relative value theorem to pharmacy practice.
5. Apply the relative value theorem to guide your personal life.

SCENARIO

James Deaux recently graduated with a Doctor of Pharmacy degree, earning a 3.9 GPA. He was a leader in Rho Chi and Phi Lambda Sigma and actively involved in several other student organizations. James performed well in his experiential rotations and generally received high marks from his preceptors.

James decided to apply for a clinical pharmacist position at The Ideal Hospital, located in the same city as his pharmacy school. He has crafted an impressive resume and was invited by Dr. Frank Stein, director of pharmacy, to interview for the position. After greetings and a few minutes of chitchat, Dr. Stein gets right to the point. "James you seem like a fine young man. Your credentials are impeccable. But we have had over 100 applicants for this position. In the interest of not wasting time and getting right to the point, I have only two questions to ask you. What do you have to offer me that the other 99 applicants do not? What are you going to do for me and The Ideal Hospital that should make me want to pay you $120,000 per year?"

How should James respond?

CHAPTER QUESTIONS

1. What is the current state of the health care marketplace?
2. What is the status of the pharmacist job market? Why is postgraduate training (residencies, fellowships, and graduate school) required for some pharmacist positions, but not for others?
3. What is the role of the pharmacist regarding management of drug therapy for individual patients? For organizations? For society? How successful have pharmacists been in these roles?
4. What is the concept of "value"? How can pharmacists add value to their patients, organizations, and society?

INTRODUCTION

The health care market place is changing rapidly. Health care reform legislation (*Summary of New Health Reform Law*, The Henry J Kaiser Family Foundation, 2011), budget deficits (Congressional Budget Office, 2010a), healthcare spending (*Healthcare Costs*, The Henry J Kaiser Family Foundation, 2009; Passel and Cohn, 2008), the patient-centered medical home model (Joint Principles of the Patient Centered Medical Home, 2007), scope of practice disputes (Kaldy, 2010), the great recession (Taylor et al., 2010), and payment model concerns (MEDPAC, 2007) have and will continue to alter the market for health care. Given the realities of the market for pharmacist positions, resource constraints, a changing landscape in health care, and the knowledge and skills that pharmacists and students gain across their education and work experience, all pharmacists and students should ask two critical questions:

1. How will I distinguish myself to get the position I want with the salary I desire?
2. How will the profession of pharmacy serve the needs of patients, health care professionals, the health care system and society?

The market for pharmacists is challenging due to economic pressures, with more graduates chasing fewer jobs (Knapp et al., 2010). Yet at the same time there are expanding new roles and opportunities for pharmacists (APhA, 2008; JCPP, 2005). Pharmacy residencies are more difficult to obtain as increasingly large numbers of graduates chase a limited number of positions (Knapp et al., 2009). Yet pharmacy students often focus much of their time and efforts mastering the clinical skills required to be a good pharmacist. Students tend to judge courses such as pharmacy management as having a lower priority than more clinically oriented courses such as pharmacology and therapeutics. It is important to remember that the key to one's success as a pharmacist is not, and never will be, what he or she knows, but rather what that pharmacist can do with what he or she knows. A critical component of learning to become a pharmacist is to do something useful with one's knowledge to create value for those who will be impacted—including their patients, coworkers, organization, profession, and society at large.

Anecdotal evidence suggests that pharmacists are not hired by employers in rank order of their pharmacy school grade point average. Factors such as past work experience, communication skills, problem solving and the ability to work effectively with others have also influence hiring decisions. This suggests that employers believe that success in the workplace requires a different set of attributes and behaviors than how success may have been measured in the classroom. The workplace requires pharmacists to translate knowledge into useful actions. Pharmacists who can do this successfully are rewarded, while pharmacists who cannot may find themselves with limited opportunities in the workplace.

An essential skill that distinguishes any individual from others is the ability to create value for those with whom they interact and serve. A pharmacist must not only create value, but also must clearly articulate their value to others to thrive as a professional in today's health care environment. This chapter will explore how to create value using an approach known as the *relative value theorem* (RVT). This approach borrows from literature in neuroscience, marketing, and economics to create a model that is simple to understand and easy to apply to decisions pharmacists make on a daily basis (Alston and Blizzard, 2011).

THE RELATIVE VALUE THEOREM

Pharmacy students and pharmacists cannot increase their value to the constituencies they serve unless they understand conceptually how value is created and utilized. Zeithaml has defined the concept of value, suggesting that value is a function of our desire to obtain high-quality goods and services that meet our needs and wants, as well as what we need to sacrifice to obtain them (usually, but not always, money or some other resource). The perceived value of a good or service has been defined as a balance between what one gets relative to what they must give up to obtain that benefit (Zeithaml, 1988). For example, the "value" of a drug product can be assessed by comparing the benefits that a patient obtains from using a drug (e.g., lower blood pressure, increased quality of life) relative to the costs of obtaining the drug (e.g., money, time, effort). The services that a pharmacist provides to a patient or an employer can be assessed in the same way. What benefits does that pharmacist bring to their patients or employer relative to what the patients or employer must pay to receive the pharmacist's services?

The RVT is a conceptual model that attempts to illuminate key factors that a "buyer" uses to decide which goods or services to select for "purchase" from a list of possible alternatives. Whether a "buyer" is buying a tangible good at a store, or agreeing to use a professional service from a health professional, the mental process used to decide whether or not to make a purchase is the same. The "buyer" can be an individual patient, another health care professional, or an organization such as a business, insurance company or government agency. This decision to purchase a good or utilize a service is made by comparing the options available in the marketplace of choices. The person or entity considering the purchase must make a choice by comparing what they get, versus what they have to give up, to satisfy their needs and wants (see Chapter 21). Understanding how value is created can guide pharmacists in their decisions of what goods to sell in their pharmacies, and in the development of patient-care services. Understanding how value is created also can assist pharmacy students in creating their own career value strategies for potential employers. By understanding how they can translate their knowledge, skills, and experience to help meet the needs of potential employers, pharmacy students can market their value in an effort to obtain a position. Because just as any consumer likes a good bargain (when the benefits obtained from a good or service outweighs their costs), any employer would hope to obtain the same from their employees (the benefits of having the employee outweigh the costs of employment).

Value, and specifically relative value (RV), can be expressed as a mathematical equation ($RV = (P + S) \times PV$) where P is price, S is service and PV is perceived value. The relationships between these concepts can also be described graphically (see Fig. 3-1).

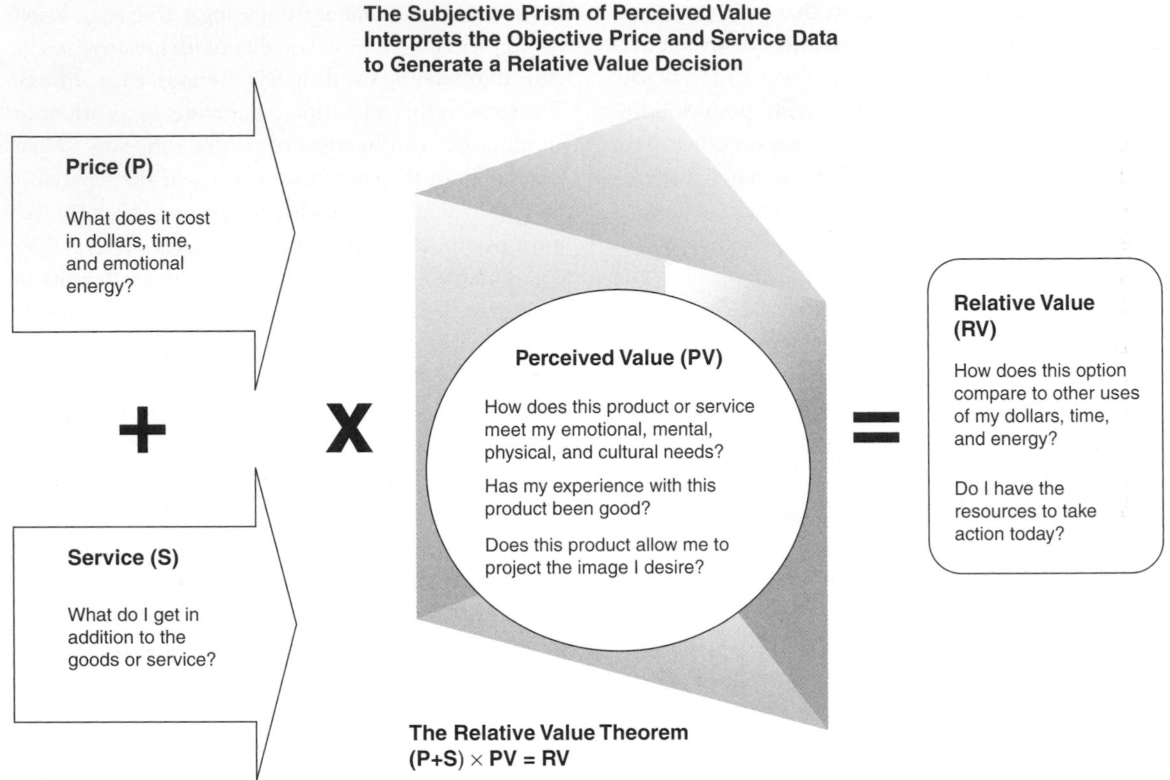

Figure 3-1. The relative value theorem. (Dr. Greg Alston Copyright 2012.)

As will be further described in Chapters 13 and 21, there are links between customer service, quality, and purchasing habits (Bloemer et al., 1999; Bolton and Drew, 1991; Caruana et al., 2000; Churchill and Surprenant, 1982; Cronin et al., 2000; Oliver, 1993). In addition, customer loyalty and profitability of a business over the long term are improved by service quality as perceived by the customer (Reicheld, 1996; Venetis and Ghauri, 2004; Woodruff, 1997). Therefore quality, customer service, as well as price matter in the mind of the purchaser of goods and services. Purchases are not just based on the amount of money sacrificed to obtain the good or service, but also on a variety of factors including the quality of the good or service, the expected outcomes associated with using the good or service, the reputation of the vendor offering the good or service, the other "costs" of obtaining the good or service (physical, social, time), and the overall benefits the consumer perceives by having the good or service. The RVT model organizes these factors into three component groups listed as price (P), service (S), and perceived value (PV). When combined in algebraic form, these components determine the overall relative value of a good or service in the mind of the 'buyer."

The relative value theorem is moderated by a fundamental question that buyers must ask themselves at some point; "Do I have the resources available to make the purchase at this time?" If the answer is yes, the buyer performs the mental calculations in determining if they are willing to sacrifice their resources given the benefits they perceive they will obtain by making the purchase. If the answer is no, the mental calculations inherent in the RVT are not altered in any way. A buyer still can consider if they would sacrifice the resources if they had them. On the other hand, the buyer must delay making an actual purchase decision until the resources are available. Note that decisions that buyers make when they have resources to make a purchase may be different from those made when they do not.

Price (P)

The first element of the RVT is the price (P) component. The pricing element of the equation is the component in which the consumer analyzes the cost to acquire a good or service. Cost can include monetary and nonmonetary factors. Since we know that a variety of products exist in the marketplace, and that not all products are identically priced, there must be something besides price alone that buyers consider (Alston and Blizzard, 2011).

Service (S)

The concept of service (S in the RVT equation) widens the consumer thought process beyond the price/cost comparison. Service factors are those things the provider could market or use to distinguish their good or service from competing products. When developing a new good or service, pharmacists should consider these distinguishing features and purposefully build them into the overall design of their product. Pharmacists can continue to highlight these extra benefits in their communications and marketing efforts to create perceptions of value in the minds of their consumers over and above a low price strategy.

Perceived Value (PV)

Perceived value (PV), the third element of the RVT equation, is defined as the cognitive tradeoff between perceptions of quality (what I get) versus the sacrifice (what I have to give up) (Drew and Bolton, 1987). Buyers considering a purchase ask themselves several questions about any good or service. They include (1) How well does this good or service meet my emotional, mental, physical, and cultural needs? (2) How well does this good or service allow me to project the image I desire to project? (3) How satisfactory has my experience with the good or service been? The more positive the responses are, the higher the perceived value created in the mind of the buyer. However, the more negative the responses are to these questions, the lower the perceived value. For example, many patients consider these questions before deciding to get a prescription filled. Positive responses to these questions increase the perceived value of the medication in the eyes of the patient, increasing the likelihood that the prescription will be filled.

The reason the (P + S) portion of the formula is multiplied by the PV component in the RVT model is to reflect the hypothesis that a buyer's perceived value of a professional service or tangible good can trump or overrule its price and service elements. Conceptually, if a buyer determines a perceived value of zero for a professional service or tangible good, then the RVT predicts that RV will equal zero and the good or service will not be purchased, regardless of its price or service elements.

Setting a lower price on a good or service does not necessarily make it better or increase the likelihood that it will be purchased. The risk in using low price as a marketing strategy is that another marketer may be able to provide a similar good or service at an even lower price. The market risk is that a good or service could become a commodity, with sales that go up or down solely on how the competition is priced. A low-price strategy is only successful if the marketer will *always* be the low-price leader, and then only if the price generated covers the costs of producing the goods and services.

An advantage to pharmacies that develop professional services is their ability to attract customers willing to pay for the benefits they receive from the service, rather than seeking out the lowest price on a commodity such as a prescription drug product. While amoxicillin 500 mg should be the same regardless of the pharmacy, the services that a pharmacy provides to accompany that product (e.g., patient counseling, prescription delivery, therapeutic drug monitoring) can help shift consumer attention away from the price of the drug and toward the benefits of the services. A high-service strategy will succeed if high-quality service is consistently delivered at a fair price. This high-service strategy allows a pharmacist to stand apart from the competition and offer a clear alternative to the low-price strategy. An additional benefit of creating a service-based business is that it is more difficult for competitors to copy a successful business model. Professional service success is based upon the service provided, not solely the price charged. The challenge for continued success in a high-service business strategy is to consistently deliver great service and promote the business to distinguish their offerings from less expensive alternatives.

There are numerous products that consumers purchase due to their personal preferences, even though less expensive alternatives exist in the market. A good example is purchasing a car. A pharmacy student may want a nice car that he or she cannot afford. If the student values paying tuition more than buying a nice car (PV), the student may shop for a lower-priced car (P) that will not break down and will be inexpensive to maintain (S), such as a Honda Civic. Once the student graduates and starts earning a higher income, the same student may prefer a vehicle that reflects his or her new status. In this situation, the perceived value of the Honda Civic may become zero if it does not reflect the image the student wishes to project. The fact that the Civic sells for $20,000 dollars less than a BMW or Lexus is not important in the eyes of a purchaser seeking status over function. Honda may offer Civics at bargain prices, but the purchaser may not buy one if he or she has graduated to a luxury car mindset. Interestingly, once the purchaser starts a family, he or she may find themselves back in the economy car mindset, as one's values often change with their priorities. The RVT does not predict the future, it simply suggests what is likely to happen using given set of conditions.

The relative value theorem predicts that any professional service must have potential for generating a high perceived value (PV) in the minds of potential buyers if it is to succeed in the marketplace. The RVT predicts that if consumers do not perceive any value for a particular good or service (PV = $0), they will not assign it a relative value regardless of the price or level of service provided, and will not make a purchase because there will be no relative value. Conversely, high perceived value not only leads to purchase behavior, but can build high customer loyalty and result in higher profitability (Reicheld, 1996). Ultimately, PV exists in the mind of the consumer. Marketers such as pharmacies and pharmacists can attempt to influence PV by offering competitive pricing, enhancing the quality of their service offering, and adding additional service elements to their offer. But the only true metric for success is sufficient marketplace response.

Given the decreased profitability associated with dispensing prescriptions to third-party payers (see Chapter 19), pharmacists are increasingly developing professional services with the intention that consumers pay to obtain the benefits they can offer. Pharmacists must note that they are not the only professionals capable of providing services such as immunizations, smoking cessation, disease state management, drug regimen reviews, or even dispensing prescription medications. Pharmacists' failure to demonstrate that they can provide services at a competitive price, with better outcomes, or with high perceived value in the eyes of consumers may find consumers turning to other providers to obtain these services (e.g., physicians, nurses, respiratory therapists, etc.) (Alston and Blizzard, 2011). If pharmacists allow their professional services to become a commodity, other providers will find a way to a similar service for a lower price.

FUTURE CHANGES TO THE HEALTH CARE SYSTEM

Recent events indicate that substantial changes in the markets for health care, including the markets for pharmacies, pharmacists, and professional pharmacy services, are about to be seen in the coming years. These events include efforts to increase the quality, decrease the costs and improve access to health care such as the passage of the Patient Protection and Affordable

Care Act (ACA) in 2010 and the movement toward the patient-centered medical home model (PCMH). At the same time, economic downturns and budget deficits at all levels of government (a major payer of health care in the United States and other countries) limit resources available to pay for health care goods and services. These events point to stakeholders in the health care marketplace demanding even more value for their dollar. Pharmacists and other health care professionals are not guaranteed a future role in our nation's health care team. Pharmacists must prove they deserve a role by demonstrating that they bring value to all stakeholders in the health care system (Kaldy, 2010). An example of where pharmacists must demonstrate their value is the issue of medication adherence.

Adherence is defined from the provider perspective as "the extent to which patients take medications as prescribed by their health care providers" (Osterberg and Blaschke, 2005). It would be natural to assume that if patient counseling is performed adequately, a majority of patients would be adherent with their medications. Unfortunately, that is not the case.

Poor medication adherence in the treatment of chronic diseases is a serious problem. The consequences of poor adherence grow as the prevalence of chronic disease grows worldwide. These consequences include poor health outcomes and increased health care costs. Improving adherence enhances patients' safety, and effective adherence interventions may have a far greater impact on the health of the population than any improvement in specific medical treatments (NCPIE, 2007).

In the United States, poor adherence affects Americans of all ages, genders, income levels, and education levels. It has been estimated that this lack of medication adherence leads to unnecessary disease progression, disease complications, reduced functional abilities, a lower quality of life, and premature death. The total cost of suboptimal medication adherence has been estimated at $177 billion annually in total direct and indirect health care costs (NCPIE, 2007).

The costs and consequences of medication nonadherence represent a wakeup call to all of health care, and particularly to pharmacy given the profession's desired role in medication therapy management (MTM). Medication adherence represents an area where pharmacists truly do add value to the health care system, yet questions exist as to just how well that benefit is perceived by other stakeholders in health care. Moreover, while pharmacists have added value, they can certainly do more to improve the adherence of their patients to their medications.

As stated earlier in this chapter, goods and services that create value are not only the keys to success for any health professional or business; they drive the success of today's economy. Pharmacists can create value by engaging with patients to such a degree and in such ways that patients embrace medication adherence as something truly "valuable". Once this has been done, patients would recognize the perceived value inherent in taking medications in an effective manner, and would therefore take their own actions to this effect. This engagement would result in improved medication adherence and health outcomes.

It is not enough for a highly trained pharmacist to know relevant clinical therapeutics and applied pharmacology. Pharmacists must be able to motivate patients to achieve desired outcomes. Clinical knowledge is important, but understanding how to create value in the eyes of each of our stakeholders is equally, if not more, important. By utilizing the RVT, pharmacists may understand how to better motivate stakeholders to "buy in" to our recommendations.

Consumer purchase decisions are driven by their perceptions of value of the goods and services they are offered. When thinking about patient decisions to accept, or "purchase" medication adherence services, pharmacists must learn to ask questions and listen to patients to understand their resistance to adherence. Are patients able or willing to spend the money, time, or effort on their medications or adherence (P)? Do they understand what they get for the expenditure of time, money, or effort (S)? Or, do they inherently value the intended outcomes of their medication therapy (PV)? While the rational mind computes the price and service components, perceived value is controlled by emotions and feelings. It is not uncommon for an adult male patient to refuse to take blood pressure medications because he believes the side effects can negatively impact his sexual performance. For some people, the perceived value (PV) of male pride can be much more of a motivator than the risk of a heart attack (S).

HOW WILL PHARMACISTS CREATE VALUE FOR HEALTHCARE STAKEHOLDERS

The process of developing patient care services that will succeed in a competitive marketplace requires pharmacists to apply the concepts inherent in the relative value theorem. Pharmacists must embrace the economic, business, and marketing concepts necessary to define the nature of the work that they are expected to perform in professional practice. Many student pharmacists, pharmacy practitioners, and even leaders in our profession have underemphasized the importance of business and management knowledge in creating value for health care stakeholders. Given the realities of a market-based economy, the transition from dispensing services to patient care services, a tightened job market for pharmacists and changes resulting from healthcare reform, all pharmacists will need to sharpen these skills to remain competitive in the marketplace. In short, to get a rewarding job or continue to get paid a competitive salary, pharmacists will need to demonstrate that they can create value and provide benefits to an employer that are worth their salaries.

HEALTH CARE INDUSTRY STAKEHOLDERS

Evidence suggests that there are five distinct groups with an economic, clinical, or humanistic stake in the health care marketplace (see Fig. 3-2). These groups each have different perspectives on their role in today's health care marketplace. Many pharmacists overlook the professional service opportunities that exist outside of direct patient care. Each stakeholder group has a unique role in the healthcare system, and entrepreneurial pharmacists can greatly expand the universe of potential market niches by designing professional services custom tailored to the targeted needs of a stakeholder tier.

First Tier Stakeholders

The first tier stakeholders are patients, their extended families, and unpaid caregivers who provide custodial assistance for daily living activities such as bathing, wound care, shopping, child care, and meal preparation. This tier's primary focus is on receiving quality care, improved health and a better quality of life for the patient at an affordable price.

Second Tier Stakeholders

The second tier stakeholders are the professional caregivers trained in a medical specialty that permits them to legally diagnose and/or treat disease or provide wellness services. This group includes physicians, pharmacists, nurses, physician's assistants, nurse practitioners, licensed caregivers, dentists, podiatrists, physical therapists, osteopaths, and chiropractors who provide direct patient care. These stakeholders seek value not only for their patients, but also for their business operations. Because their professional practices treat or prevent patient illness, their interests are aligned with those of the primary stakeholders outlined earlier but expand to include additional factors such as the profitability of their professional practice and their compliance with industry standards.

Third Tier Stakeholders

The third tier stakeholders in the health care marketplace include employers, insurers, governmental agencies and programs, and taxpayers who, through the actions of their elected representatives, ultimately decide which bills get paid. The interests of these stakeholders logically include all of the economic, clinical and humanistic outcomes of the primary and secondary stakeholders, but keep in mind that logic and practice are not always one and the same. Third tier stakeholders typically focus less on individual patient treatment and more on managing the overall costs of providing care to a group of patients. This can create situations where

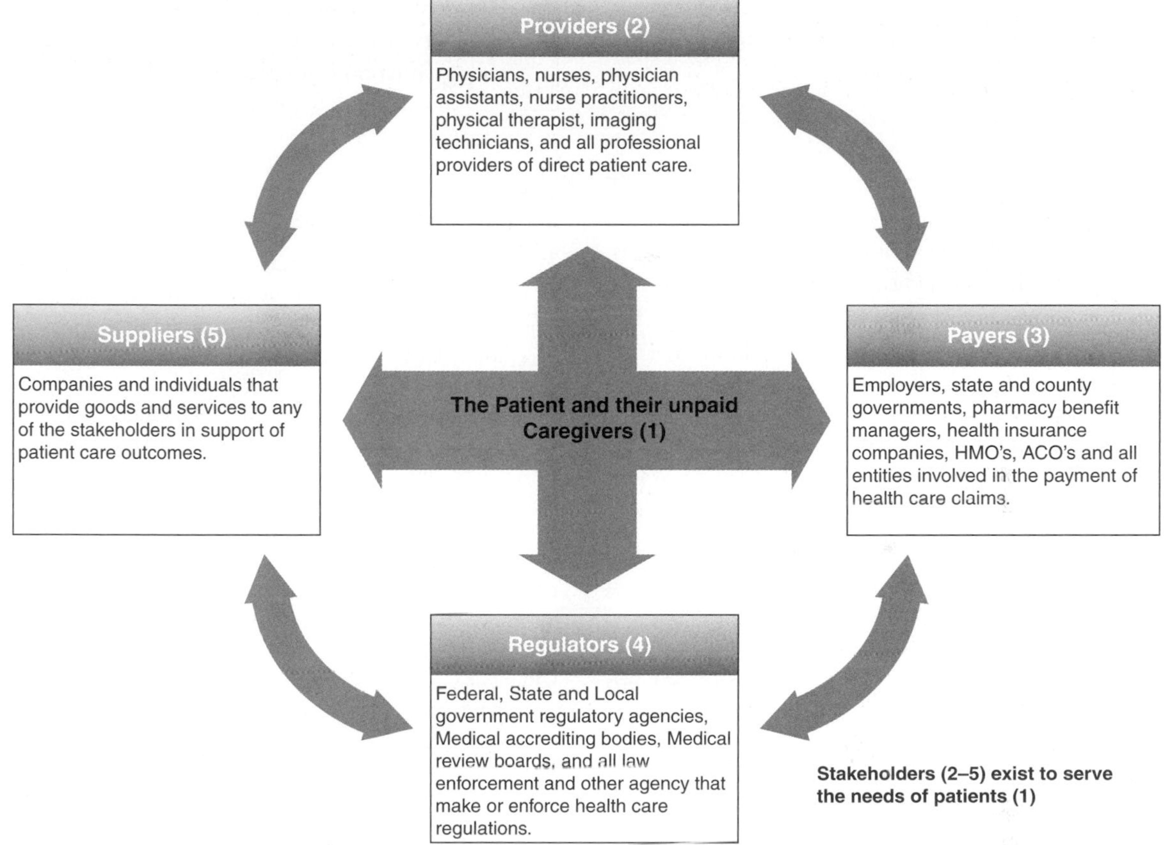

Figure 3-2. Health care industry stakeholders. (Dr. Greg Alston Copyright 2012.)

a patient's therapeutic goals and the provider's clinical plans are not perfectly aligned with the payer's budget. Payers must be concerned with utilization rates, the cost-effectiveness of outcomes, fairness, and remaining solvent.

Fourth Tier Stakeholders

The fourth tier stakeholders include state, federal, and international agencies that regulate health care. Regulators develop, write, revise, and enforce rules, regulations, and laws governing the practice of health care, the licensing of health care professionals, and the prosecution of criminal behavior. Fourth tier stakeholders typically focus on preventing fraud and abuse more than improving the quality of health care outcomes for individual patients. Their role in the health care marketplace is characteristically to protect the public interest rather than optimizing individual patient care.

Fifth Tier Stakeholders

The fifth tier stakeholders are ancillary providers of goods and services to any of the other stakeholders. This tier includes drug wholesalers, drug and device manufacturers, office equipment suppliers, payroll services, raw materials suppliers, and numerous support services that add value to the supply chain. Not traditionally considered members of the health care team, these stakeholders can affect both the cost and productivity of health care providers' work. A thoughtful analysis of all elements that increase costs and decrease effectiveness must include all links in this value chain to produce the best result possible.

CONCLUSION

The discussion of value is increasingly critical in the health care marketplace due to resource limitations, the complexities of medical practice, and health care reforms efforts as drivers of institutional change. Regardless of one's personal political philosophy, costs must be controlled, outcomes must be improved, and resources must be used wisely.

The relative value theorem is a simplified model to guide pharmacists through the process of deciding what will be valuable to a stakeholder. An individual practitioner can use the relative value theory to create value for his or her stakeholders and carve a successful niche in the American health care system.

Student pharmacists can apply the relative value theorem to help them make decisions that will impact their careers. Students should consider the price or cost of a decision (P), the benefits they receive for making the decision (S), and if making this decision allows them to project the image they wish to project (PV)? There is no insurmountable barrier to success other than one's own desire to make a difference.

QUESTIONS FOR FURTHER DISCUSSION

1. What type of professional service could you develop that would create value for a first tier stakeholder?
2. What type of professional service could you develop that would create value for a second tier stakeholder?
3. What type of professional service could you develop that would create value for a third tier stakeholder?
4. What type of professional service could you develop that would create value for a fourth tier stakeholder?
5. How could you use value creation theory to create a personal career plan for the first three years after graduation from pharmacy school?

REFERENCES

Alston G, Blizzard J. 2011. The value prescription: Relative value theorem as a call to action, research in social and administrative pharmacy. Available at http://www.sciencedirect.com/science/article/pii/S1551741111000787; accessed on August 30, 2011.

Bloemer J, de Ruyter K, Wetzels M. 1999. Linking perceived service quality and service loyalty: A multi-dimensional perspective. *Eur J Mark* 33(11/12):1082–1106.

Bolton RN, Drew JH. 1991. A multistage model of customers' assessment of service quality and value. *J Consum Res* 17(4):375–384.

Caruana A, Money AH, Berthon PR. 2000. Service quality and satisfaction- the moderating role of value, *Eur J Mark* 34:1338–1352.

Churchill GA, Surprenant C. 1982. An investigation into the determinants of customer satisfaction. *J Mark Res* 19(4):491–504.

Congressional Budget Office (CBO). 2010a. Budget and economic outlook: Historical budget data, Table F-1: Revenues, outlays, deficits, surpluses, and debt Held by the public, 1970 to 2009, in billions of dollars. Available at http://www.cbo.gov/ftpdocs/108xx/doc10871/historicaltables.pdf; accessed on April 12, 2011.

Congressional Budget Office (CBO). 2010b. Federal debt and interest costs. Available at http://www.cbo.gov/ftpdocs/119xx/doc11999/12–14-FederalDebt.pdf; accessed on April 12, 2011.

Cronin JJ, Brady MK, Hult GTM. 2000. Assessing the effects of quality, value, and customer satisfaction on consumer behavioral intentions in service environments. *J Retailing* 76(2):193–18.

Drew JH, Bolton RN. 1987. Service value and its measurement: local telephone service. In Suprenant C (ed.) *Add Value to Your Service: 6th Annual Services Marketing Proceedings*. Chicago, IL: American Marketing Association.

JCPP. 2005. Future vision of pharmacy practice statement. Available at http://www.aacp.org/resources/historicaldocuments/Documents/JCPPFutureVisionofPharmacyPracticeFINAL.pdf; accessed on October 3, 2011.

Joint Principles of the Patient Centered Medical Home. 2007. Patient Centered Primary Care Collaborative Web site. Available at http://www.pcpcc.net/content/joint-principles-patient-centered-medical-home; accessed on April 12, 2011.

Kaldy J. 2010. Medical home 101: The pharmacist's role in this growing patient-centered care model. *Consult Pharm* 25(8):468–74.

Knapp KK, Shah BM, Kim HB, et al. 2009. Visions for required postgraduate year 1 residency training by 2020: A comparison of actual versus projected expansion. *Pharmacotherapy* 29(9):1030–38.

Knapp KK, Shah BM, Barnett MJ. 2010. The Pharmacist aggregate demand index to explain changing demand over a ten year period. *Am J Pharm Educ* 74(10):189.

Medicare Payment Advisory Commission (MEDPAC). 2007. Report to the Congress: Assessing alternatives to the sustainable growth formula. Available at http://www.medpac.gov/documents/Mar07_SGR_mandated_report.pdf; accessed on February 3, 2012.

National Council on Patient Information and Education (NCPIE) 2007. Enhancing prescription medicine adherence: A national action plan. Available at http://www.talkaboutrx.org/documents/enhancing_prescription_medicine_adherence.pdf; accessed on October 3, 2011.

Oliver RL. 1993. A conceptual model of service quality and service satisfaction: Compatible goals, different concepts. *Adv Serv Mark Manage* 2:65–85.

Osterberg L, Blaschke T. 2005. Adherence to medication. *N Engl J Med* 353:487–497.

Passel JS, Cohn D. 2008. US population projections: 2005–2050. Pew Research Center Web site. Available at http://pewresearch.org/pubs/729/united-states-population-projections; accessed on April 12, 2011.

Reicheld FF. 1996. *The Loyalty Effect, The Hidden Force behind Growth, Profits, and Lasting Value.* Boston, MA: Harvard Business School Press.

Taylor P, Morin R, Kochhar R, et al. 2010. A balance sheet at 30 months: How the great recession has changed life in America. Pew Research Center Web site. Available at http://pewsocialtrends.org/2010/06/30/how-the-great-recession-has-changed-life-in-america/; accessed on April 12, 2011.

The American Pharmacists Association (APhA). 2008. Project destiny executive summary. Available at www.pharmacist.com; accessed on April 12, 2011.

The Henry J Kaiser Family Foundation. 2009. Healthcare costs: A primer. Available at http://www.kff.org/insurance/upload/7670_02.pdf; accessed on April 12, 2011.

The Henry J Kaiser Family Foundation. 2011. Summary of New Health Reform Law. Available at http://www.kff.org/healthreform/upload/8061.pdf; accessed on April 12, 2011.

Venetis AK, Ghauri NP. 2004. Service quality and customer retention: building long-term relationships. *Eur J Mark* 38(11–12):1577–98.

Woodruff RB. 1997. Customer value: the next source for competitive advantage. *Acad Mark Sci J* 25:139–53.

Zeithaml V. 1988. Consumer perception of price, quality and value: a means end model and synthesis of evidence. *J Marketing* 52:2–22.

SECTION II

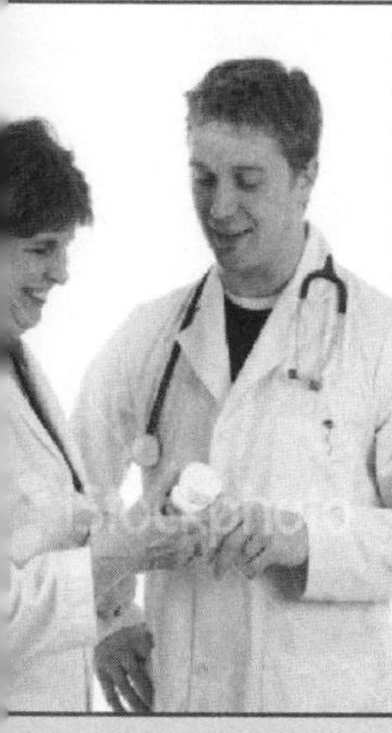

MANAGING OPERATIONS

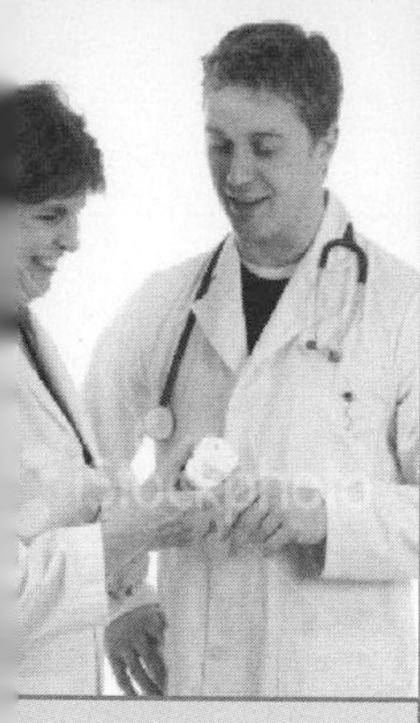

4

STRATEGIC PLANNING IN PHARMACY OPERATIONS

Glen T. Schumock, Godwin Wong, and JoAnn Stubbings

About the Authors: Dr. Schumock is a graduate of Washington State University (B.Pharm.), the University of Washington (Pharm.D.), and the University of Illinois at Chicago (MBA). He also completed a residency and a research fellowship. Currently, Dr. Schumock is director of the Center for Pharmacoeconomic Research and professor in the Department of Pharmacy Practice at the University of Illinois at Chicago. He teaches courses in pharmacy management, pharmacoeconomics, and business planning for pharmacy services. He has published over 100 articles, book chapters, and books. He is on the editorial boards of the journals *Pharmacotherapy* and *PharmacoEconomics.* He is a board-certified pharmacotherapy specialist and a fellow in the American College of Clinical Pharmacy.

Dr. Wong has been on the faculty of the Haas School of Business at the University of California, Berkeley, for over 20 years. His areas of interests are corporate strategic planning, entrepreneurship, information technology management, and venture capital. He has conducted leadership and strategic planning workshops for various health care groups, hospital administrators, and pharmaceutical companies and has lectured to executives in 20 countries. He has served on the boards of directors of several California banks, Silicon Valley companies, and international corporations. He received a B.S. from the University of Wisconsin, an M.S. from UCLA, and a Ph.D. from Harvard University.

JoAnn Stubbings is manager, research and public policy, in the Ambulatory Care Pharmacy Department at the University of Illinois at Chicago (UIC), and is clinical associate professor in the Department of Pharmacy Practice and Administration. She also has a faculty appointment in the UIC Center for Pharmacoeconomic Research. She received a B.S. in Pharmacy from the Ohio State University and Masters in Health Care Administration from the University of Mississippi. Professor Stubbings is responsible for managing and communicating pharmaceutical policy issues that pertain to outpatient pharmacy services especially to underserved populations. She teaches courses and publishes in business planning, justification, and payment for clinical pharmacy services, risk evaluation and mitigation strategies, and Medicare Part D.

LEARNING OBJECTIVES

After completing this chapter, readers should be able to

1. Provide an overview of planning activities conducted by pharmacy and health care organizations.
2. Describe the general process common to all types of planning.
3. Describe the purpose of strategic planning, and illustrate the specific steps to develop a strategic plan.
4. Differentiate a vision statement from a mission statement.
5. Highlight examples of strategic planning in pharmacy organizations.
6. Identify barriers and limitations to planning.
7. Identify and describe the different people involved in the strategic planning process, and what roles/functions they play.

SCENARIO

Ted Thompson graduated from pharmacy school magna cum laude 2 years ago with a doctor of pharmacy degree and successfully passed the licensing examination, making him a registered pharmacist. After graduation, Ted completed a pharmacy practice residency at a prestigious teaching hospital with a reputation for having an excellent pharmacy department and advanced clinical pharmacy services. Following his residency, Ted took a job as a clinical pharmacist in a community hospital in his hometown. In hiring Ted, the hospital pharmacy department fulfilled an interim objective toward their goal of developing contemporary pharmacy services.

The hospital is located in a town of approximately 100,000 people, and a large portion of the population is elderly. Partly because of both the favorable payer mix (mostly Medicare) and the fiscal savvy of the chief financial officer (CFO),[1] the hospital has done very well from clinical and economic perspectives. The pharmacy department has a good drug distribution system and a director of pharmacy (DOP) who, while not trained clinically, understands the value of these services.

The hospital is growing rapidly and, as such, has become increasingly reliant on pharmacy services. The hospital is in talks to become part of an accountable care organization (ACO), a network of hospitals and providers that deliver care and assume risk for achieving improvements in the quality of care and reductions in spending. Because of the many opportunities that confront the pharmacy department, the DOP has decided that the department should develop a plan to guide its priorities over the next 5 years. To accomplish this, the DOP has determined that over the next several months, the department will undergo a strategic planning effort. This effort will begin with a selected group of individuals from within the department, each representing key functions and constituencies. Ted was asked to be part of this group because of his clinical role and expertise and because expansion of the clinical pharmacy services provided by the department is recognized as a goal that likely will be part of this strategic plan.

Having no real management training or experience, Ted recognized the need to learn more about the purpose of strategic planning and the process that will be required to develop the departmental strategic plan.

[1] In a business or organization, the CFO is the individual who is responsible for the financial decisions and investments made by the company. In a hospital or health system, the CFO is likely to have several departments and functions reporting to him or her, including general accounting, accounts receivable and accounts payable, payroll, budgeting, procurement, and finance.

CHAPTER QUESTIONS

1. What are the different activities that pharmacies and health care organizations engage in when they plan for the future?
2. What is the purpose of strategic planning, and how is it different from other types of planning?
3. What are the steps typically taken by a pharmacy organization when developing a strategic plan?
4. What is a vision statement, and for whom is it written?
5. What is a mission statement, and for whom is it written?
6. What are the barriers or limitations associated with planning that should be kept in mind while undertaking this process?
7. Who are the people involved in the planning process, and what roles/functions do they play?

INTRODUCTION

The scenario illustrates an important activity within pharmacies and health care organizations that is rarely considered by new pharmacy graduates. In this scenario, Ted is asked to participate in the development of a strategic plan. Strategic planning is one of the most common types of planning that is conducted by health care organizations. However, strategic planning is not unique to pharmacies or health care organizations; in fact, it represents a core management activity that is employed by all businesses.

This chapter begins with a general discussion of management planning by pharmacy organizations. Pharmacies and health care organizations, like many businesses, are involved in or should be involved in, many different types of planning for different purposes within the organization. This chapter provides an understanding of where the responsibility of planning lies within organizations and the general structure or process involved in planning efforts. These general concepts are applicable to all types of planning in all different types of organizations, including pharmacies.

Next, this chapter discusses one specific type of planning—strategic planning. The intent of this discussion is to provide a general understanding of the role of strategic planning and to identify its key steps or components. While the material in this chapter is applicable to almost any type of organization, examples pertinent to the profession of pharmacy or pharmacy practice within health care organizations are provided. For readers interested in a more complete understanding of planning, there are many options for obtaining information beyond what is presented here. There are literally hundreds of textbooks addressing both general and specific topics within this field. Several good texts are included in the reference list at the end of this chapter (Allison and Kaye, 2005; Fry et al., 2005; Grünig and Kühn, 2006; Haines and McKinlay, 2007; Harrison, 2010; May, 2010; Nolan et al., 2008; Zuckerman, 2005).

PLANNING IN GENERAL

In the broadest sense, *planning* represents the purposeful efforts taken by an organization (for our purposes, a pharmacy organization) to maximize its future success. Planning, as it is referred to here, is sometimes called *management planning* because it is typically part of the duties of managers. Planning has been described as one of the four key functions of managers (along with organizing, leading, and controlling). In fact, of the four functions, planning is crucial because it supports the other three (Stoner et al., 1995). However, planning may involve more than just managers at high levels; in fact, in smaller companies or in companies with fewer levels of management, frontline employees often are involved in planning.

Many different types of planning activities occur within pharmacy organizations. The most common types include business planning, financial planning, operational planning, organizational planning, resource planning, and strategic planning. The purpose of each type of planning is different. It is not the intent of this chapter to cover all these types of planning. Instead, a brief description of the purpose and characteristics of each is outlined in Table 4-1. Some of these types of planning activities have subtypes within them. For example, one type of resource planning

Table 4-1. Types of Planning

Type	Purpose	Characteristics
Strategic planning	To ensure that the organization is doing the right things. Addresses what business the organization is in, or ought to be in, provides a framework for more detailed planning and day-to-day decisions.	Long term (5–20 years); scope includes all aspects of the organization; viewpoint is external—how the organization interacts with or controls its environment.
Operational planning	To ensure that the organization is prepared, perform the immediate tasks and objectives to meet the goals and strategy of the organization. To ensure that the organization is doing things right.	Short term (1–5 years); scope is specific to the immediate actions that need to be taken to move the organization forward; viewpoint is internal—day-to-day accomplishment of tasks.
Business planning	To determine the feasibility of a specific business or program. Business planning is used to make a decision about investing in and moving forward with a program.	Short term (1–5 years); can be used to make decisions to start a new business, expand a business, or terminate a business.
Resource planning	To ensure the resources necessary to achieve the goals and strategy of the organization. Resource planning can be comprehensive (all resources needed to achieve goals and strategic plan of the organization) or can focus on a specific type of resource.	Midterm (1–10 years); scope is specific to the resource or resources defined in the plan—specific resources may include human resources, information/technology resources, financial resources, capital and facilities, and others; viewpoint is internal—the resource needs of the organization.
Organizational planning	To ensure that an organization is organized appropriately to meet the challenges of the future. Key elements include reporting relationships, definition of responsibilities, and definition of authorities.	Midterm (1–10 years); scope specific to the structural aspects of the organization including divisions, reporting relationships, coordination, control; viewpoint is internal—how the company organizes itself.
Contingency planning	To provide a fallback option or direction should the original strategy of the organization fail or something unexpected occur. Contingency planning can occur for a specific anticipated situation, the most common of which are business-related crises (such as a labor strike), natural disasters, and changes in management personnel.	Short to long term (1–20 years); scope is specific to the particular situation that may occur; viewpoint is both external (if the situation is created in the environment) and internal.

deals specifically with human resources (Bechet, 2008; Westerling et al., 2010; Young, 2006). Another type of resource planning that has gained increasing importance is information technology planning. This type of planning focuses specifically on the present and future information needs of an organization and the technologies and systems to meet those needs (Breen and Crawford, 2005; Cassidy, 2006; Wong and Keller, 1997).

Because of the importance of effective planning, many organizations invest significant time and resources in these efforts. Ultimately, the chief executive officer (CEO) or president of a company is responsible for making certain that the organization is successful—ensuring that success largely depends on planning that occurs within the organization.[2] However, in large companies, given the scope of planning activities that must take place, much of the work involved in planning is delegated to a special department dedicated entirely to planning. Often, outside consultants are employed to assist organizations in their planning efforts.

The actual process of planning may vary by the type of planning being conducted and by the size of the organization or system. Here, the term *system* refers to the entity for which planning is being conducted. That entity may be the entire pharmacy organization or a program or function within it. Programs can be considered subunits or specific services within an organization. An example of a program within a pharmacy organization would be a clinical pharmacy service program. A *function* is an activity that cuts across different subunits of an organization. An example of a function within a pharmacy organization would be the function of information management.

Regardless of the system for which planning is being conducted, planning varies in terms of sophistication. In some cases, planning can be relatively simple and straightforward. In other cases, it may involve extensive analyses of data with complicated forecasting, decision-making models, and algorithms. Nevertheless, all planning processes share a few basic characteristics. Specifically, the eight steps shown in Table 4-2 define the general process that is followed in most planning efforts. These general steps in some cases may be expanded or condensed depending on the situation or presented in a slightly different fashion. Nevertheless, the key components of understanding the purpose, assessing the situation, establishing goals, and devising a method to accomplish those goals should be common to all planning activities.

Table 4-2. Steps in the Planning Process

1. Define or orient the planning process to a singular purpose or a desired result (vision/mission).
2. Assess the current situation.
3. Establish goals.
4. Identify strategies to reach those goals.
5. Establish objectives that support progress toward those goals.
6. Define responsibilities and timelines for each objective.
7. Write and communicate the plan.
8. Monitor progress toward meeting goals and objectives.

As shown in the table, the planning process should begin with consideration of the purpose of the organization or system and of the planning effort, itself. This is followed by an analysis of the present situation or status of the system. Next, specific future goals are determined, and then a strategy for bridging the gap between the present and future is developed. Interim objectives that measure progress toward the goals are then identified, and responsibilities and timelines for each objective are assigned. The plan then needs to be communicated, implemented, and monitored.

STRATEGIC PLANNING

The purpose of strategic planning is to ensure that the organization is doing the right things now and in

[2] The CEO is the top executive and the key decision maker of an organization, reporting only to the board of directors. The CEO, together with the Board of Directors, is responsible for the overall success of the organization.

the future. Strategic planning addresses what business the organization is in or ought to be in and helps to determine long-term goals for the organization. For example, what is the business of a particular community pharmacy? Does the pharmacy want to be in the "prescription business" or the "health care business"? Does a health system want to be in the "hospital business" or a "business that provides a continuum of care"? Obviously, how a pharmacy organization answers these questions may influence how it views itself and how it conducts its business, thus providing a framework for more detailed planning and day-to-day decisions.

Strategic planning has been defined as the process of selecting an organization's goals, determining the policies and programs (strategies) necessary to achieve specific objectives en route to those goals, and establishing methods necessary to ensure that the policies and strategic programs are implemented (Steiner et al., 1982). More broadly, strategic planning can be considered an effort that enables the optimal deployment of all organizational resources within current and future environmental constraints. The result of this optimization is to increase the likelihood that the organization will survive, and preferably thrive, in the future.

Before further discussion of strategic planning, the differences between strategic and *business planning* should be noted. These are the two most common types of planning, and while they are very different, people often confuse the two. Table 4-1 helps to clarify the differences—the most important being their purpose. While strategic planning is about achieving a long-term vision and making sure the organization is doing the things necessary to ensure overall success, business planning focuses on a the feasibility of a specific program (usually a new initiative). Business planning, like all the other types of planning listed in Table 4-1 must occur within the context of the strategic plan of the organization. As such, the strategic plan can be viewed as the overarching effort that should guide all other types of planning and even the day-to-day activities of the organization.

In evaluating the performance of a company, it is often informative to look at its strategy historically over time. While many factors can influence organizational performance, companies that engage in long-range strategic planning are often more successful than those that do not. Again, this is true for pharmacy organizations as well as other types of businesses. Strategic planning can be either reactive or proactive. Reactive strategic planning is not the ideal, but it is often necessary, especially in industries that are changing rapidly (such as health care). Preferably, proactive strategic planning enables an organization to control its environment instead of vice versa.

Beyond proactive planning, organizations that are able to think and plan in a provocative or "out of the box" manner may position themselves not only to control the business environment but also to actually create or recreate the business environment. This type of strategic thinking has been considered the pinnacle of planning efforts by organizations—ideal for companies to position themselves to be most competitive. Using strategy to create an environment that puts the company at an advantage compared with its competitors is integral to this effort (Porter, 1985). An example outside the health care industry is Apple, Inc., and its evolution of electronic products and services that respond to customer needs and reshape the digital environment, from the iMac and MacBook, to the iPod, iPhone, and now the iPad. Other examples include the social networking Web site, Facebook, and the professional networking Web site, Linkedin, and the group discount Web site, Groupon. These new businesses have developed new markets for interaction via the Internet that did not exist previously.

The time horizon of strategic planning helps to distinguish it from other types of planning. Strategic planning has also been called *long-term planning.* The actual timeline used by organizations may vary or in some cases may not be known. Because the future is unknown, it is often difficult to predict with any accuracy the amount of time it will take for an organization to reach its long-term goals. Nevertheless, a key component of strategic planning is to identify time periods within which goals are to be reached.

The time horizon for strategic planning may be as long as 10 to 20 years or as short as 2 years. In a survey conducted by the Net Future Institute, managers were asked what time period they considered to be long term (Martin, 2002). The most common response was 2 years (40.2 percent), followed by 5 years (32.7 percent) and 1 year (17.9 percent). Admittedly, many of the companies involved in this survey were in high-tech industries, where rapid change may impair longer-term planning. However, health care is also an industry of rapid change, and thus planning must be done similarly to that in other fast-growing industries, though the time horizon may be longer.

The problem with strategic planning, even in 5-year time periods, is that it is not likely to result in any truly sustainable competitive advantages or a significant organizational metamorphosis. Further, because strategic goals are based on the company's vision for the future, goals that incorporate new paradoxes or visionary changes may be difficult for employees to believe if the time period for accomplishing those goals is too short. Nevertheless, these are the types of goals that should be created in strategic planning, so it is the time period that must be congruent with these goals, not vice versa. The worst mistake would be to "dumb down" the goals to make them consistent with a shorter time period.

Vision and Mission

An important part of the process of strategic planning is to create momentum and to motivate personnel within the pharmacy organization. Strategic planning has a lot to do with defining what a company is all about and creating a "story" about the organization. The communication of the organization's story occurs across a number of different statements that may be products of strategic planning. Most essential of these statements are the vision and the mission.

The *vision* is what the pharmacy organization wants to be at some future time point. The vision may be complex and multidimensional, while at the same time it must be concise. The *vision statement* should make people think and motivate them, especially employees, to create a different and better future for the organization. For example, the vision of the national pharmacy chain, CVS Caremark, is "to improve the quality of human life" (see http://info.cvscaremark.com/our-company/our-culture/vision-mission-values). This vision clearly sets a lofty goal that serves to inspire the organization and its employees.

The vision of the organization is used in the strategic planning process as both the beginning point and the end point. That is, once the vision is set, then strategic planning is about how to reach that end point. The vision also is used to define the mission of the organization. For example, the vision statement of Mayo Clinic in Rochester, MN is to "... provide an unparalleled experience as the most trusted partner for healthcare" (see http://www.mayohealthsystem.org/mhs/live/page.cfm?pp=locations/aboutus.cfm&orgid=LM&affid=31&nav=Abo&sub=Relationship%20with%20Mayo%20Clinic). This vision drives both the mission of the organization and its values, and presumably, these together guide the daily business decisions made by Mayo Clinic.

The *mission* is the purpose of the company. The *mission statement* defines what the company does or is. It is a statement of the present going ahead into the near future. It is a document written to create a sense of purpose for customers and employees. The mission statement should be short—usually no more than two sentences. It focuses on the common purpose of the organization and may draw from the values or beliefs held by the organization. The mission statement should help to differentiate the company from others that provide the same products or services. Some organizations include in the mission statement not only what the company does but also how it does it—essentially the differentiating point. Mayo Clinic's mission statement is "to inspire hope, and contribute to health and well-being by providing the best care to every patient through integrated clinical practice, education and research."

The following elements have been suggested in developing a mission statement for a community pharmacy: the intended (or target) customers, the core values of the pharmacy (such as compassion, respect, and confidentiality), the key services and products provided by the pharmacy, the benefits incurred by customers (such as improved health and improved safety), and the desired public image of the pharmacy (Hagel, 2002).

All pharmacy organizations should have a mission statement. Kerr Drugs is a successful chain of community pharmacies in the Carolinas. The organization provides a good example of a mission statement that focuses on the company's key priorities—"providing healthcare solutions with exceptional customer service" (see http://www.kerrdrug.com/content/about-kerr-drug). The mission statement of CVS Caremark is very specific but clear. It is to "... provide expert care and innovative solutions in pharmacy and health care that are effective and easy for our customers" Similarly, the mission of pharmaceutical company Pfizer Inc. (http://www.pfizer.ie/mission_statement_and_values.cfm) is to "apply science and our global resources to improve health and well-being at every stage of life."

As noted earlier, the mission statement creates a sense of purpose for both the employees and customers of the organization. Employees of Kerr Drugs know that their customers will expect help with their medications and their health and they should strive to provide excellent customer service everyday. This chapter later discusses how pharmacies such as Kerr Drugs that have well-defined missions and that engage in strategic planning are more likely to be successful.

In addition to the mission statement, some businesses use a *company slogan* to convey a message to customers about the organization. The company slogan generally is more marketing driven than is the mission statement, but in some cases the company slogan serves a similar role. Like the mission statement, the company slogan sends a message to both customers and employees, and it must be congruent with the actions of the organization or else it will not be credible. A great example of a company slogan is that of the Nike Company. The slogan "Just Do It!" has energy and a sense of action. It is easy to see how the slogan and the company's mission, "To bring inspiration and innovation to every athlete in the world," combine to create a powerful image of what this company is all about (http://help-us.nike.com/app/answers/detail/a_id/113/~/what-is-nike%27s-mission-statement%3F). Other memorable slogans are "I'm Loving It" for McDonalds, "It's the Real Thing," for Coke, "I Guarantee It!" for Men's Wearhouse, and "Fly the Friendly Skies," for United Airlines. Kerr Drugs' slogan is "For a Healthy Relationship." Pfizer's slogan is "Working Together for a Healthier World." Again, these slogans are brief yet convey meaningful messages.

The vision, mission, and other statements that form the company story are critical elements in strategic planning. If these elements already exist in the organization, then the process of strategic planning starts with these as its foundation or modifies them as necessary. If these elements do not already exist, then the process of strategic planning must include their conception.

Process of Strategic Planning

The structuring, facilitating, and implementing the process of strategic planning is an important consideration for any organization (Fogg, 2010). The process of strategic planning does not vary significantly from the process used in other types of planning. This chapter highlights only the aspects of the steps shown in Table 4-2 that are distinctive to strategic planning compared with other types of planning efforts. It is apt to point out that sometimes companies would also do "tactical planning" which is of a much short time frame/horizon then strategic planning.

Preplanning Phase

Preplanning can be defined as the steps necessary to organize the strategic planning effort—or "planning for the planning." Strategic planning is a significant undertaking that consumes much time and energy. A pharmacy organization choosing to engage in a strategic planning effort should not take this lightly. Strategic planning is a financial investment—in the personnel time required and in the payment of consultants, if used. These costs should be weighed against the value to be gained by the effort. If strategic planning is performed correctly, its value will greatly exceed any costs. On the other hand, if strategic planning is done in a superficial or hurried manner, its costs will exceed its benefits. Preplanning should include a careful assessment of this balance.

Preplanning should define the objectives of the planning efforts and the procedures that will be used to accomplish those objectives. Preplanning will define who should be involved, where the planning process will occur, and how much time will be allotted to the effort. Preplanning should also consider any political purposes and ramifications of the undertaking. In laying out the scope of the planning effort, preplanning should orient the activity to the vision of the organization, if one exists.

Among the preplanning activities, determining who should be involved in strategic planning is most important. The type of organization and level of the strategic planning effort will dictate who should be involved. For example, if the plan is at the highest level within a large corporation then planning must start at the Board of Directors. Conversely if a plan is designed for a department within an organization, then participation may be limited to the department leaders and managers, key staff, and perhaps important stakeholders.

For example, a strategic plan for the pharmacy department of a hospital would need to include the Director of Pharmacy. He or she would also want to be sure to communicate with the senior leadership of the hospital so that the planning process includes consideration of issues pertinent to the hospital wide vision and strategic goals. Participation in the planning effort should include key managers and staff within the pharmacy department who will be involved in day-to-day implementation of the proposed plan. Other important stakeholders might also be involved. These might include influential medical staff, managers from other departments (such as nursing), and perhaps individuals from the finance department, human resources, and/or marketing. For most strategic planning of any significant scale or impact, some outside consultant or advisor will be brought in to provide and external perspectives and to ensure that the process is complete and objective. This may or may not be necessary for departmental planning.

Planning Phase

In the *planning phase* of strategic planning, ideas are actively generated for the pharmacy organization. This may be referred to as *strategizing.* As in any planning process, it is usually best to start with the destination in mind, as in planning a trip by viewing a map. Once the destination is clear, one must find the starting place on the map. The next step is to determine the different routes or options to get from here to there. Among the different routes, one should select that which best meets the needs within the constraints of limited resources. If speed is important, then one selects the quickest route. If scenery is important, then one selects the most scenic route. Besides the route, the mode of transportation needs to be determined. Options might include taking a train, driving a car, or flying in an airplane (or a combination of any of these). Once the route and method of transportation are known, one selects key milestones, or places to stop, along the way. Knowing these intermediate points helps to keep the journey on track. The process of strategic planning is very similar, except strategic planning is, or should be, a group effort involving all levels of the organization.

In strategic planning, the "destination" is the vision of the organization in the future. It also is necessary, though, to identify where, what, and how the organization is in the present. This is called *situation analysis,* and it should consider both the past performance and the current situation. This is the starting point on the journey. Based on the vision (destination), along with the present situation (starting point), planners next should identify the goals for the organization. These goals could be considered synonymous with the things considered important in the map example, such as speed and scenic beauty. Once the goals are identified, the course is plotted to get from the present to the future. For this, it is crucial to identify and select preferred strategies that will accomplish the goals. Strategies are synonymous with the routes and the modes and costs of transportation in the travel example. Last, one should determine objectives that will help to reach the goals. Objectives are like the intermediate points, or places to pass through on the map. These objectives provide a shorter-term milestone and, in

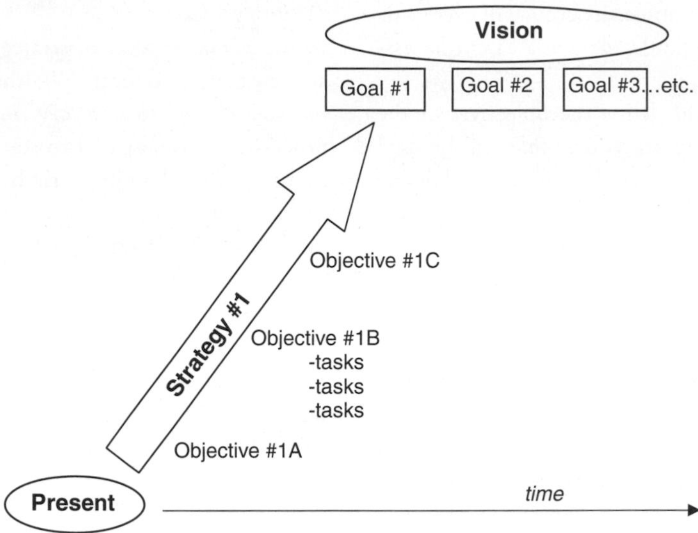

Figure 4-1. Relationship between vision, goals, objectives, strategy, and mission. To reach a certain vision, or future state, the organization must set and reach one or more goals. Each goal is associated with a specific strategy or method of reaching that goal. The strategy can be defined by the objectives that are necessary intermediate accomplishments toward the goal. A set of tasks, or actions, may be associated with each objective. Collectively, these tasks are also called *tactics* that the organization employs to meet an objective. *(Adapted from Coke, 2001, with permission from the publisher.)*

implementation, help to measure progress toward the goal. The relationship between vision, goals, strategy, and objectives is shown graphically in Fig. 4-1.

Considering the preceding overview, the steps in the planning process can be examined more closely. After crafting a vision statement, planners must analyze and define the current situation. As is the case with any system, history helps to define the present. Therefore, part of the situation analysis is to evaluate the past performance of the organization. This evaluation should include all measures of performance, including customer satisfaction and financial indicators.

The situation analysis also should define the present. A common method for conducting the situation analysis is to evaluate the internal strengths and weakness of the organization and the external opportunities and threats to the organization. This is known as a *SWOT (strengths, weaknesses, opportunities, threats) analysis.* Strengths and opportunities are generally considered to be positive attributes of the company/program or characteristics of the environment that may bode well for the success of the business. Weaknesses and threats are negative attributes or characteristics, as shown in Fig. 4-2.

	Positive	Negative
Internal	S	W
External	O	T

Figure 4-2. Conceptual diagram of the elements of a SWOT analysis. Strengths, weakness, opportunities, and threats are the elements that comprise a SWOT analysis. These elements can be characterized with respect to both their place in the environment, for example, either internal or external to organization, and based on their desirability, for example, either positive or negative from that standpoint of the organization. These relationships are shown in the figure.

Categories of internal strengths and weaknesses to consider when conducting a SWOT analysis may include profitability, quality of pharmacy service, customer service, competence and ability of pharmacy staff, and the efficiency of the pharmacy operations. Categories of external opportunities and threats to consider may include the extent of competition from other pharmacy organizations, the availability of technology, regulations that may help or hinder the business, availability of reimbursement for services provided (i.e., clinical or cognitive pharmacy services), costs incurred by the pharmacy organization, political issues having an impact on health delivery, and changes in the market and types of customers served by the organization. A more detailed example of a SWOT analysis for a pharmacy program is provided in Chapter 5.

By comparing the results of the situation analysis with the desired future state (vision), the extent and nature of the gap between the two begins to become clear. The next steps in the planning phase attempt to bridge that gap. First, strategic planning serves to define goals for the organization that are consistent with the vision. These goals should capitalize on the organization's strengths and opportunities while minimizing the threats and mitigating the weaknesses.

The last part of the planning process deals with organizing to *operationalize* the strategy. Because the goals and vision are a desired future state that may be unachievable in the short term, intermediate objectives are needed to help advance toward that target. In the planning process, the objectives pertinent to each goal are identified and usually are accomplishable in the short term (1 year), whereas goals are in the longer term (3 to 5 years). Because objectives are short term, a budget, schedule, and responsibility can be assigned to each.

There is no common or standard way to organize the written strategic plan. However, most contain the following key elements: (1) the organization's vision, (2) strategies, (3) goals for each strategy, (4) objectives required to meet those goals, and (5) tasks or action plans to compete the objectives. Examples of strategic plans for pharmacy organizations can be found in the references listed at the end of this chapter, and

Table 4-3. Example Strategic Plan

Strategy: The department will align its pharmacy services to be consistent with the hospital's initiative to become part of an accountable care organization.

Goal: Develop and implement specific clinical pharmacy services that help to deliver care, improve patient outcomes, reduce spending, and/or generate revenue.

Objectives:

- Identify gaps in care delivery, quality, and spending where pharmacy services can lead to improvements.
- Select one clinical pharmacy service to implement in the short term.

Tasks/action plans:

- Perform a situation analysis of the hospital, accountable care organization, and pharmacy department, including a SWOT analysis.
- Prepare a list of clinical pharmacy services that can be developed and implemented to meet the needs of the organization, and compare the services on the basis of feasibility and impact.
- Select the most appropriate service and develop a business plan for the service.

Table 4-3 provides an example of a strategic plan for Ted Thompson's pharmacy services scenario at the beginning of this chapter. Note that the tasks listed also should include a planned date for completion of the task and a party responsible for each task.

Postplanning Phase

Once the major pieces of the planning phase have been developed, the *postplanning phase* begins. This phase includes three vitally important steps: (1) communicating the plan, (2) implementing the plan, and (3) monitoring progress and assessing results once the plan is implemented.

While strategic planning is a process, the strategic plan is a document that communicates the plan. The strategic plan should be written such that it communicates all aspects of the plan effectively.

The actual implementation of the strategic plan requires managers and executives of the pharmacy organization to understand the long-range goals while at the same time determining and taking the steps necessary to accomplish the shorter-range objectives. The process of mapping out the actions necessary to accomplish short-term objectives is called *operational planning,* which focuses on determining the day-to-day activities that are necessary to achieve the long-term goals of the organization. One can differentiate strategic planning from operational planning by viewing the primary focus of each. Strategic planning focuses on doing the right thing (effectiveness), whereas operational planning focuses on doing things right (efficiency). In other words, strategic planning defines what to do, and operational planning defines how to do it.

The operational plan is an outline of the tactical activities or tasks that must occur to support and implement the strategic plan—sometimes called *tactics.* The relationship between tasks or tactics (operational planning) and the key elements of strategic planning is shown in Fig. 4-1. Managers in an organization focus their day-to-day work on tactics. Their perspective tends to relate to the short term. Yet it is important that, on a periodic basis, an attempt be made to step back from day-to-day activities and reorient oneself to the bigger picture (the vision, goals, and strategy of the organization). For example, a pharmacy manager may receive a request from a physician or a nurse to have the department begin to provide a new service in a hospital. Before agreeing to do so, it is important that the manager consider how this new service fits into the vision and goals of the pharmacy department.

Another key element of the postplanning phase is *monitoring.* A plan for monitoring should be created. This monitoring should evaluate the extent of implementation in comparison with the planned schedule and the effectiveness of the organization in meeting its goals, especially in the deployment of limited resources, both human and financial. In other words, have both the plan and its implementation been effective? Intrinsic to this monitoring process is the possibility that changes to the plan may be necessitated by changes in the environment or by changes in the organization. As such, the strategic plan should be considered a fluid document.

STRATEGIC PLANNING EXAMPLES IN PHARMACY ORGANIZATIONS

There are plenty of published examples and descriptions of strategic planning in pharmacy organizations, although a majority come from the hospital practice setting (Guerrero et al., 1990; Hutchinson et al., 1989; Newberg and Banville, 1989; Westerling et al., 2010). For chain drug stores, independent pharmacies, or other for-profit pharmacy organizations, it may be counterproductive to publish the company strategy and objectives. Rather, these plans frequently are guarded fiercely so that they do not fall into the hands of competitors. Nevertheless, there are some general publications designed to assist community pharmacies in strategic planning (Hagel, 2002).

A survey of 1,500 randomly selected community pharmacies found that only a small proportion (30.8 percent) of respondents reported having conducted strategic planning in their pharmacies (Harrison and Ortmeier, 1996). For those that did conduct strategic planning, an average of 5.9 (of 7) different steps in the strategic planning process were used, and 45.7 percent incorporated all seven steps (Table 4-4). The authors also reported that community pharmacies that conducted strategic planning had significantly higher self-rated performance on clinical services, dispensing services, and financial performance—suggesting that strategic planning can improve organization success. An update of the survey showed little change. As in the previous survey, increased use of strategic planning was associated with improved organizational performance (Harrison, 2005, 2006). This same author found that owners and managers of independent community pharmacies who participated in a formal strategic planning education program

Table 4-4. Steps Used in the Strategic Planning Process by Community Pharmacies

Step	Percentage[a]
Develop mission statement	76.9
Identify strengths and weaknesses	94.2
Identify threats and opportunities	90.2
Formulate and select strategies	83.8
Review pharmacy structure and systems	60.1
Implement strategies	86.1
Evaluate implemented strategies	76.3

Source: Adapted from Harrison and Ortmeier, 1996, with permission from the publisher.
[a]*N* = 173 community pharmacies that reported use of strategic planning; values represent the percentage that incorporate each specific step of the strategic planning process.

were more likely to conduct strategic planning, and had greater comprehension of strategic planning concepts, when compared to those who did not participate (Harrison, 2007).

A similar study conducted in the hospital pharmacy environment found that 63 percent of respondents (hospital pharmacy directors) conducted strategic planning in their pharmacies and followed 4.7 (of 6) steps in the strategic planning process. This supported the belief that strategic planning within hospital pharmacies is more commonplace than previously thought (Harrison and Bootman, 1994). In the hospital environment, many published descriptions of strategic planning activities have focused specifically on planning for clinical pharmacy services (Anderson, 1986; Jones and Crane, 1990; Kelly, 1986; Linggi and Pelham, 1986).

Strategic planning also appears to have merit when used by hospital pharmacy departments. A study of pharmacy directors at hospitals in the United States was conducted to determine if more sophisticated planning resulted in improved departmental outcomes (Birdwell and Pathak, 1989). Pharmacy departments were categorized into levels of strategic planning sophistication based on different steps that were employed the planning process. In departments with high levels of planning, outcomes such as satisfaction by hospital administrators, professional image among hospital administrators, number of clinical pharmacy programs, and the quality of clinical pharmacy programs were rated higher by pharmacy directors than in departments with lower levels of sophistication in planning. In other industries, strategic planning also has been shown to improve company performance and has yielded positive results (Hodges and Kent, 2006).

Consistent with these findings was another study that described the impact of strategic planning conducted in the Department of Veterans Affairs Medical Center pharmacies. Strategic planning resulted in more Veterans Affairs Medical Centers with increased pharmacist involvement in patient care, increased involvement in specific types of clinical services, more efficient drug distribution systems, and increased involvement in pharmacy education (Portner et al., 1996).

Strategic planning in pharmacy is particularly important when there are changes that occur in the practice environment. The Medicare Modernization Act (MMA) of 2003 is a good example of such a change. This legislation, which went into effect in 2006, created the Medicare prescription drug benefit (also known as Medicare Part D) and established the requirement that medication therapy management (MTM) be provided to high-risk Medicare beneficiaries (see Chapter 20). Successful pharmacy organizations used strategic planning to predict the impact of the MMA and to develop practice plans for provision of MTM (Lewin Group, 2005). Another example of change in the pharmacy practice environment is the increased emphasis on medication errors promoted by the Joint Commission, the body responsible for accrediting hospitals and other health care organizations. By monitoring the literature, successful hospital pharmacy departments were able to predict this movement and then developed and implemented plans to establish the technologic and human resources necessary to improve patient safety (Shane and Gouveia, 2000).

BARRIERS AND LIMITATIONS TO PLANNING

Effective planning requires a serious commitment of time and resources. For a variety of reasons, organizations may not be successful in their planning efforts. Lack of success may stem from failure to recognize and minimize common barriers to planning efforts or failure to understand inherent limitations in planning.

Barriers

Organizations must overcome several barriers to ensure a successful strategic planning process, as shown in Table 4-5. The most serious barrier is lack of endorsement by the top executive(s). Buy-in and participation by top corporate executives and the board of directors are critical to strategic planning. Without these, the whole planning effort could be a waste of time and resources.

A frequent barrier to effective planning is failure to commit sufficient time to the planning process. Good planning requires significant management and staff time. Ideally, some of the more creative aspects of planning should be accomplished during uninterrupted time. Pharmacy organizations commonly hold retreats, whereas those involved in the planning process meet in a location outside the usual work environment.

Table 4-5. Barriers to Effective Planning

1. Failure to commit sufficient time to the planning effort
2. Interpersonal issues such as struggles over power or politics and individual or group resistance to change
3. Lack of planning skills
4. Failure to plan far enough into the future
5. Constantly changing environment
6. Failure to implement owing to lack of time or lack of resources
7. Failure to monitor progress
8. Lack of support of top executive and/or board of directors

The time and expense associated with such events require a huge commitment on the part of both the organization and the personnel involved.

Sometimes interpersonal issues, such as organizational culture or struggles for power and politics, become barriers to effective planning. Individuals who are involved in planning or implementation may be resistant to change (for a variety of reasons) and thus consciously or subconsciously sabotage the planning effort. Likewise, if the organization or personnel lack the skills necessary to conduct planning, the results may be less than optimal and even harmful to the organization. In the same context, failure to plan far enough into the future can be problematic, especially for certain types of planning. Strategic planning in particular is intended to guide the organization over the long term.

The environment also can pose a barrier to effective planning. In an environment such as health care, where things are changing constantly or sometimes ambiguous, effective planning is more difficult and uncertain. For example, consider all the changes that may affect pharmacy organizations that make planning for the future difficult. These include changes in technology and automation, new drugs and therapies, changes in payment rates of prescriptions and availability of reimbursement for clinical pharmacy services, changes in regulations, and fluctuations in the labor market for pharmacists.

Organizations operating in rapidly changing environments may put off or avoid planning altogether. Unfortunately, failure to plan, even when it is difficult, may be even more detrimental in the long term.

Another barrier to the planning effort is failure to communicate the plan effectively to the employees of the pharmacy organization. Written plans must be drafted in such a way that the messages are communicated clearly to the appropriate audience. Plan documents sometimes have the tendency to use jargon or terminology, so-called plan-speak, that is not consistent with that which would be most beneficial to clear and accurate interpretation by the audience. Besides the written document, verbal presentations and other forms of communication are often important.

The most common barrier to effective planning is failure to implement, so-called "analysis but no action." Three causes of failure to implement plans include the unavailability of resources, lack of time, and failure to monitor or measure progress. Implementation of strategy often involves the mobilization of resources. If organizations do not have the necessary resources, or are unwilling to commit those resources, then implementation will be jeopardized. In today's ever-increasing speed of business, managers often cannot find the time to use adequately the results of planning already conducted to guide their daily activities. The term *management by crisis* is used often to describe the modus operandi of busy managers, meaning that their work is directed more by the problems they face at the immediate moment than by any careful consideration of the actual goals of the organization. In the long term, this may result in failure of the company to meet its goals (Martin, 2002). Finally, the failure to monitor, for whatever reason, the progress made toward goals developed in the planning process can be a significant barrier to success of the planning effort.

Limitations

Besides the barriers to planning just listed, certain limitations to planning must also be acknowledged. Managers often are caught up in the notion that planning is a magic bullet for the ills of an organization. They must acknowledge the fact that planning is no cure-all.

First, planning is to some degree, guesswork (but educated and experienced guesswork, hopefully). While decisions are based on evidence available about the past and the likelihood of events in the future, risk is still involved. Nothing is certain. Even with good data and good strategy, negative things may happen that were unpredictable and thus unavoidable.

Second, plans and predictions are only as good as the data and information that go into them. Poor data will result in poor strategy. What pharmacy organizations get out of the planning activity will be correlated directly with the degree of effort, creativity, time, and resources they put into it. Organizations that adopt boilerplate or "cookie cutter" approaches to planning most likely will not get the optimum results they would like to achieve.

Two additional limitations of planning deal with how an organization implements the plan. Planning is not a substitute for action. Organizations that are all about planning but neglect to take the actions dictated will not be successful. To the opposite extreme, the plan should not be considered as static or unyielding. Planning should be a continuous process, and plans should change as the environment dictates. To follow a plan blindly without consideration of changes in the environment that may make the plan obsolete is foolhardy.

CONCLUSION

The scenario of Ted Thompson that began this chapter illustrates how knowledge of planning-related concepts may be applicable to the work activities of a recent pharmacy graduate. Knowledge of concepts in the chapter should better position Ted to participate in the strategic planning initiative being organized by the DOP. Ted should now clearly appreciate the importance of this type of planning to the future of the hospital and to the pharmacy department. He should be able to anticipate the process that might be followed. Ted should also anticipate certain questions that will need to be addressed in the planning process. For example, given the pharmacy described in the scenario, what might be a suitable vision for the department? What goals and objectives might the department establish during its strategic planning exercise?

The concepts discussed in this chapter become only more important as one advances through a career and assumes higher levels of leadership and responsibility in a pharmacy or health care organization. It is also important for students and new practitioners to understand the process involved in establishing and maintaining the viability of the organization for which they work. A good understanding of management concepts, and planning in particular, will allow the pharmacy practitioner to better appreciate the context from which management operates.

This will then better enable pharmacy practitioners to have input into and be able to influence the direction and decisions of a pharmacy organization.

■ QUESTIONS FOR FURTHER DISCUSSION

1. Select a specific pharmacy practice setting (i.e., hospital practice, community practice, or managed care). What barriers do you believe would limit the ability of pharmacists and pharmacy managers to conduct effective planning in that setting?
2. Write a vision statement for a hypothetical pharmacy organization. Explain how you selected the language and message of the statement.
3. Conduct an Internet search of vision and mission statements of health care organizations. Identify and compare the statements from at least three different organizations. What are the strengths and weakness of these statements?
4. Describe changes that have occurred in the practice of pharmacy over the past 20 years. How would strategic planning have enabled a pharmacy organization to better position itself for those changes?

REFERENCES

Allison M, Kaye J. 2005. *Strategic Planning for Nonprofit Organizations: A Practical Guide and Workbook.* Hoboken: Wiley.

Anderson RW. 1986. Strategic planning for clinical services: The University of Texas M.D. Anderson Hospital and Tumor Institute. *Am J Hosp Pharm* 43: 2169–73.

Bechet TP. 2008. *Strategic Staffing: A Comprehensive System for Effective Workforce Planning.* New York: American Management Association.

Birdwell SW, Pathak DS. 1989. Use of the strategic-planning process by hospital pharmacy directors. *Am J Hosp Pharm* 46:1361–69.

Breen L, Crawford H. 2005. Improving the pharmaceutical supply chain: Assessing the reality of e-quality through e-commerce application in hospital pharmacy. *Int J Qual Reliab Manage* 22:572–90.

Cassidy A. 2006. *A Practical Guide to Information Systems Strategic Planning.* Boca Raton, FL: Auerbach Publications.

Coke A. 2001. *Seven Steps to a Successful Business Plan.* New York: American Management Association.

Fogg CD. 2010. *Team-Based Strategic Planning.* New York: AMACOM American Management Association.

Fry FL, Stoner CR, Weinzimmer LG. 2005. *Strategic Planning Made Easy.* Irvine, CA: Entrepreneur.

Grünig R, Kühn R. 2006. *Process-Based Strategic Planning.* Berlin, Germany: Springer.

Guerrero RM, Nickman NA, Bair JN. 1990. Using pharmacists' perceptions in planning changes in pharmacy practice. *Am J Hosp Pharm* 47:2026–30.

Hagel HP. 2002. Planning for patient care. In Hagel HP, Rovers JP (eds.) *Managing the Patient-Centered Pharmacy.* Washington, DC: American Pharmaceutical Association.

Haines SG, McKinlay J. 2007. *Reinventing Strategic Planning: The Strategic Systems Approach.* San Diego, CA: Systems Thinking Press.

Harrison DL. 2005. Strategic planning by independent community pharmacies. *J Am Pharm Assoc* 45:726–33.

Harrison DL. 2006. Effect of attitudes and perceptions of independent community pharmacy owners/managers on the comprehensiveness of strategic planning. *J Am Pharm Assoc* 46:459–64.

Harrison DL. 2007. Effect of strategic planning education on attitudes and perceptions of independent community pharmacy owners/managers. *Am J Pharm Assoc* 47: 599–604.

Harrison DL, Bootman JL. 1994. Strategic planning by institutional pharmacy administrators. *J Pharm Market Manage* 8:73–96.

Harrison DL, Ortmeier BG. 1996. Strategic planning in the community pharmacy. *J Am Pharm Assoc* NS36:583–88.

Harrison JP. 2010. *Essentials of Strategic Planning in Healthcare.* Chicago, IL: Health Administration Press.

Hodges HE, Kent TW. 2006. Impact of planning and control sophistication in small business. *J Small Bus Strategy* 17(2):75–88.

Hutchinson RA, Witte KW, Vogel DP. 1989. Development and implementation of a strategic-planning process at a university hospital. *Am J Hosp Pharm* 46:952–57.

Jones DR, Crane VS. 1990. Development of an organizational strategic planning process for a hospital department. *Health Care Superv* 9:1–20.

Kelly WN. 1986. Strategic planning for clinical services: Hamot Medical Center. *Am J Hosp Pharm* 43:2159–63.

Lewin Group. 2005. Medication therapy management services: A critical review. *J Am Pharm Assoc* 45:580–7.

Linggi A, Pelham LD. 1986. Strategic planning for clinical services: St Joseph Hospital and Health Care Center. *Am J Hosp Pharm* 43:2164–68.

Martin C. 2002. *Managing for the Short Term: The New Rules for Running a Business in a Day-to-Day World.* New York: Doubleday.

May GL. 2010. *Strategic Planning: Fundamentals for Small Business.* New York: Business Expert Press.

Newberg DF, Banville RL. 1989. Strategic planning for pharmacy services in a community hospital. *Am J Hosp Pharm* 46:1819–21.

Nolan TM, Goodstein LD, Goodstein J, Pfeiffer JW. 2008. *Applied Strategic Planning: An Introduction.* San Francisco, CA: Pfeiffer.

Porter ME. 1985. *Competitive Advantage: Creating and Sustaining Superior Performance.* New York: Free Press.

Portner TS, Srnka QM, Gourley DR, et al. 1996. Comparison of Department of Veterans Affairs pharmacy services in 1992 and 1994 with strategic-planning goals. *Am J Health Syst Pharm* 53:1032–40.

Shane R, Gouveia WA. 2000. Developing a strategic plan for quality in pharmacy practice. *Am J Health Syst Pharm* 57:470–4.

Steiner GA, Miner JB, Gray ER. 1982. *Management Policy and Strategy.* New York: Macmillan.

Stoner JAF, Freeman RE, Gilbert DR. 1995. *Management,* 6th edn. Englewood Cliffs, NJ: Prentice-Hall.

Westerling AM, Haikala VE, Bell JS, Airaksinen MS. 2010. Logistics or patient care: Which features do independent Finnish pharmacy owners prioritize in a strategic plan for future information technology systems? *J Am Pharm Assoc* 50:24–31.

Wong G, Keller U. 1997. Information technology (IT) outsourcing: An alternative to re-engineer your IT. In Berndt R (ed.) *Business Reengineering.* Heidelberg, Germany: Springer-Verlag.

Young MB. 2006. *Strategic Workforce Planning: Forecasting Human Capital Needs to Execute Business Strategy.* New York: Conference Board.

Zuckerman AM. 2005. *Healthcare Strategic Planning.* Chicago, IL: Health Administration Press.

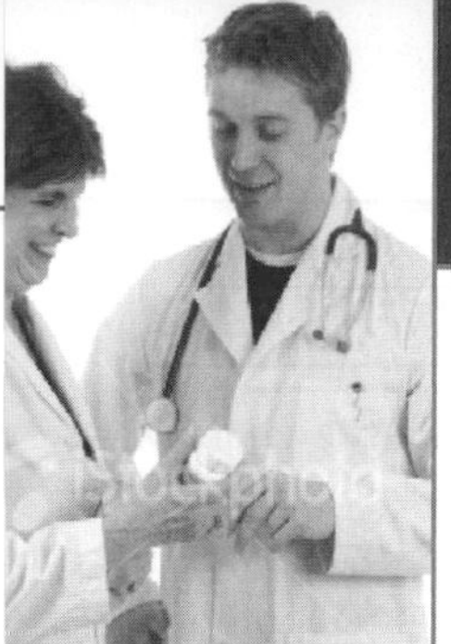

5

BUSINESS PLANNING FOR PHARMACY PROGRAMS

Glen T. Schumock, Godwin Wong, and JoAnn Stubbings

About the Authors: Dr. Schumock is a graduate of Washington State University (B.Pharm.), the University of Washington (Pharm.D.), and the University of Illinois at Chicago (MBA). He also completed a residency and a research fellowship. Currently, Dr. Schumock is director of the Center for Pharmacoeconomic Research and professor in the Department of Pharmacy Practice at the University of Illinois at Chicago. He teaches courses on pharmacy management, pharmacoeconomics, and business planning for pharmacy services. He has published over 100 articles, book chapters, and books. He is on the editorial boards of the journals *Pharmacotherapy* and *PharmacoEconomics.* He is a board-certified pharmacotherapy specialist and a fellow of the American College of Clinical Pharmacy.

Dr. Wong has been on the faculty of the Haas School of Business at the University of California, Berkeley, for over 20 years. His areas of interests are corporate strategic planning, entrepreneurship, information technology management, and venture capital. He has conducted leadership and strategic planning workshops for various health care groups, hospital administrators, and pharmaceutical companies and has lectured to executives in 20 countries. He has served on the boards of directors of several California banks, Silicon Valley companies, and international corporations. He received a B.S. from the University of Wisconsin, an M.S. from UCLA, and a Ph.D. from Harvard University.

JoAnn Stubbings is manager, research and public policy, in the Ambulatory Care Pharmacy Department at the University of Illinois at Chicago (UIC), and is clinical associate professor in the Department of Pharmacy Practice and Administration. She also has a faculty appointment in the UIC Center for Pharmacoeconomic Research. She received a B.S. in pharmacy from the Ohio State University and Masters in Health Care Administration from the University of Mississippi. Professor Stubbings is responsible for managing and communicating pharmaceutical policy issues that pertain to outpatient pharmacy services especially to underserved populations. She teaches courses and publishes in business planning, justification and payment for clinical pharmacy services, risk evaluation and mitigation strategies, and Medicare Part D.

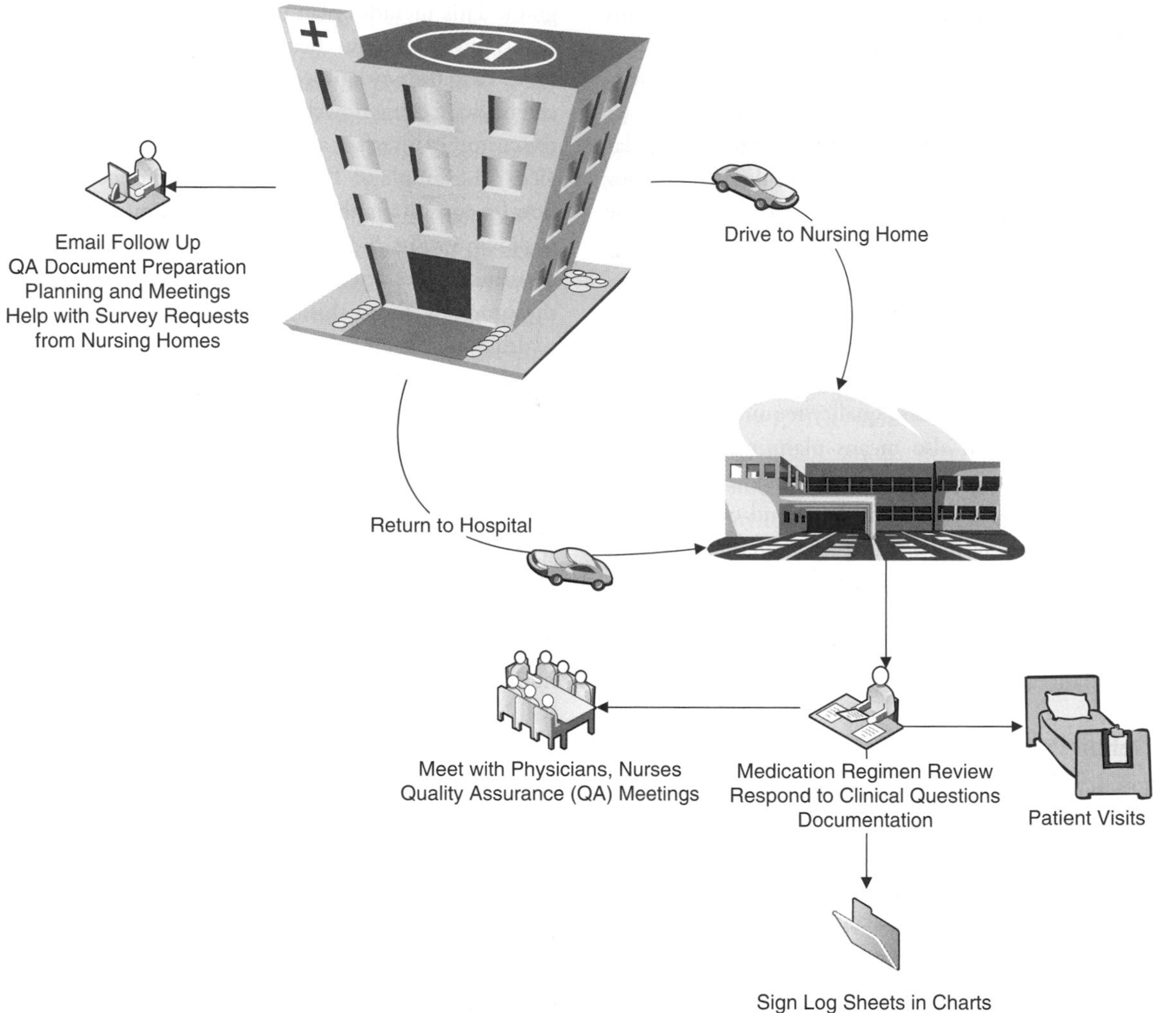

Figure 5-1. Diagram of work flow for consultant pharmacy services to nursing homes. This figure shows the workflow that might occur within the proposed consultant pharmacy services business. Pharmacists employed by the hospital would visit contracted nursing home and provide consulting service, including review of patient medical records, discussion with physicians and nursing, documentation of services provided and of clinical recommendations, and participation in quality assurance meetings. (The authors would like to acknowledge Rebecca Gatzke, Pharm.D., who is consultant pharmacist, Pharmore Drugs, Skokie, IL. Dr. Gatzke provided information used to develop this figure.)

Develop a Marketing Strategy

The second of the goal-setting steps is to define a marketing strategy. The marketing strategy should be based on information gathered in the previous steps of the business planning process, especially the market and competitor analyses. The marketing strategy should identify the target market for the program and develop a plan for gaining the business of that market. This plan should include the means of communicating to customers and the message that should be communicated to them. The strategy for a new business should be separated into the initial marketing plan and the ongoing marketing plan. The initial marketing plan defines the promotional activities and market goals for the period directly before and immediately after implementation of the new program. The ongoing marketing plan defines the promotional and market goals over the longer term. Resources are available to assist in the development of pharmacy-related marketing plans (Doucette and McDonough, 2002; Holdford, 2007).

The marketing strategy for the consultant pharmacy service (scenario) largely will depend on the current status of such services in area nursing homes. It is likely that the market comprises all the nursing homes in a limited geographic region surrounding the hospital. However, it may be Ted's wish to target the service only to the largest homes (i.e., those over 500 beds) or to those with the highest acuity (or some other target characteristic). Usually, nursing home administrators make the decision to contract with a consultant pharmacy service (with input from medical and nursing staff); therefore, the communication plan should focus on those individuals. The best method of communicating information about the program likely will be face-to-face visits by Ted with those administrators responsible for homes in the target market. The marketing plan may call for obtaining contracts with only a couple homes in the first 6 months of the program but then to increase gradually by one home every 6 months. The ongoing marketing strategy would be in accordance with this.

Develop Financial Projections

Perhaps the most critical step in the business planning process is the development of financial projections for the program. Most programs that do not have a positive benefit-to-cost ratio usually will not be approved. That is, the program must be profitable. While it is preferable that programs generate revenue, it is possible that pharmacy services are justifiable based on reducing expenditures. For example, a clinical pharmacy antibiotic dosing service in a hospital may reduce expenditures on antibiotics and reduce patient length of stay but generate no revenue. If the financial benefit of the dosing service (i.e., reduced expenditures) exceeds the costs associated with providing the program (i.e., pharmacist salary), then the program can be considered financially viable. Obviously, there may be additional benefits from the dosing service, such as improved patient outcomes, that also would favor its approval.

The business planning process must include an analysis of both the costs that will be incurred to provide the service and the financial benefits that may occur as a result of the program. More detailed descriptions of the methods to project these figures are available elsewhere (Schumock, 2000). The calculations involved in this planning process may be aided by the use of financial spreadsheets. A set of financial spreadsheets designed for creating financial projections is available to those in the position of having to develop a business plan (Schumock and Stubbings, 2007). The revenue and expense statement, which lists revenue by category, expenditures by category, and net profit each year for a 3- to 5-year period, is the most useful of these. An example of a revenue and expense projection for consultant pharmacy services (scenario) is shown in Table 5-1.

In developing the financial projections, revenue (if it exists) should be based on the anticipated volume of business, changes to that volume expected over time, and the income per unit of service. Information on billing for pharmacy services may be helpful in estimating potential revenue of the proposed service (American College of Clinical Pharmacy, 1999; Larson et al., 2000; Vogenberg, 2006). Discounts to income (contractual agreements) should be factored into these calculations, as should future increases in the amount charged for the service. Expenditures also must be projected. If the program requires significant capital investment, those expenditures should be depreciated over the life of the item and accounted for appropriately. Other investments required to initiate the program also should be shown in the financial estimates. Ongoing costs, such as salaries and benefits, minor equipment, supplies, rent, and other overhead, should be categorized and accounted for. Costs that are considered variable should be increased proportionate

Table 5-1. Example Revenue and Expense Projections for Consultant Pharmacy Services Program, Most Likely Scenario, Years 1–5

	Year 1	Year 2	Year 3	Year 4	Year 5	Total
Operating revenue						
Patient revenue	504,000	1,008,000	1,176,000	1,260,000	1,764,000	5,712,000
Deductions from revenue	0	0	0	0	0	0
Net patient revenue	504,000	1,008,000	1,176,000	1,260,000	1,764,000	5,712,000
Operating expenses						
Salaries	312,000	426,400	561,600	595,296	1,017,120	2,912,416
Employee benefits	81,100	110,900	146,000	154,800	264,500	757,300
Medical director	0	0	0	0	0	0
Medical supplies	6,000	6,890	7,420	7,950	8,500	36,760
Office supplies	0	0	0	0	0	0
Education and travel	0	0	0	0	0	0
Maintenance/repair	300	318	337	357	757	2,069
Consulting	0	0	0	0	0	0
Contracted services	0	0	0	0	0	0
Marketing	5,000	2,500	2,650	2,809	5,300	18,259
Dues and subscriptions	3,585	3,780	3,975	3,975	4,170	19,485
Rent	12,500	12,700	13,500	14,300	15,150	68,150
Postage	3,500	4,200	4,800	5,300	6,900	24,700
Equipment expense	13,000	1,272	1,348	0	1,515	17,135
Utilities/telephone	8,300	8,798	9,326	9,886	10,479	46,789
Insurance	900	1,166	1,248	1,323	1,826	6,463
Other expenses	16,500	3,090	3,285	12,423	8,894	44,192
Bad debt expense	0	0	0	0	0	0
Building depreciation	0	0	0	0	0	0
Equipment depreciation	0	0	0	0	0	0
Total operating expenses	462,685	582,014	755,489	808,419	1,345,111	3,953,718
Net income (loss)	41,315	425,986	420,511	451,581	418,889	1,758,282
Net assets at beginning	350,000	391,315	817,301	1,237,812	1,689,393	4,485,821
Net assets at end	391,315	817,301	1,237,812	1,689,393		

to the changes in volume expected. All costs should be increased annually based on inflation, the consumer price index (CPI), or other evidence of expected increases in the costs of goods or services. Additional resources are available on financial management in pharmacy organizations, which might be useful in developing the financial projects in a business plan (Carroll, 2007; Wilson, 2009)

Identify an Action Plan

The next step in the business planning process is to define major milestones and an action plan of implementation and operation of the program. This action plan should detail the start and finish dates and list responsible individual(s) for each task necessary to accomplish the objectives of the business plan. The action plan should include periodic monitoring and assessment of the performance (i.e., clinical, financial, or other) of the program. A Gantt chart is one method to depict the action plan visually. An example of a Gantt chart for long-term consultant pharmacy services is shown in Fig. 5-2.

Assess Critical Risks and Opportunities

Another key step in the business planning process is to determine the critical risks and opportunities of the proposed program. Chapter 4 introduced the concepts of a SWOT (*s*trengths, *w*eaknesses, *o*pportunities, *t*hreats) analysis. As part of the business plan such an analysis should be completed for the proposed business/service. While it may seem more reasonable to conduct the SWOT analysis earlier in the business planning process, as was done in strategic planning, because the program is in the proposal stage, some of the key considerations for this analysis must come from the previous steps, such as the financial analysis, and thus it is done later in the process.

An example of a SWOT analysis for a proposed long-term care consultant pharmacy services program is shown in Tables 5-2 and 5-3. As mentioned in Chapter 4, strengths and weakness are internal characteristics, whereas opportunities and threats are characteristics of the external business environment. A number of factors can be considered when conducting this analysis. The factors considered will vary based on the nature of the business and the business environment.

Establish an Exit Plan

The last step of the planning process is to develop an exit plan. The *exit plan* is a formal protocol for determining when and why a decision would be made to terminate the program. The exit plan also defines the steps that would be taken if such a decision were to be made.

A decision to exit a program usually is based on failure of the business to meet predetermined goals (financial, or otherwise). Typically, any new business is given a certain amount of time to meet its goals (18 to 24 months). Many organizations fail to have a mechanism in place to make a termination decision and instead let the business flounder and perhaps continue to lose money. It is much more preferable to have a definitive benchmark to which the program can be compared and a decision made promptly and decisively. This requires routine measurement of the ongoing performance of the business and comparison to those pre-established benchmarks or performance thresholds.

If a decision is made to terminate a program, then there should be clear actions for how the business will be dissolved. First, there should be a plan for when and how customers will be notified. Further, in some cases it may be important to provide customers with information about others who can provide the service and then schedule a seamless transition. Second, there should be a plan for how employees will be notified. The plan may include efforts to place employees in other areas of the organization or what, if any, compensation package may be available. Third, there should be a plan for how the facilities, equipment, and other capital (*capital* will be discussed in Chapter 18) will be sold or transferred. An exit plan for a program could involve transferring the control of the program

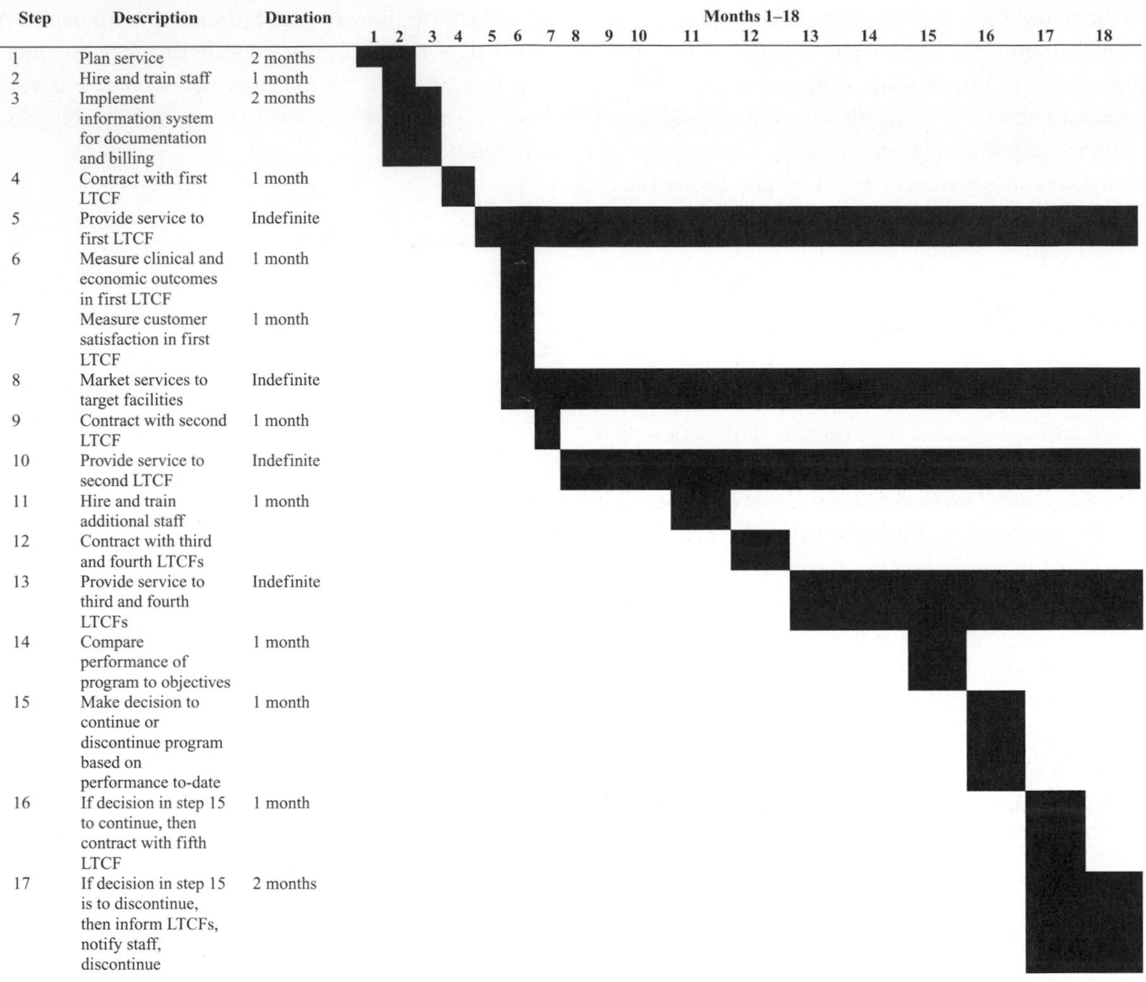

Step	Description	Duration
1	Plan service	2 months
2	Hire and train staff	1 month
3	Implement information system for documentation and billing	2 months
4	Contract with first LTCF	1 month
5	Provide service to first LTCF	Indefinite
6	Measure clinical and economic outcomes in first LTCF	1 month
7	Measure customer satisfaction in first LTCF	1 month
8	Market services to target facilities	Indefinite
9	Contract with second LTCF	1 month
10	Provide service to second LTCF	Indefinite
11	Hire and train additional staff	1 month
12	Contract with third and fourth LTCFs	
13	Provide service to third and fourth LTCFs	Indefinite
14	Compare performance of program to objectives	1 month
15	Make decision to continue or discontinue program based on performance to-date	1 month
16	If decision in step 15 to continue, then contract with fifth LTCF	1 month
17	If decision in step 15 is to discontinue, then inform LTCFs, notify staff, discontinue	2 months

Figure 5-2. Example of a Gantt chart for implementation of proposed business to provide consultant pharmacy services to nursing homes. This figure shows the steps that should be taken in order to implement the proposed consultant pharmacy service. The chart includes when (month) each step should be initiated and when it would be would be expected to be completed. Gantt charts such as this often also include the party/person responsible for completion of each step (not shown here).

from one organization or one administrative unit to another.

While the exit plan implies termination of the program, there are actually several possibilities for how a business may be disposed. These include (1) closing the program, (2) merging the business with another program, (3) selling the business/program, and (4) taking it out of its current arrangement and operating it as a separate and individualized entity.

COMMUNICATION OF THE BUSINESS PLAN

Typically, there are two key components to communicating the work accomplished in planning. The first is to create a written document—the actual business plan. The second is to present the business plan orally, usually as part of a formal decision-making process.

Table 5-2. Internal Strengths and Weaknesses of Consultant Pharmacy Services Program

Factor	Strength	Weakness
Profitability	As a new program associated with a hospital, overhead expenses will be minimal and thus profitability could be high. The program is also able to share staff with the hospital, thus reducing salary expenses.	Profitability may be limited initially due to start-up expenses and small number of nursing homes served.
Quality	Quality management is a strength of the hospital environment and this may spill-over to the nursing home program.	As a new program, the organization has limited experience specific to the long-term care environment. This may jeopardize quality initially.
Customer service	Because the program is small (at least initially) it may be able to provide more attention to customers and thus better customer service.	Because the hospital is the primary responsibility of the pharmacy department, it may not always be able to respond as quickly to nursing home customer needs.
Staff	Because the pharmacists included in the program have hospital experience, their level of clinical knowledge is beyond that of most competitors.	The pharmacists are new to the consultant pharmacy business so there may be a learning curve and lack of nursing home-specific knowledge initially.
Operations	Because the program is associated with a hospital, it can rely on the hospital pharmacy department for backup during off hours.	Because the program is small and new in this business, efficiency may be limited. It may also be difficult to get contracts with nursing homes initially due to establish competition.

Writing the Business Plan

As stated previously, writing the business plan is an extremely important part of business planning. The business plan should be informative and balanced in its presentation of the proposal. The document should be written with a specific audience in mind (the financial decision maker). It should be both easy to read and easy to understand and therefore must possess proper organization, grammar, punctuation, and sentence structure.

The contents of a business plan typically follow a sequence of items that are unique to this type of planning. An example of the table of contents of a simple business plan is shown in Table 5-4. It should be noted that the contents of the business plan will vary based on the industry, the business proposed, and the needs of the organization. More detailed plans may be required in certain industries.[3]

The business plan should begin with an *executive summary*. This summary should be short (one to two pages) but should hit the main points of the proposal.

[3]As another example, the proposed contents of a business plan for a for-profit venture could include executive summary, introduction/synopsis, venture idea, overall industry, market research/competition, production/sourcing plan, service/delivery plan, marketing/sales plan, management plan, human resources plan, ownership/organization plan, financial plan, financing plan, growth/exit plan, implementation plan, contingency plan, and assessment/evaluation plan.

Table 5-3. External Opportunities and Threats of Consultant Pharmacy Services Program

Factor	Opportunities	Threats
Competition	Because the competitors also provide pharmaceutical products, they could be considered biased in the clinical recommendations they make—this may be an advantage for the proposed service which will focus only on the consulting service.	Competitors are well established, large, and financially sound. Competitors also provide pharmaceutical products, which may be desirable to the nursing homes. New competitors may enter the local market in the future.
Technology	The competitors don't have the same access to and understanding of technology as might already exist in the hospital (electronic medical records, bar coding, and other technology) and be advantageous to the nursing homes.	Competitors have advanced information systems and experience with these systems.
Regulation	Consultant pharmacy services are mandated by state law. Thus, nursing homes must contract with a provider of these services.	There may be changes to regulations in the future that may alter the ability of the hospital/ACO to provide this service in the future.
Reimbursement	Nursing homes must contract with an outside organization to provide this service. The proposed program will provide a alternative for nursing homes to choose.	Health care reform may alter funding for nursing homes or may change the reimbursement for consultant pharmacy services.
Costs	Competitors may not be able to use pharmacists as efficiently as the proposed program.	Pharmacist salaries are rising rapidly due to a labor market shortage. These salaries will drive up costs, making it more difficult for the program to generate profit.
Market/customers	The population continues to age, and as such, there may be more nursing homes in the future.	Changes to how health care is provided may result in fewer people going to nursing homes and more cared for at home.

The executive summary needs to capture the attention of the reader. In a poorly written business plan, the reader may form a negative opinion of the program and read no further than the executive summary. This illustrates the importance of a writing style that is engaging and error free. Because of its position in the document, the executive summary is clearly the most critical section of the plan. In addition to the executive summary, the plan should also begin with a *table of contents.* This will both help the writer organize the plan and assist the reader in navigating the document.

The second section of the business plan is the *background and description.* Here, in a logical sequence, the plan should define the rationale for the program or service (i.e., the patient care need) and provide an explanation of why the organization is prepared to fill this need. The *service opportunity* provides the reader with a picture of the purpose of the proposed program

Table 5-4.	Typical Table of Contents of the Business Plan
1.	Executive summary
2.	Background and description
3.	Market analysis and strategy
4.	Operational structure and processes
5.	Financial projections
6.	Milestones, schedule, and action plan
7.	Critical risks and opportunities
8.	Exit strategy
9.	Conclusion
10.	Supportive documents (include financial pro forma statements, letters of support)

and should lead directly to a description of the formal *mission of the business.* Last, this section should provide other details that will help to illustrate the service, including data that may have been obtained from literature or other sources.

The next section of the business plan is the *market analysis and strategy.* In some cases, the market analysis is presented as a separate section from the marketing strategy. In either case, the market analysis is part of the situation analysis conducted during planning, whereas the marketing strategy is part of the goal-setting and strategy development elements of planning. In the business plan document, these are sometimes presented together because they address the same general topic.

The fourth major section of the business plan is the *operational structure and processes.* In brief, this section describes how the program will be run. This section of the document should provide details on how the service will be provided and by whom—in other words, the work processes that will occur. It should include information on how customers will interface with the program. The organizational structure, number and types of employees, and equipment and other resources used in operation of the program should be described. This section also should include definitions of the regulatory, clinical, and quality requirements that may be applicable to the business and a description of how these requirements will be met.

The fifth major section of the plan is the *financial projections* or *financial pro forma.* This section identifies the estimated expenditures and revenue over the first 3 to 5 years of the program. Investments required to begin and operate the program should be described as either startup costs or ongoing costs (or operating costs) and should be organized by cost categories (e.g., salaries, equipment, capital, etc.). The financial data are best presented in a revenue and expense statement (sometimes referred to as the *profit and loss statement*), as shown in Table 5-1.

The sixth section of the business plan defines the *milestones, schedule, and action plan* for the program. A timeline should be defined that includes the major accomplishments and goals of the program for implementation and through the first 3 to 5 years and may include long-range growth and expansions objectives. The action plan also may include responsibility assignments and is often presented as a Gantt chart. For an example see Fig. 5-2.

The next section of the business plan defines the *critical risks and opportunities* of the business. Here, the plan should outline the major strengths and weakness of the proposed business and describe the opportunities and risk associated with the program if implemented (as formulated in the SWOT analysis). This information, both positive and negative, must be presented in an unbiased manner so that an informed decision can be made about moving forward with the program.

The business plan should include a brief discussion of what will happen if the business should fail, or alternatively become very successful. This *exit strategy* or *contingency strategy* should define specifically when and how a decision would be made to exit the business. The section then should outline a plan for exiting the business. This plan might include issues such as what to do with existing patients or customers (i.e., refer to other providers), what will happen with existing staff (i.e., reassign to other divisions of the organization or terminate), and how equipment and resources may be disposed of.

The last section of the business plan is the *conclusion.* The conclusion should be brief in summarizing the document. Most importantly, the conclusion should provide a recommendation with respect to the proposed business decision. Following the conclusion are any *attachments* or *additional materials.* Supportive documentation, tables, figures, financial statements, and/or letters of support should be attached to the business plan to corroborate the written text or present the material in a more detailed fashion.

Presenting the Plan

The oral presentation of the business plan may be as important as the written document. In most organizations, those seeking to implement new programs must present the business plan before a group, usually consisting of senior leaders in the company.

A good oral presentation can go a long way toward garnering positive support for the business plan. The personal nature of the oral presentation may add dynamics to the decision-making process that do not exist with the written document. These issues, which include politics, group dynamics, and personal interactions, can be either positive or negative. In either case, these dynamics should be anticipated and either reinforced or preempted depending on the situation.

CONCLUSION

After reading this chapter, Ted Thompson should be prepared to address the charge given him in the scenario. Ted will recognize quickly that developing a business plan for the proposed consultant pharmacy services program will be a significant undertaking. Ted would be well advised to seek assistance from others as he begins this planning process. For example, he might want to establish a team that would include representatives from the hospital finance department, other pharmacists who might be involved in the program, and perhaps even a physician or nurse with experience in long-term care. The assembled team then could begin the business plan planning process as outlined in this chapter. When this process is complete, Ted and his boss (the DOP) will need to follow the appropriate administrative channels within the organization to gain approval from key hospital decision makers.

Obviously, business planning is an important tool for gaining further acceptance and penetration of contemporary pharmacy services. New pharmacy graduates must understand and be able to write business plans that will justify new or continued investments in these services. It is very likely that most new graduates will be expected to develop or help to develop a business plan for a pharmacy program at some point in their careers. Clearly, the ability to do so will benefit the pharmacist, the employer, and patients. If accepted, the new program may be an opportunity to provide new or unique services—thus heightening job satisfaction. Likewise, the new program may generate revenue or save costs elsewhere in the system—thus benefiting the employer. Patients, physicians, nurses, and others who are the recipients of the program also will benefit.

QUESTIONS FOR FURTHER DISCUSSION

1. Conduct a literature search to identify articles that may be pertinent to the business proposal described in the scenario. How many articles did you find, and how useful are they to understanding the business concept?
2. Conduct a hypothetical market and competitor analysis, and develop a marketing strategy for the consultant pharmacy services program. What are the market segments that may be important to this business? What are the strengths and weaknesses of the proposed service compared with those of its potential competitors?
3. What are important costs that would be incurred if the consultant pharmacy services program were implemented? Classify these costs as fixed or variable.
4. Explain why you think an understanding of business planning is important for pharmacists. What changes are occurring in the health care environment that make business planning even more important?

REFERENCES

American College of Clinical Pharmacy. 1994. Establishing and evaluating clinical pharmacy services in primary care. *Pharmacotherapy* 14:743–58.

American College of Clinical Pharmacy. 1999. *How to Bill for Clinical Pharmacy Services.* Kansas City, MO: American College of Clinical Pharmacy.

American College of Clinical Pharmacy, Harris IM, Baker E, Berry TM, et al. 2008. Developing a business-practice model for pharmacy services in ambulatory settings. *Pharmacotherapy* 28(2):285.

Chater RW, Moczygemba LR, Lawson KA, et al. 2008. Building the business model for medication therapy management services. *J Am Pharm Assoc* 48:16–22.

Chisholm-Burns MA, Kim Lee J, Spivey CA, et al. 2010. US pharmacists' effect as team members on patient care: systematic review and meta-analyses. *Med Care* 48:923–33.

Coke A. 2002. *Seven Steps to a Successful Business Plan.* New York: AMACOM, American Management Association.

Cooper JK, Saxton C, Cameron KA (eds.). 2004. *Developing a Senior Care Pharmacy Practice: Your Guide and Tools for Success.* Alexandria, VA: American Society of Consultant Pharmacists.

Carroll NV. 2007. *Financial Management for Pharmacists: A Decision-Making Approach,* 3rd edn. Baltimore, MD: Lippincott Williams & Wilkins.

DeThomas A, Derammelaere SA. 2008. *Writing a Convincing Business Plan.* Hauppauge, NY: Barron's Educational Series.

Doucette WR, McDonough RP. 2002. Beyond the 4Ps: Using relationship marketing to build value and demand for pharmacy services. *J Am Pharm Assoc* 42:183.

Ford BR, Bornstein J, Pruitt PT, Siegel ES. 2007. *The Ernst & Young Business Plan Guide.* Hoboken, NJ: John Wiley & Sons.

Hagel HP. 2002. Planning for patient care. In Hagel HP, Rovers JP (eds.) *Managing the Patient-Centered Pharmacy.* Washington, DC: American Pharmaceutical Association.

Hatoum HT, Akhras K. 1993. A 32-year literature review on the value and acceptance of ambulatory care provided by clinical pharmacists. *Ann Pharmacother* 27:1108–16.

Hatoum HT, Catizone C, Hutchinson RA, Purohit A. 1986. An eleven-year review of the pharmacy literature: Documentation of the value and acceptance of clinical pharmacy. *Drug Intell Clin Pharm* 20:33–48.

Holdford DA. 2007. *Marketing for Pharmacists,* 2nd edn. Washington, DC: American Pharmaceutical Association.

Larson TA, Uden DL, Hadsall RS. 2000. Practice models used by pharmacists in rural Minnesota to obtain Medicare reimbursement. *J Am Pharm Assoc* 40:554–9.

McDonough R. 2007. Writing a business plan for a new pharmacy service. *The Dynamics of Pharmaceutical Care: Enriching Patients Health,* Monograph 23. Washington, DC: American Pharmacists Association.

McKeever M. 2010. *How to Write a Business Plan,* 10th edn. Berkeley, CA: NOLO Press.

Perez A, Doloresco F, Hoffman JM, et al. 2008. Economic evaluations of clinical pharmacy services: 2001–2005. *Pharmacotherapy* 28(11):285e–323e.

Phillips CR, Larson LN. 2002. Creating a business plan for patient care. In Hagel HP, Rovers JP (eds.) *Managing the Patient-Centered Pharmacy.* Washington, DC: American Pharmaceutical Association.

Pinson L, Jinnet J. 2005. *Anatomy of a Business Plan,* 4th edn. Chicago, IL: Dearborn Trade Pub.

Plumridge RJ, Wojnar-Horton RE. 1998. A review of the pharmacoeconomics of pharmaceutical care. *Pharmacoeconomics* 19:1349–51.

Record M. 2009. *Writing a Winning Business Plan.* Oxford: How To Books.

Sellars D. 2009. Business plan project: A step-by-step guide to writing a business plan. New York: Business Expert Press.

Schneller LW, Powell MF, Solomon DK. 1998. Using the business plan to propose revenue-generating pharmacy services. *Hosp Pharm* 23:806–11.

Schumock G. 2000. Methods to assess the economic outcomes of clinical pharmacy services. *Pharmacotherapy* 20;243S–52S.

Schumock G, Butler M. 2003. Evaluating and justifying clinical pharmacy services. In Grauer D, Lee J, Odom T, et al. (eds.) *Pharmacoeconomics and Outcomes: Applications for Patient Care,* 2nd edn. Kansas City, MO: American College of Clinical Pharmacy.

Schumock G, Butler M, Meek P, et al. 2003. Evidence of the economic benefit of clinical pharmacy services: 1996–2000. *Pharmacotherapy* 23:113–32.

Schumock G, Meek P, Ploetz P, Vermeulen LC. 1996. Economic evaluations of clinical pharmacy services: 1998–1995. *Pharmacotherapy* 16:1188–208.

Schumock G, Michaud J, Guenette A. 1999. Re-engineering: An opportunity to advance clinical practice in a community hospital. *Am J Health Syst Pharm* 56:1945–49.

Schumock G, Stubbing J. 2007. *How to Develop a Business Plan for Pharmacy Services.* Lenexa, KS: American College of Clinical Pharmacy.

Schumock G, Stubbings J, McBride SJ. 2004. Business planning and marketing. In *Developing a Senior Care Pharmacy Practice: Your Guide and Tools for Success.* Alexandria, VA: American Society of Consultant Pharmacists.

Tipton DJ. 2001. A tool for corporate decision making about cognitive pharmaceutical services. *J Am Pharm Assoc* 41:91–9.

Vogenberg FR. 2006. *Understanding Pharmacy Reimbursement.* Bethesda, MD: American Society of Health System Pharmacists.

Willett MS, Bertch KE, Rich DS, Ereshefsky L. 1989. Prospectus on the economic value of clinical pharmacy services. *Pharmacotherapy* 9:45–56.

Wilson A. 2009. *Financial Management Basics for Health-System Pharmacists.* Bethesda, MD: American Society of Health-System Pharmacist.

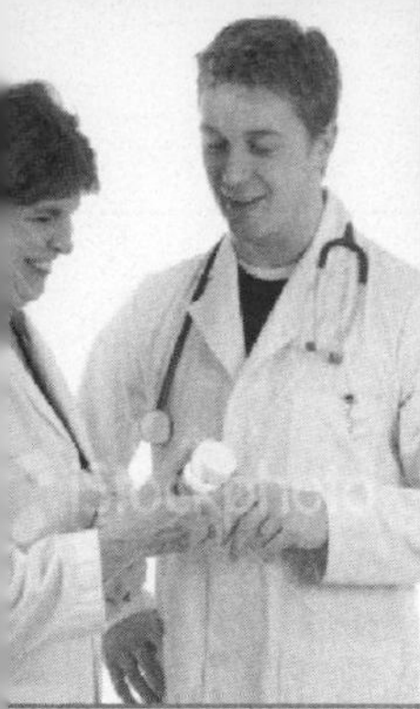

6

OPERATIONS MANAGEMENT

Greg L. Alston and Wesley R. Haltom

About the Authors: Dr. Alston is an associate professor of pharmacy management and assistant dean for assessment at Wingate University School of Pharmacy in North Carolina. He has over 30 years of experience in community pharmacy management, both as a chain-pharmacy administrator and an independent pharmacy owner. He earned a Doctor of Pharmacy degree from the University of the Pacific while simultaneously becoming a credentialed K-12 teacher through their School of Education. He teaches courses in pharmacy management, community health outreach, and pharmacy communications skills. His main research interest is in quantifying and qualifying the processes required to create viable professional niche business models.

Dr. Haltom is an assistant professor of pharmacy and director of introductory pharmacy practice experience (IPPE) at Wingate University School of Pharmacy. He earned his Doctor of Pharmacy degree at Wingate. His background includes community pharmacy practice with an interest in custom compounding. Dr. Haltom is course leader for IPPE discussion courses as well as Wingate's electronic mentor interaction course. He also teaches in community health outreach, pharmacy communications skills, and problem-based learning courses. His research interest is in understanding the predictors of failure to achieve competence.

■ LEARNING OBJECTIVES

After completing this chapter, readers should be able to

1. Define the role of the business in society and the role of profits in business.
2. Define the role of operations management within a business.
3. Describe the concept of command intent.
4. Describe how operations managers accomplish the command intent of an organization.
5. Describe the essential operations management tasks.
6. Illuminate differences between a production worker and a knowledge worker.
7. Describe Human Sigma as a model for customer service operations.

SCENARIO

Trey Smith, Pharm.D., is the pharmacy manager at Smith's Drug, a small independent pharmacy. His pharmacy performs regular dispensing, custom compounding, and sells a line of durable medical equipment. Trey has recently lost one of his senior technicians to a competitor and has since hired a new associate, Lisa. It is Trey's responsibility to ensure that every member of Smith's Drugs staff is adequately trained in the pharmacy's workflow. Lisa has no prior experience in pharmacy, but is willing to give a great effort and wants to be well trained so that she can be an asset to the pharmacy team. Trey has outlined a plan with Lisa to get her up to speed on how to count and label prescriptions, how to compound medications, and bill patients' insurance. One of the most experienced technicians at Smith's Drug, Bill, often handles the position in the pharmacy that offers the greatest challenge—that is, where the patients drop off their prescriptions for entry into the computer system. As part of the training plan for Lisa, Trey has decided to let her train at the drop-off position on Wednesday afternoons when the pharmacy's business is slower so that she can work on inputting prescription and insurance information. This plan has worked quite well for the past 2 weeks, but on this particular Wednesday there happens to be a festival going on just up the street from the pharmacy. This had led to an influx of customers, and prescriptions are beginning to pile up at Lisa's station. Customer waiting time for prescriptions has increased from 10 minutes to 25 minutes. What is the most appropriate course of action for Trey to take to ensure the success of his business?

CHAPTER QUESTIONS

1. What is the role of a business in society?
2. What is the role of profits in a business?
3. What do operations managers do to help their business achieve its goals?
4. What is command intent? How can it be applied to pharmacy operations?
5. What is Human Sigma? How can it be applied to pharmacy operations?

INTRODUCTION

The first two chapters of this book described the domains of patient-oriented pharmacy practice and its intersections with the managerial sciences. This chapter will deal with the domain of business management and the science of operations.

When most people think of the concept of management and what it is that managers do, they are envisioning operations managers. Operations managers are often referred to as "front-line" managers, as they typically are involved in directly overseeing a business' major functions (e.g., dispensing prescriptions in a community pharmacy, preparing medication orders in a hospital). While operations managers typically have input with the executive team on all phases of the management of a company, this chapter will focus on those functions that are the primary responsibility of the operations manager.

After the executive team creates the vision and mission statements for a business, it is the responsibility of operations managers to execute the vision and mission in compliance with the values of the organization. Operations managers must make the daily decisions required to keep the business moving in the right direction. Operations management involves a variety of tasks that managers perform to control, organize, and lead the work team to fulfill the goals and objectives of the organization.

All business processes require that management effort be routinely applied to remain effective. Pharmacy dispensing and professional services are no different. Whether you see yourself in a formal administrative position (e.g., chief pharmacist, pharmacy director, assistant or associate director, clinical coordinator) or as a staff pharmacist, the reality is that the highest ranking pharmacist on duty must play the role of the professional operations manager to ensure the provision of quality patient care.

THE ROLE OF BUSINESS IN SOCIETY AND THE ROLE OF PROFITS IN A BUSINESS

It is important to first discuss the role of a business in society, especially a professional business such as pharmacy. The profession of pharmacy exists in society to provide a variety of goods and services related to the appropriate management and use of medications. These goods and services provide an array of benefits to patients, health care providers, and society at large.

The primary role of any pharmacy in society should be to benefit those that they serve, not necessarily to make money for pharmacy owners. Yet, if *any* pharmacy fails to bring in enough revenue to cover their expenses, the pharmacy will not be able to continue to provide goods and services that create benefits for others. And for a for-profit organization in a market-based economy (e.g., most community pharmacies in the United States), pharmacies must be able to generate a profit (the excess of revenues over expenses) large enough to justify an owner's investment in the organization. If pharmacies cannot generate profits, owners will lack incentives to invest in pharmacies, leaving patients and society without the benefits they provide.

Management expert Peter Drucker echoes this idea of businesses existing to serve society. A company should focus on serving its customers, and profits are simply a required resource for the company to continue to serve society (Drucker, 1973). Money and profits do play a role in a pharmacy, and that is to keep the pharmacy solvent so that it can continue to provide its highly needed goods and services to society.

A good way to demonstrate how this principle works is to ask the following question.

Why Did You Choose Pharmacy as a Career Path?

While interviewing for admission to a Doctor of Pharmacy program, students are often asked why they would like to become pharmacists. Prospective students are afraid to mention money and income as a motivator to enter the profession because they fear this motivation will appear unprofessional. The typical response from a prospective student is something like, "I want to help people" in an effort to appeal to the sense of altruism commonly found among health care professionals.

Now ask another question. If pharmacists were paid only minimum wage, would people still be so inclined to enroll in pharmacy school? Over the course of their professional education (not including prepharmacy studies), the average pharmacy student will accumulate over $107,000 of student loan debt (AACP, 2010). Even if minimum wage was $10 an hour, a full-time pharmacist working 2080 hours per year would only earn a little over $20,000 per year. $107,000 of student loans paid back at 7% interest over 10 years would cost over $14,900 a year in student loan payments alone. That would leave a pharmacist making a minimal wage with less than $500 a month to live on. Most pharmacists, like almost everyone who pursues a higher education, would like to seek a greater return on their investments of time, effort, and financial resources.

What this points out is that there are economic and financial realities to any business and any profession. There is a public mission, to serve society, and there is a private mission, to provide income for the operators of the business. It is not just the business owners that benefit from an organization's profits. Society benefits by having a valuable service provided. And all employee salaries, benefits, and career advancement are paid out of the income generated by any business. Whether the business is a for-profit organization (like most community pharmacies) or a not-for-profit organization (like many hospitals and organizations which provide care as a charity), the rules do not change, someone has to pay the bills.

The Role of Operations Management within a Business

It is the role of operations managers in any business to ensure the smooth functioning of the business unit to achieve both its public and private missions. This sentiment was expertly outlined by Peter Drucker (1973):

> And the manager in public-service institutions faces the same tasks as the manager in a business: to perform the function for the sake of which the institution exists; to make work productive and the worker achieving; to manage the institution's social impacts and to discharge its social responsibilities [p. 32].

An operations manager must understand the vision, mission, and goals of the organization to direct his or her workforce. The management structure of an organization requires multiple roles to be played. Typically large public corporations will have a chief executive officer (CEO) whose responsibility it is to direct the strategic planning of the organization, a chief financial officer (CFO) who directs the budget and financing activities of the organization, and the chief operating officer (COO) who is responsible for the day-to-day operations of the business. In a small business (e.g., an independent community pharmacy, a consulting firm), single person (e.g., a pharmacy owner, a consultant) may play all of these roles.

The operations manager focuses the energy and intent of the organization on what must be done today to accomplish the long-term goals of the business. These focused activities must also behave in alignment with the vision, mission, and values of the organization. The executive team creates the goals or "marching orders" for the organization. An operations manager must understand the intent of the orders and the results of potential actions to avoid disaster and ensure success.

At the most basic level, operations managers decide:

1. What must be done right now?
2. Who needs to be doing it?
3. What resources do they need?
4. When is the work finished?

It may be helpful to think of operations management in terms of the critical decisions that need to be made by operations managers. The ten decisions under the purview of operations management are described by Heizer and Render (1999) in Table 6-1.

Not all tactics and directives employed by operations managers are equally successful. However, operations managers are ultimately responsible for modifying their directives until the results are successful. All business tactics and directives must occur within the framework of the values held by the business. Tactics and directives that contradict the company's ideals even though they achieve financial results are not acceptable. For example, suppose that a pharmacy condoned the selling of cigarettes to teenagers without identification. The pharmacy could make a lot of money selling cigarettes to teenagers. But at the same time, this tactic would be illegal as well as contradict the health and wellness missions held by most pharmacies.

The Theory of Command Intent

It could be argued that the most challenging component of managing a pharmacy's operations is managing its human resources. A manager cannot supervise what every employee is doing all day long. The manager must find a way to ensure that employees are working on the right tasks at the right time. In addition to understanding the fundamentals of human resources management (see Chapters 10–16), operations managers must develop plans and communicate them effectively. The business has no hope of achieving its goals without a clearly communicated plan of action.

A useful strategy to ensure that this is accomplished is known as *command intent* (Shattuck, 2000). The U.S. Army has determined that the most successful battlefield commanders are the ones who are able to think critically and change tactics during a mission, while still working toward the ultimate goal of capturing a strategic location, cutting off a supply line, or achieving a military objective. Good leaders are aware of the command intent of their orders and understand that circumstances constantly change while in battle.

Command intent gives a description of what the desired outcome is in relation to the current mission. That is, the command intent focuses on the endpoint, and does not summarize how to achieve that endpoint. The idea being that it will focus subordinates on what needs to get done, even when monumental change is

Table 6-1. Decisions under the Purview of Operations Managers

Designing goods and services	What should be offered for sale and at what price? How should the business arrange the price and service component of the product to maximize perceived value using the relative value theorem?
Process strategies	What is the best workflow methodology to ensure productivity?
Managing quality	How do we provide sufficient productivity while maintaining impeccable quality?
Location strategies	Where is the best location for this service to be offered?
Layout strategies	What is the best physical layout to ensure productivity? Does this layout fit with the pharmacy's workflow process?
Human resources	How do you motivate and inspire people to do excellent work? How can you develop engaged employees that represent your brand and develop relationships with your customers?
Scheduling	When and where should each employee be when our customers need service?
Supply chain management	Which suppliers will best help the company meet the needs of our customers?
Inventory management	How does the business insure that it will have enough without having too much or too little inventory?
Maintenance	How can the business keep all the equipment and facilities in good working order?

encountered on the battlefield and the original plans are no longer able to be applied. The U.S. Army General George S. Patton summarized this philosophy by stating, "Never tell people how to do things. Tell them what to do and they will surprise you with their ingenuity." The commander who gives very precise battle plan orders, but does not communicate the command intent to his or her subordinates is at risk of exposing soldiers to disastrous consequences. The battle never goes exactly as planned, so if the troops are not able to adjust to the constantly shifting tide of battle, they could be more easily defeated.

The concept of command intent can be applied to pharmacy operations management. An example of a vision statement for a community pharmacy may be "To be a recognized leader in customer service by providing affordable, timely, and effective drug therapies to improve our patients' lives." There are many tasks involved in the day-to-day operations of a pharmacy to strive to accomplish its vision and achieve success. These include ordering medications and supplies, stocking shelves, receiving and entering patients' prescriptions, printing labels and filling vials, final verification, checking out customers, counseling patients, and offering a variety of services. These tasks should be accomplished as efficiently and effectively as possible. But how does a manager know when to change the priority of the tasks? In a busy pharmacy circumstances may change at any given moment, making it difficult for technicians and service employees to know the best task to perform at any given moment.

To continue this example, assume that the pharmacy's warehouse order of medications and over-the-counter goods normally arrives on Tuesday mornings. The pharmacy manager may plan to have additional clerks scheduled to work Tuesday mornings, ensuring that technicians have clear access to shelves, preventing delays in filling prescriptions and improving inventory control. If on any Tuesday morning one of the additional clerks calls in sick, the priorities of the pharmacy manager and other employees may need to shift. Even if the pharmacy manager is off duty and is not directly supervising associates, the command intent of his or her orders needs to be followed. If the pharmacy manager has communicated his or her command intent properly, the employees will immediately recognize the priority of customer service and cease putting away the order to help meet customer demand. The staff should be able to adjust the command from "put away the order" order to "serve the customers" without facing discipline.

Managers who give orders without providing a command intent context may unintentionally imply that putting away an order from the warehouse is more important than customer service. This type of rigid top down order giving can make employees feel powerless to make changes regarding how key tasks are accomplished. It also psychologically relieves employees of any responsibility that they might have felt to rectify a faulty directive and do what they know to be the real mission of the business. This ultimately creates inefficient operations. When an operations manager communicates command intent to associates and subordinates, the statement should be brief, and it should promote flexibility so that resources can be most efficiently utilized to accomplish tasks.

How do Operations Managers Carry out Command Intent?

Once the operations manager knows the command intent and how to communicate it, how do they use this knowledge to guide their daily actions? An operations manager must set specific goals for what needs to be accomplished at the pharmacy. These goals must be set in real time based on an accurate assessment of the situation.

Examples of operational goals might include the following:

1. Improving the speed and efficiency of patient service.
   a. Are there bottlenecks in the workflow? Is the pharmacist's time being used efficiently? Is the business meeting its productivity goals?
2. Offering more services to patients.
   a. Is there a service that a pharmacy's customers want or need that they are not currently providing? Can they provide this service at their traditional standard of quality? Do they have the expertise and talent to make it work?
3. Creating and maintaining a collegial work environment for employees.
4. Do employees enjoy working at the pharmacy? Are they challenged to excel? Does the team work well together when it matters?
5. Improving the knowledge of health care team members.
   a. Can the pharmacy staff use their talents to improve the efforts of others? By identifying problem areas and resolving those problems, can the pharmacy improve their efficiency?

Regardless of the work environment, any list of operational goals should be formulated with feedback from employees, customers, and management. The list should be clear, concise, and align with the overarching vision of the business.

Executive-level management sets the vision and mission for the long-term value strategy of an organization. Operations managers use this guidance to create the goals or command intents of the business. The operations manager then must turn these goals into actions that create results. While the executive team views the mental process as "set the goals to direct the actions," the frontline employees view the process as "complete the actions to achieve the goals." The primary challenge for operations managers is to bridge the two points of view to create success.

In the context of the military, if the commanding officer is unable to continue in command, the next highest ranking officer takes over to ensure continuity of command. In the pharmacy world, if the pharmacy supervisor is not present or able to provide guidance at a particular time, a staff pharmacist must perform the operations management roles for the organization to be successful. This is a very common occurrence in pharmacies, in that there is no practical way in which an administrator can oversee or direct every event in a pharmacy. This is another of the many reasons why all pharmacists, from administrators to staff pharmacists, must have some degree of management skills (see Chapter 2).

When the official pharmacy supervisor is off duty, it must be clear to the work team who is in charge. In health care professions, the professional authority bestowed upon practitioners (e.g., pharmacists, physicians) will not allow them to abdicate their authority over the patient care process. When choices must be made to keep the daily activities (e.g., appropriate care of patients) aligned with the command intent of the organization (e.g., maximizing sales), the pharmacist on duty should have the authority to make that call. For example, pharmacists must have the authority to refuse to fill a prescription if the prescription would harm the patient, even though the command intent of maximizing sales may not be met in this particular case. Good pharmacists and operations managers realize that there are alternative methods to meet the command intent that do not put patient care at risk.

What Tasks Do Operations Managers Actually Perform?

Once a list of goals is established for the pharmacy, operations managers are charged with coming up with specific plans of action to meet these goals. Each goal is likely to have a number of tasks associated with it. These tasks drive what pharmacy managers do on a day-to-day basis. These tasks will change depending on the circumstances of the day, and the ways to accomplish these tasks can change. The tasks are what employees must complete to accomplish the command intent of the pharmacy.

For example, the list of operational goals previously mentioned can be expanded into specific action tasks for a pharmacy manager to use to direct his or her staff. By focusing on action steps, in the context of the business mission, the command intent of the organization can be clarified for employees. General goals such as "improving sales" do not belong on an action list. When the action list items are completed, a natural consequence will be an increase in sales.

Action steps are clear, concise, and can be acted upon in a short period. Read the following example action steps. Do you think the command intent is clear and unambiguous?

Goal #1: Improving the speed and efficiency of patient service.

Many different tasks can be derived from this goal. These might include

1. Cross train staff members to do each other's jobs.
2. Redesign the workflow to smooth out bottlenecks.
3. Upgrade the computer systems.
4. Add an additional computer terminal.
5. Take shorter lunch breaks to cover a staffing shortage.

Goal #2: Offering more services to patients.

There are many different services that customers may want or need. Are there services that a pharmacy could add that would provide a good return on their investment?

1. Develop a customer survey to identify unmet needs.
2. Conduct a customer focus group with ten customers.
3. Ask every employee to identify profitable opportunities.
4. Get all pharmacists immunization certified.
5. Create a layout plan for a new private counseling room.

Goal #3: Creating and maintaining a collegial work environment for employees.

There are many simple things that a manager can do to make work more enjoyable:

1. Create a career advancement plan for each employee.
2. Take one employee out for a private lunch each week.
3. Catch employees doing something well and praise them immediately.
4. Develop a corrective action plan for the employee who is always late.
5. Rotate job assignments during slow afternoon hours.

Goal #4: Improving the knowledge of health care team members.

One low-risk strategy for expanding a pharmacy manager's sphere of influence as a professional is to devote time and energy to improving the functional knowledge and skills of other providers:

1. Provide educational seminar on new drug developments.
2. Provide educational seminar on Medicare Part D annual plan changes.
3. Provide a lunch meeting for physician office staff to explain formulary changes.
4. Create a drug chart to assist prescribers in selecting the preferred drug for their patients.
5. Work with prescribers to apply for federal grant funding.

These are just a few examples of the types of tasks that pharmacy operations managers can develop. The tasks will change depending on the circumstances. The daily activities must change to meet the command intent of the organization. Operations managers must get the job done irrespective of the previously determined corporate plan.

For a business to operate successfully its employees must operate in alignment with the mission, vision, and values of the organization. Historically, management practices were built upon the industrial factory model that came into vogue with the development of the industrial revolution in the nineteenth and early twentieth centuries. As the economy moved from one of industrial production to one based on service jobs, Peter Drucker (1973) formalized the concept of a new type of worker distinct from a production worker that he called a knowledge worker:

> The basic capital resource, the fundamental investment, but also the cost center of a developed economy, is the knowledge worker who puts to work what he has learned in systematic education, that is, concepts, ideas, and theories, rather than the man who puts to work manual skill or muscle. [p. 32]

Drucker envisioned the importance of the knowledge worker in today's society. He hypothesized that the knowledge worker cannot be productive unless he or she is allowed to figure out how they work best, and to modify their routine accordingly.

There are some key differences between a production job and a knowledge worker job. Factory production lines are optimized to control every step of the process to produce identical products of consistent quality. Knowledge jobs typically revolve around customer service. Customer service "production" is different from factory line production because the end product is different depending on the customer.

To manage a customer service "production line," the employee must be empowered to figure out what the customer needs, and then modify the process to deliver the correct product. Knowledge workers now far outnumber factory workers in the United States economy. Knowledge workers need to be managed differently than production line employees (see Chapter 2).

Health care in general, and pharmacy in particular, cannot be effectively managed using production line management techniques because health care is essentially a customer service business. While many of the activities that pharmacists perform on a daily basis mimic a factory production line, there are critical distinctions that must be made. These distinctions are not based on the processes used, as the dispensing activities performed in pharmacies physically resemble a process-driven assembly line. Nevertheless, pharmacists do not just assemble prescriptions accurately; they are also responsible for knowing when prescriptions should not be filled, how medications should be appropriately used, and what to tell patients and their caregivers to help them get the most from their medications. The critical distinctions are that a pharmacist's professional license demands that they evaluate whether the prescription order is appropriate for the end-user and that they modify the order to achieve the intended outcome. Practically speaking, they must use their professional knowledge to deliver, or refuse to deliver, the proper product to the correct patient.

This professional knowledge component to what pharmacists do is the personification of knowledge worker. Even though prescriptions are written and dispensed correctly the vast majority of the time, the time one is not could lead to potentially devastating complications. One of the roles of the pharmacist is to ensure that medication errors and their sequelae are avoided. The efficient production of prescriptions must always be tempered with a healthy dose of professional judgment.

Pharmacy is not simply a production job where the same product has to be provided in the same fashion to every customer. The command intent of any pharmacy will involve providing high-quality patient care. Pharmacy is a customer service-driven profession that requires tailored approaches to each individual. A pharmacist needs to be able to apply their years of advanced training and knowledge to ensure that the right patient receives the right dose, of the right medication, at the right time, and in the right way.

Principles of Human Sigma

As mentioned earlier, it would not be difficult to argue that the most important aspect of managing a pharmacy is managing the people who work there. The employees are the ones who provide the myriad of goods and services to patients and customers. Many service-oriented industries have tried to apply quality control principles that were designed for production line models. Perhaps the most famous of these models is the Six Sigma program originated by the Motorola Corporation. Six Sigma assumes that output quality improves by eliminating defects in the production of the product (Pyzdek, 2003). The primary approach to performance improvement is based on the model known as DMAIC (Gygi et al., 2005):

1. *D*efine
2. *M*easure
3. *A*nalyze
4. *I*mprove
5. *C*ontrol

The intent of the Six Sigma approach is to create high quality, identical outputs from standardized inputs. Many hospitals and health care systems use the Six Sigma approach to improve the quality of patient care. However, recent evidence suggests that this type of quality improvement process breaks down in a customer service enterprise. Unlike a production line, consumers of services desire and need different outputs, and those desires and needs are framed by the circumstances of that specific encounter. For example, no two patient encounters are identical, even if they are getting the same medication for the same condition.

The Gallup organization recognized this potential inability of Six Sigma to address a customer service environment effectively, and consequently spent a great deal of time and energy researching customer service encounters. The insights gathered from their research led to the development of the Human Sigma project.

The Human Sigma is based on the following fundamental principles (Fleming and Asplund, 2007):

1. "E pluribus unum"—Employee and customer experiences should be measured and managed under the same department. The employee–customer experience is directly linked, and to manage them separately would be inefficient.
2. "Feelings are facts"—Gallup's research has found that the customers that contribute the most loyalty, and therefore the most business, to a company are the ones that feel an emotional connection with it. Customers that passionately advocate for the company through word-of-mouth advertising are the backbone of any successful business. Employees should be managed to develop this kind of deep relationship with customers, and performance metrics should be oriented toward measuring these emotional connections.
3. "Think globally, measure and act locally"—In an environment where there are multiple locations run by the same management, it would be easy to assume that all locations will achieve the same results. This assumption could not be farther from the truth. Even if all locations have the same process strategies, policies, regulations, and expectations, there will still be a significant variance between their

outputs. This is primarily due to differences in the "who" factor. Who is managing the location that is not performing? Who is working there as the face of the brand to the public? Engaging these people and giving them the command intent that they need will improve local performance.

4. "There is one number you need to know"—Gallup's vast quantity of data surrounding their Human Sigma project suggests that there is one performance metric that strongly predicts the success and future organic growth of a company. It is known as the Human Sigma metric, and it involves the levels of customer and employee engagement. The evidence has shown that when combined together, high levels of customer and employee engagement achieve synergy. The sum of the two is greater than the parts. Just having high levels one or the other will provide a degree of success, but balance between the two should be striven for.
5. "If you pray for potatoes, you better grab the right hoe"—Managers should gather the correct data in order to efficiently evaluate their company's performance and set goals. Improvement strategies should be custom tailored to each department's (or individual's) level of engagement. Finally, rewards and recognition should be designed to promote an increased sense of pride in employees' responsibilities and encourage improvement.

The Human Sigma data helps explain why scripting employee and customer relations does not work well and has the potential to backfire. Consider the following example of a production line Six Sigma management style mistake made at a pharmacy operation:

> John is a pharmacist at a large chain pharmacy. The company has a library of training resources that are provided to each new hire. Among these resources are scripted strategies to deal with a customer when a prescription error has been made. The scripts are designed to placate the customer and decrease the likelihood of losing them as a patron. A key script involves waiving the patient's co-payment and providing them with a gift card as compensation.
>
> Marie calls the pharmacy after noticing that her new prescription looks different from previous orders. John takes Marie's call, and after some research, discovers that Marie's prescription was filled for hydralazine 25 mg instead of hydroxyzine 25 mg. John follows the steps outlined in his training manual, explaining the mistake and letting Marie know that he would call her doctor. John then follows his corporate script and offers to refund her co-pay and give her a gift card.
>
> However, Marie does not respond the way the corporate script outlines and anticipates. She becomes offended by the suggestion that her problem can be bought off with a gift card. She didn't want money, she just wanted for someone to fix the mistake and deliver it to her home. The mechanical use of the script made her feel like the company was trying to buy her off. She was insulted and transferred all of her prescriptions to another pharmacy.

This connects back to the earlier discussion of command intent in pharmacy management. It is important that pharmacy operations managers emphasize the desired outcome and not try to micromanage every aspect of pharmacy associates' jobs, especially the encounters they have with customers. Fleming and Asplund (2007) mention that inefficiencies can be learned by employees when too much of their ability to engage customers is taken away:

> Once an employee becomes accustomed to ignoring customer comments or behaviors because they don't conform to the steps in the script the employee is required to follow in a given situation, employees will be primed to ignore customers in all situations. [p. 178]

If John had been given more freedom, he could have found out what Marie preferred and made the effort to fix the mistake for her in a more engaging manner. Even though an error had been committed and Marie was displeased, John had an opportunity to take care of her and through the outcome, instill a sense of deeper connection between Marie and the pharmacy. When training associates on customer service, operations managers should emphasize flexibility and the outcome desired, and then let the employee with the most intimate knowledge of the situation develop the best approach to achieve the desired outcome.

The Human Sigma data suggests that to form long-lasting relationships with customers and make them value a company above its competitors, the company must go beyond simply trying to achieve customer satisfaction. Companies must try to engage their customers on a deeper level. Engaging customers on an emotional level is what will gain their trust and loyalty.

How could a pharmacy operations manager engage his or her pharmacy's customers at a deeper, emotional level? Operations managers should start by recognizing that most customer engagement occurs at the level of their frontline employees, those that directly interact with customers. Employees that are also engaged directly with a company will want the company to succeed, and will more actively pursue tactics and directives to achieve mutual success. In addition, they will have a more thorough understanding of a company's short- and long-term goals.

The quality of the local operations manager is a critical ingredient in creating a highly productive workplace. Managers who consistently keep their employees engaged produce superior results for their organization. The Human Sigma project defined four key dimensions of employee engagement (Fleming and Asplund, 2007):

1. What do I get?
   a. Do I know what is expected of me at work?
   b. What materials and equipment do I get to use?
2. What do I give?
   a. Do I get to do what I do best every day?
   b. Have I received any recognition in the last week?
   c. Does my supervisor care about me?
   d. Do they encourage me to develop my skills?
3. Do I belong?
   a. Do my opinions matter?
   b. Do I agree with the mission or purpose of the company?
   c. Are my coworkers committed to quality?
   d. Does my best friend work with me?
4. How can we grow?
   a. Has my career progressed in the last 6 months?
   b. Do I have opportunities to learn and grow?

As a manager, what you do and how you act is more important than what you say. If a manager tells employees what he or she are going to do for them, but then they never get around to doing it, they have unintentionally communicated to their employees that they are not important. If a manager threatens to discipline an employee who is always late, but the manager never gets around to it, the manager has unintentionally communicated that he or she do not really care if employees are always late. If a manager criticizes employees when they do something wrong, but does not praise them when they do something right, the manager has unintentionally communicated that giving extra effort is not important. However, if a manager treats everyone fairly, refuses to accept less than everyone's best effort, and delivers on his or her promises, the manager and their organization are much more likely to be successful.

REVISITING THE SCENARIO

As the prescriptions start to back up at the drop off station, Trey must recognize that the operational goals have suddenly shifted, and he must compose and deliver new command intent to his associates. Trey needs associate tasks with the goal, and determine which tasks should be delegated to Bill and Lisa. Bill and Lisa should both recognize the new directive, and Bill should reassume the spot where he has more expertise than Lisa. This will ensure that customers are taken care of in a timely fashion. It is important that Trey not try to manage how his technicians handle the situation. Once he gives the new tasks, Trey must trust Bill and Lisa to do what is necessary in the way that best suits their individual strengths and weaknesses. When they are given the freedom to make decisions and direct their own success, Trey's employees will develop a closer connection and sense of pride in their jobs. This is especially true if the appropriate recognition is provided for a job well done. An increase in the quality of customers' experiences and their engagement level with Smith's Drug is to be expected once Trey's employees become more concerned with the pharmacy's success.

■ CONCLUSIONS

The primary role of operations managers in a pharmacy environment is to manage the human resources and tasks derived from the pharmacy's goals to produce quality customer service. This transformation of human resources and physical goods into a custom solution for each individual patient is what distinguishes pharmacy from most "production worker" styles of business. Goals should be derived from the overarching vision of the pharmacy, and daily tasks are developed from these goals. Tasks should be clear, concise, and measurable. Operations managers must prioritize tasks for completion, realizing that not everything can simultaneously be accomplished and that circumstances may change the order in which tasks need to be approached. Operations managers should communicate clear and unambiguous command intent to employees and allow them appropriate flexibility to best accomplish these specific tasks. Finally, the operations manager should understand that inspiring engaged employees is the key to creating engaged and loyal customers.

The daily work of the operations manager is to:

1. Get it done right
2. In a timely fashion
3. Consistent with the values of the organization
4. In a way that creates long-term value for all the stakeholders in the business

■ QUESTIONS FOR FURTHER DISCUSSION

1. Write an imaginary mission statement that outlines the reasons that your pharmacy exists.
2. As the pharmacist manager, come up with a command intent statement to deliver to your staff in order to accomplish the following goal: Educate local prescribers on the various compounding services offered at the pharmacy.
3. Identify specific tasks that can be derived from the following operational goal: Increase the efficiency of the pharmacy's drive-through service.
4. Identify operational strategies that can be used to more deeply engage customers.
5. Identify operational strategies that can be used to more deeply engage employees.

REFERENCES

American Academy of Colleges of Pharmacy. Graduating Student Survey. 2010. All schools nationwide. http://www.aacp.org/resources/research/institutionalresearch/Pages/GraduatingStudentSurvey.aspx Page 3; accessed on June 2, 2011.

Drucker PF. 1973. *Management: Tasks, Responsibilities, Practices.* New York: Harper & Row.

Fleming JH, Asplund J. 2007. *Human Sigma: Managing the Employee – Customer Encounter.* New York: Gallup Press.

Gygi C, DeCarlo N, Williams B. 2005. *Six Sigma for Dummies.* Hoboken, NJ: Wiley Publishing, Inc.

Heizer J, Render B. 1999. *Operations Management*, 5th edn. Upper Saddle River, NJ: Prentice-Hall.

Pyzdek T. 2003. *The Six Sigma Handbook.* New York: McGraw-Hill.

Shattuck L. 2000. Communicating intent and imparting presence. *Military Review* 66–72.

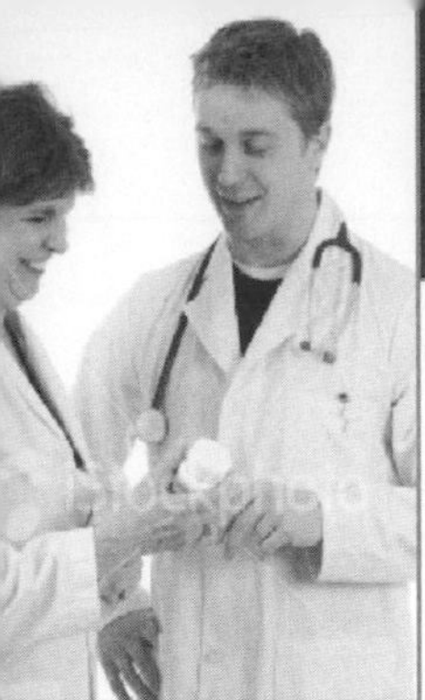

7

MANAGING MEDICATION USE PROCESS SUPPORTING TECHNOLOGIES AND AUTOMATION

Brent I. Fox and Mark H. Siska

About the Authors: Brent I. Fox is assistant professor of Pharmacy Care Systems at the Harrison School of Pharmacy at Auburn University. He received a Pharm.D. from Auburn and then worked in the software development industry prior to returning to Auburn, where he earned a PhD. Brent's education, outreach, and research efforts focus on improving medication use through health information technology.

Mark Siska is the Assistant Director of Informatics and Technology for Pharmacy Services at Mayo Clinic Rochester. Mark is the past chair of the American Society of Health System Pharmacists Section of Informatics and Technology and has served or continues to serve on a number Healthcare IT advisory committees and workgroups most recently the Pharmacy e-Health Collaborative. He received his Bachelor of Science in Pharmacy Degree from the University of Illinois, College of Pharmacy in 1980, completed his Hospital Pharmacy Resident training at Mayo Clinic Rochester in 1981 and completed his MBA in technology management in 2007.

■ LEARNING OBJECTIVES

After completing this chapter, readers should be able to

1. Describe key drivers for technology and automation in pharmacy practice.
2. List and describe the domains of the pharmacist's role in health information technology.
3. List the technologies involved at each step in the medication use process.
4. Describe the goal of closed-loop medication management systems.
5. List the elements of a request for proposal as it relates to vendor selection for procuring health information technology resources.
6. Describe four ways to manage change related to health information technology.
7. Describe the types of backup options for pharmacy information management systems.
8. List five questions to consider when planning a backup procedure for a pharmacy information management system.

9. Describe the role of best practices for pharmacy information management systems.
10. Describe the role and future implications of interoperability for pharmacy practice.

SCENARIO

Charlie Chodavarapu completed his Pharm.D. training several years ago and accepted a staff pharmacist position with a local community pharmacy. Charlie recently started spending some of his free time working at the local hospital. Charlie has been reminded of the distinct differences found between his primary practice in the community and his periodic practice experiences in the institutional setting. The most obvious difference is that his role at the hospital does not involve addressing insurance coverage issues. When he is in the hospital, Charlie distinctly misses the opportunity to directly interact with his patients as he does on a daily basis in the community. Despite these and many other differences, Charlie has been most surprised by the similarities found across the two practice settings.

The similarities that Charlie did not expect were found in the use of technology in both practice settings. Charlie's community practice is completely reliant upon information technology (IT) and automation to perform administrative, clinical, and distributive functions. Through his work in the hospital, Charlie has had the opportunity to look closely at the daily workflow of hospital pharmacists, opening his eyes to the fact that institutional pharmacy practice is equally reliant upon technology and automation to perform core practice responsibilities. Charlie's experiences in these two settings cause him to reflect on the relationship between the pharmacist, the patient, and technology and automation.

CHAPTER QUESTIONS

1. What is the pharmacist's role in health information technology management?
2. What are the primary health information technologies at each step of the medication use process?
3. How can health information technology positively impact pharmacy practice?
4. How can the pharmacist actively improve the medication use process through their use of health information technology?
5. What is the pharmacist's role in the technology vendor selection process?
6. How can pharmacy leaders minimize resistance to health information technology-related change?
7. How can pharmacists use downtime and backup policies and procedures to support patient care and administrative functions?
8. How can pharmacy leaders utilize best practices to positively impact health information technology use?
9. What does the future hold for pharmacists and their use of health information technology?

KEY DRIVERS FOR AUTOMATION AND TECHNOLOGY IN PHARMACY PRACTICE

The use of automation and information systems in pharmacy practice evolved in the early 1960s and 1980s, respectively. Limited resources, regulatory and legal requirements, customer satisfaction, the need to streamline operational costs, financial reimbursement, and point of sale prescription benefit adjudication were the predominate drivers for early adoption of technology and automation in pharmacy practice. Changes in the professional practice model, primarily the transition from traditional distributive and dispensing roles to patient-centered pharmaceutical care and medication therapy management (MTM) in the early

1990s, dramatically increased the demand for utilizing automation and technology to improve productivity as pharmacists continued to look to technology to free them up from legacy roles.

An Institute of Medicine (IOM) report significantly changed the medication management technology and automation landscape (Kohn, et al., 1999). Although operational efficiency remained an important driver for utilizing technology, the IOM report heightened the awareness, of technology's importance for enabling medication use process continuous quality improvement and safety. The report noted that medication errors represented 19 percent of adverse events in hospitals, accounting for more than 7,000 deaths annually. In the ambulatory environment, errors with potentially serious risk to patients were documented to occur on 1.5 to 4.0 percent of prescriptions (Bates et al., 1995). According to a 2005 Food and Drug Administration (FDA) report, medication errors result in at least one death per day and 1.3 million injuries per year in the United States (Figge, 2009). The report made it clear that to improve medication safety pharmacies must "implement proven medication safety practices" to reduce reliance on memory, standardize terminology, minimize data handoffs, and utilize constraints and forcing functions, protocols, and checklists. The report referenced several emerging technologies and systems that may be used to effectively reduce medical errors. It called for automation of patient-specific clinical information within the context of an electronic health record (EHR) and integrated with computerized prescriber order entry (CPOE) systems, drug distribution and medication administration systems. These systems ideally would work together within and across organizational boundaries, share real time patient specific clinical information, provide timely relevant clinical decision support at the point of care, and create data-mining capabilities (Kohnet al., 1999).

The American Recovery and Reinvestment Act (ARRA) of 2009 and the Health Information Technology for Economic and Clinical Health (HITECH) Act provided financial subsidies for those using health information technology (HIT) and required providers who wish to participate in Medicare to obtain HIT by a specified date or pay a penalty. To be eligible for these payments, hospitals and physicians are required to demonstrate *meaningful use* of HIT, exchange electronic health information to improve the quality of care, and report on key quality measures. The recommendations of the IOM reports to improve safety and quality and the federal government's financial commitment through the HITECH Act have become important drivers for advancing HIT in pharmacy practice (111th Congress, 2009).

ROLE OF THE PHARMACIST IN HEALTH INFORMATION TECHNOLOGY

Pharmacists are responsible for patient safety throughout the medication use process and should take a leadership role at all levels of health care to ensure that HIT supports safe medication use. This includes the following:

- Data, information, and knowledge management
- System selection, development, and design
- Implementation, maintenance, and optimization
- Education and research

Data, Information and Knowledge Management

Pharmacy practice is a data and information intensive discipline requiring the best evidence. Pharmacists must take a leadership role in assuring that medication data, information and knowledge management best practices (i.e., processes that lead to a desired result) are utilized across all supporting systems (Table 7-1). The most common approach for effectively managing medication content in the HIT environment is through the use of a commercial drug database vendor (e.g., First Databank, Multum, and Micromedex). Medication management supporting systems are able to leverage the content provided by these vendors to enable essential clinical decision support, including drug–drug interaction checking, drug disease alerts, duplicate therapy alerts, and dose range checking. Although the commercial drug database vendors' approach is

Table 7-1. Information and Knowledge Management Best Practices

- Adoption of standard formats, human and machine interpretable
- Readily and rapidly understood and accessed in the context of the workflow
- Centrally managed, collaboratively developed, and easily disseminated and maintained
- Platform independent
- Controlled terminology for interoperability
- Assign responsibility for different content areas to individuals with domain expertise
- Validation and audit trail maintenance
- Measurement and evaluation of content
- Tools to support data, information, and knowledge management

Data Quality Management Best Practices

- Accessibility—easily obtainable
- Accuracy—correct and valid values
- Comprehensiveness—all applicable data are included
- Consistency—the value of data are reliable
- Recency—the data are current
- Definition—clear definitions, following a standard vocabulary
- Granularity—attributes and values of data are defined at the correct level of detail for the application
- Precision—data values should be large enough to support the application
- Relevancy—data are meaningful to the performance of the process
- Timeliness—data are used in appropriate context

commonplace in the electronic environment, pharmacists should continue to evaluate their efficacy and consistency and identify shortcomings and opportunities for optimizing these systems in clinical practice.

System Development and Selection

When new medication management supporting technologies are being discussed and/or evaluated, the pharmacist should be a part of the request for proposal (RFP) process to ensure the technology supports safe medication use, but more importantly, is effectively aligned with the ideal HIT-enabled medication use process. The RFP process allows potential vendors to submit formal proposals detailing information about their company, the cost, and other requested information pertaining to the purchase, installation, and support of a medication management technology. The pharmacist should work closely with vendors, application programmers, and medication management system users to develop system requirements while understanding system capabilities and limitations. Pharmacists must translate clinician requirements into specifications for clinical information systems, identify and prioritize system enhancements, and design safe and effective medication workflows across the medication use continuum (American Society of Health-System Pharmacists, 2007).

Implementation, Maintenance and Aptimization

The pharmacist should lead or colead medication management supporting system deployments, maintenance, and optimization efforts. Leadership efforts begin with active involvement in creating the project charter, identifying the project vision and objectives along with scope, deliverables, organizational structure, roles and responsibilities, budget, and risks. The pharmacist should serve in a project leadership role across the entire project life cycle including project initiation, planning (analysis, design), execution (build, test, train, activate) and closure. They should take responsibility for expected system benefits, integrity of the process design, information and knowledge management, risk management, trouble shooting, and production maintenance. They must collaborate with stakeholders to assist with system analysis, identifying opportunities for optimization (American Society of Health-System Pharmacists, 2007).

Education and Quality Improvement

Pharmacists should assist with providing HIT educational road maps and competencies for colleges of pharmacy and pharmacy staff development programs. Core curriculum should center on the role of technology and automation in medication management, how it can improve medication safety and quality, and the inherent risks and negative aspects of implementing medication use technologies. Other sets of courses should focus on (American Society of Health-System Pharmacists, 2007):

- Best practices surrounding the storage, retrieval, and analysis of health information
- Key issues affecting human–computer interaction
- IT-enabled closed-loop medication management
- Principles for the development of decision support tools to solve patient related problems
- The structure and key elements of an EHR
- The impact of alerts on workflow and patient outcomes
- Project and change management principles and best practices for technology projects

Pharmacists have responsibility for performing quality improvement activities that involve the core issues of medication management supporting systems. Quality improvement efforts should include the use of controlled medication vocabularies, usability, interoperability (the ability to meaningfully exchange information in electronic format) and demonstrate value involving efficiency, safety, and quality (see Chapter 8). The pharmacist should assist in determining the balance of clinical informatics and health care system reengineering needed to optimize the medication use process and improve patient safety (American Society of Health-System Pharmacists, 2007).

Pharmacists must utilize their overarching knowledge of safe and effective use of medications and medication management systems. They are able to efficiently and effectively translate and communicate the language of medication use bidirectionally at transitions in care. They are able to decipher system requirements into sound medication ordering system designs, assuring effective electronic exchange of prescription and prescription related information. Their understanding of core pharmacy operations and skills to manage the business as well as clinical aspects of medications across the continuum of care make them an invaluable resource for system development and ongoing system maintenance (American Society of Health-System Pharmacists, 2007).

MEDICATION USE PROCESS-SUPPORTING TECHNOLOGIES

The medication use process as depicted in Fig. 7-1 consists of six domains: (1) selection and procurement, (2) storage, (3) ordering and transcribing, (4) preparation and dispensing, (5) administration, (6) patient monitoring and assessment. The processes within these domains are exceedingly complex, involving numerous handoffs and regulations in widely diverse health care arenas including pharmaceutical manufacturing, insurers, community pharmacies, long-term health care facilities, hospitals, and clinics. These processes also involve numerous stakeholders, including physicians, nurses, pharmacists, and other allied health care workers. They frequently require multiple methods of

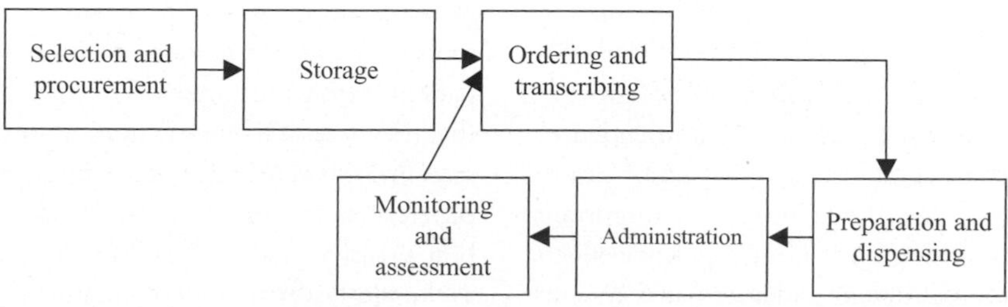

Figure 7-1. Medication use process.

Table 7-2. Medication Use Process Errors

Medication Use Step and Common Type of Error	Distribution of Errors by Step	Errors Intercepted
Prescribing	39%	48%
• Wrong dose		
• Wrong choice		
• Known allergy		
Transcribing	12%	33%
• Wrong dose		
• Wrong frequency		
• Missed dose		
Dispensing	11%	34%
• Wrong dose		
• Wrong drug		
• Wrong time		
Administering	38%	2%
• Wrong dose		
• Wrong choice		
• Wrong drug		

Adapted with permission from: Bates et al., 1995; Leape et al., 1995.

Table 7-3. Medication Use Process Technology and Automation Strategies

Prescribing
- Computerized prescriber order entry systems
- Clinical decision support systems

Transcribing
- Order management systems
- Pharmacy information management systems

Preparation and Dispensing
- Solid dosage form robotics
- Workflow management systems
- Inventory management systems
- Automated dispensing devices
- Tablet counters
- Bar code packagers
- Sterile compounding robotics

Administration
- Electronic medication administration records
- Bar code medication administration systems
- Smart pumps

Adapted with permission from: California Healthcare Foundation, 2001.

communication, documentation, and manual as well as automated sources of data with the goal of providing safe and effective MTM (California HealthCare Foundation, 2001).

Leape et al. (1995) outlined where errors are most likely to occur and their corresponding rates for being detected prior to reaching the patient (Table 7-2). Pharmacists should use this research as a roadmap for developing medication management technology strategic plans. Table 7-3 provides a list of automation and technology solutions that address common causes of medication errors within the medication use process. Although this list is not exhaustive, it is intended to present those technologies recently adopted by health care organizations across the country. It is important for pharmacists to understand both the positive effects and limitations for technology and automated systems and the variability in their actualized benefits from one organization to the next.

The core medication use process supporting technologies include:

- CPOE and clinical decision support systems
- Pharmacy information management systems
- Preparation and dispensing systems
- Medication administration systems

CPOE is an integrated application allowing clinicians to create orders with the benefit of decision support tools that provide guidance within the context of a patient's electronic medical record (EMR) ensuring that they receive the most appropriate medication therapy. The software incorporates a variety of tools to help physicians, including alerts, checks, reminders, and best practice guidelines. CPOE is generally regarded as the most difficult to implement and the most costly;

however, it is considered one of the most important HIT investments an organization can make to improve safety and quality (California HealthCare Foundation, 2001).

An e-prescribing or ambulatory CPOE system provides a standardized, secure, and safe vehicle for transporting and sharing information across the health system and community pharmacy environment. E-prescribing allows for the transmission of prescription or prescription-related information between prescriber, pharmacies, and pharmacy health plans. By adopting a nationally established electronic messaging standard (NCPDP SCRIPT) and a third-party pharmacy health information exchange network (e.g., Superscripts), e-prescribing allows medication use process stakeholders to access secure, low-cost electronic prescription fill and history information from payers and pharmacies across the country. This connection offers the needed technical framework to improve medication communication failures at interfaces and transitions in care, and assists providers in making more informed MTM related decisions. Conversely, community pharmacy practices will have the potential to receive pertinent medication related information from health systems including laboratory data, allergy, and diagnosis information. This information allows pharmacists to more effectively manage medicines and unlocks the door to developing convergent pharmacy practice models (Siska, 2011). Features of CPOE and e-prescribing systems that contribute to safety and quality include:

- Legibility
- Structure menu driven orders
- Real-time patient information at the point of care
- Embedded drug information including dose checking, drug–drug interaction checking and allergy alerts

Pharmacy information management systems (PIMS) have been in place for more than two decades and are often considered the backbone of medication use process technologies. These systems can function as independent ordering systems requiring transcription, or they ideally can be tightly integrated with CPOE systems to reduce the potential for errors in verification and transcription. These systems effectively control access to medications prior to administration, and through their integration with medication documentation systems, they direct the creation of the electronic medication administration record (eMAR). PIMS can also be used to assist in managing inventory, point of sale, and prescription benefit reimbursement (Siska, 2006). Features of PIMS that contribute to safety and quality include the following:

- Verification of prescribed orders
- Structured ordering
- Online drug information support (dose checking, drug interactions, allergy alerts)

Preparation and dispensing automation is widely utilized in both the hospital and community pharmacy environments. The goals for use of automation include improving patient care, customer service, and resource utilization. Technologies include the following:

- Drug purchasing and supply chain management systems
- Automated drug distribution systems
    - Automated dispensing cabinets
    - Robotic cart filling systems
    - Automated medication storage systems
- Preparation systems
    - Sterile compounding devices
    - Unit dose and bar code packaging systems
    - Medication counting and labeling devices

The key benefits of pharmacy automation in the dispensing and preparation processes go well beyond safety. The advent of computer-controlled equipment to automate processes that were traditionally performed by pharmacists has allowed technicians to play a more active role in medication dispensing. This allows pharmacy administrators to maximize their resources and move pharmacists into patient care roles.

This redesigned practice model will enable hospitals and community pharmacies to utilize the pharmacist's expertise in drug therapy management and the provision of patient centered pharmaceutical care.

Point-of-care medication administration systems sustained by data produced from upstream-integrated CPOE and pharmacy systems provides important medication information at the bedside and allows nurses to electronically document medications administered. Bar code medication administration (BCMA) technologies combine a number of hardware and software components to perform important safety checks within a process that is highly vulnerable to error. BCMA systems perform a number of safety checks that include the five rights: right patient, right medication, right dose, right time, and right route. Before administering a medication to a patient, the nurse scans a bar code on their identification badge, a second bar-code on the medication package, and a third bar-code on the patient's wrist band. These three scans allow the nurse to verify that the medication they are about to administer is intended for that patient. Nurses are alerted of any discrepancies via a visual or audible alert that requires acknowledgement prior to administration (California HealthCare Foundation, 2001).

Electronic medication administration records manage data throughout an organization and provide valuable, accurate, real time medication information for all health care providers. The eMAR is a multidisciplinary application that provides an important solution for medication documentation, therapeutic assessment and treatment, monitoring, and quality and compliance measurements. Of all the electronic tools currently used in the medication use process, the eMAR is most likely to be utilized by virtually every member of the health care team. Pharmacists should ensure an eMAR is integrated clearly and concisely with the organization's primary order entry and pharmacy systems including any automated dispensing cabinets (ADCs), point-of-care BCMA systems, infusion pumps, or other divergent medication documentation applications. The eMAR also must have the capability of integrating with the organizations billing and financial services systems as linking administered medication records can improve compliance with billing regulations (Siska, 2005).

Medication infusion devices play an important role in delivering medication infusions to patients in both inpatient and outpatient settings. Intravenously (IV) administered medications pose the greatest risk to patients and often result in medication related events causing harm. Smart infusion devices provide precise delivery of medication, and when configured with clinical decision support guidelines, they have the potential to prevent severe or even fatal medication errors. The pump can be programmed with user-defined soft and hard lower and upper limits for each medication visible to the clinician before final confirmation is requested. These hard and soft limits are at the heart of the pump's ability to avert fatalities.

■ CLOSED-LOOP MEDICATION MANAGEMENT

A closed-loop medication management system (Fig. 7-2) is developed to feed outcomes from medication processes back into the system to enable the deployment and development of improved practices and effectively monitor patient care across the continuum. Through the automation of all medication-related processes, closed-loop medication management reduces many steps in the complex process, significantly reducing the number of opportunities for error (Kilbridge and Classen, 2002). The transition between each step in the process is seamless, information is exchanged and used by all systems involved and it remains intact as it is handed off from one application to the next. Closed-loop medication management technologies help prevent medication errors by organizing information and making it easily available, it links discrete pieces of information, and performs repetitive tasks including monitoring for problems. The closed-loop system includes technologies that enable clinicians to make the most appropriate decisions about patient care at each step of the process. Ideally, a closed-loop system would have a succession of systems that are all interconnected

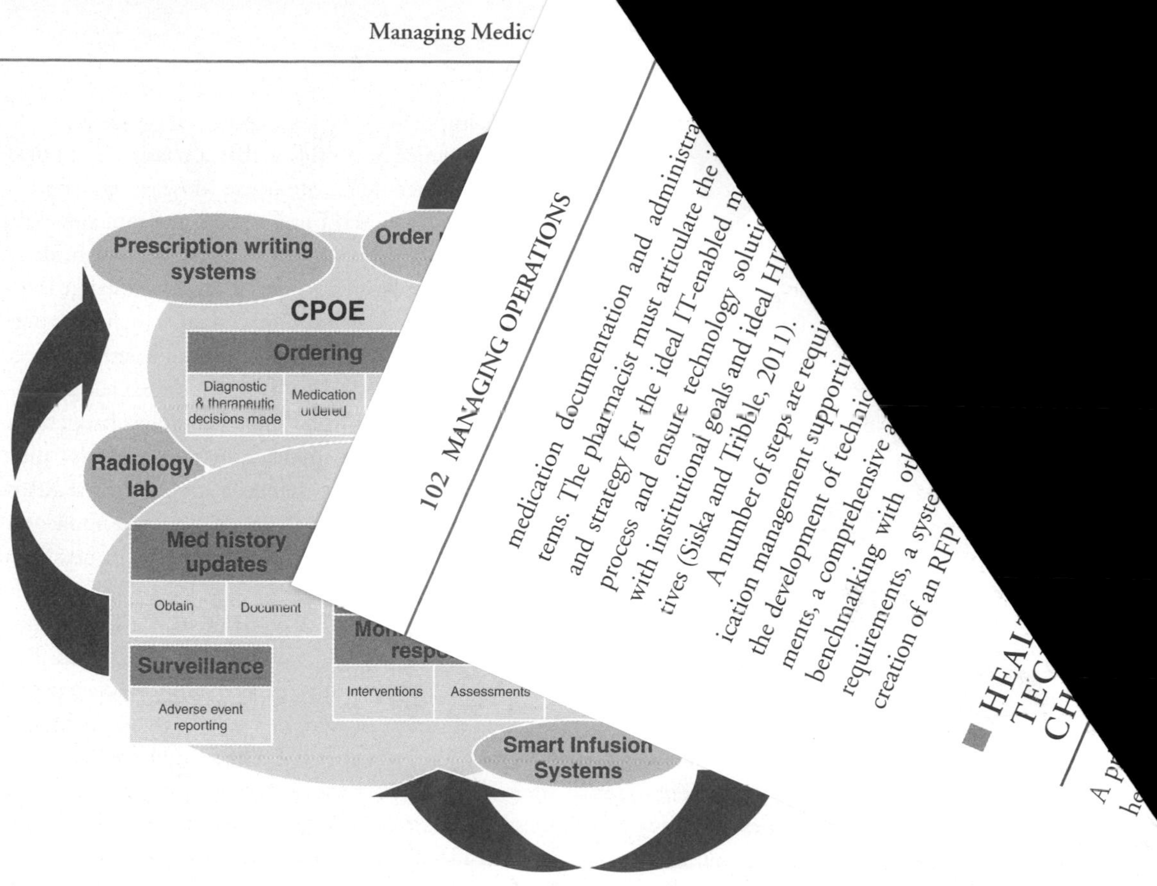

Figure 7-2. Closed-loop medication management. (Adapted with permission from: Kilbridge and Classen,

and can share data fully in real time. Such an automated infrastructure should minimally consist of:

- An electronic patient health record
- A provider order entry process
- Clinical decision support systems that evaluate not only orders as they are entered, but also evaluates all orders as changes in patient condition may demand.
- A preparation and distribution automation infrastructure that uses automatic identification and other information technologies to verify that medications selected and/or prepared in response to specific orders were appropriately selected and/or prepared.
- Computer-based bedside verification of medications at administration that is tolerant to the variety of products and dose forms that might be used to deliver a medication dose (ASHP Section of Pharmacy Informatics and Technology Executive Committee, 2009).

PHARMACISTS AND TECHNOLOGY VENDOR SELECTION

In the era of system integration and its known complexities, the vendor selection process for medication management related technologies and automation has moved beyond sole individuals or departments to multidisciplinary selection teams of pharmacists, IT experts, nurses, and physicians. However, because of their expertise and knowledge of best medication management practices, the pharmacist is responsible for ensuring that proper selection takes place. Pharmacists are the most qualified to perform a proper assessment of the potential clinical, operational, and safety features and functionalities available in a system. Pharmacists must participate in the vendor selection processes for all medication management-related systems including ordering and prescribing as well as

tion sys-
deal vision
edication use
ons are aligned
T strategic objec-

ed in selecting a med-
g technology including
al and functional require-
nalysis of potential vendors,
her organizations, contractual
n readiness assessment, and the
(Bucki, 2011).

TH INFORMATION HNOLOGY-RELATED ANGE MANAGEMENT

imary driver of HIT use in pharmacy and other alth-related disciplines is to improve patient care and, most importantly, patient outcomes from the care they receive. HIT supports clinician decision-making, workflow, and medication management. However, HIT is similar to the consumer electronics market in that change is constant. In both fields, innovation occurs at a rapid rate, although for different reasons. Due to this rapid rate of change, pharmacists and pharmacy staff members can expect to experience considerable—almost constant—change in the IT they use in their daily operations.

There are unavoidable challenges from staying current with technology, including the often expensive cost of replacing outdated technology or upgrading to completely new technology. Technical challenges also exist when moving to a new technology and frequently present as difficulties getting disparate technologies to "speak" to each other. This type of challenge is often beyond the skill set of most pharmacists and requires the expertise of a technology vendor and/or specially trained personnel; thus, it is not a focus of this chapter. A decidedly different challenge is the personnel aspect; that is, how to help people deal with technological change.

A simplistic way to view the difference between clinical practice and HIT is that a change in clinical practice impacts medication use (dose, etc.), whereas implementation of HIT impacts the way someone does their job. New technology can actually change the daily workflow of a pharmacist, and it can even change their responsibilities. This type of change can have a significant impact on job satisfaction and performance. Adding potentially more difficulty to the change process is that decisions regarding technology changes can often occur without input from the person(s) ultimately impacted by the change. For example, ARRA is having and will continue to have substantial impact on the implementation of new technologies in hospitals and community pharmacies.

From a management perspective, the significance of HIT-related change should not be overlooked. Resistance to change is to be expected, but managers can draw on a variety of resources to help manage change. The research and experiences of many have produced several consistent themes in managing change, and these themes can be applied to managing change related to IT:

1. Leadership is critical to navigating any type of change. Leaders should be effective communicators that establish the need and a vision for change, convene a group to lead the change, and empower others to implement change. Leaders should identify anticipated tangible improvements due to change and should acknowledge those involved in the improvements. The connection between changes experienced and achievement of organization goals should be articulated by leadership (Kotter, 1995).
2. End-users should be involved in technology design and implementation decisions, since they know what best fits their workflow.
3. Training is critical to acceptance of new technology. Training should be available in a variety of formats (in-person, written materials, video tutorials, etc.) and should be available throughout the day. Training should be tailored to the specific needs of the trainee and conducted in a nonthreatening environment.

4. Theories of change demonstrate that users' acceptance of new technologies is strongly influenced by their perceptions of usefulness of the technology. Accordingly, users are more likely to adopt technologies that prove useful in their jobs (Davis et al., 1989; Venkatesh et al., 2003; Kijsanayotin et al., 2009).
5. Resistance to change is inevitable, should be expected, and can be overt and covert. Resistance is due to a sense of loss of control. Change that is more appealing leads to less resistance (Luo, 2006).

Pharmacists faced with leading technology adoption should consider the importance of their role as leader, the importance of staff involvement, and the use of training as an opportunity to demonstrate the positive impact of change. In reality, technological change will likely bring about both positive and negative implications. Social influences within the pharmacy may also provide positive (and negative) support for acceptance.

Health Information Technology Essentials: Downtime and Backup

In August 2005, Hurricane Katrina devastated the Louisiana and Mississippi gulf coasts. Images of flooded homes in New Orleans and cement foundations where homes once stood on the Mississippi coast are vivid reminders of the power of the storm. Unfortunately, natural disasters do not intentionally bypass health care facilities, as evidenced by reports from the aftermath of Katrina. Hospitals in New Orleans were flooded. Pharmacies in coastal Mississippi were washed away. Most hospitals relied on paper-based medical records, and although pharmacies in hospitals and the community rely on electronic patient records, records stored on computers submerged under water were not retrievable.

Hurricane Katrina provides a picture of the worst-case scenario regarding pharmacy downtime and the loss of patient records. Fortunately, the devastation from such a storm does not occur very often. However, pharmacies are faced with the potential for downtime (a temporary outage of computing systems) and data loss (the permanent inability to access data) due to failed computing equipment, theft, fire, floods due to faulty plumbing, power surges, and a variety of other causes. Scheduled maintenance is another cause of downtime.

Scheduled downtime is most often seen in hospital pharmacies as community pharmacy downtime occurs when the pharmacy is closed or not busy. Unscheduled downtime occurs in both settings and is more likely to negatively impact pharmacy operations. To minimize the impact of either type of downtime, pharmacies should have a downtime policy in place that clearly defines how the pharmacy will transition to a manual process. Key concepts related to downtime planning and recovery are addressed below.

Downtime planning should focus on ensuring uninterrupted pharmacy services in both planned and unplanned outages. A downtime *policy* designates who to call in the event of an outage. That person then determines what aspects of the downtime policy to enact. In general, downtime policies should clearly describe who is responsible for pharmacy operations, such as maintaining patient records, overseeing existing medication orders, handling new orders—including clinical review, label preparation, communicating with other providers and patients, and any differences in responsibilities across shifts. Downtime *procedures* describe the progressive steps that are to be followed to comply with the downtime policy, including recovery. Recovery is a challenging, critical step that can lead to additional confusion due to uncertainty about the process and timing for reverting back to the original, electronic system. Therefore it is important that downtime policies and procedures include the recovery phase (Miller, 2009; Lockwood, 2010). A sample downtime policy can be found at http://www.hosp.uky.edu/pharmacy/departpolicy/PH18–04.pdf (accessed June 15, 2011).

One of the most effective methods to minimize the impact of unplanned downtime is to have a backup procedure in place that routinely copies pharmacy files to another location. There are several approaches to backups. The local backup occurs when personnel within the pharmacy make a copy of their data on physical media that remains on site. Several years ago, this was the customary practice for backing up pharmacy records. After a predetermined period of time, the media was cycled through to overwrite a previous backup. As an example, a backup policy could call for having the last 6 days worth of data available on external media.

Today's advancements in networking and storage provide additional options for performing backups. Two primary backup procedures today are: (1) off-site backup with data stored internally, and (2) data stored and backed up externally. In the first backup method, the PIMS vendor remotely connects to the pharmacy system and transfers data to an external location. This method provides a second backup location in case a backup made and stored locally in the pharmacy is not available. The second backup method is actually a result of a pharmacy's use of software as a service (SaaS), an approach to computing in which a technology vendor (PIMS, in this case) uses a secure network connection to provide software and manage associated data. The advantage of SaaS is that the pharmacy bears little responsibility for computing hardware and software because it is maintained by the vendor. From a backup perspective, data are already stored external to the pharmacy.

Considering that there are several backup methods, what are the desirable features? The primary goal of backing up is to safely and securely store critical data in an easily retrievable manner. At a minimum, backup processes should safely store patient data, including demographic data, allergy lists, medication histories, and insurance information (in the community) in compliance with Health Insurance Portability and Accountability Act (HIPAA) regulations. Other features that managers should consider include the following:

1. How frequently do backups occur? Does pharmacy management have input into the frequency of backups?
2. How are patient data secured? Data should be encrypted for transmission to and storage at the backup location.
3. To where are data backed up? Off-site backups should store data on robust media in multiple locations that are protected from fire, water, and temperature damage. Data centers should have redundant power supplies and 24/7 security. Backups that occur within the pharmacy using physical media should also be stored in locations protected from fire, weather, and temperature damage.
4. How quickly can a backed-up date be accessed in the event of an outage?
5. Does the backup process include application and/or operating system software, in addition to patient data?
6. Are automated notifications available to inform key personnel when backups occur, or more importantly, when scheduled backups do not occur?
7. Can incremental backups be performed to capture changes since the most recent backup?
8. For SaaS models, how reliable are network connections between the pharmacy and vendor for both backups and day-to-day operations?
9. For multisite pharmacies that share data, are data backed up such that a failure of the central server does not prevent access to backed-up data by one or more pharmacies?
10. In the case of a catastrophic event at the pharmacy or hospital, is remote access to backed-up data available from other sites?

Downtime and backup procedures are likely not considered to be the most critical aspects of pharmacy operations. However, recent weather events clearly demonstrate the need for diligent downtime planning (iHealthBeat, 2011). Once a planned or unplanned downtime event is over, restoration of pharmacy data from backups becomes critical to resumption of activities.

■ BEST PRACTICES

Although infrequent, the impact of downtime or the loss of data due to the absence of a backup storage method can have far reaching consequences on a pharmacy. The questions above address proven ways (i.e., best practices) to minimize the impact of downtime and perform secure backups. Best practices often are developed through a combination of research and real-world experience. In the domain of HIT, best practices define ways to use HIT to improve the quality of care as well as to enhance business functions. An important characteristic of best practices is that they are not legislated or regulated. Instead, best practices are benchmarks for self-assessment to attain a desired outcome, focusing on quality.

Best practices in HIT often focus on workflow, system design, and usage. For example, in hospital settings, medication reconciliation remains a challenge and is the subject of a consensus statement that calls for best practice research and dissemination (Greenwald et al., 2010). Siska and Tribble (2011) called for best practices to guide clinical decision support within clinical information systems. They also identified a need for best practices to guide deployment of clinical information systems within hospitals. ADCs are frequently encountered in hospitals and are intended to increase the efficiency and safety of medication distribution. Due to the importance of ADCs in the medication use process, the Institute for Safe Medication Practices (ISMP) published guidelines on ADC use, specifically focusing on safety (2008).

In community pharmacies, eleven best practices have been suggested for e-prescriptions (Rupp and Warholak, 2010). These best practices—that apply to both pharmacies and prescribers—focus primarily on workflow and include:

1. Physicians should enter electronic prescriptions or closely review prescriptions entered by other providers.
2. Decision support software should be enabled for prescribers.
3. The receipt of an electronic prescription in the pharmacy should trigger an obvious notification in the PIMS.
4. Pharmacy procedures should eliminate the process of printing and then reentering prescriptions into the PIMS.
5. Electronic prescribing systems should allow pharmacists to request additional information from prescribers and for prescribers to respond to these requests.

This sample of e-prescribing best practices includes steps that likely logical and reasonable for anyone who has worked in a community pharmacy. While these best practices do focus on workflow, the underlying goal is to improve patient care. For example, enabling decision support is a workflow change for prescribers. The intent of this change in workflow, however, is to assist physicians in making more informed prescribing decisions, resulting in medication use that is safer and more efficacious.

Best practices can be found for various aspects of HIT use in pharmacy practice. However, due to the wide range of HIT use and the variety of pharmacy practice environments, there is no single source for best practices. Accordingly, pharmacy managers who are tasked with implementing best practices within their pharmacy (hospital or community) have several potential sources to consider. In general, these sources include internal documents, published literature, HIT vendors, professional associations, patient safety groups, accrediting bodies, foundations, and other groups. Table 7-4 includes suggested resources for best practices.

THE FUTURE: PHARMACY PERSPECTIVES ON NATIONAL INITIATIVES FOR INTEROPERABILITY

Interoperability

Not too many years ago, PIMS operated in silos both in hospitals and in the community. In today's health care environment, significant emphasis is being placed on the ability of disparate computer systems to exchange data in a manner that allows the data to be used in a meaningful way (Brailer, 2005). This type of exchange is known as *interoperability.* Pharmacists are responsible for ensuring safe and effective medication therapy. Prescription drug utilization continues to grow in the United States and is an important component of the overall health care system (Kaiser Family Foundation, 2010). Due to the importance and widespread use of medications in patient care and the responsibility of pharmacists to manage medication therapy,

Table 7-4. Sample Best Practices Resources for Pharmacy Managers

Resource	Web URL
American Pharmacists Association	www.pharmacist.com
American Society of Health-System Pharmacists	www.ashp.org
Leapfrog Group	www.leapfroggroup.org
Markle Foundation	www.markle.org/health
National Governor's Association Center for Best Practices	www.nga.org
The Joint Commission	www.jointcommission.org
The Office of the National Coordinator for Health Information Technology	www.healthit.hhs.gov

pharmacists should be aware of and involved with interoperability efforts related to medication management.

The inability to use clinical and administrative information—including information related to medication use—that has been generated or is stored in another location leads to a variety of problems. These problems take the form of unnecessary repeat procedures, errors and delays in care, and providers making less than optimal decisions because they do not know the full story. There are obvious financial implications from repeating procedures or tests that were previously performed. One report projects an annual savings of over $77 billion due to interoperability between providers and laboratories, radiology centers, pharmacies, payers, public health departments, and other providers. This interoperability avoids repeat procedures or tests, the associated administrative work for such activities, and errors due to oral reporting of results (Walker et al., 2005). There are also costs to patients who undergo an unnecessary repeat procedure or test. In addition, it is difficult to measure the financial impact of delays in care. We do know, however, that a lack of access to pertinent information does hamper clinical decision making (Leape et al., 1995).

With over 60,000 community pharmacies, 500,000 practicing physicians, 5,000 hospitals, and 16,000 nursing facilities, there are, unfortunately, an abundance of opportunities for patient-related information to be created in one location but not be available in another location (Brailer, 2005; National Association of Chain Drugs Stores, 2010; National Community Pharmacists Association, 2009). The practice of pharmacy provides a great example. A patient can have their prescription filled at Pharmacy A. If they then go to Pharmacy B, the pharmacists at Pharmacy B will not know about any medications filled at Pharmacy A unless the patient tells them. If this patient is then admitted to the hospital, there is a strong likelihood that their complete medication list will not follow them into the hospital. Consider the number of physician offices, hospitals, and hospital pharmacies, and the magnitude of the problem can be appreciated. Polypharmacy and drug interactions are two obvious outcomes of not sharing medication-related information across pharmacies. Due to the financial and humanistic significance of this problem, the federal government has devoted substantial resources to the creation of a nationwide interoperable health information network. The goal of this network is to allow patients' medical records to follow them wherever they receive care.

E-Prescribing and Electronic Patient Records

Interoperability efforts took a major step forward with nationwide implementation of e-prescribing. The ability of Surescripts and other networks to connect prescribers, payers, and pharmacies to electronically exchange prescription-related information addresses safety and efficiency issues on both the prescribing and dispensing ends of the process. Within pharmacies, e-prescribing primarily impacts pharmacy workflow by creating a new method for prescription receipt and entry into the PIMS, and by providing a new method for requesting prescription refills. These are important areas of training for pharmacy staff. Patients should be informed that the use of e-prescriptions does not necessarily decrease the time to fill their prescription. A variety of unrelated factors impact filling time, and pharmacists should be careful to educate their patients to temper expectations. An important consideration for any independent community pharmacy manager is that the pharmacy is responsible for a transaction routing fee for each e-prescription. This fee varies across e-prescribing prescribing networks, but it is usually less than 40 cents.

EMRs are software applications that are owned by a care delivery organization (e.g., hospital) or by a provider (e.g., physician) and serve to house the electronic history of the care that patients receive in that location. EHRs are also repositories for patient care information, but EHRs pull a patient's information from multiple EMRs to create a comprehensive record of all their care. Federal interoperability efforts focus on EMR design and functionality for physician offices and hospitals to ensure that information exchange can occur across EMRs to create EHRs for US citizens. If achieved, EHRs will provide a complete medical history for a patient. A key term in the EMR/EHR domain is "meaningful use," which signifies that hospitals and providers must be able to demonstrate that their use of EMRs meets specific functional and technical benchmarks. Hospitals and providers who are able to demonstrate achievement of meaningful use will be eligible for financial incentives to support the adoption of this new technology. A sample functional benchmark is that a minimum percentage of orders in the hospital setting must be entered using CPOE.

Medications are an important part of patient records and are addressed in current federal EMR, and EMR development efforts that include standards for medication and allergy information access, e-prescribing, formulary and benefits checking, and other transactions related to medication prescribing and dispensing (Hansonet al., 2012). Current federal efforts are largely focused on physicians and hospitals, not recognizing other health care professionals who play a significant role in the patient centered multidisciplinary model of care. Recognizing this deficiency, nine pharmacy organizations formed the Pharmacy e-Health Information Technology (e-HIT) Collaborative in 2010. The purpose of the collaborative is to ensure the inclusion of pharmacist's patient care services (community and institutional) in national EHR efforts. The Collaborative developed a roadmap that defines pharmacy's priorities for HIT.

The roadmap lays out a vision for HIT as it relates to pharmacy in the coming years. The roadmap includes specific pharmacy services and activities that should be included in meaningful use criteria for EMRs and EHRs, with the goal of pharmacists being recognized as providers eligible for meaningful use incentives in the near future. The second goal of the roadmap is the development of the Pharmacist/Pharmacy Provider her (PP-EHR), which is a functional profile for an EHR where pharmacists document their activities. For example, pharmacists are increasingly providing immunization services in community pharmacy settings. The pharmacist meaningful use criteria for EHRs, according to the roadmap, should include documentation and bidirectional exchange of data related to immunizations administered by pharmacists. This information exchange should occur between pharmacists' and other health care providers as well as public health agencies. Pharmacists' provision of MTM services in a variety of practice settings represents another example. The roadmap specifies that adoption of the PP-EHR will ensure (1) the inclusion of MTM in pharmacists' workflow, (2) that pharmacists have access to the EHR, and (3) that pharmacists' MTM documentation is exchanged with other providers, patients, and payers (Mackowiak, 2011).

These two examples highlight the potential for exciting change on the horizon. The examples also reflect the importance of pharmacists' independent clinical activities to patient care. Documentation of these activities should be incorporated in patients' EHRs, informing other providers. Similarly, pharmacists need access to EHRs to have a complete picture of their patients to enhance decision making. These changes will bring new practice roles for pharmacists. Pharmacists' documentation will become widely visible, increasing awareness of pharmacists' contribution to patient care. Challenges will exist. Professional and pharmacy business models will require significant reengineering to change the MTM delivery process. Community pharmacists could benefit from something as simple as a diagnosis, but the opportunity to review a patient's medical history can inform the pharmacist's activities. Unfortunately, today's community pharmacies face daunting prescription volumes that may not allow pharmacists to fully utilize the available information. Readers also might consider the opportunity for pharmacists to document the care they provide, especially in the community setting. This may be even more challenging than reviewing newly available information.

If the coming role of EHRs in pharmacy practice can pull pharmacists away from actual reimbursable activities (i.e., dispensing), then how can these new activities be adopted? There is a growing movement in health care to focus reimbursement on the quality of care. For example, hospitals are facing decreasing reimbursement if patients are readmitted for a condition that they recently received treatment. In many of these readmission events, poor adherence to medication regimens leads to the readmission. The Collaborative's efforts are intended to lead to—among many other things—community pharmacists having access to medication discharge information, allowing them to help ensure patients take the appropriate medications in an appropriate manner. This positions the pharmacist to be recognized for bringing quality to medication management by preventing readmissions. Unfortunately, pharmacists are not currently recognized as providers by Centers for Medicare and Medicaid Services (CMS), so they are not eligible for reimbursement from the government. The Collaborative's approach is to use meaningful use incentives (Collaborative goal #1 above) to provide the financial support to change pharmacy practice since pharmacists are not currently recognized as providers by CMS. Then, over time, documentation of pharmacists' activities within the EHR will demonstrate the pharmacist's impact on quality, leading to recognition of pharmacists as providers by CMS (Mackowiak, 2011).

The approach described above represents a significant change in pharmacy practice. At the time of this writing, the future is uncertain regarding what will ultimately happen for pharmacists' documentation in the EHR. If the changes above occur, everyone in the pharmacy will be impacted. New workflows will need to be established. Training will need to address responsibilities and policies for EHR use. New relationships between pharmacy staff and other providers will likely be established. Patients will need education regarding the changing dynamic between providers, as well as the patient's role as a contributor to their own EHR. Pharmacists will need to adapt to the changing health care landscape, focusing on safe and effective medication use.

REVISITING THE SCENARIO

Charlie's experiences in community and hospital pharmacy practice settings have caused him to realize the potential impact that fully interoperable HIT systems could have on his practice, and more importantly, on his patients' care. These systems support the administrative and clinical aspects of his practice, but are not fully optimized until they can meaningfully exchange information. Charlie recognizes the significant wave of change that is coming and how it will impact both of his practice settings. He is encouraged by the potential of having critical lab values when filling prescriptions in the community and of having accurate, up-to-date medication lists while working in the hospital. Charlie also recognizes the significant change that these systems can have on how people work and the importance of leadership in guiding people through the change. Ultimately, pharmacy managers, supervisors, and other leaders will be responsible for implementing policies, procedures, and workflow to fully benefit from future HIT advancements.

CONCLUSION

A variety of HIT systems exist in today's pharmacy practice environments, and the role of HIT is going to continue to grow. Pharmacists are experts in medication management systems and in medication therapy use. As such, pharmacists should be involved in any efforts impacting the medication use process, whether or not HIT is involved. When considering HIT, pharmacists should carefully evaluate the impact of HIT on pharmacy workflow and patient care, and provide leadership within all practice settings. Leadership can involve developing RFP documents, planning system implementation, developing new policies due to emerging practice models, formalizing adoption of best practices related to medication management, and managing personnel respective to change. Pharmacists should follow national efforts related to HIT, as these efforts will impact practice. Furthermore, pharmacists should become directly involved in these efforts whenever possible.

QUESTIONS FOR FURTHER DISCUSSION

1. How has the role of technology and automation in pharmacy changed over the last several years? What future changes do you anticipate?
2. What can pharmacy managers do to support the emerging role of pharmacists in health information technology?
3. What is the PIMS vendor's role in assisting pharmacy leaders establish downtime procedures and backup services?
4. What are the potential negative consequences of not having pharmacy fully involved in national efforts for interoperability?

REFERENCES

111th Congress of the United States of America. 2009. American Recovery and Reinvestment Act of 2009—Title XIII: Health Information Technology. Available at: http://frwebgate.access.gpo.gov/cgi-bin/getdoc.cgidbname=111cong_bills&docid=fih1enr.pdf; accessed on June 15, 2011.

American Society of Health-System Pharmacists. 2007. ASHP statement on the pharmacist's role in informatics. *Am J Health-Syst Pharm.* 64:200–203.

Brailer DJ. 2005. Interoperability: The key to the future health care system. *Health Aff* (Suppl Web Exclusives):W5-19–21.

Bucki J. 2011. The successful vendor selection process. Available at: http://operationstech.about.com/od/vendorselection/a/VendorSelectionHub.htm; accessed on June 16, 2011.

Bates DW, Cullen DJ, Laird N, et al. 1995. Incidence of adverse drug events and potential adverse drug events: Implications for prevention. *JAMA.* 274:29–34.

California HealthCare Foundation. 2001. Addressing medication errors in hospitals: A framework for developing a plan. Available at: http://www.chcf.org/publications/2001/07/addressing-medication-errors-in-hospitals-a-practical-toolkit; accessed on June 16, 2011.

Davis FD, Bagozzi RP, Warshaw PR. 1989. User acceptance of computer technology: A comparison of two theoretical models. *Manag Sci* 35(8):982–1003.

Greenwald JL, Halasyamani L, Greene J, et al. 2010. Making inpatient medication reconciliation patient centered, clinical relevant and implementable: A consensus statement on key principles and necessary first steps. *J Hosp Med* 5(8):477–85.

Hanson A, Levin BL, Scott DM. 2012. Informatics in health care. In McCarthy RL, Schafermeyer KW, Plake KS (eds), *Introduction to health care delivery: A primer for pharmacists (5th edition)*, pp.315–35. Sudbury, MA: Jones & Bartlett Learning.

Higge HL. 2009. Reducing medication errors using technological innovations. US Pharm 34(3):HS-15–16.

iHealthBeat. 2011. Tornado-hit hospital had data held on EHR system. Available at: http://www.ihealthbeat.org/articles/2011/6/3/tornadohit-hospital-in-missouri-had-data-held-on-ehr-system.aspx; accessed on June 8, 2011.

Institute for Safe Medication Practices. 2008. Guidance on the interdisciplinary safe use of automated dispensing cabinets. Available at: http://www.ismp.org/tools/guidelines/ADC_Guidelines_Final.pdf; accessed on June 15, 2011.

Kaiser Family Foundation. 2010. Prescription drug trends (May 2010). Available at: http://www.kff.org/rxdrugs/upload/3057-08.pdf; accessed June 8, 2011.

Kijsanayotin B, Pannarunothai S, Speedie SM. 2009. Factors influencing health information technology adoption in Thailand's community health centers: applying the UTAUT model. *Int J Med Inform.* 78(6):404–16.

Kilbridge P, Classen D. 2002. Surveillance for adverse drug events: History, methods, and current issues. *Voluntary Hospitals of America* 3:1–35. Irving, TX: VHA Inc. Research Series.

Kohn LT, Corrigan JM, Donaldson MS, eds. 1999. *To Err is Human: Building a Safer Health System.* Washington, DC: National Academy Press.

Kotter JP. 1995. Leading change: Why transformation efforts fail. *Harv Bus Rev.* 73(2):59–67.

Leape LL, Bates DW, Cullen DJ, et al. 1995. Systems analysis of adverse drug events. *JAMA.* 274:35–43.

Lockwood WA. 2010. Automation of ambulatory care pharmacy operations. In Fox BI, Thrower MR, Felkey BG (eds), *Building Core Competencies in Pharmacy Informatics,* Washington, DC: American Pharmacists Association, pp.299–310.

Luo JS, Hilty DM, Worley LL, et al. 2006. Considerations in change management related to technology. *Acad Psychiatry.* 30:465–69.

Mackowiak L. 2011. The Pharmacy eHIT Collaborative: Its purpose and progress to date. Presentation at the American Society of Health-System Pharmacists Summer Meeting, Denver, CO.

Miller AS. 2009. Planning for downtime. In Dumitru D (ed), *The Pharmacy Informatics Primer,* Bethesda, MD: America Society of Health-System Pharmacists, pp. 195–219.

National Association of Chain Drugs Stores. 2010. NACDS 2010-2011 chain pharmacy industry profile. Alexandria, VA.

National Community Pharmacists Association. 2009. 2009 NCPA digest. Alexandria, VA.

Rupp MT, Warholak TL. 2008. Evaluation of e-prescribing in chain community pharmacy: Best-practice recommendations. *J Am Pharm Assoc.* 48(3):364–70.

Section of pharmacy informatics and Technology executive committee. 2009. Technology-enabled practice: A vision statement by the ASHP Section of pharmacy informatics and Technology. *Am J Health-Syst Pharm.* 66(17):1573–7.

Siska MH. 2005. Organizational and functional requirements for eMAR selection. In *Pharmacy Purchasing & Purchasing.* Available at: http://www.pppmag.com/article/96/September_2005/Organizational_and_Functional_Requirements_for_EMAR_Selection/; accessed on June 16, 2011.

Siska MH. 2006. Functional requirements for pharmacy information management systems. In *Pharmacy Purchasing & Purchasing.* Available at: http://www.pppmag.com/article/107/November_2006/Functional_Requirements_for_Pharmacy_Information_Management_Systems/; accessed on June 16, 2011.

Siska MH. 2011. E-prescribing: One giant leap toward pharmacy practice integration. *Am J Health-Syst Pharm.* 68(5):380–81.

Siska MH, Tribble DA. 2011. Opportunities and challenges related to technology in supporting optimal pharmacy practice models in hospitals and health systems. *Am J Health-Syst Pharm.* 68(12):1116–26.

Venkatesh V, Morris MG, Davis GB, et al. 2003. User acceptance of information technology: Toward a unified view. *MIS Q* 2003:425–78.

Walker J, Pan E, Johnston D, et al. 2005. The value of health care information exchange and interoperability. *Health Aff* (Suppl Web Exclusives):W5-8–10.

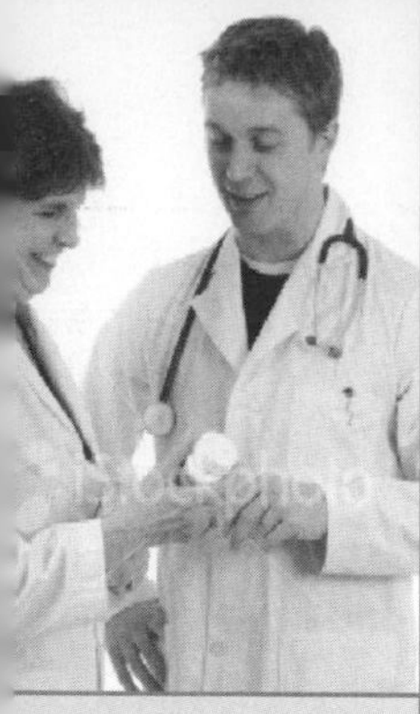

8

ENSURING QUALITY IN PHARMACY OPERATIONS

Terri L. Warholak

About the Author: Dr. Warholak is assistant professor at the University of Arizona College of Pharmacy. She earned a B.S. in pharmacy and an M.S. and Ph.D. in pharmacy administration from Purdue University. Her professional experience encompasses practice in both hospital and community pharmacies, including 5 years as a commissioned officer in the U.S. Public Health Service (Indian Health Service). In addition, she completed a short tour of duty with the Food and Drug Administration (FDA). Dr. Warholak has been recognized as winner of the American Association of Colleges of Pharmacy Council of Faculties Innovations in Teaching Competition for her work titled "Application of Quality Assurance Principles: Reducing Medication Errors in 30 Pharmacy Practice Settings." This work formed the basis of a national quality improvement educational program for students and pharmacists. Dr. Warholak's teaching and research interests include medication error reduction, health information technology evaluation, questionnaire development, and bringing pharmaceutical care to underserved populations. As such, she has substantial experience collaborating with pharmacists and other health care providers. She has participated in studies evaluating the quality of patient care, techniques for reducing medication errors, and health information technology assessment.

LEARNING OBJECTIVES

After completing this chapter, reader should be able to

1. Discuss the importance of quality in pharmacy practice.
2. Describe how quality is measured in pharmacy practice.
3. Justify the use of successful quality practices employed by other industries in pharmacy practice.
4. Explain the differences between quality assurance, quality control, and continuous quality improvement.
5. List three methods for ensuring quality in pharmacy practice.
6. Outline the steps necessary for a successful continuous quality improvement plan.

7. Prioritize areas/functions most suitable for conducting a quality analysis.
8. Identify sources for additional information about quality assessment and improvement.

SCENARIO

Anita Katz was promoted to "pharmacy manager" at a community pharmacy last week. She was excited and wanted to make some positive changes. Among the charges assigned her was to implement quality improvement programs in the pharmacy to decrease errors, increase efficiency, and improve store performance on pharmacy quality measures so as to maximize service, avoid mistakes that had cost the pharmacy in the past, and also to more easily pass accreditation processes. However, she was overwhelmed and did not know where to start the quality improvement process. Some questions she asked herself were: How should I begin? Who should I involve? How should I decide which quality issue to address first? What type of interventions have been successful in the past? Are there quality improvement programs available that I could use? What stakeholders do I need buy-in from? Anita began to do researching on the Internet but also began to recall key concepts from her Quality Improvement and Medication Error Reduction class in pharmacy school. Armed with this information, she began the planning that would make her pharmacy truly exceptional.

CHAPTER QUESTIONS

1. How is *quality* defined within the context of pharmacy practice?
2. Define *health care quality* in layperson's terms.
3. How can the need for quality improvement be justified to decision makers?
4. How can quality be measured?
5. What can pharmacy organizations learn from other industries concerning quality?
6. List the steps of a continuous quality improvement (CQI) model.
7. List four practical CQI suggestions for the pharmacist.

WHAT IS QUALITY?

Quality may appear to be a nebulous term. We know what quality is when we see it, but its definition might be subjective. In fact, there are quite a few definitions of quality. For example, *Webster's Dictionary* defines *quality* as a "degree of excellence" (Merriam-Webster, 2003). While this definition provides a framework for quality in general, it is also helpful to examine the definitions of quality specific to health care.

The U.S. Office of Technology Assessment (OTA) has defined the *quality of medical care* as "evaluation of the performance of medical providers according to the degree to which the process of care increases the probability of outcomes desired by patients and reduces the probability of undesired outcomes, given the state of medical knowledge" (Congress of the United States, Office of Technology Assessment, 1988).

The Institute of Medicine (IOM), in a report entitled, "Medicare: A Strategy for Quality Assurance," stated that "quality of care is the degree to which health services for individuals and populations increase the likelihood of desired health outcomes and are consistent with current professional knowledge" (Lohr, 1990a), whereas Ovretveit (1992) simply states, "A quality health service/system gives patients what they want and need."

An amalgamation of these definitions may provide the best explanation of the concept of quality in health care. The OTA definition implies that the care offered to patients should increase the probability of positive outcomes (e.g., getting rid of an infection) and decrease negative outcomes of care (e.g., death). The care offered to patients should be the most current. While the broadened perspective from Ovretveit has merit, patients may not be the best judges of the quality of medical care because even though they may know what they *want* from medical care, they may not have well-defined notions of what they *need* from medical care. Thus, it is up to the medical provider to offer quality care to benefit the patient even when the patient does not know what he or she needs. While this may appear paternalistic, it seems reasonable that any person who is not an expert in a field may not know all the best alternatives.

So what is quality in pharmacy practice? Extrapolating from the preceding discussion, it can be said that quality in pharmacy practice

- Represents a degree of excellence
- Increases the probability of positive outcomes
- Decreases the probability of negative outcomes
- Corresponds with current medical knowledge
- Offers the patient what he or she wants
- Provides the patient with what he or she needs

Understanding these aspects of quality will help Anita explain pharmacy quality to patients and will serve as the basis for pharmacy improvement.

HOW IS QUALITY MEASURED?

Historically, pharmacy practice quality has been measured by assessing its structure, process, and outcomes (Donabedian, 1969, 1991). Simply put, for a good or service,

- *Structure* refers to the raw materials needed for production.
- *Process* is the method or procedure used.
- *Outcomes* are the end result.

Each of the preceding (i.e., structure, process, and outcomes) has been used to measure quality. Traditionally, quality in pharmacy practice has been measured by structure and process methods. This relies on a premise that a quality outcome is not possible without appropriate structure or process. Moreover, it is much simpler and less controversial to measure structure and process than it is to measure outcomes. Recently, however, outcomes quality measurement has become more prevalent.

In the realm of pharmacy, the raw materials or structure necessary for quality care are many and varied. Examples include number of pharmacists per shift, counter space, pharmacist credentials or licensing, pharmacy square footage, medication reference books, medication stock, and counseling facilities.

Because pharmacists are responsible for all phases of medication use, processes in the pharmacy can refer to any phase of the medication use process (e.g., prescribing, dispensing, administering, or monitoring). Examples of process measures include, but are not limited to, adherence to clinical guidelines or pathways, percent of prescriptions assessed for appropriateness, and percent of patients counseled.

Outcomes are the driving force behind medication therapy management, which has pharmacists participating in patient education, medication review, and disease management. Through such activities, pharmacists have been able to improve patient care by (1) increasing patients' control of their medical conditions (Clifford et al., 2005; Cranor et al., 2003; Garrett and Bluml, 2005; Kiel and McCord, 2005; Leal and Herrier, 2004; Ragucci et al., 2005; Sadik et al., 2005; Scott et al., 2006; Schnipper et al., 2006; Sookaneknun et al., 2004); (2) decreasing use of health care resources (Cordina et al., 2001; Dedden et al., 1997; Garrett and Bluml, 2005; Rupp et al., 1997); (3) increasing patients' knowledge of their conditions, treatments, and medications (Mangiapane et al., 2005; Schulz et al., 2001); (4) increasing adherence to and persistence with medication regimens (Krass et al., 2005; Lee et al., 2006; Mangiapane et al., 2005; Sookaneknun et al., 2004; Vrijens et al., 2006); (5) increasing patients' satisfaction with their care (Cranor et al., 2003; Garrett and Bluml, 2005; Weinberger et al., 2002), (6) saving payers money (Cranor et al., 2003; Fertleman et al., 2005; Garrett and Bluml, 2005; Ragucci et al., 2005); and (7) improving patients' quality of life

(Cordina et al., 2001; Mangiapane et al., 2005; Rupp et al., 1997; Sadik et al., 2005; Scott et al., 2006; Schulz et al., 2001).

The systems engineering for patient safety (SEIPS) model expands Donabedian's process concept from direct patient care to processes that support patient care (i.e., housekeeping) and indicates that these processes must also be designed to support safety. SEIPS is a multidisciplinary initiative applying systems engineering, human factors engineering, and quality engineering approaches. The research supporting this model examines systems design, quality management, job design, and technology implementations that affect safety-related patient and organizational and/or staff outcomes (Carayon et al., 2006).

Pharmacists' ability to identify, resolve, and prevent medication-related problems, as well as take responsibility in disease management, is well documented (Bluml et al., 2000; Cranor et al., 2003; Fertleman et al., 2005; Hansen et al., 2006; Nolan, 2000; Schnipper et al., 2006). Thus, outcomes describe the ultimate goal of the care or therapy and answer the question, "What are we trying to accomplish?"

There are different ways to look at outcomes. One method, the ECHO model, purports three basic types of outcomes: economic, clinical, and humanistic (Kozma et al., 1993). Economic outcomes include direct costs and consequences, both medical and nonmedical, and indirect costs and consequences. For example, when assessing outcomes from a patient perspective, a medication co-payment would be a direct medication cost, whereas gas money to pick up the medication from the pharmacy would represent a nonmedical direct cost. Lost wages from missed work could be regarded as an indirect cost.

Clinical outcomes measures can include morbidity and mortality, event rates, and symptom resolution (Ovretveit, 2001). These measures are a direct measure of quality but may be difficult to assess, especially in pharmacy, where their onset could be years following a treatment or intervention (Chassin and Galvin, 1998; Shane and Gouveia, 2000). In these cases, indicators or markers can be used to assess outcomes. These indicators can be condition-specific (e.g., HgA1c) or procedure-specific (e.g., rate of postoperative infection after hip surgery) or address an important issue of patient care. For example, blood pressure may be used as a marker to assess susceptibility to stroke because it is not practical, safe, or ethical to wait and measure the occurrence of stroke.

Humanistic outcomes include measures of the "human" aspects of care. Specific types of humanistic outcomes include patient satisfaction and health-related quality of life (HRQoL). For example, a survey concerning patient satisfaction with pharmacy care services could be used to assess humanistic outcomes for patients receiving these services. Alternatively, an HRQoL assessment may be useful to assess the impact medication therapy has on the patient's life as a whole.

Measuring outcomes can seem to be a daunting task. Thus, the remainder of this chapter will present these concepts in an easy-to-understand manner and will include simple implementation tips.

WHAT CAN PHARMACY LEARN FROM OTHER INDUSTRIES?

Health care traditionally has lagged behind other industries in quality improvement. It has been suggested that medicine should follow the lead of the airline and other industries by using quality management to decrease unnecessary variation and improve quality (Leape, 1994). An IOM report supported this contention when the authors suggested that the American health care system can improve the quality of care by borrowing techniques used in other industries to standardize processes (Kohn, 2000). Many of these techniques are based on systems theory.

Systems theory, developed by von Bertalanffy (1968), has been used in engineering, medicine, and education (Nagel, 1988; Sheridan, 1988). A systems approach involves defining the purpose and performance expectations of the system, examining the characteristics of the input, considering alternative mechanisms for achieving the stated goals, implementing the system, and adjusting the system based on feedback (Park, 1997; Sheridan, 1988).

Various organizations and regulators have turned to a systems view of quality improvement termed *human factors principles* (FAA, 1993; Leape et al., 1998a). The human factors view of quality focuses on the relationship between quality problems and the system in which they occur (Rasmussen et al., 1994). "Human factors principles are concepts about the design of work that take advantage of the strengths and weakness of the human mind and compensate for its limitations" (Leape et al., 1998a). Human factors principles include (1) reducing reliance on memory, (2) simplifying and standardizing, (3) using protocols and checklists, (4) using mechanisms to physically prevent error (constraints and forcing functions), (5) improving access to information, (6) decreasing reliance on vigilance, (7) differentiating, and (8) implementing automation (Kohn, 2000; Leape et al., 1998a).

In pharmacy practice, decreased reliance on memory can be accomplished by using decision-support systems. Most community pharmacies now use in-store computer systems to assist with Omnibus Budget Reconciliation Act of 1990-mandated (OBRA 90–mandated) prospective drug utilization review (DUR). However, decision-support systems should be used wisely because they are not intended to supplant the pharmacist's clinical decision-making skills (Leape et al., 1998a; Nolan, 2000).

Standardization is thought to be one of the most powerful tools for improving quality (Leape et al., 1998b). If a person does something the same way every time, the chances that he or she will perform the activity incorrectly are greatly reduced (Leape et al., 1998b). Industry has long known that quality and variation are inversely related; quality improves as variation is reduced (Deming, 1986). In pharmacy, standardization is the simplest, most broadly applicable, and most effective method for quality improvement (Leape et al., 1998b). In fact, the move to standardization has created the impetus for critical pathways that focus not only on error prevention but also on optimization of outcomes, cost reduction, and satisfaction (Clearinghouse, 2000; American Pharmacists Association, 2003). These decision support systems can also be used to decrease reliance on vigilance through alerting the pharmacist of potential problems.

Another mechanism for decreasing reliance on memory and reducing variation is the use of protocols and checklists. Protocols and checklists serve as reminders of critical tasks, especially when an omission can have serious consequences, and are often recommended as mechanisms for increasing quality (Boeing, 1993). Policies and protocols decrease confusion, thus improving overall dispensing quality (Agency for Healthcare Research and Quality, 2001). A constraint that "prevents further action until some condition is met" (Leape et al., 1998a) can also be written into protocols to provide a quality check in a system. For example, protocols usually preclude prescriptions from being dispensed until they are approved by the pharmacist's final check.

Improving access to information leads to improved quality (Abelson and Levi, 1985; Weinstein and Fineberg, 1980). One study indicated that pharmacists make more appropriate prospective DUR decisions when they have access to more complete patient information, such as medication profiles, allergy information, patient age, and diagnosis (Warholak-Juarez et al., 2000). Therefore, medication orders should not be processed without the pharmacist considering these and similar pieces of information.

Moreover, improved quality produces a corresponding increase in productivity because less rework is needed and less waste is produced (Deming, 1986). In pharmacy, quality improvements may produce improved clinical and humanistic outcomes such as improved QoL and customer satisfaction. Improved customer satisfaction can help make the workplace more pleasant and may produce a corresponding increase in employee satisfaction. This ultimately may lead to the pharmacy having a competitive edge and an image as a provider of high-quality pharmaceutical care and may allow the business to recruit and maintain the most highly qualified and desired personnel.

METHODS FOR ENSURING QUALITY IN PHARMACY PRACTICE

Quality Assurance

Quality assurance (QA) has been defined as "the systematic monitoring and evaluation of the various aspects of a project, service, or facility to ensure that standards of quality are being met" (Merriam-Webster, 2003). Basically, a check is performed to ensure that a good or service meets a certain quality standard. Problems are addressed after they occur (Godwin and Sanborn, 1995).

Quality Control

Quality control (QC), as defined by *Webster's Dictionary*, is "an aggregate of activities (as design analysis and inspection for defects) designed to ensure adequate quality" (Merriam-Webster, 2003). Quality control improves product or service design to improve the level of quality; it can be thought of as defect prevention.

Continuous Quality Improvement

Continuous quality improvement (CQI) is "a philosophy of continual improvement of the processes associated with providing a good or service that meets or exceeds customer expectations" (Shortell et al., 1998). CQI has been referred to as *quality improvement process, total quality management,* and *total quality control* (Lohr, 1990b).

CQI introduced two important ideas that transcend QA and QC. First, CQI represents a total systems perspective concerning quality; all workers within the health care system are interconnected (Godwin and Sanborn, 1995). When examined from a systems perspective, every action of the health care professional is performed to benefit the patient (Shortell et al., 1998). Therefore, all actions must be planned to improve care and should not focus on correcting individual mistakes after the fact (Godwin and Sanborn, 1995; Shortell et al., 1998). Thus, quality problems are not examined (or blamed) on an individual level (Blumenthal and Kilo, 1998). CQI promotes identification of the cause of problems via "fact-based management and scientific methodology, which make it culturally compatible with the values of health care professionals" (Shortell et al., 1998, p. 605).

Second, CQI demands that the quality improvement process is continuous or never-ending (Blumenthal and Kilo, 1998). Improvement occurs by integrating information concerning quality into the cyclic redesign and improvement of care (Godwin and Sanborn, 1995). The changes can be quick and on a small scale but should be occurring constantly. In this manner, CQI empowers health care providers to improve quality on a daily basis (Shortell et al., 1998).

CQI is more than looking for things that could be wrong; it is a systematic process for continuously improving the quality of every aspect of a pharmacy practice setting from patient care to managerial responsiveness. In this manner, CQI is a much more positive process than QA or QC because the focus is on constantly making things better for all who work in and have contact with the practice. CQI is a method for constantly striving for improvement in every facet, every portion of the medication use system.

A CQI IMPROVEMENT MODEL

Many CQI models exist. Examples of specific models include the plan, do, check, and act (PDCA) model and the find, organize, clarify, understand, select, plan, do, check, and act (FOCUS-PDCA) model and six sigma (Lazarus and Butler, 2001; Lazarus and Stamps, 2002). Most models include elements that reflect the following core concepts: (1) plan, (2) design, (3) measure, (4) assess, and (5) improve (Coe, 1998a).

CQI has been described as a practical application of the scientific method (Blumenthal and Kilo, 1998). Planning in both processes is similar. In this manner, one can think of the steps in the CQI cycle as parallel to the sections of a scientific article: background, methods, results, conclusions, and recommendations. Considering CQI in this manner diminishes the need to memorize additional terminology. See Fig. 8-1 for a flowchart representation of the process.

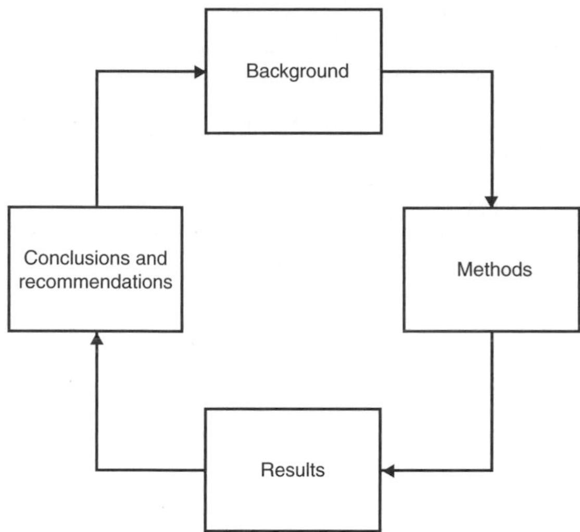

Figure 8-1. The CQI measurement cycle.

The steps to CQI discussed in this chapter are included in the CQI Cycle Checklist and Planning Worksheets in Appendices 8A and 8B, respectively. The CQI Cycle Checklist includes an abbreviated list of the actions needed for a successful CQI cycle. The Planning Worksheets are more detailed forms to assist in CQI cycle implementation. Worksheet 1 is intended for use during the first team meeting, Worksheet 2 should be used for the second meeting through completion of data collection, and Worksheet 3 begins with data analysis and guides the user through the remainder of the CQI cycle.

Recruiting the CQI Team

The planning phase of quality improvement is essential. The first step in developing a cohesive plan is to assemble an expert panel. This panel should be interdisciplinary and include representatives of those who are part of or will be affected by the quality plan. The team also should include subject matter experts, decision makers, and frontline personnel. In a pharmacy setting, the entire staff should be invited to participate. This will stress the importance of the quality process and help to get staff support for the quality improvement project. It is important to note that while buy-in will be increased by inviting staff participation and opinions, this effect will be lost quickly if staff members do not perceive that their participation is beneficial.

CQI Cycle Background

Focus Selection

The CQI cycle begins with the selection of a quality improvement focus. Selection may be based on mandate, or the choice may be left to the team. If the team is given the latitude to choose, one of several processes may be used to facilitate this decision. The team could brainstorm possible areas for study. In this case, all team members should provide ideas freely, and each idea should be recorded. Ideas then may be ranked, and team consensus can be used for system selection. Examples of systems that have been shown to provide quality improvement opportunities in health care settings include identifying and measuring the incidence of medication errors, implementing methods to reduce medication errors, measuring medication filling time, analyzing satisfaction with pharmacy services, evaluating the effect of pharmacists' interventions, analyzing adherence to requirements for documentation, documenting the incidence of medication allergy, auditing patient-controlled analgesia pumps, assessing patient-specific medication errors in cart filling, and analyzing hypertension control and guidelines compliance.

Alternatively, processes such as failure mode and effects analysis or root cause analysis can be used to identify systems ripe for quality improvement activities. Failure mode and effects analysis is a prospective procedure used to identify areas for quality improvement before they become a problem (Cohen et al., 1994; DeRosier et al., 2002; NCPS, 2011a). Once possible areas are identified, the investigators decide if the results will be tolerable or intolerable (Cohen et al., 1994).

Root cause analysis is a systematic process used to identify the exact or root cause of a problem (Coe, 1998b). It is used after a quality problem has been discovered (a retrospective procedure) to prevent recurrence (Coe, 1998c; NCPS, 2011b). The process begins with "triage questions" that help the team decide what

Table 8-1. Two Tools for Identifying Quality Improvement Priority Areas

Prospective: Failure mode and effects analysis (FMEA)

The Veterans Administration National Center for Patient Safety (NCPS) has translated this industrial and engineering procedure for health care. The NCPS has termed its adaptation *healthcare failure mode effects analysis* (HFMEA), and it offers live and videoconference training courses on use (DeRosier et al., 2002). Before doing FMEA, obtain a copy of the video course and/or articles and worksheets that have been developed as a process guide (available from NCPS at www.patientsafety.gov/pubs.html#cogaids). HCFMEA can be performed for general processes (e.g., use of medications on the night shift) or for specific medications. Steps include

Step 1: Define the scope or topic to be studied.

Step 2: Assemble a multidisciplinary team that includes a subject matter expert.

Step 3: Describe and narrow the focus.

Step 4: Conduct a hazard analysis.

Step 5: Select necessary actions and outcome measures and assign activities to specific persons and dates for follow-up.

Retrospective: Root cause analysis (RCA)

A comprehensive "flip card" root cause analysis guide is also available from NCPS (see Web site as listed above). This card set walks the pharmacist through every step of a comprehensive root cause evaluation of a quality problem. For example, the cards begin with triage questions such as

- Was the error a criminal act?
- Was it a violation (intentional) or an error?
- Were human factors an issue?
- Was staff training or competency an issue?
- Was equipment involved?
- Was information lacking/misinterpreted?
- Was communication an issue?
- Were policies/procedures/rules an issue?
- Did a protective barrier fail?

Once these questions are answered, the user is led to more detailed questions that address the specific situation. These more detailed questions cover areas such as human factors, communication, training, fatigue, scheduling, environment, equipment, rules, policy, procedure, or barriers to quality.

issues (e.g., staff training, competency, human factors, equipment, and information) could have contributed to the quality problem (Gosbee and Anderson, 2003). Once these questions are answered, more detailed, specific questions are considered in order to identify ways to improve systems to reduce the chance of it recurring. The investigators create an action plan for implementing system improvements and improvements evaluation (Anonymous, 2002; Bagian et al., 2001). A more detailed account of these two processes is included in Table 8-1.

Focus Description

After the focus for quality improvement has been chosen, it is important to make sure that it is clear to each team member. This can be accomplished by providing a detailed description of the area chosen for study, the setting in which the focus occurs, the portion of the medication use process affected, and baseline data, if applicable.

Flowcharts that explicitly represent all portions of the process can be helpful for system description. Flowcharts use standard symbols that represent all process steps (represented as rectangles), as well as decision points (represented by diamond shapes) and the direction of progression from one subprocess to the other (Coe, 1998a). Flowcharts are also useful because they can help the team recognize if the process chosen is too broad (i.e., represented by an unwieldy flowchart). An example of a flowchart is given in Fig. 8-1.

Focus Importance

Next, the team should state why the focus is important. The selected focus should be important to the organization and have the potential to lead to improvement. It should be considered high priority, high volume, high cost, or high risk. For example, a community pharmacy may choose to focus on prescription order-entry error if anecdotal evidence suggests that this may be an error-prone step in its dispensing process.

Literature Review

Relate the focus to the literature by investigating what is known and not known about similar situations. This step can save the team an enormous amount of time in the long run. A brief literature search will help the team to discover techniques, interventions, and other tools that have been successful in improving quality in similar situations.

Goals

Once the focus (i.e., process or problem) is chosen, the team should *determine the overall goal* (Leape et al., 1998c). Common overall goals include (1) discovery, (2) frequency estimation, and (3) measuring a change (Leape et al., 1998c). For example, after a pharmacy's CQI team has decided that it wants to focus on prescription order-entry error, team members must then decide *what* they want to know about it. They may decide that since this is their first CQI cycle, they will focus on frequency estimation of the problem. This will serve as baseline data for the assessment of improvements. The overall goal can be used to *choose specific goals for the cycle* (Leape et al., 1998c). Note that it is important to assess the practicality of the specific goal. The CQI team should examine the specific goal carefully to determine whether it is realistic. If the goal is not realistic, then it may need to be scaled back (Leape et al., 1998c). Choosing something reasonable for the first CQI cycle will provide the team with experience, improve its chances for success, and thus bolster team members' confidence for the next cycle.

CQI Cycle Methods

Intervention

Interventions discovered through a literature review should be included on a list of possible interventions. These may include quality improvement techniques such as reducing reliance on memory, simplifying, standardizing, or automating processes.

Process and Outcomes Measured

Next, the CQI team must determine how progress will be measured (Leape et al., 1998c). Team members should list process and/or outcome measures necessary to determine if the goals were met. Usually, a mix of process and outcome measures is recommended (Leape et al., 1998c). Many measures have been developed, so keep the following in mind: Do not invent a new measure if a good one exists; measure what is important—not easy; and do not measure things you cannot change or interpret (Ovretveit, 2001). Table 8-2 provides additional resources on selecting and developing measures.

Data-Collection Procedures

If the required data are not already being collected, the CQI team should devise a plan to collect the appropriate data. The team can choose from several different data-collection methods (Leape et al., 1998c), including inspection points, focus groups, monitoring for markers, and observation.

Data-Analysis Plan

The planned statistical analysis should be thought out in detail to make sure that all necessary information will be gathered. It can be frustrating and time-consuming to gather forgotten data at a moment's notice. This

Table 8-2. Health Care Process and Outcome Measurement Resources

Need help selecting a measure?

Many process and outcome measures exist, so there may be no need to develop one of your own. Measure selection can be expedited by examining the core critical literature, soliciting expert opinion, or using recognized guidelines such as those from JCAHO, HEDIS, or Healthy People 2010.

Other resources include the National Quality Measures Clearinghouse (NQMC). NQMC provides information on health care quality measures and measure sets and includes a glossary of terms and information on how to select, use, apply, and interpret a measure. Available at www.qualitymeasures.ahrq.gov. Ready-to-use quality tools can be accessed via www.qualitytools.ahrq.gov/.

seems self-evident but is a mistake that many people make.

CQI Cycle Results

Analyze Data

Most descriptive statistics (e.g., mean, median, and percentages) often suffice for data analysis. Some analyses can be performed simply by plotting data onto charts or graphs. Which can help to determine patterns and trends. For more sophisticated analysis or hypothesis testing, outside assistance may be required. If there is not a statistician on the CQI team, it may be beneficial to refer to statistics books to make sure that the chosen analysis is appropriate. Asking for outside help is also an option; the team should not hesitate to call the local college of pharmacy for a referral.

CQI Cycle Conclusions, Implications, and Recommendations

The final section in the process is describing the conclusions, implications, and recommendations that the team reached after examining the results. Since this is the "bottom line" of the process, it is important that this section be understandable to those outside the CQI team. This section should concisely explain the conclusions and detail the actions that need to take place. The CQI process is iterative; thus, the team's recommendations for *this CQI cycle* and for the *next CQI cycle* must be included (Leape et al., 1998b). This will be good news to pharmacist Pat. Because CQI is a continuous improvement process, an understanding of the iterative nature of the process will take the pressure off him to "fix" all pharmacy system problems at once.

ACCREDITATION/ COMPLIANCE WITH QUALITY STANDARDS PROMULGATED BY AGENCIES OR ASSOCIATIONS

Often quality improvement activities are necessary for accreditation. Earning accreditation indicates that an organization has met predefined standards. The accreditation process provides a framework to help organizations focus on providing safe, high-quality service and requires that the organization demonstrate to outside reviewers its commitment to continuous improvement (Ovretveit, 2001).

The Joint Commission

The Joint Commission is a nonprofit organization founded in 1951 by the American Medical Association and the American College of Surgeons (O'Malley, 1997). The Joint Commission was established to "continuously improve the safety and quality of health care provided to the public through the provision of health care accreditation and related services that support performance improvement in health care organizations" (Joint Commission on Accreditation of Healthcare Organizations Web site a). The Joint Commission's focus is organization-wide (O'Malley, 1997).

The Joint Commission survey process is largely process-oriented but gradually is moving toward more of an outcomes measurement model in an effort to provide organizations with information they can use to improve patient care (Anonymous, 2003b). Although Joint Commission compliance is voluntary, many organizations view it as mandatory (O'Malley, 1997). Not obtaining Joint Commission accreditation can adversely affect an organization's prestige and reimbursement status (Coe, 1998c; O'Malley, 1997). Key dimensions of performance evaluation include efficacy, appropriateness, availability, timeliness, effectiveness, continuity, safety, efficiency, respect, and caring (Coe, 1998a).

The Joint Commission's annual safety goals often involve medication use and thus pharmacists can use these goals to help improve the quality of medication use throughout the health care system. For example, one of the Hospital National Patient Safety Goals for 2011 is "Check Patient Medications" which includes identifying the patient's home medications, making sure new medications are appropriate to add the patient's regimen, providing a medication list to the patient's next caregiver during their health system stay, and then providing the medication to the patient's regular physician and the patient upon discharge. The medication list should be explained to the patient (Joint Commission on Accreditation of Healthcare Organizations Web site 2011b). These are roles the pharmacist is uniquely suited for and a pharmacist who can contribute in this way to the health system will not only improve the quality of patient care but will also help better integrate him- or herself into the interprofessional medical team.

National Committee for Quality Assurance

The National Committee for Quality Assurance (NCQA, 2011) is a nonprofit organization established in 1979 by a managed-care trade association in response to a perceived need to provide standardized quality measurement and reporting (NCQA, 2003). The NCQA reviews and accredits all types of managed health care organizations (NCQA, 2007).

Quality Measurement

While health care accreditation organizations have existed for quite a while, quality data were not readily available to the general public until recently. These quality measurements (sometimes called "report cards") make health care quality indicators readily available to the public. This encourages health care organizations to compete on the basis of quality and creates markets where quality, not just cost containment, is rewarded (Blumenthal and Kilo, 1998; O'Malley, 1997).

HEDIS

The Health Plan Employer Data and Information Set (HEDIS) is a health care report card created by NCQA that is used by more than 90 percent of America's health plans to measure performance (NCQA Web site). HEDIS standardizes health plan performance data and disseminates this information publicly so plans can be compared (O'Malley, 1997). This allows health care purchasers and consumers to compare plans and make informed decisions and provides plans with data on where they could focus to improve quality. HEDIS's performance domains include effectiveness of care, access and availability of care, health plan stability, use of services, cost of care, informed health care choices, satisfaction with the experience of care, and health plan descriptive information. Many HEDIS measures involve medication management thus providing an opportunity for pharmacists to help improve the quality of patient care.

Leapfrog Group

The Leapfrog Group was formed by a coalition of Fortune 500 companies and leading health care purchase organizations (Leapfrog, 2003). The Leapfrog Group was developed to create a market that rewards quality, not just the lowest-cost provider, by providing quality information to consumers (Leapfrog, 2003). The Leapfrog survey includes process and outcome measures (Leapfrog Web site).

Deciphering Quality Measures

Quality measures such as those just mentioned are developed for consumer use. However, many patients have difficulty understanding these measures and reports well enough to use them for rational health care decision making. Patients and health care providers can get assistance from a U.S. government Web site called *TalkingQuality.* (www.talkingquality.ahrq.gov/default.aspx). TalkingQuality was developed to help patients understand the concept of health care quality and to give practical suggestions for choosing health care coverage and providers (Anonymous, 2003a). Sites such as this one are also useful for pharmacists who want to better understand quality improvement in health care.

The Future

Since establishment of the Joint Commission, the scope of health care organizations that are eligible for accreditation has widened from hospitals to encompass health systems and now even pharmacy benefit managers (URAC, 2006). In some countries, such as Australia, pharmacies are accredited (Pharmacy Guild of Australia, 2011). The National Association of Boards of Pharmacy (NABP) has announced a plan to develop and implement a community pharmacy accreditation program. The program would focus on issues such as patient counseling, patient medication adherence, and patient safety. As part of the proposed program, pharmacies would have to implement and maintain continuous quality improvement programs (NABP 2010).

Groups such as the Pharmacy Quality Alliance (PQA) are developing pharmacy-specific quality indicators (PQA, 2011a). These measures assess gaps in patient medication therapy, dosing for specific conditions such as diabetes, suboptimal treatment of conditions such as hypertension, drug–drug interactions, and inappropriate medication use in the elderly (PQA, 2011b). PQA has sponsored demonstration projects to test measures and measure reporting to pharmacists (report cards). PQA is also active in helping pharmacists learn how to improve quality. They have sponsored several educational programs including the self-contained, three-credit QI class titled Educating Pharmacy Students and Pharmacists to Improve Quality (EPIQ) that is available upon request to pharmacists and pharmacy schools (PQA, 2011c).

In the future, the quality improvement process may become more focused on outcomes measurement. Eventually, health care report cards may be more accessible and easy to understand, thus helping to produce a market for quality. Some discussion of adjusting copayments to encourage patients to use providers that meet the standards purchasers have set has already occurred (Lovern, 2001). In some cases, pharmacy quality improvement may be mandated by state and local governments. For example, a new law in the state of Arizona requires that every pharmacy participate in a CQI program, although the State Board of Pharmacy rules have yet to be implemented (Arizona Revised Statutes, 2007).

So what does this mean for pharmacy practice? More pharmacists must understand continuous quality improvement and be able to develop, implement, and measure the outcomes of such a plan. This could provide an opportunity for a community pharmacy report card (quality measurement) system on which pharmacies can compete on the basis of quality. Such a system may provide a great opportunity for pharmacies to advertise quality outcomes to payers and patients. If such a system is successful, quality could drive patient choices and payer decisions. Ultimately, the pharmacies with the highest quality may get more market share or obtain higher reimbursement rates for certain services (pay-for-performance).

REVISITING THE SCENARIO

There are several things that Anita can do to improve quality in her pharmacy. First, she can promote a "systems view" of errors within their organization (Hume, 1999). Systems changes should be implemented only when the organization is ready for change and has capable leadership that supports a systems view of "no finger-pointing" (Shortell et al., 1994). Everyone in the organization should be informed of and invited to participate in any quality systems changes (i.e., the quality team). Personnel evaluations (i.e., performance appraisals) should comprise a quality improvement component so that employees are rewarded for their efforts in such matters (Shortell et al., 1994).

Second, Anita and the quality improvement team she creates should focus on high-leverage important systems changes (Hume, 1999; Shortell et al., 1994). For medication safety, this could involve focusing on high-alert medications (e.g., fast movers, narrow-therapeutic-index medications, and medications that are available in multiple strengths), high-risk populations (e.g., pediatrics or geriatrics), or problem processes (e.g., e-prescribing). Significant opportunities for improvement can be gleaned from an analysis of intervention data, medication errors that get identified before they leave the pharmacy (near misses); medication error incident reports, patient comments, or employee feedback (Johnson et al., 2002; Rogers, 1997).

Third, Anita and her team should implement small changes in quick improvement cycles (Hume, 1999). The quality improvement team should be given the opportunity to learn about quality by attempting small changes; it may be too frustrating to take on a large project for the first cycle. Team members should be allowed to experience a success and see how much improvement can be made with a relatively small change; then their enthusiasm will redouble.

Fourth, Anita and her quality improvement team should implement interventions that have worked elsewhere (Hume, 1999). This improves the likelihood of success and reduces the amount of effort required in the process. It is worth noting that the most successful interventions changed *systems*, not *people* (Nolan, 2000; van Bokhoven et al., 2003).

If Anita's pharmacy organization does not want to develop its own CQI plan, help is available. Pharmacy Quality Commitment (PQC) has developed the Sentinel System for community pharmacies. This system, which incorporates best practices, risk-management techniques, and systematic procedures to increase quality, is ready to use and is available from the National Alliance of State Pharmacy Associations at www.pqc.net.

It is important to remember that quality improvement in pharmacy is far reaching and that quality improvement projects may take many shapes. That is, the pharmacist can be involved in many different type of quality improvement projects such as the following: decreasing prescribing errors by educating physicians on principles of safe prescribing; improving patient medication compliance by providing a lower-cost alternative; decreasing mortality by helping prescribers select appropriate antibiotics; decreasing medication dispensing errors by implementing dispensing technology; improving the identification of e-prescribing drop down menu selection errors by having prescribers transmit the diagnosis with prescriptions; helping patients better adhere to anticoagulant therapy by providing education; using "show and tell" patient counseling as a method to identify medication errors before they leave the pharmacy; or improving quality of medication use by adding pharmacist-performed medication reconciliation to an accountable care organization. The list—and the ways in which pharmacists can improve the quality of patient care—is endless.

CONCLUSION

Quality is an essential component of competent, professional pharmacy practice. Increasing quality can have many beneficial effects on any practice, such as minimizing rework and increasing productivity. Many quality improvement changes are simple and can be implemented quickly but may have a large impact on the quality of patient care.

Health care quality finally has achieved a position of high visibility on the national agenda. Thus pharmacists will be called on increasingly to ensure quality in all portions of the medication use system.

QUESTIONS FOR FURTHER DISCUSSION

Anita has begun to address quality in her pharmacy practice setting.

1. What other steps should she take?
2. How can a quality improvement plan be sustained continuously?
3. How can the pharmacy use the quality improvement plan for marketing?
4. Where can Anita go for additional information about quality improvement?

ACKNOWLEDGMENT

I would like to thank Dr. Tom Reutzel for his guidance and support in helping to write this chapter.

REFERENCES

Abelson RP, Levi A. 1985. Decision making and decision theory. In *Handbook of Social Psychology*, p. 231. New York: Random House.

Agency for Healthcare Research and Quality (AHRQ). 2001. *Medical Errors: The Scope of the Problem.* Rockville, MD, AHRQ.

American Pharmacists Association (APhA). 2003. *American Pharmacists Association Catalogue.* Washington, DC: APhA.

Anonymous. 2002. *Root Cause Analysis.* Washington, DC: VA National Center for Patient Safety.

Anonymous. 2003a. *The Big Picture.* Talkingquality.gov.

Anonymous. 2003b. *Performance Measures in Health Care.* Washington, DC: Joint Commission on Accreditation of Healthcare Organizations.

Arizona Revised Statutes. 2007. Amending Title 32, Chapter 18, Article 3, Arizona Revised Statutes, by adding 32–1973, relating to the state board of pharmacy.

Bagian JP, Lee C, Gosbee J, et al. 2001. Developing and deploying a patient safety program in a large health care delivery system: You can't fix what you don't know about. *Joint Comm J Qual Improv* 27:522.

Blumenthal D, Kilo CM. 1998. A report card on continuous quality improvement. *Milbank Q* 76:625.

Bluml BM, McKenney JM, Cziraki MJ, et al. 2000. Pharmaceutical care services and results in project ImPACT: Hyperlipidemia. *J Am Pharm Assoc* 40:157.

Boeing. 1993. *Accident Prevention Strategies: Removing Links in the Accident Chain.* Seattle: Boeing Commercial Airplane Group.

Carayon P, Schoofs-Hundt A, Karsh BT, Gurses AP, et al. 2006. Work system design for patient safety: the SEIPS model. *Qual Saf Health Care* 15 Suppl 1:i50–8.

Chassin MR, Galvin RW. 1998. The urgent need to improve health care quality. Institute of Medicine National Roundtable on health care quality. *JAMA* 280:1000–5

Clearinghouse NG. 2000. Evidence-based clinical practice guidelines. Agency for Healthcare Research and Quality. Available at www.qualitymeasures.ahrq.gov/; accessed on May 28, 2011.

Clifford RM, Davis WA, Batty KT, et al. 2005. Effect of a pharmaceutical care program on vascular risk factors in type 2 diabetes: The Fremantle diabetes study. *Diabetes Care* 28:771–6.

Coe CP. 1998a. An overview of the Joint Commission's improving organizational performance standards. In *Preparing the Pharmacy for a Joint Commission Survey*, p. 189. Bethesda, MD: ASHP.

Coe CP. 1998b. Overview of the Joint Commission's Sentinel Event Policy. In *Preparing the Pharmacy for a Joint Commission Survey*, p. 200. Bethesda, MD: ASHP.

Coe CP. 1998c. Joint Commission on Accreditation of Healthcare Organizations. In *Preparing the Pharmacy for a Joint Commission Survey*, p. 1. Bethesda, MD: ASHP.

Cohen MR, Senders J, Davis NM. 1994. Failure mode and effects analysis: A novel approach to avoiding dangerous medication errors and accidents. *Hosp Pharm* 29: 319.

Congress of the United States, Office of Technology Assessment. 1988. *The Quality of Medical Care: Information for Consumers*, p. x. Washington, DC: U.S. Government Printing Office.

Cordina M, McElnay JC, Hughes CM. 2001. Assessment of a community pharmacy-based program for patients with asthma. *Pharmacotherapy* 21:1196–203.

Cranor CW, Bunting BA, Christensen DB, 2003. The Asheville Project: Long-term clinical and economic outcomes of a community pharmacy diabetes care program. *J Am Pharm Assoc* 43:173.

Dedden P, Chang B, Nagel D, 1997. Pharmacy-managed program for home treatment of deep vein thrombosis with enoxaparin. *Am J Health-Syst Pharm* 54:1968.

Deming WE. 1986. *Out of the Crisis.* Cambridge, MA: Massachusetts Institute of Technology, Center for Advanced Engineering Study.

DeRosier J, Stalhandske E, Bagian JP, et al. 2002. Using health care failure mode and effect analysis: The VA National Center for Patient Safety's prospective risk analysis system. *Joint Comm J Qual Improv* 28:248.

Donabedian A. 1969. Quality of care: Problems of measurement: II. Some issues in evaluating the quality of nursing care. *Am J Public Health Nations Health* 59:1833.

Donabedian A. 1991. Quality assurance: Structure, process, and outcome. *Nurs Stand* 7:4.

Federal Aviation Authority (FAA). 1993. Human Factor Policy. Washington: US Department of Transportation.

Fertleman M, Barnett N, Patel T, 2005. Improving medication management for patients: The effect of a pharmacist on post-admission ward rounds. *Qual Saf Health Care* 14:207–11.

Garrett DG, Bluml BM. 2005. Patient self-management program for diabetes: First-year clinical, humanistic, and economic outcomes. *J Am Pharm Assoc* 45:130–7.

Godwin HN, Sanborn MD. 1995. Total quality management in hospital pharmacy. *Am Pharm* NS35:51.

Gosbee J, Anderson T. 2003. Human factors engineering design demonstrations can enlighten your RCA team. *Qual Saf Health Care* 12:119.

Hansen LB, Fernald D, Akaya-Guerra R, et al. 2006. Pharmacy clarification of prescriptions ordered in primary care: A report from the Applied Strategies for Improving Patient Safety (ASIPS) collaborative. *J Am Board Fam Med* 19:24–30.

Hume M. 1999. Changing hospital culture, systems reduces drug errors. Exec Solutions *Healthcare Manag* 2:1.

Johnson ST, Brown GC, Shea KM, 2002. Reengineering a pharmacist intervention program. *Am J Health-Syst Pharm* 59:916.

Joint Commission on Accreditation of Healthcare Organizations a. 2011a. Facts about the Joint Commission on Healthcare Organizations. Available at www.jointcommission.org/about_us/about_the_joint_commission_main.aspx; accessed on June 13, 2011.

Joint Commission on Accreditation of Healthcare Organizations a. 2011b. Hospital: 2011 National Patient Safety Goals. Available at http://www.jointcommission.org/hap_2011_npsgs/; accessed on June 13, 2011.

Kiel PJ, McCord AD. 2005. Pharmacist impact on clinical outcomes in a diabetes disease management program via collaborative practice. *Ann Pharmacother* 39: 1828–32.

Kohn L. 2000. To err is human: An interview with the Institute of Medicine's Linda Kohn. *Joint Comm J Qual Improv* 26:227.

Kozma CM, Reeder CE, Schultz RM, 1993. Economic, clinical and humanistic outcomes: A planning model for pharmacoeconomic research. *Clin Ther* 15:1121.

Krass I, Taylor SJ, Smith C, et al. 2005. Impact on mediation use and adherence of Australian pharmacists' diabetes care services. *J Am Pharm Assoc* 45:33–40.

Lazarus IR, Butler K. 2001. The promise of six sigma, part 1. *Manag Healthcare Exec* 10:22.

Lazarus IR, Stamps B. 2002. The promise of six sigma, part 2. *Manag Healthcare Exec* 1:27.

Leal S, Herrier RN, Glover JJ, Felix A. 2004. Improving quality of care in diabetes through a comprehensive pharmacist-based disease management program. *Diabetes Care* 27:2983–4.

Leape LL. 1994. Error in medicine. *JAMA* 272:1851.

Leape LL, Kabcenell A, Berwick DM, et al. 1998a. Change concepts for reducing adverse drug events. In *Reducing Adverse Drug Events: Breakthrough Series Guide*, p. 49. Boston: Institute for Healthcare Improvement.

Leape LL, Kabcenell A, Berwick DM, et al. 1998b. Achieving breakthrough improvement in reducing adverse drug events. In Reducing Adverse Drug Events: Breakthrough Series Guide, p. 79. Boston: Institute for Healthcare Improvement.

Leape LL, Kabcenell A, Berwick DM, et al. 1998c. A step-by-step guide to reducing adverse drug events. In *Reducing Adverse Drug Events: Breakthrough Series Guide.* Boston: Institute for Healthcare Improvement, p. 13.

Leapfrog. 2003. *The Leapfrog Group for Patient Safety: Rewarding Higher Standards.* The Leapfrog Group. Available at www.leapfroggroup.org/about.htm; accessed on 23 May 2003. www.leapfroggroup.org/about_us

Leapfrog Web site. Leapfrog Hospital Survey. Available at www.leapfroggroup.org/about_us; accessed on June 13, 2011.

Lee JK, Grace KA, Taylor AJ, 2006. Effect of a pharmacy care program on medication adherence and persistence, blood pressure, and low-density lipoprotein cholesterol: A randomized, controlled trial (see Comment). *JAMA* 296:2563–71.

Lohr KE. 1990a. Health, health care, and quality of care. In *Medicare: A Strategy for Quality Assurance.* Washington, DC: National Academy Press, p. 19.

Lohr KE. 1990b. Concepts of assessing, assuring, and improving quality. In *Medicare: A Strategy for Quality Assurance.* Washington, DC: National Academy Press, p. 45.

Lovern E. 2001. Minding hospitals' business: Purchasing coalition pushes hospitals to improve patient safety through process measures, but industry says standards are too expensive. *Mod Healthcare* 31:30.

Mangiapane S, Schulz M, et al. 2005. Community pharmacy-based pharmaceutical care for asthma patients. *Ann Pharmacother* 39:1817–22.

Merriam-Webster. 2003. *Merriam-Webster Dictionary.* Springfield, MA: Merriam-Webster.

Nagel DC. 1988. Human error in aviation operations. In Nagel DC (ed), *Human Factors in Aviation*, p. 263. New York: Academic Press.

National Association of Boards of Pharmacy (NABP). 2010. NABP Community Pharmacy Accreditation Program to Focus on Patient Care Available at www.nabp.net/news/nabp-community-pharmacy-accreditation-program-to-focus-on-patient-care/; accessed on June 13, 2011.

National Center for Patient Safety (NCPS). 2011a. Healthcare failure mode and effect analysis. Available at www.patientsafety.gov/CogAids/HFMEA/index.html#page=page-1; accessed on June 13, 2011.

National Center for Patient Safety (NCPS). 2011b. *NCPS Triage Cards for Root Cause Analysis.* Available at www.patientsafety.gov/CogAids/Triage/index.html# page=page-1; accessed on June 13, 2011.

National Committee for Quality Assurance (NCQA). 2003. *NCQA Overview.* Washington, DC: NCQA.

National Committee for Quality Assurance (NCQA). 2007. Accreditation, certification and recognition. Available at http://web.ncqa.org/tabid/58/Defalt.aspx; accessed on June 25, 2007.

National Committee for Quality Assurance (NCQA). 2011. HEDIS & Quality Measurement. Available at http://www.ncqa.org/tabid/59/Default.aspx; accessed on June 13, 2011.

Nolan TW. 2000. System changes to improve patient safety. *Br Med J* 320:771.

O'Malley C. 1997. Quality measurement for health systems: Accreditation and report cards. *Am J Health-Syst Pharm* 54:1528.

Ovretveit J. 1992. *Health Service Quality.* Oxford, England: Blackwell Scientific.

Ovretveit J. 2001. Quality evaluation and indicator comparison in health care. *Int J Health Plan Manag* 16:229.

Park KS. 1997. Human error. In Salvendy G (ed), *Handbook of Human Factors and Ergonomics.* New York: Wiley-Interscience, p. 150.

Pharmacy Guild of Australia. 2011. Quality Care Pharmacy Program. Available at; www.guild.org.au/NSW_Branch/Professional_Services/Quality_Care_Pharmacy_Program/Quality±Care±Pharmacy±Program.page; accessed on June 13, 2011.

Pharmacy Quality Alliance (PQA). 2011a. PQA. Available at www.PQAAlliance.org; accessed on June 13, 2011.

Pharmacy Quality Alliance (PQA). 2011b. PQA Measures Available at www.pqaalliance.org/measures.htm; accessed on June 13, 2011.

Pharmacy Quality Alliance (PQA). 2011c. EPIQ Flier. Available at www.pqaalliance.org/files/EPIQ-Flyer_MAR 2010.pdf; accessed on June 13, 2011.

Ragucci KR, Fermo JD, Wessell AM, et al. 2005. Effectiveness of pharmacist-administered diabetes mellitus education and management services. *Pharmacotherapy* 25:1809–16.

Rasmussen J, Pejtersen AM, Goodstein LP, 1994. *Cognitive Systems Engineering.* New York: Wiley.

Rogers B. 1997. Preventing medication errors. *Healthplan* 38:27.

Rupp MT, McCallian DJ, Sheth KK, 1997. Developing and marketing a community pharmacy-based asthma management program. *J Am Pharm Assoc* NS37:694.

Sadik A, Yousif M, McElnay JC, 2005. Pharmaceutical care of patients with heart failure. *Br J Clin Pharmacol* 60:183–93.

Schnipper JL, Kirwin JL, Cotugno MC, et al. 2006. Role of pharmacist counseling in preventing adverse drug events after hospitalization. *Arch Intern Med* 166:565–71.

Schulz M, Verheyen F, Muhlig S, et al. 2001. Pharmaceutical care services for asthma patients: A controlled intervention study. *J Clin Pharmacol* 41:668–76.

Scott DM, Boyd ST, Stephan M, et al. 2006. Outcomes of pharmacist-managed diabetes care services in a community health center. *Am J Health-Syst Pharm* 63:2116–22.

Shane R, Gouveia WA. 2000. Developing a strategic plan for quality in pharmacy practice. *Am J Health-Syst Pharm* 57:470.

Sheridan TB. 1988. The system perspective. In Nagel DC (ed), *Human Factors in Aviation.* New York: Academic Press, p. 27.

Shortell SM, Bennett CL, Byck GR, 1998. Assessing the impact of continuous quality improvement on clinical practice: What it will take to accelerate progress. *Milbank* Q 76:593.

Shortell SM, O'Brien JL, Hughes EF, et al. 1994. Assessing the progress of TQM in U.S. hospitals: Findings from two studies. *Q Lett Healthcare Lead* 6:14.

Sookaneknun P, Richards RM, Sanguansermsri J, et al. 2004. Pharmacist involvement in primary care improves hypertensive patient clinical outcomes. *Ann Pharmacother* 38:2023–8.

URAC. 2007. Pharmacy Benefit Management. Available at www.urac.org/programs/pbm.aspx; accessed on June 13, 2011.

van Bokhoven MA, Kok G, Vander Weijden T, 2003. Designing a quality improvement intervention: A systematic approach. *Qual Saf Health Care* 12:215.

Vrijens B, Belmans A, Matthys K, et al. 2006. Effect of intervention through a pharmaceutical care program on patient adherence with prescribed once-daily atorvastatin. *Pharmacoepidemiol Drug Saf* 15:115–21.

von Bertalanffy L. 1968. *General Systems Theory: Foundations, Development, Application.* New York: George Braziller.

Warholak-Juarez T, Rupp MT, Salazar TA, et al. 2000. Effect of patient information on the quality of pharmacists' drug use review decisions. *J Am Pharm Assoc* 40:500.

Weinberger M, Murray MD, Marrero DG, et al. 2002. Effectiveness of pharmacist care for patients with reactive airways disease: A randomized, controlled trial (see Comment). *JAMA* 288:1594–602.

Weinstein MC, Fineberg HV. 1980. *Clinical Decision Analysis.* Philadelphia: Saunders.

APPENDIX 8A. CQI CYCLE CHECKLIST

Cycle Background

Focus description
Should describe practice setting, the portion of the medication use process where the focus occurs, and baseline data (if possible).

Focus importance
State why the focus is important.

Literature review
Relate the focus to the literature.

Goal
Global and specific goals should be clearly stated and relate to the focus described in background.

Cycle Methods

Intervention
Describe and justify the intervention made (if any) for this cycle.

Processes and outcomes measured
Describe and justify the processes and outcomes measured (should relate to goal).

Data-collection procedures
Measurement methods should be clearly described and appropriate.

Data analysis
Planned statistical analysis should be clearly described and appropriate.

Cycle measurement

Cycle results

Sample description
Type and size of sample should be clearly described.

Results presented
Results should be reported for each stated goal. Result presentation should include graphs and/or charts.

Cycle Conclusions and Recommendations

Conclusions
Describe the conclusions your team came to after examining the data.

Implications
Describe why these results are important and what actions need to take place.

Recommendations
Recommendations for additional CQI cycles in this area.

APPENDIX 8B. CQI PLANNING WORKSHEETS FOR A REASEARCH PROJECT

Research Planning Worksheet 1

Date of meeting: ________

Name and contact information of each team member present:

1. ______________________ 2. ______________________
3. ______________________ 4. ______________________
5. ______________________ 6. ______________________

Introduction

1. Brainstorm possible areas of study (list here). ______________________

2. Rank and select an area of focus from the list above.
3. Provide a detailed description of the area chosen for study.

Area or project: ______________________
Setting: ______________________
______________________ *Portion of the medication use process involved:*

Baseline data (if available): ______________________

4. State why the proposed project is important.

5. Relate the proposed project to the literature.

6. State the global goal of the project [*Hint:* Some options may include (1) discovery, (2) frequency estimation, and (3) measure of a change or a combination.] *Note:* Goal should relate to project stated in 3 above.

7. State the specific goal(s) of the project.

Methods

8. List possible interventions (some options may include reduce reliance on memory, simplify, standardize, use constraints or forcing functions, use protocols of checklists, improve access to information, decrease reliance on vigilance, reduce handoffs, differentiate, or automate).

9. Select best intervention to accomplish goals (listed in 7 above).

10. List process and/or outcome measures necessary to determine if goals were met.

11. Determine what data are all ready being collected and what measures exist.

12. Plan data collection methods [*Hint:* May choose from (1) inspection points, (2) focus groups, (3) monitoring for markers, (4) chart review, (5) observation, and (6) spontaneous report.]

13. Plan statistical analysis. Make sure you will collect all information needed.

14. Break the project into steps and detail practical considerations.

Step	Who	What	Where	When	How

15. Sketch preliminary timeline for project.

Timeline										
	Week									
Step	1	2	3	4	5	6	7	8	9	10

16. List challenges to be addressed before the next meeting

17. Assign a responsible party to address each challenge listed above.

Challenge	Person Responsible	Due Date
1.		
2.		
3.		

18. Set date for next team meeting. ______________________

Research Planning Worksheet 2

Date of meeting: ___________

Name and contact information of each team member present:

1. ______________________ 2. ______________________
3. ______________________ 4. ______________________
5. ______________________ 6. ______________________

Introduction/Methods Revision

1. Review materials from last meeting.
2. Review progress made.
3. Indicate plan changes, if needed.

____
____
____

4. Add additional steps and detail practical considerations, if needed:

Step	Who	What	Where	When	How

5. Discuss challenges solved during this report period.

Challenge	How It Was Solved	Lesson Learned

6. List challenges to be addressed before the next meeting.
   1. ______________________
   2. ______________________
   3. ______________________
   4. ______________________

7. Assign a responsible party to address each challenge listed above.

Challenge	Person Responsible	Due Date
1.		
2.		
3.		
4.		
5.		
6.		
7.		

8. Update the timeline for project.

Timeline										
	Week									
Step	1	2	3	4	5	6	7	8	9	10

9. Set date for next team meeting. ____

Note: This worksheet can be used for several team meetings. Proceed to Worksheet 3 when data are collected.

Research Planning Worksheet 3

Date of meeting: __________

Name and contact information of each team member present:

1. ______________________ 2. ______________________
3. ______________________ 4. ______________________
5. ______________________ 6. ______________________

Measurement

1. Just do it!

Results

2. Analyze data.
3. Describe sample type and size.

4. Describe a result for each specific goal.

Conclusions and Recommendations

5. Describe conclusions the group reached after examining the results.

6. Why are these results important, and what actions need to take place?

7. What are the team's recommendations for this project?

8. What are the team's recommendations for the next project?

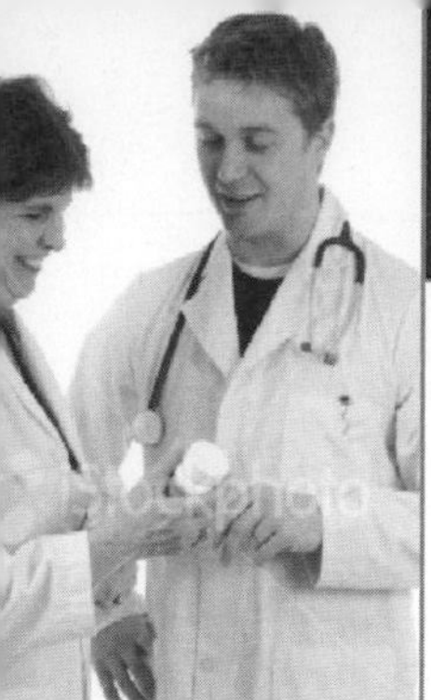

9

OUTCOMES EVALUATION OF PHARMACY OPERATIONS

Michelle A. Chui

About the Author: Dr. Chui is currently an assistant professor at the University of Wisconsin in Madison, Wisconsin. She earned a B.A. in biological sciences from the University of California—Davis, a Pharm.D. from Creighton University, and an M.S. and Ph.D. in pharmacy administration from Purdue University. Her research centers on applying human factors approaches and utilizing a systems perspective to characterizing community pharmacy practice and its practitioners to understand processes that impact medication safety and quality of care.

LEARNING OBJECTIVES

After completing this chapter, readers will be able to

1. Discuss the different facets of the ECHO model and their application to evaluating existing and proposed pharmacy goods, services, and operations.
2. Describe differences among the five types of economic analyses as tools for managerial decision-making.
3. List the advantages and disadvantages of the various methods of measuring humanistic outcomes, and describe the role that humanistic outcomes play in evaluating goods, services, and operations.
4. Identify the objectives of a service and determine the types of outcomes a pharmacist would need to measure in a pharmacy-related service.
5. Identify the advantages and disadvantages of the various methods used to collect data when evaluating services.
6. List and describe the uses of various outcomes evaluations and assessments.

SCENARIO

Cynthia Marshall is a pharmacist who works at a closed-staff-model health maintenance organization (HMO) pharmacy. Pharmacists at this clinic have access to patient charts that can be used to supplement information given by the patient to the pharmacy staff and what is written on the prescription. Cynthia enjoys working at this pharmacy because she feels that the added information is helpful when she is assessing and counseling her patients. She also believes that the HMO she works for values high-quality health care and is seeking to improve its ratings on some of its quality indicators.

Cynthia sees a number of heart failure patients every month. These patients see their physicians (including primary care physician, cardiac specialist, and frequently one or two other specialists) annually. Many times, these physicians do not coordinate care or know about the other medications that her heart failure patients are taking. She notices that these patients can improve or deteriorate quickly, have a difficult time remembering the complicated medication regimen they are on, and that their health conditions frequently change from month to month. They occasionally complain that their symptoms get so bad that they have to go to the emergency room. She thinks that these patients could have better outcomes if they were better educated about their conditions and monitored more closely.

Cynthia approaches the cardiologists in her clinic with an idea that she could start a heart failure clinic to provide additional education and monitoring for these patients. While the physicians would oversee the clinic, she could conduct monthly educational seminars about heart failure for patients, order and assess laboratory tests, order medications and adjust dosages under physician-approved protocols, and communicate with patients' other physicians about concurrent medications to prevent medication errors.

The HMO is also supportive, as their administrators recognize that Cynthia's clinic may contribute to higher scores on their quality indicators ratings related to heart failure. Given the HMO's patient load, Cynthia figures that she would have to spend 50 percent of her time with the heart failure clinic. Because the pharmacy is always busy, the HMO would have to hire an additional part-time pharmacist to take care of her dispensing duties.

CHAPTER QUESTIONS

1. Why is it important to measure baseline data for individual patients and/or a cohort of patients before initiating a new service?
2. How can outcomes be used to prove the value of your service?
3. How do pharmacists use outcomes measures to assess the success of their services?
4. What type of economic analysis would be appropriate to evaluate the service described in the scenario? How should the costs and outcomes be measured?
5. Why is it important to choose a perspective for the analysis prior to starting a project? How do perspectives differ?

INTRODUCTION

Pharmacists make many contributions that improve the lives of their patients on a daily basis. These contributions range from catching a drug–drug interaction, counseling a patient about his or her medication, or providing immunizations. To keep up with a transitioning profession and evershrinking margins, pharmacies must persistently evaluate its services and the resources that they use to provide those services (e.g., automated dispensing system, bar code scanning) to determine if they contribute to patient satisfaction, allow pharmacists to provide optimal care, and are cost-effective. In addition to evaluating the services and programs that pharmacists are already typically offering, pharmacists frequently conceptualize opportunities to provide a new service, such as the heart failure clinic proposed by Cynthia Marshall in the scenario.

While many pharmacists would like to offer services that would improve the quality of care to their patients, they can have upfront costs that cannot be ignored. How can pharmacists provide these services and show that they both help their patients and actually decrease the overall cost of care? Many studies have been conducted that show that pharmacists can make a difference both in cost and in the quality of their patients' lives (Perez et al., 2009; Boyd and Briggs, 2009). How can Cynthia Marshall do the same in her situation?

FRAMING THE QUESTION

How does one begin documenting the value of a pharmacy program or service? The first step is to define the problem being addressed. Stating the problem upfront seems rather obvious, but it is not always done. Many pharmacists waste time and energy trying to answer poorly defined questions. For example, one can start with a very broadly defined problem such as heart failure, which arises from a combination of factors and results in numerous health outcomes. Evaluating all the possible causes and effects of heart failure may be an overwhelming task, so the problem should be narrowed. One could evaluate the effect of medication adherence in patients with heart failure or even one particular outcome of heart failure (e.g., blood pressure or quality of life). The more narrow the problem, the easier it will be to address. Once having identified one or more worthy problems, the pharmacist will need to prioritize which one should be the focus of the service. These criteria may be useful in determining which service or program will provide the most impact and demonstrate success.

- Impact: Is the service properly aimed to help the greatest number of high-risk heart failure patients?
- Improvability: To what extent will the service improve the most appropriate aspects of care in a heart failure patient?

After the problem has been stated, the next step is to define the objectives. A very broad problem will result in broadly defined objectives. If heart failure is broadly identified as the problem, an objective could be to reduce the number of patients with heart failure. However, no specific method of reducing heart failure is addressed, and heart failure itself has many potential outcomes. On the other hand, if the problem is addressed more narrowly, a more specific objective could be studied. For example, one may look to reduce the number of heart failure exacerbations related to nonadherence with medications. In addition, other specific objectives may be included, such as increasing the quality of life of patients with heart failure, reducing the number of medications used by patients with heart failure, or making patients more aware of behavioral and dietary modifications related to heart failure.

All objectives, regardless of whether they are broad or narrow, must be measurable. While this also may seem obvious, many objectives (especially if they are broadly defined) can be difficult, if not impossible, to measure. The broad objective of reducing heart failure may be difficult to measure because so many factors must be considered when arriving at a diagnosis of heart failure. On the other hand, specific objectives such as reducing blood pressure or improving quality of life in patients with heart failure are much easier to quantify and measure.

The third step is to establish a framework to evaluate the question. When establishing the framework, pharmacists need to know some basic facts about the programs and diseases they are studying. Pharmacists undertaking these projects first should prioritize their objectives by determining what interventions and outcomes most need to be evaluated. For example, Cynthia Marshall may wish to determine the effect of her monitoring program on cost of care (an economic outcome), blood pressure or adherence to heart failure medication (clinical outcomes), and quality of life (a humanistic outcome).

These steps are not dissimilar from evaluating more common or "traditional" services and resources such as an automated dispensing system, or a refill reminder or patient satisfaction program. That is, the pharmacist must determine the objectives, or main outcomes of the program, determine the number of patients involved, or who could be involved, and appropriate parameters for estimating its impact.

SELECTING THE VARIABLES TO MEASURE

Many health care organizations make the mistake of focusing on only one area of care when trying to reduce the overall cost of health care. Evaluating the cost of a single aspect of patient care in isolation from all other aspects is commonly known as *component management.* Examples of component management include focusing on the costs of drugs or laboratory tests without looking at the impact of these costs on overall health care costs or outcomes. Unfortunately, many studies have focused on just one type of cost without considering the overall care of patients. Studies have suggested that while organizations can reduce drug use and costs used for chronic conditions, these reductions may be accompanied by an increased use of other health care services (Austvoll-Dahlgren et al., 2008). For instance, Kaiser-Permanente of Northern California compared the clinical and economic outcomes of beneficiaries whose annual drug benefit was capped at $1,000 with those with unlimited drug benefits. A cap on drug benefits was associated with lower drug consumption but poorer adherence and control of blood pressure, lipid levels, and glucose levels. Savings in drug cost was offset by increases in costs of emergency department visits and hospitalizations (Hsu et al., 2006).

Disease management strives to consider all individual components of health care for a specific disease with a view toward an outcome that is important for successful management of that disease. Instead of dealing with one element at a time (such as prescription costs, only), disease management attempts to control the disease by integrating the components of health care to provide the best total patient outcomes at the most reasonable cost. As a result, the number of variables measured in this paradigm is greater and more global. When making changes to one component of health care, other components are considered as well (Armstrong and Langley, 1996; Patterson, 1995; Zitter, 1994).

When identifying economic, clinical, and humanistic variables to be measured, it is important to integrate elements from all components of health care. In our example, Cynthia is trying to manage her patients' heart failure medications. Because she is a pharmacist, she may identify only medication-related variables to measure, such as cost of the drug or number of prescriptions filled. When evaluating this project with an eye toward disease management, one could also measure hospitalizations, emergency department visits, laboratory costs, physician visits, and other factors related to the care of these patients if those variables are available to her.

Because the heart failure clinic may require more work and personnel hours, and because other pharmacy staff may be impacted by the clinic, Cynthia could also include variables that would measure employee productivity and satisfaction. For example, all pharmacists working in the pharmacy may feel that a heart failure clinic would improve patient care, but if pharmacists perceive that their workload is high, they may not be able to effectively or happily help Cynthia recruit patients or cover her while she is working in the clinic. Cynthia, not wanting to assume that current services and programs (such as a refill request program) may be working as originally conceptualized, could also assess the effectiveness of current services and programs to determine if both patients and pharmacy staff have responded well to their implementation, and if they are achieving their goals (e.g., increase patient satisfaction and loyalty, increase prescription count, add to the variety of challenging work that pharmacists do) and if they might positive or negatively impacts the success of her clinic.

It is also important to be cognizant of the quality indicators that might be related to your service of interest. In this case, the HMO that Cynthia works for is interested in improving their heart failure indicator scores. The indicators that they would like to see improved are:

- Greater proportion of heart failure patients taking an angiotensin-converting enzyme inhibitor (ACEI)
- Evidence of disease management education for all heart failure patients
- Greater proportion of heart failure patients taking a beta-blocker
- Reduced proportion of heart failure patients taking a calcium-channel blocker
- Reduced proportion of heart failure patients taking a Type I antiarrhythmic agent
- Regular monitoring for digoxin toxicity
- Appropriate anticoagulation for patients with heart failure and atrial fibrillation (Fonarow, 2001).

At the point where one is determining which outcomes will be measured, one also should be keeping in mind the perspective of those to whom the outcomes of the intervention will be of value. While practically any disease management project can be evaluated from the perspective of the patient (e.g., Did the patient's health and quality of life improve? Did the patient save money?), there are other important perspectives whose outcomes could be considered as well (Drummond et al., 1986). These perspectives include that of the health care provider (e.g., Did the job satisfaction of the pharmacist improve as a result of providing the service?), the department (e.g., Did the program result in lower drug costs to the pharmacy?), the organization (e.g., Did the program result in decreased costs of caring for heart failure patients for the HMO?), and even society (e.g., Did the program reduce the prevalence of heart failure in the community?). Not every outcome from every perspective needs to be considered in each evaluation. Pharmacists should revisit their original question, objectives, and framework when determining which variables from which perspectives should be measured.

IDENTIFYING CONFOUNDING VARIABLES THAT CAN AFFECT OUTCOMES

After identifying a question, objectives, and variables to evaluate, pharmacists also need to think about other variables that may affect the results of the study. For example, Cynthia Marshall may wish to evaluate the impact of her monitoring service on the cost of caring for these patients from the perspective of the HMO, her employer. The results may show that patients who used her service had much lower costs of care compared with those who did not. Based just on this finding, one might jump to the conclusion that the service is an effective way to reduce the cost of caring for heart failure patients. However, on further examination, it may be discovered that many of the patients receiving the service had mild-to-moderate heart failure and only had one to two other disease states. In comparison, those who declined to participate may have had moderate-to-severe heart failure and multiple disease states.

Does this mean that the service did not have a positive effect? Actually, it means that the results are unclear. The severity of heart failure and number of disease states may have clouded the results of the study. For example, the service may not have saved the HMO any money, but the fact that those who used the service (less severely ill patients) generally had lower costs of care than those who did not use the service (more severely ill patients) may have made it look that way.

AN EARLY REVISIT TO THE SCENARIO

Cynthia would like to implement a new service that would manage the medications taken by the HMO's heart failure patients. The questions that the HMO is asking include, "How much will the service cost?", "Will hospitalizations and emergency department visits be reduced?", and "Will this improve our rating/score on related quality indicators?" Cynthia has additional questions: "Will I be able to increase my patients' health-related quality of life?" and "Will my patients be better satisfied with the quality of pharmacist care than with the care they currently receive?"

Cynthia's objectives are to reduce hospitalizations and emergency department visits by increasing adherence to heart failure medications and educating patients about their disease state and how to make diet and behavioral modifications, as well as improve patients' health-related quality of life and satisfaction with care.

Her examination of the literature about heart failure has given her some information about what types of information she should collect. Patients with heart failure show symptoms of decreased exercise tolerance, shortness of breath, increased fatigue, and fluid buildup in the lungs and tissues. Patients with heart failure are classified clinically by their level of disability so that they may be followed longitudinally and provide a reference point when compared with other patients (New York Heart Association [NYHA, Criteria Committee, 1973]).

Cynthia also has discovered that heart failure is the most common hospital discharge diagnosis in individuals over age 65. Median survival rate from the time of diagnosis is 1.7 years in men and 3.2 years in women (Ho et al., 1993). Cynthia knows that she also will have to collect some demographic data that could impact the results of her program, such as age, gender, marital status, ethnicity, income level, and mental status.

ECHO MODEL

Outcomes evaluations attempt to identify, measure, and evaluate the end results of health care services. Outcomes evaluation examines not only the clinical effects of health care services but also the economic and humanistic impact of these services, such as quality of life and satisfaction (Bootman et al., 1996). From an increasing consumerism perspective, and with regard to resources becoming more scarce, evaluation of these types of outcomes are increasingly important. The economic, clinical, and humanistic outcomes (ECHO) model assumes that the outcomes of medical care can be classified along the three dimensions of economic, clinical, and humanistic outcomes (Kozma et al., 1993). *Clinical outcomes* are defined as medical events that occur as a result of disease or treatment. *Economic outcomes* are defined as the direct, indirect, and intangible costs compared with the consequences of medical treatment alternatives. *Humanistic outcomes* are defined as the consequences of disease or treatment on patient functional status or quality of life. All three of these outcomes need to be balanced simultaneously to assess value.

Economic Outcomes

Traditional cost-containment measures are not always consistent with improved patient care. Thus attention has turned toward demonstrating the value of health care, overall. A full evaluation of relevant costs and consequences would provide significantly more information that simply looking at traditional cost-containment strategies. *Costs* are defined as the value of the resources consumed by a program or treatment alternative. These include direct costs, or the resources consumed in prevention, detection, or treatment of a disease, nonmedical costs such as transportation to medical facilities or special diet considerations. Indirect costs include loss of productivity at work (such as when a patient is absent from work because of a migraine, or working but is suffering from depression), and intangible costs are things like pain, suffering, and grief. *Consequences* are defined as the effects, outputs, and outcomes of the program or treatment alternative (Eisenberg, 1989).

The economic evaluation of medical care may occur from many perspectives. These perspectives, or viewpoints, will influence the costs and consequences identified, measured, and compared for a program or treatment alternative. An economic evaluation can be conducted from a single perspective or multiple perspectives. Common perspectives are those of the patient, health care professional, insurer, and society. There are subtle differences between perspectives. A patient may be extremely concerned with his or her quality of life, level of pain, ability to see health care professionals, or how much time is spent in the hospital or nursing home, in addition to the actual direct costs of health care. However, an insurer may be interested only in the direct costs of health care to its organization. In fact, while a patient who is at the end of his or her life may be interested in extending life as long as possible, an insurer may see this as an expensive prospect.

There are also differences between the insurer's and societal perspectives. Many insurers assume that patients will not be covered on their plans throughout their lifetime, so expensive interventions that provide benefits in the very long term tend to be discouraged (i.e., screening programs for diseases that manifest in the elderly). However, from a societal perspective, these screenings may be appropriate because they identify patients at risk earlier. In the long run, such screenings are beneficial to society.

Types of Economic Evaluations

The basic task of economic evaluations is to identify, measure, value, and compare the costs and consequences of the alternatives being considered. Therefore, a full economic evaluation must have two features: a comparison of two or more alternatives and both the costs and consequences of the alternatives being examined.

Cost-minimization analysis is a tool used to compare two or more treatment alternatives that are assumed to be equal in efficacy. It simply compares the direct and indirect costs of treatment alternatives in dollars and does not consider the outcomes of the treatments (because they are assumed to be the same). Examples could be to compare the costs of intravenous versus oral dosage forms of the same drug or hospital versus home administration of intravenous pain management.

Cost-benefit analysis is used when outcomes can be expressed in monetary terms, such as in the amount of money an HMO might save if it implements a new program. The direct and indirect costs of a program or intervention are measured as they occur, and the benefits accrued from the program or intervention are identified and converted into dollars in the year in which they occur. These two values are then expressed as a ratio of the dollar value of the costs of the program or intervention to the dollar value of the outcomes that arose as a result of the program or intervention. For example, if the cost associated with new heart failure monitoring service were $100 per patient and, as a result of the service, the HMO saved $1,000 in hospital care per patient, the cost-benefit ratio would be expressed as the benefit, $1,000, divided by the cost, $100, or as 10:1. This ratio would be interpreted such that the service produces $10 of benefits for every $1 that is spent. The results may also be interpreted by subtracting the costs from the benefits or, in our example, as a $900 net benefit per patient.

Cost-effectiveness analysis is used when the treatment alternatives are not therapeutically equivalent or when outcomes cannot be expressed in monetary units. Cost is measured in monetary units, and outcomes are expressed in terms of obtaining a specific therapeutic objective, such as cases cured, lives saved, or millimeters of mercury drop in blood pressure. Cost-effectiveness analysis allows researchers to summarize the health benefit and resources used by two or more competing programs so that policymakers can choose among them (Detsky and Nagiie, 1990; Doubilet, 1986). For example, pharmacy director, anticipating an increase in prescription count, may want to consider adding another technician or purchasing an automatic dispensing system (i.e., dispensing robot). The pharmacy director can estimate the number of prescriptions, and other duties that a technician can perform and compare those duties to what a dispensing robot can perform. Clearly there are more upfront costs to a robot (i.e., purchasing the equipment and training the staff), whereas the costs for a technician are variable and can change (i.e., the director can hire the technician part-time with the potential for more hours, if needed). Using a cost-effective analysis, the pharmacy director can create a ratio of the prescriptions filled to the hourly cost of the technician or the extrapolated hourly cost of the robot to determine which would be more cost effective for the pharmacy. Another example that Cynthia might consider is whether hospitalizations and emergency department visits would be reduced more with a heart failure clinic or an asthma clinic. The therapeutic objective in this example would be a decrease in hospitalizations or emergency department visits, and the costs would primarily be Cynthia's personnel time at work.

Cost-utility analysis is used when quality of life is the most important outcome being examined. This is common in disease states in which how one feels or what one can do is more important than a clinical laboratory value or economic outcome (e.g., chronic diseases such as heart disease, diabetes, arthritis, cancer, or HIV/AIDS). Cost-utility analyses compare the direct and indirect costs of an intervention with some measurable level of humanistic outcome, such quality of life or level of satisfaction. Quality of life often is measured in quality-adjusted life years (QALYs).

ANOTHER VISIT TO THE SCENARIO

To determine what type of analysis to conduct, Cynthia must identify all the costs related to her project. She created a table to identify all possible costs from every perspective (see Table 9-1).

Table 9-1. Costs of Heart Failure

Direct Medical Costs	Direct Nonmedical Costs	Indirect Costs	Intangible Costs
Medications	Special food	Missing work	Pain
Hospitalizations	Transportation	Lost productivity	Suffering
Physician visits	Burden on family	Premature death	Grief

When determining which method of economic analysis she should use, she eliminated cost-minimization analysis because the treatment alternatives (service versus no service) will not result in equivalent outcomes. A cost-effectiveness analysis would not be appropriate because she is interested only in one particular program. A cost-utility analysis is also not appropriate because quality of life, while included in the project, is not the focus of her project. A cost-benefit analysis could be appropriate. A cost-benefit analysis requires that both the interventions and outcomes be valued in monetary units. She can determine the direct medical and/or nonmedical costs for each patient from data captured by her HMO. The HMO is very interested in costs, both those to implement the service and those it may save as a result. Cynthia decides that the most understandable analysis to present to the HMO is a cost-benefit analysis.

Uses of Economic Outcomes

Many benefits can be realized by applying pharmacoeconomic principles and methods to evaluating pharmacy services and programs. Economic assessments can assist in balancing cost and outcome when determining the most efficient use of health care goods and services. Economic assessments are helpful in optimizing clinical decision making. Decisions involving formulary management, practice guidelines, drug policy, individual patient treatment, and resource allocation are all amenable to economic assessments.

Decision analysis is a technique used in economic evaluations to structure the analysis. It is a systematic way of describing decision problems, identifying possible courses of action, assessing the probability and value of outcomes, and making a calculation to select the optimal course of action. A tool used in decision analysis is a decision table or decision tree. A *decision tree,* shown in Fig. 9-1, allows you to display graphically all treatment alternatives being compared, the relevant outcomes associated with these alternatives, and the probabilities of these outcomes occurring in a patient population. It can allow for the algebraic conversion of all these variables into one summary measurement, often a cost-effectiveness ratio, to allow for a meaningful comparison of two or more treatment alternatives (Barr and Schumacher, 1994; Crane, 1988).

In economic evaluations, there is a need to make assumptions about the variables in the analysis. For instance, assumptions that are made commonly include the incidence of adverse effects, the drug's efficacy (in clinical trials) and effectiveness (use in actual practice), and the costs of drugs or other direct medical costs. Assumptions that you might make about a current pharmacy service (such as a prescription delivery service, or an adherence program in which you put a patients' prescription in pill boxes) might be how many patients will use a service, what patients might be willing to pay for a service, or how much pharmacist time will need to be allocated to the service. It is important to keep in mind that assumptions are simply *predictions* about what might happen as a result of a

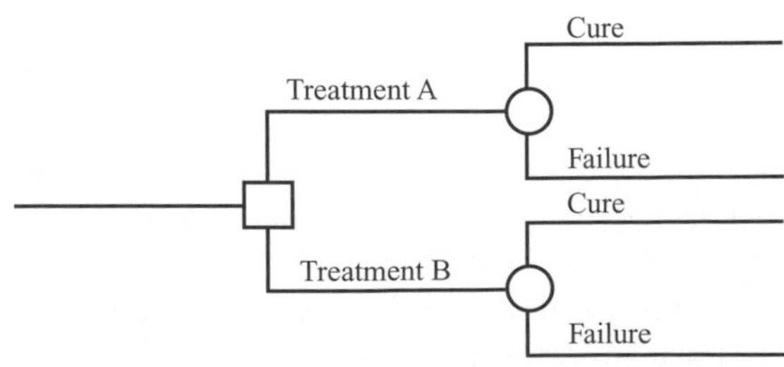

Figure 9-1. Decision tree.

program or intervention. To account for the variety of outcomes that may arise in any intervention, one might use a technique known as *sensitivity analysis.* a sensitivity analysis, identifies one parameter, hold other evaluation parameters constant, and recalculate the results using a range of the chosen parameter. The results of a sensitivity analysis can determine if the outcome of the study is "sensitive" to ranges in the chosen parameter. If changing the values of specific variables does not substantially alter the results, there is more confidence in the original findings.

For example, if the pharmacist decided to promote and add food tours in a grocery store pharmacy to patients with diabetes, he or she might want to measure if patients transfer their prescriptions to your pharmacy and continue to use your pharmacy. It is estimated that 80 percent of the individuals given food tours will start filling their prescriptions in the pharmacy. That would increase prescription count, which would be used to justify the amount of time required to provide the food tours. In a sensitivity analysis, one might test whether your service would still be cost effective if only 60 percent of food tour recipients start coming to your pharmacy.

Clinical Outcomes

To health care professionals, the most obvious variables that should be addressed when evaluating any medical intervention are clinical outcomes. Any program or service can assert that patients will receive better care if given that service. Clinical outcomes vary with each disease state but should include any pertinent medications [e.g., prescription, over-the-counter (OTC), and herbal], any side effects or adverse effects from the disease state or medications, any laboratory values used, the documented physical state, and any use of other health care professionals or services.

■ BACK TO THE SCENARIO

At Cynthia's pharmacy, patients with heart disease are usually on several medications for their heart disease: a diuretic, a beta-blocker, and an angiotensin-converting enzyme (ACE) inhibitor. Patients with more severe disease may also be on an aldosterone inhibitor such as spironolactone, digoxin, hydralazine nitrate, and/or an angiotensin receptor-blocker (ARB). Some patients are also on oxygen. Patients are also required to submit to frequent laboratory testing for potassium and serum creatinine levels. They are assessed for blood pressure, weight, level of edema, and shortness of breath and then are assigned a NYHA classification (I, II, III, or IV). For the pharmacy's heart failure service, each of these pieces of clinical data would be recorded at baseline and at each subsequent visit by the pharmacist. Other clinical markers that Cynthia would like to measure include the incidence of medication side effects and adverse drug reactions.

Humanistic Outcomes

Quality of life refers to an evaluation of all aspects of our lives, including where we live, how we live, how we play, and how we work. Health-related quality of life (HRQoL) encompasses only those aspects of life which are dominated or influenced significantly by personal health or activities performed to maintain or improve health. HRQoL is defined as a multidimensional concept referring to a person's total well-being, including physical symptoms, functional ability, and perceptions. Advances in medical science have encouraged attention to HRQoL because medical care is no longer limited to providing only death-averting treatments (Coons and Kaplan, 1993). Indeed, if a pharmacist can provide information to a physician regarding an improvement in quality of life for his or her patients, the pharmacist could earn trust and loyalty, and build a collaborative relationship with a physician, which could then lead to further collaborations to improve patient care.

To evaluate aspects of HRQoL that are specific to a particular disease or condition, specific measures also may be used. Specific measures include only important aspects of HRQoL that are relevant to the patients being studied, such as the loss of function in asthma patients or the amount of pain in arthritis patients. Disadvantages of using specific measures are that they are not comprehensive and cannot be used to compare across conditions. They also cannot measure unforeseen side effects or conditions.

Another area of humanistic outcomes that may be even more important when measuring outcomes of pharmacy services is patient satisfaction. *Satisfaction* is defined as the extent to which individuals' needs and wants are met. This is linked with attitudes toward the health care system, as well as expectations and perceptions regarding the quantity and quality of care received.

During the last decade, the health care industry has begun to recognize the importance of satisfaction with services as patients became increasingly recognized as consumers. Consumer or patient satisfaction surveys have evolved from marketing tools to measures of quality. In fact, the level of satisfaction with medical care has been shown to be associated directly with willingness to adhere to medical recommendations, rates of switching medical care providers, and disenrollment from prepaid health plans (Cvengros et al., 2007). In addition, the degree of patient satisfaction has been negatively correlated with a willingness to initiate malpractice lawsuits, meaning that people who are less satisfied with their health care are more likely to sue their health care professionals (Stelfox et al., 2005).

Surveys specifically measuring both traditional pharmacy dispensing and counseling services, as well as disease state and medication management services provided in community pharmacies also have been developed. These surveys can be adapted for one or more specific programs that a pharmacist might want to implement and evaluate (MacKeigan and Larson, 1989; Tinelli et al., 2011; Van Geffen et al., 2011; Moczygemba at al., 2010).

Although economic and humanistic analyses usually have been conducted using the perspective of the insurance company, the perspective of patients' employers also have become more prevalent, particularly if an employer is working directly with a pharmacy to manage his employees' medications or providing immunizations or other wellness programs. To meet the evaluation needs of employers, work functioning can be measured as a humanistic outcome. Traditionally, work functioning has been measured as lost days from work (absenteeism). However, this measurement has become more specific and can be measured as reductions in productive capacity ("presenteeism"). Diseases that may cause reductions in work productivity include migraines, allergic rhinitis, and depression.

REVISITING THE SCENARIO

Cynthia has found that patients with heart failure report a number of physical symptoms that affect HRQoL, such as dyspnea, fatigue, anorexia, cachexia, edema, sleeplessness, attention deficit, and memory impairment. Functional abilities such as problems with social interactions, depression, and poor psychosocial adjustment also may affect this patient population. Furthermore, perceived health status has been found to be lower in the heart failure population when compared with other patient populations with chronic disease states (Juenger et al., 2002).

In addition to the analysis requested by the HMO, Cynthia is interested in measuring humanistic outcomes and thinks that it would be important to collect information on her patients' HRQoL, as well as clinical and economic measures. She chooses to use the SF-12 and the Chronic Heart Failure Questionnaire found in the literature to assess HRQoL (Guyatt et al., 1989). She also chooses to adapt some of the questions from a patient satisfaction survey developed by Tinelli et al. (2011) that measured satisfaction for a community pharmacy medication therapy management service in patients with coronary artery disease.

Cynthia is interested in measuring actual absenteeism from work as well as decreases in productivity owing to shortness of breath and fatigue. However, she acknowledges that these data would be difficult to obtain from patients and their employers, so she chooses not to collect data on these outcomes at this time.

DATA COLLECTION

Once the question, objectives, variables, and methods of analysis have been identified, one must determine how data will be collected for each of their variables.

While researchers can use a variety of sources and methods of data collection, health care professionals often can obtain most of their data from records they already maintain.

Partnerships with Other Health Care Entities

As pertinent variables are identified, it will become clear that some data will be easily obtainable, whereas information on other variables will be extremely difficult to acquire. Pharmacy-related data often are easily retrievable because much of the information can be obtained directly from the pharmacy's prescription computer program (and the patient profiles). Patient demographic information such as gender and age generally is also stored on the pharmacy computer. However, depending on the question, data from other areas of the health care system may need to be collected as well. For instance, one hypothesis could be that a pharmacy service may result in a reduction in emergency department visits. Unless pharmacists have access to an electronic medical record, they often do not have access to data on emergency department visits.

To obtain disease-related health data, it is helpful to develop partnerships with physician groups and hospitals that serve patients participating in a clinical pharmacy service. A partnership with physicians may allow pharmacists access to patient charts to collect disease-related health data (with patients' permission). A patient chart contains progress notes, laboratory values, referrals to specialists, and any other pertinent information about the patient. A patient chart could provide a complete picture of the patient and serve to show how a patient has improved under a pharmacist's care.

Another partnership that would be helpful is with insurers for health services. Insurance companies, HMOs, pharmacy benefits managers (PBMs), and government agencies such as Medicaid and the Veterans Administration generally maintain health care expenditure data for the patients for whom they pay for health services. Pharmacist interventions can be correlated with these health care expenditure data to determine the effectiveness of the intervention. For example, the numbers and costs of hospitalizations and emergency department visits for patients enrolled in a pharmacist-managed health program can be examined prior to the start of the program and again 1 year later.

ECONOMIC EVALUATION

Costs of goods and services seem intuitively simple to quantify. However, a number of potentially complicated issues must be considered. When identifying the goods or services, will the actual cost (wholesale cost) to the pharmacy or health care organization be measured, or will the charge to the patient or payer (retail cost) be measured? Sometimes access to cost data may be limited, or the data may be entirely unavailable. For instance, if Cynthia Marshall was using a hospital database to collect hospitalization and emergency department information for the HMO's heart failure patients, it may be impossible to isolate the actual costs related to heart failure, particularly if a patient was admitted for multiple reasons.

There are advantages and disadvantages to using different data sources. Primary data collection, in which data are collected solely for purposes of the project, are the best sources of data because one can request and generate exactly the information that is needed for the program. This is also helpful when it is important to see how a particular patient behaves or uses the health care system. For instance, if Cynthia changes a patient's drug regimen, she will want to collect data to determine if the patient becomes more compliant with his or her medications or has a better quality of life as a result. The disadvantage of primary data collection is that the data have to be collected manually as opposed to simply retrieving them from a database that already houses the information. Primary data collection can be time consuming and expensive.

A secondary data source, such as a hospital or HMO database, can be a useful resource. Secondary data sources are particularly useful when gathering economic data because there is usually a direct correlation with how much an insurance company is charged and how much the product or service actually costs to provide. A researcher or clinician also can examine the data on a large number of patients to see if an intervention

Table 9-2. Characteristics of HMO Heart Failure Patients Prior to the Start of the Heart Failure Clinic

	Number	Cost	Average Length of Stay
Hospitalizations	5/year	$500/day	5.6 days
Emergency room	7/year	$1000/visit	
Heart failure medications	3/month	$40/Rx	

actually affects a population of patients. A disadvantage of data such as these is that they are completely anonymous. There are no patient identifiers, and the data cannot be linked to individual patients. As a result, if one sample of patients patronizing one pharmacy is provided an intervention and another sample of patients is not, there is no way to detect economic change through the secondary data source.

BACK TO THE SCENARIO

Cynthia is using a secondary data source to conduct her cost-benefit analysis. After she has identified her variables of interest, she asks the HMO to provide her with baseline information on all heart failure patients prior to implementing her service. The HMO is able to stratify the data by diagnosis, so Cynthia asks for annual numbers and costs of hospitalizations, emergency room visits, and medications for their heart failure patients (see Table 9-2). She also asks for the data used to calculate the HMO's quality indicators on heart failure.

Cynthia forges ahead and begins her heart failure clinic. She successfully enrolls 250 patients in her service over the course of 1 year. At the end of the year, she conducts her cost-benefit analysis and asks the HMO for the same information that she collected at baseline (see Table 9-3).

Cynthia also must determine how much the clinic costs the HMO so that she can factor those costs into her analysis. She includes the salary and benefits of a part-time pharmacist to manage the service ($50,000) and the laboratory tests, supplies, and space costs necessary to monitor the patients ($72,000). Therefore, the direct cost of the clinic was $122,000 that year. The benefits of this service included decreases in the number of hospitalizations and average length of stay. Taken together, the total number of hospital days was reduced by an average of 7.2 days [(5 × 5.6) – (4 × 5.2)] for each of the 250 patients enrolled in the HMO and monitored by the service. If hospitalizations are assumed to cost the HMO $500 per day, the service saved the HMO $900,000 in hospitalizations (7.2 days × 250 patients × $500/day). The service also decreased the number of emergency department visits, resulting in savings of $250,000 ($1,000 × 1 visit × 250 patients). However, when Cynthia started to properly manage her heart failure patients, she found that they typically needed more medications to better manage their disease. The average number of prescription drugs for her patient population rose from three to four prescriptions per month, resulting in an increased expenditure of $10,000 ($40 × 1 prescription × 250 patients). When the costs and benefits are summed, the annual total cost of providing the service is $122,000, and the

Table 9-3. Characteristics of HMO Heart Failure Patients after the First Year of the Heart Failure Clinic

	Number	Cost	Average Length of Stay
Hospitalizations	4/year	$500/day	5.2 days
Emergency room	6/year	$1000/visit	
Heart failure medications	4/month	$40/Rx	

Table 9-4. Changes in Clinical Outcomes of Heart Failure Clinic Patients after One Year

	Showed Improvement	Remained Stable	Symptoms Worsened
Level of edema	45%	35%	20%
Blood pressure	24%	68%	8%
Patient weight	13%	84%	3%
NYHA classification	15%	79%	6%
Shortness of breath	67%	19%	14%

total benefits are $1,140,000 ($900,000 + $250,000 – $10,000). These results can be expressed as either a benefit-cost ratio of 9.3:1 ($1,140,000:$122,000) or a net benefit (cost savings) of $1,018,000. From this analysis, it appears that this service is valuable to the HMO.

Cynthia realizes that her analysis is only as strong as the variables that she has chosen to include. As a result, she decides to conduct a sensitivity analysis to ensure that her conclusions are sound. Some of the variables that she thinks may change the results of the project are the decreased number of hospitalizations, decreased length of stay, and decreased number of emergency department visits. She reexamines the data by taking half the difference in the number of hospital days and half the number of emergency department visits to see if the results change. The average number of hospital days per patient was decreased from 7.2 to 3.6 days, and the average of emergency department visits per patient was decreased from 1 to 0.5. As a result, hospitalizations cost savings were $450,000 (3.6 days × 250 patients × $500/day), and emergency department visits cost savings were $125,000 (0.5 visits × 250 patients × $1,000). This sensitivity analysis shows the total benefit to equal $565,000 ($450,000 + $125,000 – $10,000). The benefit-cost ratio drops to 4.6:1, and the net benefit is $443,000, but the service still clearly appears to be valuable to the HMO.

CLINICAL EVALUATION

Pharmacists have the ability to assess patients for general signs and symptoms of many disease states. In many states, pharmacists are also able to check blood glucose and lipid levels. They are able to measure peak flows in pulmonary patients and can assess minor skin abnormalities and wound care. All these clinical variables may be recorded at baseline and at each subsequent visit to chart changes and/or improvements in the patient's condition.

REVISITING THE SCENARIO

Cynthia has decided to collect information on each patient's level of edema, blood pressure, weight, NYHA classification, and shortness of breath. She also will record laboratory values where appropriate. When patients are enrolled in her clinic, she records baseline values of the variables listed. She sees each patient every month for the first 3 months. Patients continue to be seen monthly until both Cynthia and the patient agree that the patient is stable, and then they will see Cynthia every 3 months thereafter. At each clinic visit, Cynthia recorded the same values in the electronic medical record. At the end of the year, she compiled the data to show that her medication management and education program have provided clinical benefits to her patients (see Table 9-4). She also asks the HMO for the same data on all heart failure patients (not just the ones that enrolled in her clinic) in order to calculate the quality indicators for heart failure.

HUMANISTIC EVALUATION

Humanistic outcomes generally are obtained directly from patients in the form of standardized questionnaires. There are two steps when collecting humanistic information. First is to identify the best and most appropriate survey or surveys to use (general or specific), and second is to decide how to administer the HRQoL instruments or surveys.

The four main ways to administer surveys are self-administered, face-to-face, mail, and telephone. When patients self-administer the surveys, they can answer the questions on their own. They are sometimes more willing to be truthful with sensitive information, such as income. This method is the least expensive method. The downside of self-administered surveys is that patients sometimes do not finish the surveys and that some disease states make it difficult for patients to self-administer (e.g., glaucoma, rheumatoid arthritis, and Parkinson disease).

Mail surveys generally have the same advantages as self-administered surveys and can effectively reach a large number of people. However, it is often difficult to motivate people to complete the survey and return it without some form of incentive, and it is also more logistically complicated for the pharmacist who needs the data. Face-to-face interviews are effective in eliciting narrative responses and can be used with patients who lack good reading or writing skills, whose first language is not English, or who have difficulty seeing. The interviewer can gauge how the survey is going and can determine if the respondent is having difficulty understanding the items. On the other hand interviews take more time and the process can be very costly.

Telephone surveys have the same advantages of face-to-face interviews but tend to be less expensive. Researchers can survey individuals from a large geographic area, and data can be linked to a record management system that can track respondents. Unfortunately, researchers cannot reach respondents who do not have a telephone and whose first language is not English, and they cannot verify the identity of the respondent. Multiple calls may be needed to contact the individual, and visual aids cannot be used unless they are mailed to respondents in advance.

The advantages and disadvantages of each method of administration are important as the study is designed and the patient population is identified. If an indigent population is being studied, the telephone format may not be appropriate because that population may not have access to telephones. If a predominately Spanish-speaking population is being surveyed, face-to-face interviews with bilingual interviewers may be appropriate.

REVISITING THE SCENARIO

Cynthia feels that health-related quality of life and patient satisfaction are important aspects of her clinic. She thinks that these outcomes can serve to complement the economic and clinical outcomes that she is reporting to the HMO and can further prove her case that the clinic is a valuable service to the heart failure patients.

When patients enroll in the clinic, Cynthia assists them in completing the surveys. Most patients prefer to read the surveys and complete them at their own pace. Cynthia reads and records the survey information for those who are uncomfortable filling out the surveys individually. Through statistical analysis, she determines that there has been statistically significant change in all three quality-of-life measures over the course of the year (i.e., the SF-12, the Heart Failure Questionnaire, and the PSQ) and concludes that the clinic provides benefits from the patients' perspective.

DATA ASSESSMENT

After the data collection is completed, the data must be analyzed and assessed to interpret the results and reach meaningful conclusions. There are several ways to compile data so that they are easy to read and understand.

First, the service needs to be evaluated to determine if it provided a positive intervention for the patients. Prior to implementing the intervention, demographic, clinical, and humanistic information should have been collected. These are called *baseline data* because collection is done at the beginning of the intervention, prior to any changes. Collecting baseline data is extremely important, a task that health care professionals routinely forget to do prior to starting new programs or services.

After the program ends or has reached a predetermined point, the same pieces of information that were collected at baseline should be collected again. The data then are analyzed to determine if patient outcomes changed after enrolling in the clinic. Again, if baseline data were not collected, it becomes impossible to determine if changes in the values collected after the intervention were due to the intervention or to some other factor. For example, assume that a patient comes into a pharmacy and suggests that a new herbal remedy has caused her diabetes to get better. She says that she knows this because her blood sugar level is below 140 mg/dL. However, on further examination, she admits that she is not aware of what her blood sugar was prior to starting the herbal remedy. As a result, it is unclear whether the patient may have had blood sugar levels below 140 mg/dL prior to the remedy and to what extent, if any, the remedy provided any benefit.

Second, the financial impact of the service must be determined, keeping in mind the perspective of the analysis. For example, were the dollars saved from averted emergency department visit and hospitalization costs greater than the cost of implementing the clinic? Was the financial benefit to the patient worth the extra money he or she spent on the clinic? To perform these analyses, a sample of patients who participated in the clinic (intervention group) and a similar sample of patients (control group) who did not participate are needed. The total costs of health care between the two groups are compared to determine if there are differences. Total health care costs would include all hospitalizations, emergency department visits, physician visits, prescription medications, laboratory costs, and visits to the new clinic. To determine the benefit to the patient, various outcome variables are identified that measure change in patient status (e.g., humanistic outcomes such as HRQoL and decreases in side effects) and increases in patient satisfaction and/or clinical outcomes (e.g., blood pressure, edema, and blood sugar levels). These variables can be evaluated separately or compiled to form an outcome measure.

USES OF OUTCOMES EVALUATION

Assessment of Success or Failure of a Program or Service

After conducting an evaluation, the results may not be strongly in favor of a service. This does not necessarily mean that the service will be, or was a failure. There are many reasons why the results may be equivocal.

First, there may not have been enough patients for a complete evaluation. If the changes that are sought are small but clinically and economically significant, a larger number of patients may have been needed to detect statistically, or even clinically significant changes. The number of subjects needed to detect the impact of the interventions should be determined prior to starting the clinic. In biostatistics, this concept is commonly referred to as *power*.

Second, many outcomes depend on how much time passes since the intervention. Many changes, particularly for clinical outcomes, take time to occur. A literature review of similar interventions may help to identify how much time may be needed to detect a clinically significant change. For instance, patients with asthma can see almost immediate relief when they are provided appropriate education and long- and short-acting medications to treat exacerbations. Conversely, comparisons between patients being educated with smoking-cessation classes and those not receiving education will be much more long term. Decades may be required to determine if some interventions provide economic, clinical, and humanistic benefits.

If the clinic was implemented and the analysis was conducted only to find that the outcomes were not as anticipated, what should a pharmacist do? While some outcomes can be disappointing, it is important to seek explanations for what was found in the results. Was the appropriate amount of time spent developing the clinic? Was there appropriate marketing to the patients? Was there buy-in by other employees in the pharmacy? Even though these objective results are important, other intangible benefits may be equally or even more important. Developing a trusting relationship with physicians, promoting goodwill among patients or patient organizations, and encouraging patient loyalty to the pharmacy are equally important. Individuals in management, although focused on the numbers, should recognize that some benefits are not seen right away or directly. It is incumbent upon the pharmacist to be able to convey these benefits to management so that they recognize the value that your services and programs provide.

Contributing to the Quality Improvement Programs

Health care organizations, insurance companies, and health care professionals are now being rated for the quality of health care that they are providing. These ratings are made public so that patient can make informed choices, and are used by corporations and employers to choose which health care organization they want to use to provide health care to their employees. Many of the quality indicators that are being used are related to appropriate medication use and medication safety. So, pharmacists are in a unique position to provide value to a health care organization and their physicians seeking to improve their scores.

Development of Additional Services

Once a successful service has been developed, it becomes easier to develop a new service in the future. The skills necessary to evaluate the outcomes of a service can be leveraged to start a new service. Perhaps a similar service with a different disease state would be a good next step. Be careful when thinking of starting new projects that are not directly similar to the one already implemented. For instance, the skills gained with the heart failure clinic may not apply directly to starting a compounding specialty or wound care clinic.

To develop a new service, identify additional resources that will be required. More personnel, both for dispensing and for clinical functions, may be needed. More space for counseling, compounding, conducting classes, or placing diagnostic instruments or durable medical equipment also may be needed. Lastly, the way the pharmacy is perceived and marketed to the public may need some rethinking. If the pharmacy previously has dispensed only medications, the new services should be showcased, and the pharmacy can be marketed as a pharmacy with expanded patient care services.

A pharmacist will need to gain buy-in from management, fellow pharmacists, and physicians (see Chapters 4 and 5). Including the feedback and perspectives from colleagues and one's supervisor is essential to communicating the value of existing services and developing new ones. These individuals will have opinions about what went well, and what could use improvement. They also may have their own ideas of new services that could be offered. It is important to remember that those individuals with decision-making authority (i.e., pharmacy corporation, district manager, pharmacy owner) may prioritize ideas in terms of how consistent the idea might be to their overall market plan, organizational mission, and potential for profitability, rather than strictly improvement in patient care. It is incumbent upon the pharmacist to frame the importance of the program in terms that make sense to these decision makers and to speak to the performance indicators by which they are judged by (e.g., profitability of one store in a chain organization)

Reassessing the Service Objectives

As pharmacists who implement programs and services evaluate all they have accomplished, it is wise to do a little continuous quality improvement. They should identify the mistakes that they made along the way and think about how they can avoid making them again. They can also identify how they could have streamlined the process and created a better workflow for the service. Lastly, they may have conducted the project as a pilot project. These pharmacists will need to think about how they will expand the project in a seamless manner.

Pharmacists should seek the advice of those around them—their employees, supervisors, patients, and others affected by their services—to see if they have different viewpoints to share. Their input and constructive criticism may be as valuable as the economic, clinical, and humanistic results that were calculated.

FINAL VISIT OF THE SCENARIO

After performing her analyses, Cynthia shared her results with her administrators at the HMO. They were very happy to see these results and asked Cynthia about other types of pharmacy services she might be able to develop. Cynthia said that she would look into expanding her heart failure clinic to become a more generalized cardiology clinic that included lipid management, anticoagulation management, and blood pressure management.

CONCLUSION

The objectives and goals of any service should guide the outcomes data that are collected and how those data are analyzed. A common goal of any evaluation is to show the value of the program or service. It must be remembered that value can have numerous meanings (e.g., clinical, economic, and humanistic) and can be measured from a number of perspectives (e.g., patient, provider, organization, insurer, and society). The desired outcomes and perspective of the analysis should drive the data collection process and how the outcomes are assessed.

QUESTIONS FOR FURTHER DISCUSSION

1. What are some outcome measures that you can collect at your current practice?
2. How can you develop a relationship with a payer or physician group for the purpose of conducting economic analyses on your patients?
3. Based on Cynthia's objectives, what variables might she add to her evaluation?
4. Consider a pharmacy with which you are familiar, in any setting. List direct and indirect and medical and nonmedical costs and outcome measures for both an existing service and one that might be considered for addition to that pharmacy's repertoire.
5. Given what you have learned in this chapter, what are some existing services, or programs at your pharmacy you might take into a more formal evaluation to determine effectiveness? How might these concepts apply to current processes and technologies at this pharmacy? What are some new programs or services you might consider for their potential?

REFERENCES

Armstrong EP, Langley PC. 1996. Disease management programs. *Am J Health-Syst Pharm* 53:53.

Austvoll-Dahlgren A, Aaserud M, Vist G, et al. 2008. Pharmaceutical policies: effects of cap and co-payment on rational drug use. *Cochrane Database Syst Rev* 23:CD007017.

Barr JT, Schumacher GE. 1994. Applying decision analysis to pharmacy management and practice decisions. *Topics Hosp Pharm Manag* 13:60.

Bootman JL, Townsend RJ, McGhan WF. 1996. *Principles of Pharmacoeconomics.* 2nd edn. Cincinnati: Harvey Whitney Books.

Boyd KA, Briggs, AH. 2009. Cost-effectiveness of pharmacy and group behavioural support smoking cessation services in Glasgow. *Addiction* 104:317–25.

Coons SJ, Kaplan RM. 1993. Quality-of-life assessment: Understanding its use as an outcome measure. *Hosp Formu* 28:486.

Crane VS. 1988. Economic aspects of clinical decision-making: Applications of clinical decision analysis. *Am J Hosp Pharm* 45:48.

Criteria Committee, New York Heart Association, Inc. 1973. *Diseases of the Heart and Blood Vessels: Nomenclature and Criteria for Diagnosis,* 7th edn. Boston: Little, Brown.

Cvengros JA, Christiensen AJ, Hillis SL, Rosenthal GE. 2007. Patient and physician attitudes in the health care context: attitudinal symmetry predicts patient satisfaction and adherence. *Ann Behav Med* 33:262–68.

Detsky AS, Nagiie IG. 1990. A clinician's guide to cost-effectiveness analysis. *Ann Intern Med* 113:147.

Doubilet P. 1986. The use and misuse of the term "cost-effective" in medicine. *N Engl J Med* 314:253.

Drummond MF, Stoddart GL, Torrance GW. 1986. *Methods for the Economic Evaluation of Health Care Programmes.* Oxford, England: Oxford University Press, p. 18.

Eisenberg JM. 1989. Clinical economics: A guide to the economics analysis of clinical practices. *JAMA* 262: 2879.

Fonarow GC. 2001. Quality indicators for the management of heart failure in vulnerable elders. *Ann Int Med* 135:694–702

Guyatt GH, Nogradi S, Halcrow S, et al. 1989. Development and testing of a new measure of health status for clinical trials in heart failure. *J Gen Intern Med* 4:101.

Ho KKL, Pinsky JL, Kannel WB, Levy D. 1993. The epidemiology of heart failure: The Framingham Study. *J Am Coll Cardiol* 22:6A.

Hsu J, Price M, Huang J, et al. 2006. Unintended consequences of caps on Medicare drug benefits. *N Engl J Med* 22:2349.

Juenger J, Schellberg D, Kraemer S, et al. 2002. Health related quality of life in patients with congestive heart failure: comparison with other chronic diseases and relation to functional variables. *Heart* 87:235–41.

Kozma CM, Reeder CE, Schultz RM. 1993. Economic, clinical, and humanistic outcomes: A planning model for pharmacoeconomic research. *Clin Ther* 15:1121.

MacKeigan LD, Larson LN. 1989. Development and validation of an instrument to measure patient satisfaction with pharmacy services. *Med Care* 27:522.

Moczygemba LR, Barner JC, Brown CM, et al. 2010. Patient satisfaction with a pharmacist-provided telephone medication therapy management program. *Res Soc Adm Pharm* 6:143–54.

Patterson R. 1995. Disease management. *Case Rev* 1:59.

Perez A, Doloresco F, Hoffman JM, et al. 2009. ACCP: economic evaluations of clinical pharmacy services: 2001–2005. *Pharmacotherapy*29:128.

Stelfox HR, Gandhi TK, Orav EJ, Gustafson ML. 2005. The relation of patient satisfaction with complaints against physicians and malpractice lawsuits. *Amer J Med* 118:1126–33.

Tinelli M, Blenkinsopp A, Bond C. 2011. Development, validation, and application of a patient satisfaction scale for a community pharmacy medicines-management service. *Int J Pharm Pract* 19:144–55.

Van Geffen EC, Philbert D, van Boheemen C, et al. 2011. Patients' satisfaction with information and experiences with counseling on cardiovascular medication received at the pharmacy. *Patient Educ Coun* 83:303–9.

Zitter M. 1994. Disease management: A new approach to health care. *Med Interface* 7:70.

SECTION III

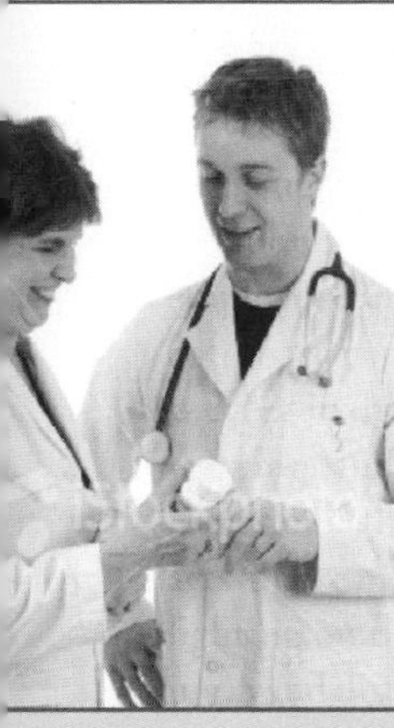

MANAGING PEOPLE

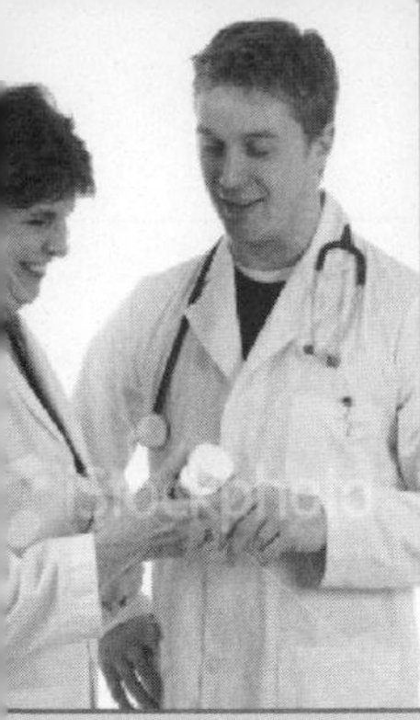

10

TIME MANAGEMENT/ ORGANIZATIONAL SKILLS

Dana P. Hammer

About the Author: Dr. Hammer is the Director of the Bracken Pharmaceutical Care Learning Center and Teaching Certificate Program in Pharmacy Education for the University of Washington School of Pharmacy. Dr. Hammer received a B.S. in pharmacy from Oregon State University, worked in hospital and community independent pharmacies, and then returned to school to earn M.S. and Ph.D. degrees in Pharmacy Administration with an emphasis on education from Purdue University School of Pharmacy. Her teaching responsibilities include an introductory pharmacy practice course series, and electives in pharmacy education. Her research involves assessment of students' educational outcomes and professional development, and interprofessional education. Dr. Hammer has served on the editorial boards of several pharmacy education, practice and research journals, and has won awards for teaching, innovations in teaching and education, and educational research. She practices her time management skills balancing a faculty position, relief work in an independent pharmacy, and parenthood of two children.

LEARNING OBJECTIVES

After completing this chapter, readers should be able to

1. Determine if they need to improve their time management skills.
2. Critically analyze the choices they make in how they spend their time.
3. Describe common myths or pitfalls with regard to time management.
4. Take action to avoid time management pitfalls.
5. Discuss various theories and approaches to time management.
6. Apply concrete suggestions, through a series of steps, to improve their time management skills.
7. Explain how time management techniques apply to pharmacy practice.
8. Recognize the relationship between poor time management and stress.

SCENARIO

Revisit the Krista Connelly scenario from Chapter 2. It appears as though Krista is a good time manager—she seems to attend all her classes, prepares for classes ahead of time and reviews material with professors, holds down a part-time pharmacy job, and even is able to squeeze in routine home activities and downtime with friends and family. Granted, Krista may not be taking very good care of herself with regard to diet, exercise, and sleep, but all in all, she seems to have her act together. One question remains, however, after reading about Krista: When does she study? Perhaps she is one of the "genius" students who does not seem to have to study very much but is still able to achieve high grades. Consider a different scenario below.

Tom Chan is also a second-year pharmacy student. Tom describes himself as a busy pharmacy student, although he would not necessarily say that he is stressed out most of the time. Tom tries to get out of bed by 7 a.m. so that he can get to class by 8 a.m., but he often oversleeps and misses his first class. He realizes that he should go to bed earlier, but it seems that the only time he can find to study or maybe watch some TV to unwind is between 10 p.m. and 2 a.m. Tom's normal day consists of attending classes, getting in an hour of basketball, and then heading to work at his pharmacy intern job at a local chain pharmacy. In between classes, he usually hangs out with friends, eats, or attends extracurricular activities and meetings. Tom finds it hard to try to get in any quality study time during the day and usually puts off studying for major exams or completing large assignments until the night before they are due. Because of this, he usually pulls all-nighters once every week or two. During midterm and finals weeks, he sometimes will stay up all night on several occasions. Tom averages B's and C's in school, although he got a D in pharmacology last year and had to repeat the course.

Tom usually works about 20 hours per week to help pay his tuition and other school-related expenses, as well as costs related to his cell phone, cable TV, and Internet subscriptions; car payment and insurance; rent; and other living expenses. He usually manages to have a little left over each month to buy music, go to movies, and go out on the town with friends, but he also maintains some credit-card debt from furniture and apartment supplies he bought when he started pharmacy school. The local chain that employs Tom as a pharmacy intern has an intern development program that helps interns to learn chain pharmacy management and administrative skills. At a recent employee annual review, Tom's preceptor shared his disappointment with Tom's tardiness to work, his inability to prioritize work tasks very well, and his lack of desire to want to improve or become engaged in management functions. Tom was discouraged with his preceptor's observations and is not sure what to do.

Do you have classmates like Krista and Tom? Do their lives sound similar to yours? Read on to find out how applying some simple time management and organizational skills can make you a better pharmacy student, better future pharmacist, and a more productive, healthy person.

CHAPTER QUESTIONS

1. How do I know if I need to manage time better?
2. What can I do to better manage time?
3. What are some resources I can use to help me better manage time?
4. What are some of the common pitfalls with regard to time management?
5. How does personal time management relate to time management in pharmacy practice?
6. How can time be better managed in pharmacy practice?
7. How does poor time management affect stress levels?

THE NEED FOR TIME MANAGEMENT AND ORGANIZATIONAL SKILLS

There are 24 hours in a day. Research tells us that for a person to be healthy, roughly 7 to 8 hours of that time should be used for sleeping. That leaves 16 to

17 hours to accomplish everything else we need and want to do in a day: go to school and/or work (usually 3 to 10 hours per day), study (rule of thumb for lecture courses is 2 hours outside class for every 1 hour in class, so let's say approximately 6 hours per day), eat (approximately 1 hour per day), shower and get ready (0.5 to 1 hour per day), exercise (0.5 to 1 hour per day), routine maintenance (e.g., pay bills, pick up room, etc.—1 hour per day), participate in a nonschool or nonwork interests (1 hour per day), relax and have fun (0.5 to 1 hour per day), and spend time with family and/or friends (face-to-face, or via e-mail or phone—0.5 to 1 hour per day). Not all of us participate in all these activities each and every day, but if we did, we are looking at spending anywhere from 14 to 23 hours per day engaged in them. And this estimate does not even include time spent on transportation or unexpected events.

Time is one of the most valuable resources we have. Several philosophies have been iterated about time:

- The gift of your time is the most valuable gift you can give.
- If you want to know what people's *real* values are, look at how they spend their time and their money.
- Time is money.
- Time management is *not* about managing time; it is about managing yourself.

Many advances in technology and other areas are all about saving time. Think about computer programs for word processing, spreadsheet creation, and statistical analyses. Think also about personal digital assistants, cell phones, microwaves, airline travel, and overnight mail. All these inventions were created to make our lives easier and allow us to be more productive and spend the time we save through their use on other activities. It has been written, however, that we can never *save* time—we can only *spend* it—so we must make wise decisions about how we choose to spend our time (Ensman, 1991).

Time management and organizational skills are important both personally and professionally. Poor time management can lead to frustration, stress, and a failure to complete daily tasks or achieve personal and professional goals. We already know that frustration and stress can be physically detrimental. Poor time management can also cause others to lose respect for and faith in us—we may be considered less reliable and dependable, less likely to follow through on commitments, and less responsible. If others feel this way about us, we are less likely to be involved in committed relationships or receive promotions at work. Safety can also be compromised—personal safety, for example, if one is constantly late and so feels compelled consistently to drive over speed limits. Patient safety certainly can be compromised if pharmacists practice in a manner that is hurried, disorganized, and haphazard. Conversely, good time management skills can lead to a higher quality of life for most people because they affect so many aspects of our lives, both personal and professional. The reasons to become a better time/self-manager are compelling and important—readers of this chapter should be motivated to improve their time management skills.

COMMON MYTHS/PITFALLS

"I don't have time . . ."

How often do you hear this phrase or utter it yourself? The truth is that we *all* have 24 hours in every day to accomplish what we need and want to do, so saying that you don't have time is actually a lie. The difference is how we *choose* to spend our time. Thus, unless you are in prison or some kind of work camp where you do not make the decisions on how your day is spent, most of us consciously decide how to spend our time. It was your choice to apply to pharmacy school. It is your choice to go to class. It is your choice to study. It is your choice to get a part-time job. It is your choice to read this book. No one is forcing you to do these things. Granted, there may be significant consequences if you do *not* choose to do these things, but the bottom line is that you *choose* how to spend your time. The next time that you feel compelled to say, "I don't have time to _____ [fill in the blank]," rephrase it to, "I can't take the time to _____ [fill in the blank]." At least that way you will not be lying.

"I'm too busy . . ."
Once again, you *choose* how to spend your time. If you feel that you are too busy to maintain your personal health, achieve your personal and professional goals, or be as successful in all your tasks and responsibilities as you would like to be, then *change your schedule.* Do not take on as many tasks. Find your success limit, and maintain it! Contrary to popular belief, the busier people are, the more productive they are, and the more they accomplish. Think about the last time that you had a week without appointments or without deadlines. How much did you get done? Granted, you may have caught up on some needed rest and relaxation, but you may not have attended to many other items on your to-do list because you were in relaxation mode and were not feeling the subtle pressure of "something needs to be done." Deadlines creep up once again and cause stress when the realization occurs that you do not have as much time to meet that deadline as you would like. It is certainly important to recharge your batteries once in awhile, but the quote "If ever the going seems easy, check to see if you are going downhill" should be heeded. Although it was stated that busy people are more productive, it is not necessarily true to say that *all* busy people are productive. Many folks spend their time working on tasks and activities that could be better handled by others. They may not be able to prioritize their responsibilities very well or may be easily distracted or consistently interrupted. And it is certainly true that some folks are just *too* busy. You know that your plate is too full when your health begins to fail, your personal relationships begin to fail, and you cannot follow through reliably with all your responsibilities. You begin to forget things. You miss meetings and deadlines. You may feel consistent stress, and guilt if you relax at all or "get off task." These are not healthy feelings and can escalate to the point of illness and exhaustion. It is important to find that balance of where you feel like you are able to stay on top of things and are getting things accomplished but not that your schedule is so easy that you are wasting your potential to achieve higher goals.

"My personal time management skills have nothing to do with how I manage time at work."
It is plausible to think this way because we are *proactive* at home—*we* determine when we want to fix dinner, do laundry, pay bills, and the like. Pharmacy practice, however, is often *reactive*—we help patients when they ask for it/need it, fill medication orders as they come in, and answer the phone when it rings. These different situations give the impression that personal and professional time management differ from each other. It is possible that a person might be completely organized at home and a train wreck at work, but this is a rare and unusual case. Most people who have a good sense of organization and time allocation know when to say "no" and how to apply those skills at home and at work. We do not usually purposefully apply different criteria for how we manage our time at home versus work; these skills usually are unconscious, routine, habit. The good news is that these skills *can* be learned.

"I need time to focus in order to . . ."
The ability to multitask is an absolute necessity for any pharmacist or pharmacy student. This does *not* mean doing several things simultaneously—if that were the case, you would never get anything fully accomplished, and patient safety certainly would be compromised. What it *does* mean, however, is that it is important that you have the ability to "switch gears" easily and maintain a sharp mind so that you can give your undivided attention for a few moments to the task at hand and then move on to the next task or back to the original task. Rarely will you have full days without any appointments or activities scheduled so that you can spend the entire day on one task.

"I'm a perfectionist . . ."
It is certainly important to do your best and to always "put your best foot forward," but as a pharmacy student or pharmacist with many demands on your time, it is critical that you discern which tasks must be perfect and which can be less than perfect. Dosing and preparation of chemotherapeutic agents, for example, should be as close to perfect as possible—it is crucially important that enough time be spent on these tasks to make sure that they are correct because people's lives are at stake. Revising a term paper five times for a three-credit course, however, does not have such severe consequences, and the time spent in the

extra three revisions could have been spent studying for an examination that is worth twice the number of points as the paper. It is okay not to be perfect all the time, unless, of course, the consequence of *not* being perfect is severe. In other words, sometimes we have to "choose our battles" in order to win the time management war.

"They didn't teach time management in my curriculum."

Some pharmacy schools provide regular workshops for students or parts of courses devoted to time management, study skills, stress management, and other pharmacy school and life survival skills. If your school is not one of those, however, this chapter is here to help get you on your way to being a better time manager. In addition, there are books and articles referred to throughout this chapter that can serve to help you become a successful time manager.

THEORIES AND PRACTICES OF TIME MANAGEMENT

In 1675, R. T. wrote a letter to a Mr. R. A. describing "the art of good husbandry, or the improvement of time: being a sure way to get and keep money."[1] In this letter, R. T. discusses several rules for merchants, shopkeepers, "mechanicks," tradesmen, and others to follow in order to use time to their advantage for themselves and families. He describes the loss of a man's time, which includes time spent in taverns, coffeehouses, or alehouses, as "the sole cause of poverty in this city and nation." This citation possibly may be one of the earliest that begins to describe the importance of time management.

Fast forward to the 1950s, where the industrial revolution had long been in place, Americans were enjoying postwar success, and management as a business discipline was evolving. Peter Drucker, well-known business management guru, wrote *The Practice of Management* in 1954, which helped to put the art and education of management on the map. Within his text, he put forth the philosophy and practice of "management by objectives" and described time as "the scarcest resource, and unless it is managed, nothing else can be managed" (as paraphrased in Applebaum and Rohrs, 1981). In a subsequent book, Drucker articulated four suggestions for helping executives to better manage their time (Drucker, 1967, pp. 26–28):

1. Find out exactly how you actually use your time.
2. Determine what does and does not have to be done (and discontinue doing the latter).
3. Delegate work to others who are equally or better qualified than you are.
4. Stop wasting other people's time.

Moving into the 1980s and 1990s, Stephen Covey became a national hero with *The Seven Habits of Highly Effective People* (Covey, 1989). Covey focuses on character development through the practice and internalization of seven habits, two of which relate directly to time management: (1) Begin with the end in mind, and (2) put first things first. Both tenets center on determining what is really important to you and then finding ways to make sure that those goals are achieved. Covey states that the essence of time management is to "organize and execute around priorities." Covey created a time management matrix (Table 10-1) to help us categorize our daily activities and understand how we can maximize our time by doing so. Covey says that we are the most effective personal managers when we are operating primarily in quadrant II. In the section on putting first things first, he also offers suggestions for long-term organizing, weekly organizing, and how to say no.

Julie Morgenstern describes a different approach in her book, *Time Management from the Inside Out* (Morgenstern, 2000). Morgenstern, founder and

[1]R. T. 1675. The art of good husbandry, or The improvement of time. A copy of the original reference is available via Microfilm from the University of Michigan, Ann Arbor, MI (1991). Also available at http://eebo.chadwyck.com/search/full_rec?SOURCE=pgthumbs.cfg&ACTION=ByID&ID=99830667&FILE=../session/1210961294_2335&SEARCHSCREEN=CITATIONS&SEARCHCONFIG=var_spell.cfg &DISPLAY=AUTHOR; accessed on June 28, 2011.

Table 10-1. Time Management Matrix

	Urgent	Not Urgent
Important	*Quadrant I* *Activities:* Crises, pressing problems, deadline-driven projects	*Quadrant II* *Activities:* Prevention and "principle-centered" activities, relationship building, recognizing new opportunities, planning and recreation
Not important	*Quadrant III* *Activities:* Interruptions, some calls, some mail, some reports, some meetings, proximate and pressing matters, popular activities	*Quadrant IV* *Activities:* Trivia and busy work, some mail, some phone calls, time wasters, pleasant activities

Source: Used with permission from Covey, 1989.

owner of Julie Morgenstern's Professional Organizers in New York City, draws a comparison between time and space and describes each day as "a container, a storage unit that has definite capacity you can reach." Her book through four phases:

1. *Laying the foundation*—thinking about creating a time management system that works for you.
2. *Analyzing*—defining your personal style, preferences, needs, and goals.
3. *Strategizing*—mapping your ideal schedule and staying on track.
4. *Attacking*—putting your plan into action.

Morgenstern's book was featured in a *Pharmacy Student* article entitled, "Yes, You Can Find the Time" (English, 2003). It also contains helpful appendices with lists of time management resources and additional references.

Marilyn Paul, author of *It's Hard to Make a Difference When You Can't Find Your Keys* (Paul, 2003), offers a "seven-step path to becoming truly organized". She claims that unlike other self-help organizational books, hers takes a more holistic approach and incorporates mental, physical, emotional, and spiritual aspects of one's life into the context of getting organized and thus living a better life.

All the books discussed thus far offer meaningful and valuable advice related to time management and other life challenges. Additionally, a comprehensive Internet-based resource can be found at http://www.effective-time-management-strategies.com/index.html. Whatever approach you choose to use to improve your time management skills, it is important to find strategies that are compatible with your personality and that will be effective for your personal and professional lives.

REAL TIME MANAGEMENT—HOW TO DO IT

There are many resources on time management. Some sources focus specifically on the busy professional and go into detail about how to manage meetings, phone calls, interruptions, and other activities that potentially can waste time in a busy professional's day. Other sources address time management as a subset of the "whole" person—personal and professional goals or mission in life, personality, communication style, and other traits because all these affect how we use our time. Although discussions about each of these subjects are beyond the scope of this chapter, this section highlights many of the principles from these references because they apply to all of us, no matter what our full-time job or personal characteristics.

Care has been taken to distill the most common themes from a variety of references that would apply to the busy pharmacy student. The steps/themes involved in practicing better time management are

- Recognize the need for improvement.
- Conduct an honest analysis of how you currently use your time.
- Establish your "mission" and set goals.
- Get organized (sort through tasks, create a master list, schedule tasks, use a system).
- Take action.
- Review, revise, and modify.

These themes are described more fully as follows along with a variety of helpful tips from many different sources.

Recognize the Need for Improvement

Almost all literature that describes successful behavioral change programs, such as 12-step programs, start at the same point: the recognition that one's behavior needs to change or that a person desires to change his or her behavior. Hopefully, you have decided already that your time management skills could use some improvement. If you have not decided this, then the chances of your being able to improve are much less. If you are in this latter category, then the next section may just convince you that you could benefit from changing some of your current habits.

Conduct an Honest Self-Reflection or Analysis of How You Currently Use Your Time

Conducting a thorough review of how you currently spend your typical day or week can be very helpful in determining how to best proceed with improving your time management. Asking yourself some key questions can also help to identify problem areas and how you should best plan your time based on your personal preferences and style. One of the most useful tools to help you diagnose the areas that could use some improvement is to keep a *time journal.* On a detailed calendar, document how you spend your time in blocks of 15 minutes. The most accurate way to do this would be to keep your calendar with you at all times and document an activity and the time you spent on it each time you change activities. Do this for an entire week, and *be honest,* for example, 75 minutes surfing the Internet for fun, 15 minutes day dreaming, 30 minute power nap, and so on. After a week, analyze those areas where you think your time could have been better spent, and evaluate factors that could have contributed to wasting time. For example, Tom Worrall, ambulatory care clinical pharmacy specialist for the Ralph H. Johnson Veterans' Affairs Medical Center in Charleston, South Carolina, explained that as a student he chose to study in the city library instead of the school's library so that he could get more done. "What takes 4 hours at the student center can take 2 hours at the city library because of fewer distractions" (English, 2003). Another author suggests asking a coworker (or significant other or roommate, for that matter) to observe your habits for 1 week and provide some constructive feedback (Wick, 1997). Be sure not to be too hard on yourself—it is important to reward hard work. Vida Farrar, a former graduate student in medicinal chemistry, indicated that "3 to 4 hours of straight studying deserves a 15- to 20-minute break. And the second round gets a half-hour to an hour break" (Dance, 1991).

When conducting the analysis of how you spend your time, Bond (1996, p. 51) suggests asking yourself these questions with regard to each activity:

- Why am I doing this?
- What is the goal?
- Why will I succeed?
- Is what I am doing at this minute moving me toward my objective?
- What will happen if I choose not to do it?

Bond continues with a few general questions about how your time is spent:

- What am I doing that does not really need to be done?
- What am I doing that could be done by someone else?
- What am I doing that could be done more efficiently?

- What do I do that wastes others' time?
- If I do not have time to do it right, do I have time to do it wrong?

Douglass and Douglass (1993) advocate creating a pie chart to depict where your time was spent. They also suggest asking yourself 12 questions when reviewing a day in your time log to better determine how well you are managing your time (Douglass and Douglass, 1993, p. 44):

1. What went right today [with regard to spending your time wisely]? What went wrong? Why?
2. What time did I start my top-priority task [assuming that you have identified your top-priority task; see the section on getting organized]? Why? Could I have started earlier in the day?
3. What patterns and habits are apparent from my time log?
4. Did I spend the first hour of my [work] day doing important work?
5. What was the most productive part of my day? Why?
6. What was the least productive part of my day? Why?
7. Who or what caused most interruptions [or what kept you from staying on task]?
8. How might I eliminate or reduce the three biggest time wasters?
9. How much of my time was spent on high-value activity and how much on low-value tasks?
10. Which activities could I spend less time on and still obtain acceptable results?
11. Which activities needed more time today?
12. Which activities could have been delegated? To whom?

While not all these questions are applicable to the typical pharmacy student, many of them do provide good food for thought with regard to self-evaluation of how you use your time.

Morgenstern offers a more thorough approach to analyzing your "personal relationship to time" and suggests that readers complete four miniexercises. The first exercise is to determine "what's working," and the author suggests that you ask yourself 12 questions, including, "No matter how busy I get, I always find time for _____ [fill in the blank]," "I never procrastinate about _____ [fill in the blank]," and "I have no problem tackling difficult projects when _____ [fill in the blank]" (Morgenstern, 2000, p. 47). The second exercise suggests nine questions to ask yourself to determine "what's *not* working," including, "I never have time to _____ [fill in the blank]," "I am usually late for _____ [fill in the blank]," and "One thing I wish I could do every day is _____ [fill in the blank]" (p. 51). The third exercise involves identifying your time management preferences. Morgenstern advocates circling each preference in a set of 12 opposites, such as "working independently versus collaboratively," "concentrating in short bursts versus long stretches," and "tight deadlines versus long lead times" (p. 54). The last exercise in her self-analysis, which consists of two parts, helps the reader to identify personal energy cycles and sources. The first part asks the same set of two questions for each period of the day (mornings, afternoons, evenings, and late night): "(Mornings) are the best times for me to _____ [fill in the blank] and the worst time for me to _____ [fill in the blank]." The second part asks you to identify what helps you "recharge" from a potential list of 13 items. Douglass and Douglass also include mini-diagnostic quizzes throughout their entire text to help readers determine their strengths and weaknesses with regard to several areas of time management (Douglass and Douglass, 1993).

Woodhull (1997) suggests that identifying your time management style will help you to better know how to use your unscheduled time, or "white spaces." She states that workaholics often have no white spaces in their schedules, which is unhealthy. She describes the four basic types of time managers:

- "*Leaders*, above all, value getting the job done and moving forward . . . . Their communication style is direct and succinct. Their motto is 'be brief and be gone.' Say what you have to say in 10 words or less. They are experts at making quick decisions" (Woodhull, 1997, p. 43).

- "*Analytics* value getting tasks done with precision and accuracy. They pay a lot of attention to detail. Their style is systematic. They use facts, logic, and structure. When communicating with them, make sure you tie new ideas to old concepts and make sure you provide a thorough explanation" (Woodhull, 1997, p. 45).
- "*Relaters* believe that getting along with others is the most important thing. Nourishing the primary relationships in their life is of utmost importance to them. They dislike making decisions that affect others. Sometimes they feel overburdened by all the things they have agreed to do for others" (Woodhull, 1997, p. 45).
- *Entertainers.* "Once considered too offbeat for the normal world of work, these types are now the ones who generate new ideas that are keeping companies alive. Unlike the other three types, entertainers do not like having a precise, predictable schedule. Instead, they enjoy a great deal of variety and flexibility" (Woodhull, 1997, p. 46).

If you are unsure of which type of time manager you are, Woodhull (1997, p. 47) offers a quiz you can take to find out. She advocates, however, that better time managers incorporate features of each style in order to be more flexible and adaptable to a variety of situations.

Now that you have thoroughly analyzed your time management style, preferences, and current use of time, you are ready to move on to the next step of becoming an improved time manager.

Establish Your "Mission" and Set Goals

While this step and the diagnostics just described are not necessarily critical to becoming a better time manager, completing them will help you to improve your time management. Setting short- and long-term personal and professional goals *is* critical to help determine priorities and stay focused. Covey (1989) and Douglass and Douglass (1993) each advocate writing your personal mission statement; from this, all your goals and priorities should flow. According to Covey, a personal mission statement is "the most effective way I know to begin with the end in mind" (Covey, 1989, p. 106). Your personal mission statement, or philosophy or creed, "focuses on what you want to be (character) and to do (contributions and achievements) and on the values and principles upon which being and doing are based" (Covey, 1989, p. 106). Covey provides several examples of people's mission statements and guidance on how to write such statements. Douglass and Douglass describe a personal mission statement as focusing "directly on your roles, relationships, and responsibilities . . . where you really figure out who you are and why you are here, . . . carefully consider your relationships with [a higher power, significant other, loved ones], friends, community, employers, and self. What kind of a person do you really want to be? What should the sum total of your life add up to? Write out your rough ideas, then edit and refine them" (Douglass and Douglass, 1993, p. 179). Some authors advocate writing your obituary as a way to help define how you want to be known and what you want to accomplish in your life. Although these ideas may seem irrelevant to practical time management, many experts say that without thinking these ideas through and setting goals, many of us will not achieve our potential in our lifetimes. And remember, there are only 24 hours in each day!

Once you have thought through these deeper questions, it is much easier to identify long- and short-term goals and priorities. Douglass and Douglass (1993, pp. 16–17) describe how to write SMART (*s*pecific, *m*easurable, *a*chievable, *r*ealistic, and *t*imed) goals:

1. *Goals should be specific.* The more specific a goal, the more direction it provides, and the easier it is to measure progress. For example, you may have a goal of studying more, which is stated very broadly. However, if you were to say, "I will increase my study time by 1 hour every day or at least 6 hours a week," this goal is more specific and clearly defined.
2. *Goals should be measurable.* Similar to the preceding comments, it is easier to determine if you are making progress toward your goal if you can somehow try to quantify the specifics in your goal. The

preceding example would be easy to quantify if you were keeping track of how your time is spent each day.

3. *Goals should be achievable.* "Goals should make you stretch and grow," but they should not be set so high that they are realistically unachievable. For example, a person may want to be a famous singer, but if that person has no previous musical training or talent, this goal may be unachievable. Goals "should be set at a level at which you are both able and willing to work. In general, your motivation increases as you set your goals higher. But if a goal is so high that you don't believe it can be achieved, you will probably never start."
4. *Goals should be realistic.* Closely related to achievability, goals should be realistic—take into account available time, resources, and skills. The preceding example illustrates this case well.
5. *Goals should be timed.* You are much more likely to achieve a goal if it has a target date by which it should be accomplished. Assigning target dates for accomplishing goals increases motivation, commitment, and action. Goals without time schedules quickly become daydreams under the pressure of daily affairs. For each step along the way, you should set a realistic target date that can, and should, be adjusted if conditions change.

Douglass and Douglass go onto to describe three additional recommendations to help you achieve your goals: *Goals should be compatible*—because if they are not, working to achieve one goal may prevent you from accomplishing another; *goals should be your own*—otherwise, your motivation to achieve them is much less—you should take ownership of at least *part* of the goal if it is not your own; *goals should be written*—writing helps to clarify goals and makes them more real—our commitment to goals improves if they are written and posted in a place where they can be seen regularly.

If you have a lot of goals, some people find it easier to focus on them if they categorize them into personal versus professional and short-versus long-term. It is important, however, to keep your goals posted somewhere, perhaps in multiple places, so that you will look at them regularly. The more often you are reminded of your goals, the more likely you are to continue working toward them. Morgenstern (2000, pp. 71–72) tells readers to classify their "big picture" goals into one of six categories: self, family, work, relationships (such as spouse and friends), finances, and community (such as making contributions and getting involved). She goes on to say that it is much easier to determine specific activities and then daily tasks that help to achieve each goal in each category. Often some daily tasks can be used to help achieve more than one goal, such as exercising with a good friend.

With regard to tackling one's goals, Woodhull (1997, p. 221) advocates using the Benjamin Franklin approach—do not try to accomplish all your goals in the same time frame, or you will become overwhelmed and discouraged. Instead, work on one or two at a time. Franklin also believed that it took 21 days for a new behavior to take root and become a routine habit; he would carry a card in his pocket with his goal for at least 21 days to constantly remind him of it.

Get Organized (Sort Through Tasks, Create a Master List, Prioritize and Schedule Tasks, and Use a System)

You have now come to the meat of time management—*getting organized.* Organizing your life and keeping it that way are the absolute best ways to save time and feel good about how you use your time. There are several steps that many authors take readers through when helping them to get organized. First, you need to sort through what you already have. This refers to tangible items such as possessions, papers, e-mail messages, bills, and tasks that need to be accomplished. There are numerous resources to help people get their possessions organized. One need only think about closet-organizing companies and "storables" stores. A complete discussion of these is beyond the scope of this chapter. However, this section will provide you with some tips about organizing some of the other parts of your life that are more difficult: papers, e-mails/texts, computer documents, and tasks that lie before us.

Sort through Tasks

You probably have heard the statement "Handle each piece of paper once." This is a very good rule of thumb for most of us that literally means that each time we get a new piece of mail, an assignment handed back, or a memo of some sort, we need to decide how we are going to use that piece of paper and do something with it—file it, recycle it, or read it later. This implies that we need to set up a filing system that works for us. Also, it is not bad to have a "read it later" pile as long as you make sure that you *schedule some time* somewhere in your calendar to actually read through the papers. Perhaps this is a task that you can work on once a week. These same ideas apply to e-mail messages, text messages, and computer documents. Most of us have some sort of computer file system set up on our hard drives that allows us to keep computer documents organized. Similar to handling paper, as you receive new e-mail/text messages or computer documents, you need to determine whether to file them, delete them, or read them later. Most e-mail programs allow users to create files in which to store e-mail messages in a place other than one's inbox. Just like paper, however, e-mails and computer files take up space on a server and/or hard drive that has limited capacity. With both paper and computer files, it is important to go through them periodically, at least once or twice a year, to clean them out and make sure that you are not running out of space.

Create a Master List

Organizing and prioritizing your tasks are often more difficult than organizing papers and e-mails. Many authors advocate creating a master list of all the tasks you need to do and then prioritizing and scheduling them. You can create your master list on your computer, on paper, in your planner (different planner options are discussed below), or by other means as long as it is on something that you can refer to regularly and are unlikely to misplace. Some folks have more than one master list, such as a "work list" and a "home list." Whatever system works best for you, the main idea is to document *all* tasks that you need to complete at some time or another. This includes any new tasks that may come your way after reviewing your mail, e-mail, phone calls, and conversations. Make sure that you keep your list(s) in a place that is easily accessible so that you can add to it when the need arises, as well as cross off tasks as you complete them.

Prioritize Tasks

Creating a master list is not too challenging as long as you remember to document everything. The more difficult task is determining how to approach the multitude of tasks on your list. Where do you start? Sometimes it can be overwhelming to think about if you have a variety of tasks that all seem very important. Thankfully, experts in the field have helped us determine how best to prioritize tasks and responsibilities so that we can be most effective and satisfied. Three general approaches to prioritizing tasks are (1) the goal-achievement approach, (2) the deadline approach, and (3) the consequences approach. Using a combination of these three will be help you to prioritize the tasks in your life effectively.

Briefly, the goal-achievement approach advocates prioritizing tasks that you know will directly help you achieve your goals as most important. For example, if one of your goals is to achieve a grade-point average (GPA) of 3.5 or higher, then the task of studying at least 4 hours a day should be high on your priority list. As another example, if you are seeking a certain internship position, then completing the paperwork and other tasks necessary to get hired should be high on your priority list. The deadline approach is relatively self-explanatory—when are your tasks due? Often others provide the deadlines for tasks such as assignments, examinations, and birthdays. Using the deadline approach is easy when the deadlines have been set by others as long as you allocate yourself enough time to complete the task. The deadline approach is not as effective, however, when certain tasks have no externally assigned deadlines, so that you have to set a deadline yourself. Regular exercise, for example, is easy to put off because it does not have a deadline (unless you are training for an athletic event). The deadline approach is also not very effective in helping you to achieve your goals. The consequence approach is somewhat related to the deadline approach and essentially asks the question, "What will happen if this task is not completed or not completed on time?" The more detrimental the consequences, the higher the priority of the task. For example, if the brakes on your car are beginning to fail, it is extremely important that you get them fixed right away, or the consequences could be fatal. On the other hand, if the penalty for turning in a late assignment is only a loss of 5 points out of 100, then completing that assignment on time may have a lesser priority than getting your brakes fixed. Some people also consider the number and importance of people who would be affected if the task or project were not completed or not completed on time—the higher the number of people or the more "important" they are, the higher is the priority of the task.

There are additional ways to prioritize activities and tasks. Many of them are similar to the goal, deadline, and consequence approaches. Covey (1989, p. 150) tells us that activities in our lives can be classified into four quadrants (see Table 10-1). Two factors that define any activity are how urgent it is and how important it is. *Urgency* refers to activities that require immediate attention, such as a ringing phone. These activities usually are visible, popular or pleasant, easy, and "in front of our noses." Often, however, these activities may be unimportant. They may be important to others but not necessarily to you. Urgent activities require us to be *reactive. Importance,* on the other hand, requires us to be *proactive.* Brushing your teeth is an example. This activity may not be urgent, but it is certainly important, and you must motivate yourself to complete this task regularly.

Covey advocates using his quadrants approach as a way to categorize and prioritize tasks and activities. Go through your master list and try to classify each task as quadrant I, II, III, or IV. How many tasks do you have in each quadrant? For those whose tasks are primarily in quadrant I, Covey explains that this is a crisis-driven, problem-minded approach that leads to stress and burnout. He says that many folks who feel that they are in quadrant I are actually in quadrant III, which can lead to short-term focus, a feeling of lack of control, and continual operation in crisis mode. They may feel like most of their tasks are urgent and important, but usually these impressions are based on the priorities and expectations of others. This is where the consequence approach may be helpful—ask yourself and others exactly what the consequences are if this task is not completed or not completed on time. This will help to determine if certain activities should be in quadrant I or in quadrant III. People whose tasks are primarily in quadrant III or quadrant IV "basically lead irresponsible lives" and often are fired from jobs and are dependent on others for the basics (Covey, 1989, p. 153). Optimally, Covey advocates that most of our tasks and activities should be in quadrant II—activities such as exercising, preparation, and preventative maintenance—these are all very important in helping us to be happy and healthy, but because they frequently do not seem urgent, they do not always get done. The results that come from primarily operating in quadrant II, however, are vision and perspective, balance, discipline, and control, and few crises arise (Covey, 1989, p. 154).

Bond (1996, p. 54) also advocates the "important and urgent" categorization process and describes the categories in this way:

- *Important* and *urgent (priority 1).* These tasks are yours alone and must be planned into your day. They consist of the most important steps to "completing your priority" (i.e., achieving your goals, avoiding negative consequences). They generally must be done well and immediately.
- *Important* not *urgent (priority 2).* Importance outweighs urgency. Important things are those which only you can do or which can advance you toward your life goals.
- *Urgent* not *important (priority 3).* Priority 3 tasks and paperwork are delegated, if possible, or assigned a small time slot and made part of a routine.
- Neither *important* nor *urgent (priority 4).* Priority 4 tasks get the least, if any, attention and are worked on in spare time or when all other tasks are completed.

Another approach to prioritization is to employ the *Pareto principle.* Commonly known as the

"80/20 rule," this principle was first discussed by Italian economist Vilfredo Pareto in the nineteenth century when studying the distribution of wealth in a number of countries. He observed that about 80 percent of the wealth in most countries was controlled by a consistent minority—about 20 percent of the people.[2] This principle suggests that we should focus on those few tasks that produce the most significant results (Petersen and Halstead, 1983). When applied to the "important and urgent" prioritization scheme, the 20 percent of the most fruitful activities fall into quadrant II or priority 2, and it is on these activities that we should focus most of our effort (Douglass and Douglass, 1993, pp. 28–29).

Similar to these approaches is the "big rock" approach. You may have heard the story about the time management seminar speaker who was presenting to a class of business students one day.[3] He had a large glass jar and proceeded to fill it up with large rocks. He asked the class if the jar was full.

"Yes," the students responded.

He then took a bag of gravel and proceeded to add it to the jar and shake it down—the gravel filled up space among the large rocks in the jar. "Is the jar full?" he asked the class.

"Probably not," replied one student.

"Good!" the speaker responded. Then he added a bag of sand to the jar, which filled up any remaining space among the rocks. "Now?" he asked the class.

"No!" the students emphatically responded.

Then the speaker brought out a pitcher of water and proceeded to pour the entire amount into the jar without causing the jar to overflow. "What's the point of this illustration?" the speaker asked.

One student responded, "The point is, no matter how full your schedule is, if you try really hard, you can always fit some more things in it!"

"No," the speaker replied, "that's not the point. The truth this illustration teaches us is: If you don't put the big rocks in first, you'll never get them in at all." He goes on to explain that the big rocks in our lives are time spent with family and friends, taking care of ourselves, our faith, and time spent on other worthy causes. The sand and water are "fillers" in our lives, and although some quantity is important, if we fill up our jars with these activities first, then we will have no room left for the big rocks.

Lastly, you probably have observed that some of these approaches discussed delegating certain tasks. As you review your master list, especially the tasks that are of lesser priority and importance, ask yourself if any of those tasks could be done by someone else or if someone else could help you with them? Would it be appropriate to enlist the help of a significant other, a roommate, a friend, a family member, or another person to complete a task? This is a very important question to ask so that you can avoid getting bogged down in activities that detract from your higher-priority tasks. One pharmacy student who was active in student organizations described delegation in this way: "You have to ask yourself if an activity suits you personally or your role as a member of an organization. You must ask, 'Is this something I need to do? Is this something the president of a corporation would do, or would someone else benefit from this experience?' Depending on the answer, you delegate. It frees your schedule and gives someone else an opportunity to have some responsibility" (Dance, 1991, p. 12).

Establishing priorities, both in your professional and personal lives, can have a significant impact on your overall time and stress management skills. By focusing on what is most important to achieving your personal goals and practice responsibilities, you should be able to have more time to focus on these activities and less stress in worrying about how you will be able to get everything done. More discussion about this can be found in the subsequent sections of Time Management in Pharmacy Practice

---

[2]Pareto principle. 2011. Available at http://en.wikipedia.org/wiki/Pareto_principle; accessed on June 28, 2011.

[3]Gerald Nash. 2011. "The Rock Parable." Available at http://www.psybersquare.com/work/parable.html; accessed on June 28, 2011. The story has also been described as filling up the jar last with beer instead of water, with the moral being, "no matter how full your life gets, there's always room for a beer."

and Stress as a Primary Consequence of Poor Time Management.

Schedule Tasks
This is not without its own set of challenges because it is often difficult to know how much time a particular task will take—especially if it is a task that you have not done before. It is best to take a conservative approach and allow yourself *more* time than you think you will need to complete a task. It is always better to undercommit and overdeliver (e.g., telling your boss that you will have a particular project done by a date later than you actually think it will take for you to complete and then turning the project in early *or* telling a patient that her prescription will be ready in 15 minutes when you are positive that it will only take 5 to 10 minutes) than to overcommit and underdeliver. Convince yourself of the phenomenon that "things always take longer than I think they will" to allow for unexpected interruptions and other unscheduled events. Then, when you finish a task early, you can reward yourself with a break or fun activity that you had not scheduled previously.

Morgenstern (2000, pp. 143–149) advocates timing yourself and then using a mathematical approach to estimating how much time tasks will take. For different activities that you work on at any given time, ask yourself how long you think it will take you to complete the task, and then keep track of how long it actually takes. The more often you do this, the better you will be at accurately estimating the amount of time tasks will take. Morgenstern tells the story of her brother who had 10 weeks to study for his medical board examination. Based on his experience as a medical student, he knew he could effectively study 10 pages of material per day. Since he had 420 pages of material to review, he calculated that it would take him 7 weeks of going through the material the first time if he studied 6 days per week. This left him with 3 weeks to review any weak areas and also served as a buffer if for some reason he was not able to study 6 days a week for 7 consecutive weeks. This schedule put him at ease and helped him to relax more about the test.

It is also important to break larger tasks into smaller ones with their own deadlines. If you are working on a semester-long research paper for a class, for example, you are much more likely to do a better job and save yourself a lot of stress if you set some deadlines for yourself to complete the paper:

Month 1: Complete literature search and reading about the topic; draft outline of paper.
Month 2: Complete rough draft of paper; turn in to instructor voluntarily for feedback.
Month 3: Revise first draft based on instructor's feedback; turn in final paper.

Breaking down large tasks also makes them seem less daunting and less overwhelming. Setting intermediate deadlines and sticking to them helps you not to procrastinate.

Lastly, it is important to schedule *all* tasks if not on paper at least in your mind; otherwise, they will not get done. Some doctors make weekly appointments with *themselves* to make sure that they can squeeze in some personal or downtime without being interrupted by another appointment. This is not to say that you need to be so rigid that you have every activity in your life entered into a master schedule, but at least allocating time for quadrant II activities is vital to make sure that they are accomplished (e.g., family time, working out, and personal time). It is also important to review your schedule and master list several times a week to make sure that you are prepared for tasks that are coming up. Some authors advocate doing this each night before going to bed.

Use a System
You have the tasks on your master list prioritized and scheduled—but how are you going to keep track of all this? Many people have found that the busier they are and the more tasks they need to complete, the more they rely on some sort of planner system to stay organized. There are a wide variety of daily, weekly, monthly, and yearly planning systems available. While a comprehensive discussion of such systems is beyond

the scope of this chapter, several useful approaches are described:

- *Paper calendar.* Many people use a simple portable calendar on which they can document scheduled tasks as well as their master or to-do list. If this system sounds appealing, make sure that the squares on the calendar are large enough so that you can legibly write down all your tasks and appointments. You also want to make sure that your master list can be attached easily to the calendar so that you can keep track of unscheduled tasks that need to be completed. The written calendar system has the advantage of allowing you to easily review daily tasks as well as others coming up in the week or month.
- *Paper-based planner/ organizer systems.* You may have heard of the Franklin–Covey planner system or the Day Runner system or seen them in stores. These are just two examples of popular paper-based organizing systems that go beyond the traditional calendar. These systems help the user to prioritize and schedule tasks and to keep a detailed calendar, master to-do list, and address book. They allow the user to customize it so that you only include the types of pages you use most. They come with instructions on how to best use their systems in order to get the most out of them.
- *Personal digital assistants (PDAs)/phones and computer programs.* In this technological age, more and more people are opting for digital systems. Many pharmacy students already own PDAs for their ability to store drug information references as well as keep a daily schedule and check e-mail, or they have applications for these on their cell phones. These systems have the ability to sound an alarm to alert you of an upcoming meeting or event. Another advantage is that many of them can be backed up to a computer system, or they exist in "the cloud" so that if either system crashes or is lost, you do not completely lose everything. One challenge of these systems, however, is that it is difficult to look at multiple pages easily. The master list may be kept in a different place than the daily schedule, and the weekly schedule may not show up in much detail. Many of the paper-based organizer programs are now available as computer programs or phone apps. The former works well for those who work on a primary computer most of the time, but if you are not able to download the information onto something that you can carry, such programs may not be as useful.

Morgenstern (2000, pp. 109–134) devoted an entire chapter in her book to "selecting a planner that works for you." She mentions that many of us probably have tried to use a particular planner system but then abandoned it for one or more of these three reasons:

1. You did not pick a planner that was right for you.
2. You did not take time to master its features and make it yours.
3. You did not make it the one and only place to record. Your appointments and to-dos, so you never came to rely on it.

She advocates determining your style and preferences first (refer to the earlier section of this chapter on self-reflection and analysis) and then considering whether you prefer visual/tactile options (such as paper-based calendars and appointment books) or linear/digital options (such as computer programs, cell phone applications and PDAs). She also warns that no system is perfect. Whatever your choice, Morgenstern recommends that you customize it, use it to its fullest, and accept its imperfections.

Take Action

You are ready! On paper or computer you are extremely organized and ready to hit the ground running. In order to help you be successful in accomplishing all your well-organized tasks, Douglass and Douglass (1993, pp. 22–23) feel that it is important to review some of the realities of human nature and how we normally spend our time—not all of which are bad. Some highlights from their 21-item list are noted:

1. We do what we like to do before we do what we do not like to do.

2. We tackle what we know how to do faster than we tackle what we do not know how to do.
3. We do activities that we have resources for.
4. We do things that are scheduled before we do non-scheduled things.
5. We respond to the demands of others before we respond to demands from ourselves.
6. We wait until a deadline approaches before we really get moving on projects.

Being aware of some of these patterns can better help you to avoid them and to stay on track in accomplishing your tasks. Always keep the big picture in mind—think of the goals that you want to achieve and how completing a task will help you do that. A great slogan for dieters who are having trouble with self-discipline is "Nothing tastes as good as thin feels." Constant self-motivation is important when you are trying to change your behavior.

Morgenstern (2000, p. 195) says, "Plan your work, and then work your plan." She recommends three actions to help you stay focused and disciplined so that you can overcome bad habits and achieve more each day (p. 196):

1. Minimize interruptions (i.e., unexpected events) and their impact.
2. Conquer procrastination and chronic lateness.
3. Overcome perfectionism.

She goes on to provide helpful suggestions on how to do all these things because they sound much easier than they are (pp. 196–210). In the end, if you are able to "containerize" your activities, you will be able to get your to-dos done and move through your day "feeling energized, optimistic, and satisfied" (p. 195).

General Tips from the Experts

Although many parts of this chapter contain helpful hints to improve your time management skills, you may have missed a few, and they are worth mentioning again:

- Take care of yourself. It is extremely difficult to be productive and successful if you subsist on junk food, get less than 7 hours of sleep per night, or only exercise when you walk from your apartment to the bus stop.
- Most people do their best work in the morning, so tackle the tough projects at that time.
- Schedule meetings and less intensive activities in the afternoon.
- Check your e-mail, text and phone messages only twice a day, once in the morning and once in the afternoon or evening.
- Cluster tasks and activities together when possible. For example, if you have a class or meeting in building A, what other tasks or activities can you accomplish that need to be done in or near building A before you trek across campus to building Z?
- Quantity does not equal quality.
- Busy does not equal productive.
- Working harder does not equal working smarter.
- Reward yourself. It gives you something to shoot for and look forward to. Besides, all work and no play is unhealthy and no fun!

Douglass and Douglass (1993, pp. 184–186) offer 39 tips for becoming a "top time master." They have even created a poster with these tips that they offer free to anyone who contacts one of the authors (contact information is included in their book). They describe it as "an excellent way to keep reminding yourself to develop good time management habits" (p. 186).

Review/Revise/Modify

Now that you are working on your plan in full swing, it is important to review periodically all the steps that you went through to determine if your system is working well. Are you accomplishing tasks and goals to your satisfaction? Are you feeling less stressed? Do you procrastinate less often? Have your preferences or your style changed in any way? Do you want to try out a new organizational system? Have your goals or priorities changed? What major changes have occurred in your life to modify your goals and priorities? When you ask yourself these questions, especially the first three, remember to cut yourself a little slack. Real change takes time, and old habits are hard to break. It is okay if you did not follow your plan to a tee. Celebrate your successes, learn from your failures, and keep striving to improve.

Bond created a 43-item questionnaire to help us review our goals and priorities to see if they have changed (Bond, 1996, pp. 89–92). Questions include

- Do you feel as strongly about your priority (goal) as you did when you set it?
- Do you reward yourself for daily or weekly successes?
- Are you adhering to your priority (goal) deadline?
- Do you spread yourself too thin and run out of time?
- Do you review your activities to determine which ones can be shortened, reorganized, or terminated?
- What are the most important factors in your success?

Analyzing your responses to these questions, along with what contributed to or detracted from your success, is an important process to help you make adjustments and corrections. As long as you are making progress toward your goals, *that* is what is most important. Remember, slow and steady wins the race. It is also helpful to remember that as much as we might like to, we will never have complete control over all our time. Douglass and Douglass (1993, p. 147) remind us to recall the Serenity Prayer:

> God, grant me the serenity to accept the things
> I cannot change,
> The courage to change those things I can,
> And the wisdom to know the difference.

■ TIME MANAGEMENT IN PHARMACY PRACTICE

So how does all this information about personal time management relate to pharmacy practice? As mentioned earlier, it is unlikely that a person who is extremely disorganized at home will be very organized in his or her work environment, and vice versa. Certainly, however, time management skills in practice depend on the type of job you have. If you have a position that is more administrative, project-based, or appointment-based, you will have more control over how your time is spent, and you can better use many of the skills described in this chapter. For example, White (1996) wrote a helpful article that describes how pharmacy managers can better control their time. She updated this piece in 2007 and offered several strategies that any pharmacist could use to improve work efficiency (Table 10-2) (White, 2007). In most pharmacy environments, however, we do not get to determine how we spend our time—the nature of the job involves responding to the demand of medication orders and questions from patients, health care providers, and others. Rarely do we have the luxury of planning our daily work activities.

Table 10-2. General Strategies for Working More Efficiently
Determine the cost of your time
Understand your responsibilities
Log your activities
Plan for productive time
Avoid time-wasting behavior
Develop reminders
Prioritize your goals
Assign times for your tasks
Manage e-mail
Manage clutter
Manage retrieval of information
Employ other time savers, such as templates for regular reports

Source: White, 2007.

Time management in practice is based on two issues: how organized you are personally at work (e.g., Can you work well in a scattered, chaotic environment, or must you work in a very structured and systematic fashion?) and what the workflow is like in your environment. Most of us have some control over the first issue but not always the second. If you do have some say, however, in yours' and others' duties and how the workflow progresses, there are numerous recommendations about how to improve efficiency and patient safety. A full discussion of these is beyond the scope of this chapter, but a few specific recommendations are shared below.

Mark Jacobs, pharmacist for Shopko Pharmacy in Beloit, Wisconsin, published his thoughts about making more time for patients in the pharmacy in the book *101 Ways to Improve Your Pharmacy Worklife* (as noted in Jacobs, 2002). He suggests six specific tasks for handling the volume of phone calls in practice that can help to improve your professional satisfaction and ability to care for patients (a few of which apply specifically to outpatient and community practices):

1. *Make full use of pharmacy technicians.* If you work with capable technicians, use them as fully as the law will allow. One example is never to answer the phone yourself unless it is a prescribers' line. Jacobs mentions that no other professionals (e.g., doctors, lawyers, etc.) answer their own phones.
2. *Respond to questions on the phone through your pharmacy technicians whenever possible.* This does not mean that you should avoid talking with patients on the phone at all possible costs, but by training your technicians to ask the caller the proper "triage" questions, you can avoid calls where the patient wants to talk to the pharmacist and then goes on to give you a prescription number to refill. Doctors most often respond to patients on the phone through their nurses.
3. *If a patient insists on speaking with a pharmacist, explain that the pharmacist is busy with another patient right now.* Jacobs advocates having the technician take down the patient's name and phone number and the reason for the call so that the pharmacist can prepare for the call prior to calling back, which also saves time.
4. *Find out when and where would be the best time to call the patient back.* Jacobs states that this will help "condition" patients to realize that you are a busy health care professional and that you may not always be available on-demand. In addition, if they really need help right now, they may be willing to ask the technician.
5. *Gracefully exit the conversation after 2 minutes* "by explaining to the patient that you have time for one more question. They will either ask it or thank you for your time."
6. *Have the technician take down all the information for prescription transfers* (depending on what the law will allow). At the very least, the technician can pull up the prescription on the computer or pull the hard copy before handing the phone to the pharmacist.

For some patients and phone calls, it may not be appropriate to adhere to all these suggestions, but for many calls, these tips can help a busy pharmacist to save time each day. Other efficiencies that many practices are implementing include a variety of dispensing technologies and robotics, automated refill phone lines and Web sites, and reconfiguring technicians' and pharmacists' job descriptions so that technicians perform most technical duties and pharmacists can concentrate on reviewing and monitoring patients' drug therapy, as well as engaging in patient and provider education. All these suggestions can be implemented relatively easily so as to better manage time in the pharmacy. Jeff Rochon, Pharm.D., Chief Executive Officer of the Washington State Pharmacists Association, reminds us that above all, we must make time to communicate with patients and other health care providers (Rochon, 2003).

Remember that priorities should be based on what is most important and urgent, then important but not urgent (remember Covey's Quadrant's 1 and 2), to achieving one's goals, whether they be personal or the goals of the practice site. An earlier part of the chapter discussed the importance of delegating tasks to help better manage your time. When delegating tasks to others, particularly technicians and others you are supervising, good managers help *them* to prioritize their tasks so that they can function effectively. One strategy to do this is *matching employee abilities and interests to the job.* As a manager, if you have the ability to create "specialized" tasks for certain technician positions, then find out who among your staff is good at and interested in those tasks, then delegate accordingly. Examples might include inventory control (i.e., ordering, tagging, stocking, processing returns, etc), billing (i.e., handling third-party claims and issues), customer service (i.e., has excellent people skills), compounding, and others.

Another strategy to help employees manage their priorities is discussing their job functions with them periodically. Simply engaging individual employees in a discussion about what they feel their work priorities are and how they best accomplish them can be very enlightening for the both of you. It can provide you as the manager an opportunity to clarify any confusion about what the employee's work priorities should be, and how s/he can best accomplish those tasks. These kinds of conversations are usually conducted during employee performance reviews, but they can happen any time that works for you and the employee.

A third strategy for helping employees managing priorities is to engage them in a time management course. Ideally any workshop or seminar they attend would focus on both work-life and personal-life strategies, in hopes that one will complement the other. When employees become good time managers, they can be more productive at work and at home and hopefully come closer to achieving work-life balance.

STRESS AS A PRIMARY CONSEQUENCE OF POOR TIME MANAGEMENT

Research has shown that individual characteristics related to job stress include balance between work and personal life, a person's outlook on life, the stressfulness of family life, and various aspects of personality (Stress at Work, 1999). The issue of balance, in all aspects of one's life, is the crux of this chapter. Effective use of time management strategies should help to reduce the probability that a person will feel overly stressed.

Interestingly, it has been shown that pharmacy students reported higher stress levels as students than they did as practicing pharmacists (Ortmeier et al., 1991; Wolfgang and Ortmeier, 1993). Another study indicated that stress among pharmacy students was partially related to "excessive study load" (Dutta, 2001). A more recent study (Marshall et al., 2008) reported that the top five triggers of stress for a group of pharmacy students were:

1. Family and relationships
2. Examinations and tests
3. Monday morning examinations
4. Outside of class assignments
5. Financial concerns.

Table 10-3. Consequences of Job Stress for Pharmacists

- Job dissatisfaction
- Lower commitment to one's organization
- Job turnover (leaving one's job)
- Lower commitment to pharmacy as a career
- Substance abuse potential
- Burnout

Source: Gupchup and Worley, 2005.

Research on consequences of pharmacists' job stress could be informative for students (Table 10-3). It is logical to conclude that what is considered "job stress" for pharmacists could be "school stress" for students or a combination of work and school. Thus, if students feel stressed about school and perhaps their internship, they likely might suffer similar consequences as pharmacists: dissatisfaction with their Pharm.D. program or internship, lower commitment to completing one's degree program or even pharmacy as a career, quitting school or the internship or both, and the potential for substance abuse and burnout.

Thankfully, coworker social support, or the material and emotional support received from one's coworkers, has been shown to buffer the impact of job stress on job dissatisfaction (Wolfgang, 1994). For students, this applies to coworkers and classmates. It is presumed that most pharmacy students probably have a network of friends in their academic class experiencing the same "stress" (at least related to the Pharm.D. program), so a natural buffer exists. How one copes with stress also makes a difference; problem-focused coping strategies, where one attempts to tackle the problems at hand, are most effective in reducing the impact of job stress on job dissatisfaction (Gupchup and Worley-Louis, 2005). Implementing time management strategies could be an example of a problem-focused coping strategy, and could certainly help to reduce of stress related to excessive study load. Emotion-based coping strategies, such as distancing oneself from the problem or trying to avoid the problem, are unsuccessful (Gupchup and Worley-Louis, 2005). Other strategies to combat stress include meditation and relaxation (e.g., yoga and massage), biofeedback, and physical exercise (Gupchup and Worley-Louis, 2005). Wick and Zanni (2002) suggest a number of strategies for pharmacists, such as:

- Keep a journal and assess your automatic emotional reactions. Ask others for feedback and try to identify new patterns.
- Keep things in perspective. Laugh often and laugh hard.
- Try to connect with people compassionately.
- Recognize that you are not perfect or superhuman.
- Focus on the positive; count your blessings.
- Recognize situations that are beyond your control; act accordingly.
- Identify your successful stress-reducing strategies and avoid stress triggers.
- Manage your environment as well as you can.
- Pay attention to diet, sleep, and exercise.
- Adopt a pet.

Marshall et al. reported that the top five coping strategies pharmacy students used to cope with stress were:

1. Exercising (running and working out)
2. Time with family and friends
3. Napping/sleeping
4. Watching TV
5. Drinking alcohol.

The study prompted investigators to help students use healthy coping strategies versus those that can have negative consequences.

REVISITING THE SCENARIO

This chapter has presented a lot of tips and ideas that Tom may heed so that he can improve his time management skills. While Tom may have a routine, he definitely does not have a system. At the very least, Tom must ask himself some important questions and establish some goals and priorities. He may also consider the use of a master list and implement the use of technology such as a PDA to help him focus on the tasks at hand. We certainly would not want to see him lose his job or have to resign from the school of pharmacy.

CONCLUSION

The goal of this chapter was to raise awareness about the importance of time management in one's personal and professional lives. Readers should have come away with concrete strategies about how to improve their skills so that they can achieve their full potential. Remember, time management is not about managing time, it's about managing yourself—and all of us can use some improvement so that we can be more effective in all that we do.

QUESTIONS FOR FURTHER DISCUSSION

1. After applying the techniques described in this chapter, are you better able to accomplish your goals?
2. Are you healthier? Why or why not?
3. Are you happier? Why or why not?
4. How can you help others to learn and employ these skills?
5. How can these skills help you as a practitioner?
6. What kinds of time management techniques can you employ in your practice to help improve the process of health care delivery?
7. In addition to time management, what strategies would you employ to reduce your stress level?

REFERENCES

Applebaum SH, Rohrs WF. 1981. *Time Management for Health Care Professional.* Rockville, MD: Aspen Systems.

Bond WJ. 1996. *Managing Your Priorities from Start to Success.* Chicago: Irwin Professional.

Covey SR. 1989. *The 7 Habits of Highly Effective People: Restoring the Character Ethic.* New York: Simon & Schuster, p. 151.

Dance B. 1991. Managing time means managing yourself. *Pharm Stud* 21:11.

Douglass ME, Douglass DN. 1993. *Manage Your Time and Your Work Yourself: The Updated Edition.* New York: AMACOM.

Drucker PF. 1954. *The Practice of Management.* New York: Harper & Row.

Drucker PF. 1967. *The Effective Executive.* New York, NY: Harper and Row.

Dutta AP. 2001. Measuring and understanding stress in pharmacy students. Published dissertation, Virginia Commonwealth University.

English T. 2003. Yes, you can find the time: Experts present time management for dummies. *Pharm Stud* 33: 16.

Ensman RG. 1991. Time test: How well do you manage time? *Consultant Pharmacist* 6:61.

Gupchup GV, Worley-Louis MM. 2005. Understanding and managing stress among pharmacists. In Desselle S, Zgarrick D (eds.) *Pharmacy Management.* New York: McGraw-Hill, pp. 52–62.

Jacobs M. 2002. Time management in the pharmacy: Efficient use of your time will leave more time for your patients. *Washington Pharm* Autumn:17.

Marshall LL, Allison A, Nykamp D, Lanke S. 2008. Perceived Stress and Quality of Life Among Doctor of Pharmacy Students. *Am J Pharm Educ* 72:137.

Morgenstern J. 2000. *Time Management from the Inside Out: The Foolproof System for Taking Control of Your Schedule—and Your Life.* New York: Holt, p. 11.

Ortmeier BG, Wolfgang AP, Martin BC. 1991. Career commitment, career plans, and perceived stress: A survey of pharmacy students. *Am J Pharm Educ* 55:138.

Paul MJ. 2003. *It's Hard to Make a Difference When You Can't Find Your Keys: The Seven-Step Path to Becoming Truly Organized.* New York: Viking Books.

Petersen DJ, Halstead EG. 1983. The ABC's of effective time management. *Top Hosp Pharm Manage* 3:47.

Rochon J. 2003. Developing relationships is an essential aspect of your practice. *Washington Pharm* Summer:9.

White SJ. 1996. High-touch human resource management: Finding the time. *Pharm Pract Manag Q* 15:75.

White SJ. 2007. Working efficiently. *Am J Health Syst Pharm* 64:1587.

Wick J. 1997. Time management tips. *Consultant Pharmacis* 12:1042.

Wick JY, Zanni GR. 2002. Stress in the pharmacy: Changing the experience. *J Am Pharm Assoc* 42(1): 16–20.

Wolfgang AP. 1994. Job stress and dissatisfaction: The role of coworker social support and powerlessness. *J Pharm Mark Manage* 9:19.

Wolfgang AP, Ortmeier BG. 1993. Career commitment, career plans, and job related stress: A follow-up study of pharmacy students as pharmacists. *Am J Pharm Educ* 57:25.

Woodhull AV. 1997. *The New Time Manager.* Brookfield, VT: Gower.

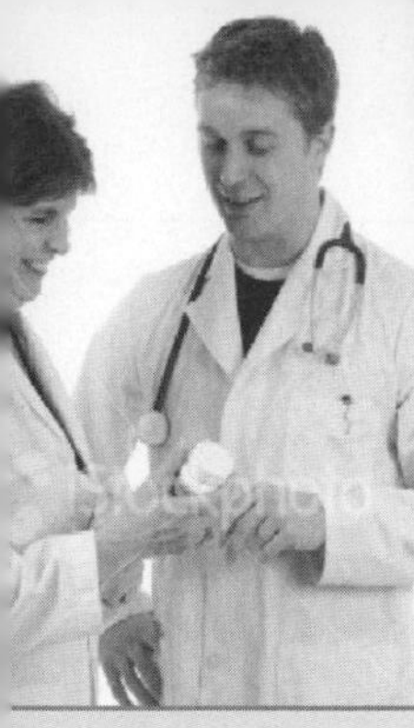

11

ORGANIZATIONAL STRUCTURE AND BEHAVIOR

Caroline A. Gaither

About the Author: Dr. Gaither is professor and assistant dean for pharmaceutical education at the University of Minnesota college of pharmacy. She received a B.S. in pharmacy from the University of Toledo and an M.S. and Ph.D. in pharmacy administration from Purdue University. Her teaching interests include the health care workforce, professionalism, career management, work-related attitudes and behaviors, interpersonal communication, and service learning. Her research interests include understanding and improving the work life of pharmacists, specifically focusing on individual-level (organizational and professional commitment, job satisfaction, job stress, role conflict, turnover, and gender and race/ethnicity effects) and organizational-level (culture and empowerment) factors. She also examines the psychosocial aspects of patient and provider decision-making regarding the management of chronic illness. She recently completed a sabbatical leave focusing on assessing pharmacy's role in addressing health disparities.

LEARNING OBJECTIVES

After completing this chapter, readers should be able to

1. Discuss the field of organizational behavior and its development over time.
2. Describe the basic components of traditional and newer organization forms.
3. Compare and contrast different elements of formal and informal organizational structure.
4. Understand the role of teams in organizations and how to build effective ones.
5. Discuss the basic incompatibilities between organizational and professional models of structure.
6. Identify influences on pharmacists' job satisfaction, organizational commitment, job stress, and job turnover intention and organizational identification and how they affect organizational behavior and performance.
7. Describe the role of emotions in organizational behavior.
8. Describe different leadership theories and how they can be applied to pharmacy practice.

SCENARIO

Joe Smart, a newly hired pharmacy intern, just completed his first week at the ambulatory pharmacy at State University Health System. Having worked previously in an independent community pharmacy, he wanted to get some hospital experience before graduation. Now he is not so sure. He really liked working with the customers that came into Sam's Pharmacy, but frequently he and the pharmacist who worked there were so busy that neither had much time to do anything other than dispense prescriptions. His first week at the ambulatory pharmacy also was quite busy. There were many more people working here than at Sam's. He was overwhelmed by it all. During orientation, he received a copy of the policy and procedure manual that detailed the health system's mission and organizational chart. He was very impressed with all this but could not figure out why it was important to know about the rest of the organization. He was going to be a pharmacist and, as such, was only interested in things that pertained to the pharmacy. Also, he could not understand why the pharmacy staff was so uptight. At his old job, Sam, the owner, would always notice if an employee was distressed or unhappy about something. Sam had an "open door" policy and was always ready to talk. He really felt like part of the team. Joe only saw his new boss, the director of the ambulatory pharmacy, once, and that was at orientation. The pharmacists he worked with were very concerned with showing him the tasks he needed to complete and not much else. Joe began to wonder if this was what it would be like to work for a large health system. He remembered that in his management class, the professor talked about working for large organizations, but he did not pay much attention. Joe thought that it was the responsibility of the manager to make sure that things ran smoothly and that he did not need to be concerned with details unrelated to patients' drug therapy. Anyway, he was new and thought that maybe he should give the place more time. In the back of his mind, however, he had this nagging feeling that things could be better, but he just did not know how to get there.

CHAPTER QUESTIONS

1. What is organizational behavior, and how has it developed over time?
2. Why do pharmacists need to understand how an organization works?
3. What is some basic terminology used to describe organizations?
4. What is the typical organizational structure among common employers of pharmacists? How do newer organizational structures differ from more traditional ones?
5. What factors should be taken into consideration when designing the most appropriate organizational structure?
6. What are the various types of teams found in organizations and how can they be structured for maximum effectiveness?
7. How does a professional work within a bureaucratic organization?
8. What are some of the typical organizational attitudes and behaviors of pharmacists?
9. What are some ways in which a leader is different from a manager?
10. What types of leaders do pharmacy organizations need?

WHAT IS ORGANIZATIONAL BEHAVIOR?

An *organization* can be defined as a group of individuals working to reach some common goal. Organizations can be very small in numbers of personnel (fewer than three) or very large (more than 5,000). Personnel can include staff (e.g., ward clerk, cashier, technician, pharmacist, nurse, or physician) and management and administrators (e.g., owner, president, vice president, manager, director, or supervisor). Both staff and administrators are important to the overall functioning of any organization. It is not enough for pharmacists to understand only the technical and professional aspects of their job (i.e., dispensing, monitoring, and counseling); they also must understand how the organizations for which they work function and how the people within them work. This is something that Joe Smart has yet to figure out on his own. An examination of certain tenets in the field of organizational behavior will provide valuable insight into this area.

Organizational behavior is the systematic and scientific analysis of individuals, groups, and organizations; its purpose is to understand, predict, and affect human behavior to improve the performance of individuals, which ultimately affects the functioning and success of the organizations in which they work (Tosi et al., 1994). To be effective, managers must be able to understand why people in their organizations behave in certain ways. This allows them to take corrective action if problems arise. Managers also must be able to predict how employees will react to new technologies and changes in the marketplace (e.g., implementation of robotics in a pharmacy department or moving from a drug-product orientation to a people orientation). Organizations exert control over their employees through rewards or sanctions to encourage fulfillment of organizational goals and objectives.

Organizational behavior draws on a number of different behavioral science disciplines. Psychology, sociology, social psychology, anthropology, and political science all provide insights into how best to organize work (Robbins, 2005). Psychology allows us to understand individual behavior and focuses on such aspects as motivation, job satisfaction, attitude measurement, and work design. Sociology contributes by helping us to understand how individuals fulfill their roles within a larger system through organizational structures, behavioral norms, and bureaucracies. Social psychology focuses on the influence of individuals on one another and helps us understand communication patterns, attitude change, and group functioning. Anthropology provides understanding of the environment in which the organization functions. Political science provides insight into organizational politics and informal organizational structures that greatly influence the functioning of an organization.

Understanding the functioning of organizations was not so important when the profession of pharmacy began. As noted in Chapter 1, most pharmacists started out as apprentices of apothecaries, from whom they learned the practice of pharmacy, and then went on to become practitioners who owned their own pharmacies and trained other apprentices. As the roles of the pharmacist have changed over time, so has their training and places of employment. Currently, a doctor of pharmacy degree requires 6 or more years of formal education. Unlike in the past, today most employers of pharmacists are large organizations. These organizations can be chain pharmacies (several stores under one owner or publicly traded on the stock market); integrated health systems that incorporate inpatient and outpatient pharmacies, ambulatory care clinics, and managed-care and mail-order operations; and even pharmaceutical manufacturers.

Other professions are following a similar trend, wherein their practitioners are transitioning from employers to employees. Very few graduates of medical or law school operate independent practices immediately after graduation (Stoeckle and Stanley, 1992; Williams et al., 2002). Many physicians are salaried employees of managed-care organizations, integrated health systems, or group practices. Ownership of an independent community pharmacy or a private medical practice is still a viable employment option for many, but they too will operate in an increasingly complex environment. Understanding how organizations function will enhance health professionals' employment experiences and increase their chances for a rewarding professional career.

Why is this shift from independent practitioner to salaried employee so important? This shift may appear to be in conflict with one of the hallmarks of a professional occupation—autonomy. "The major distinction between a profession and an occupation lies in legitimate organized autonomy—a profession is distinct from other occupations in that it has been given the right to control its work. Professions are deliberately granted autonomy including the exclusive right to determine who can do the work and how it should be done" (Friedson, 1970, p. 73). Given that pharmacy and medicine are professional occupations, the status of practitioners as employees could result in conflict between the professional and the employing organization.

In many cases, professionals' primary allegiance is to their work or patients and not to their employer. These practitioners also share a desire to exert at least some control over their work environments. If this desire is not met, job dissatisfaction and stress can result (Gaither et al., 2008b; Kuiper et al., 2011; Williams et al., 2002). Even as an intern, Joe Smart is questioning the autonomy afforded the pharmacists at State University Health System. His initial frustration, however, may be compounded by a lack of knowledge of how operations and communication channels differ in a large organization compared with a much smaller one.

This chapter will help you gain a greater understanding of how organizations function by introducing basic organizational behavior principles, describing the structure of organizations, discussing the roles of employees within organizations, examining specific pharmacist organizational behaviors, and elaborating on the concept of leadership.

ORGANIZATIONAL PRINCIPLES

Chapter 4 discussed strategic planning and the development of mission statements and organizational goals and objectives. To understand an organization requires knowledge of its purpose or reason for being. Organizations do not function in isolation. They are created to meet some need in the external environment. As shown in Fig. 11-1, at the center of any organization is a set of values that form the reason for existence, the philosophy, and the purpose of the organization (Jones, 1981). Articulations of these values often are represented as the goals of the organization. Some organizations will lose

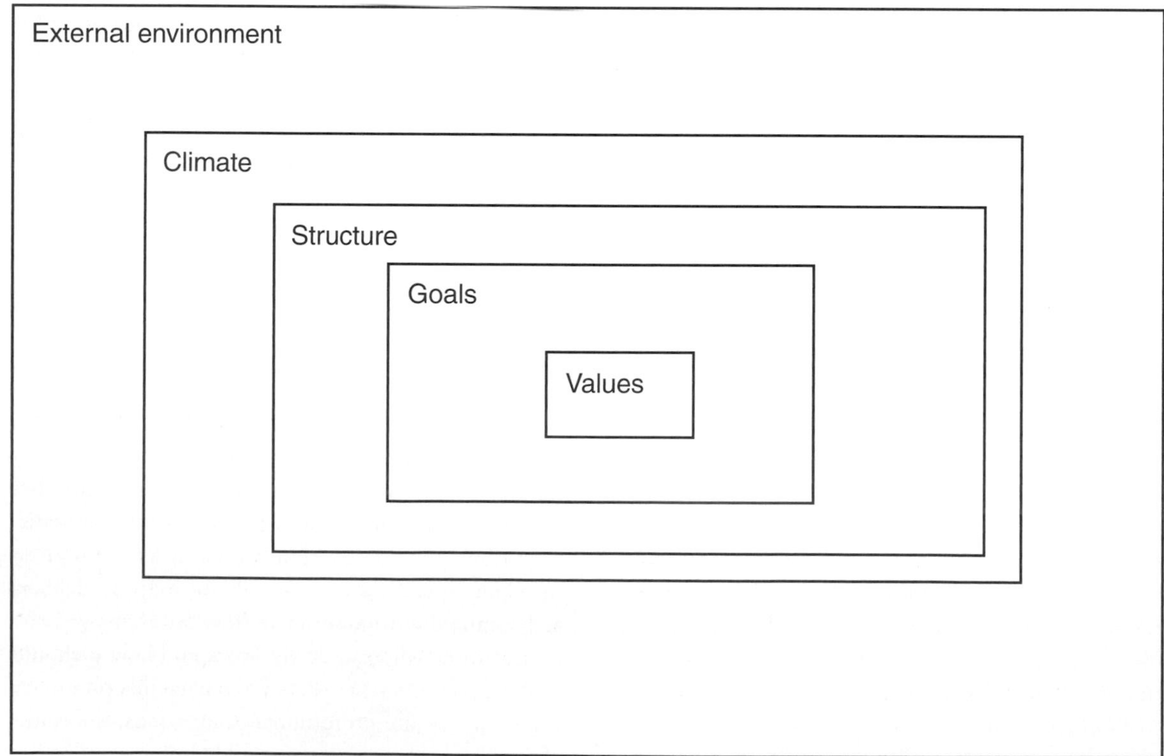

Figure 11-1. The organization.

focus if the goals they set are at odds with the core values of the organization. To make the goals of the organization a reality, a structure must be put in place to make the organization operational. Typically, the structure includes such concepts as reporting relationships, communication patterns, decision-making procedures, responsibility/accountability, norms, and reward structures.

Structure produces the climate, or the psychological atmosphere of the organization (Jones, 1981). The climate of an organization consists of such factors as the amount of trust, the levels of morale, and the support employees experience (Gibb, 1978). Organizational climate is often confused with organizational culture (Schein, 1985). *Organizational culture* is defined as the system of shared meaning held by members that distinguishes one organization from another (Robbins, 2005). *Culture* refers to the understandings and beliefs regarding how "things are done around here" (Schein, 1985). Once the culture is in place, practices within the organization act to maintain it by exposing employees to a set of similar experiences (Harrison and Carroll, 1991). The very specific and methodical training that Joe Smart is receiving is somewhat a reflection of the organization's culture.

Organizational culture affects climate. A strong culture is characterized by the organizations' core values being both intensely held and widely accepted (Weiner, 1988). A weak culture is characterized by just the opposite—vagueness, ambiguity, and inconsistency. A strong culture will have a greater effect on the climate than a weak one because the high degree of sharedness and intensity creates an internal climate of high behavioral control (Robbins, 2005). Problems in the climate can be traced back to problems in the organization's culture and structure. When improvements in the climate are needed, some managers may only monitor employees' overall job satisfaction and stress levels. While it is important to do this, managers should also determine if there are problems with communication patterns, reward structures, and decision-making procedures within the organization and focus on problem solving in these areas. Has the organization stayed true to its values? If not, the shared meaning that employees hold with management will be confused. Managers are essential in creating the culture, which influences interactions among coworkers and relationships with patients (Fjortoft, 2006). An unhealthy climate can hinder employee productivity and ultimately affect the overall effectiveness of the organization.

Organizations exist in an environment that is constantly in flux. This is particularly the case in health care. Organizations that employ health professionals and the health professionals themselves must be flexible enough to cope with the unexpected (Jones, 1981). Leaders and managers of these organizations must assess the core values of the organization regularly to determine if they are being challenged or if they need revision (Dye, 2000). Assessing an organization's culture will assist in determining how the organization is responding to both its internal and external environments.

Assessing Organizational Culture

A wide range of tools exist to assess organizational culture, including techniques ranging from observation, informal interviews, and attending meetings to the administration of carefully developed survey instruments. These instruments are designed to measure and compare the key cultural characteristics of a single organization or a number of different organizations. An example of such an instrument is the Competing Values Framework (Fig. 11-2) developed by Quinn and Rohrbaugh (1983; Quinn, 1988). Depending on the degree of flexibility or control in the structure of the organization and a focus on either the internal dynamics or external environment, four types of cultures are derived: hierarchical (i.e., internal focus, high control), group (i.e., internal focus, low control), rational (i.e., external focus, high control), and developmental (i.e., external focus, low control). An overemphasis on any of the cultures can result in a dysfunctional organization (Quinn, 1988); therefore, organizations need to embrace some elements of each culture. The most effective organizations embrace the dimensions that are most important and relevant to their goals and values (Cameron and Freeman, 1991).

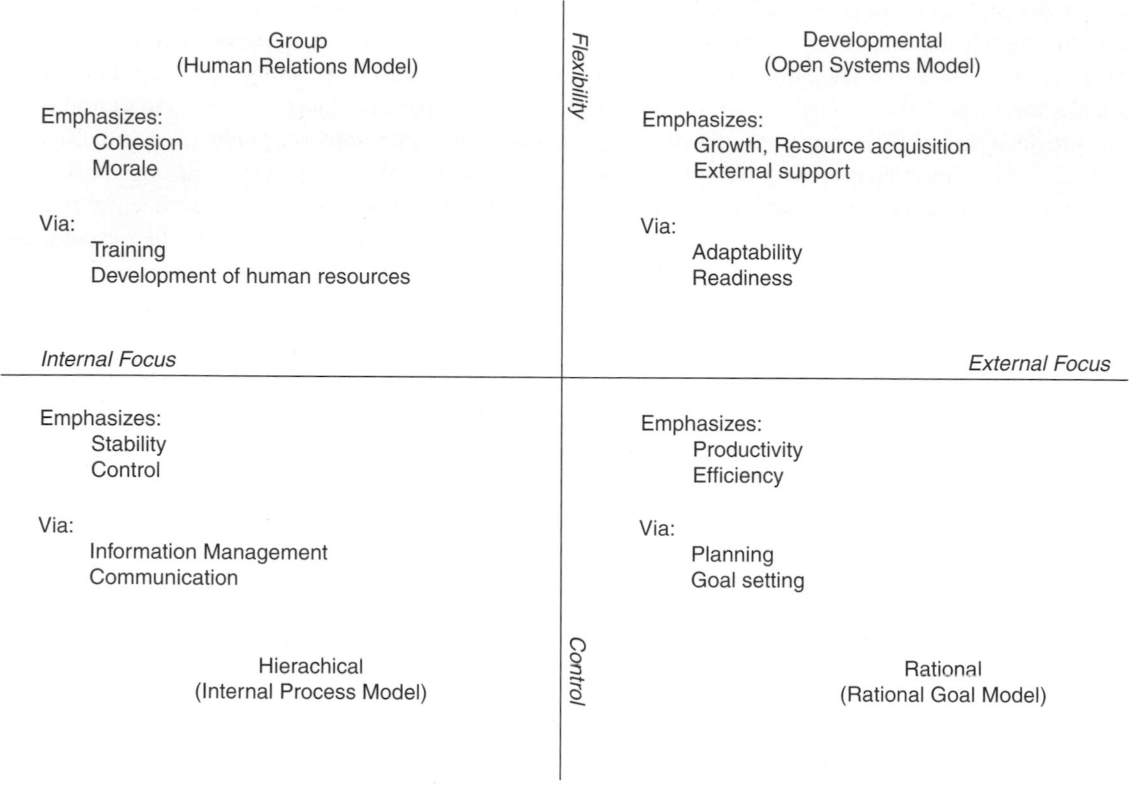

Figure 11-2. The competing values framework. (*Adapted from Quinn, 1988.*)

To determine the type of organizational culture, employees are given an instrument that contains brief statements in which they are asked to rate out of 100 points how closely their organization reflects these dimensions. Using this instrument, a recent study of health-system pharmacists indicated that the majority of study participants felt that their organization had a hierarchical organizational structure (Lane et al., 2010). When asked about the type of culture they desired in their organization, staff pharmacists (those whose work activities involved overseeing drug distribution) were more likely to indicate they desired a hierarchical culture, while clinical pharmacists (those whose work involves no drug distribution activities) and administrative pharmacists desired a group culture. These results are similar to a study of 77 intensive care units from 41 hospitals (Speroff et al., 2010). The dominant culture was a hierarchical one, and nurses were more likely to view their culture as hierarchical in comparison to physicians. Hierarchical cultures rate lower on staff job satisfaction, working conditions, and stress recognition. Quality improvements in these cultures have also been harder to implement (Speroff et al., 2010).

Other studies have demonstrated important implications of culture on pharmacy, pharmacist, and patient outcomes. Clark and Mount (2006) demonstrated that certain types of pharmacies had more of a culture toward providing patient-centered care than others. Similarly, it has been suggested that corporatization of community pharmacies may affect pharmacists' professional autonomy, yet a mixed market (i.e., various types of ownership) may be required to maintain a comprehensive range of public health services that provide maximum benefit to all patients (Bush et al., 2009). Other reports have shared that even beyond type of ownership, the culture instilled in an organization may have implications for pharmacist job satisfaction and turnover (Seston et al., 2009), effectiveness of the implementation of new policies (Tan et al., 2005), building capacity and establishment of policies for new cognitive services to patients (Feletto, 2010), the quality of care provided by pharmacists to patients (Skomo and Desselle, 2010), and even the rate of medication incident reporting among pharmacies Boyle et al., 2011). The importance of organizational culture simply cannot be understated.

Organizational Structure

Organizational theorists suggest that the structure of an organization encompasses three major aspects: differentiation (also known as *complexity*), formalization, and centralization (Robbins, 2005). *Differentiation* refers to the degree to which units are dissimilar. *Formalization* refers to the degree to which jobs in the organization are standardized, and *centralization* refers to extent to which decision-making is concentrated at a single point in the organization. Differentiation can occur either horizontally, vertically, or spatially.

Horizontal Differentiation

Horizontal differentiation describes the degree of differentiation based on how many different types of either people or units are included in the organization. Do all the employees of the organization have the same training and education? This is definitely not the case in pharmacy. Many pharmacy organizations focus not only on providing pharmacy services but also on merchandizing non pharmacy-related items. If all personnel had the same training, managing the organization would be easier because everyone would have a similar orientation. Since this is not the case in pharmacy, coordinating the work among people in the different units can be more difficult. Horizontal differentiation can also take the form of multiownership of a variety of related industries. A health system can own several hospitals, long-term care facilities, and a managed care business (Sahney, 1996).

Vertical Differentiation

Vertical differentiation refers to the depth of the organizational hierarchy. One key feature of an organization is the chain of command, or the number of levels between the owner or president of the organization and the staff. Vertical differentiation typically is represented by what is known as an *organizational chart.*

An organizational chart depicts the reporting relationships and the hierarchy of authority in an organization. An example of a typical organizational chart is given in Fig. 11-3. Authority usually flows from top to bottom, with those at the bottom of the chart holding the least authority. *Authority* is the rights given to a certain position in an organization to give orders and the expectation that those orders are carried out. Along with these rights, the responsibility for making sure work is completed is accepted. The solid lines represent direct reporting relationships important to the overall objectives of the organization (line authority). Line-authority positions include vice presidents, directors, managers, supervisors, and staff. The dashed lines in the figure represent advisory positions that supplement and support the line-authority positions (staff authority). Examples of staff-authority positions include chief personnel officer or vice president of personnel, finance, legal, real estate, information systems, etc. The degree of staff authority varies with the size of the organization. The smaller the size, the fewer are the number of positions needed to support the line authority. Many independent community pharmacies started out this way. One person (the owner) was responsible for numerous activities. As pharmacies grew and expanded, owners hired individuals to supervise different areas or functions of the store. As owners branched out into running additional stores at various locations, more personnel were needed to run the day-to-day operations of the organization.

If an organization represents a for-profit company (i.e., portions or shares of the company are sold on the stock exchange), the top position in the organization belongs to the stockholders. Typically, stockholders do not have a say in day-to-day operations but are very concerned about the profitability of the company and will sell their stock if earnings are not up to par. If the

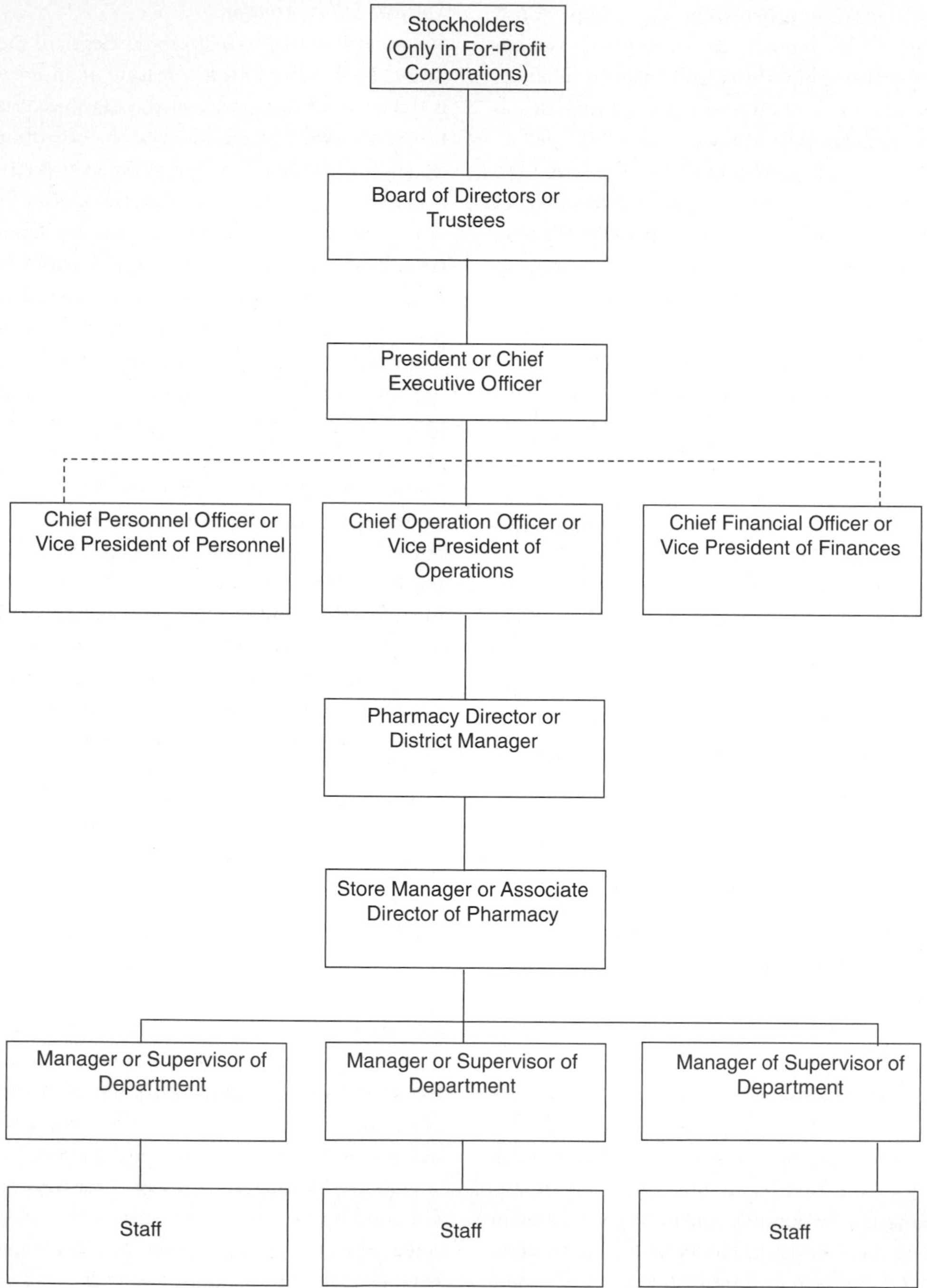

Figure 11-3. The organizational chart.

company is a not-for-profit organization, the top level will not be stockholders but may represent a board of directors or trustees who oversee the entire operation. This group also is not involved in day-to-day operations but will meet periodically to either review or make important decisions regarding the entire company. The next level represents the chief executive officer (CEO) or president. If the organization is an independent community pharmacy, the owner will occupy the top position in the organizational chart. Depending on the size of the company, a chief operations officer (COO) or the owner of the independent pharmacy will run the day-to-day operations of the organization. If the company is national or international, regional officers responsible for the operations in different areas of the country may assist this person. Under these officers are usually department directors or district managers. Departments in a health system can include nursing, medicine, quality assurance, managed care, long-term care, and so on. Each of these departments will have managers or supervisors who oversee staff who carry out the day-to-day responsibilities. Examples of specific pharmacy organizational charts are presented in Chapters 32 and 33.

Spatial Differentiation

Spatial differentiation is the degree to which the location of an organization's units is in one place or spread across several locations. An independent community pharmacy may have only one location that has all operations in one place. A large health system or chain pharmacy operation can have multiple units spread across a city, state, or entire regions of the country. Spatial differentiation also can occur when different departments are located in different areas. A pharmaceutical manufacturer may have all its research and development departments in one city or state and the sales and marketing divisions in other areas of the country or the world. As organizations spatially differentiate, more coordination between these units is necessary. Spatial differentiation is also related to the amount of horizontal and vertical differentiation. The more complex the organization, the greater is the extent each of these will exist.

Formalization

Formalization can include the presence of rules (the degree to which the behavior of organizational members is subject to organizational control), procedural specifications (the extent to which organization members must follow organizationally defined techniques in dealing with situations they encounter), technical competence (the extent to which organizationally defined "universal" standards are used in the personnel selection and advancement process), and impersonality (the extent to which both organization members and outsiders are treated without regard to individual qualities) (Hall, 1968). If a job is highly formalized, the employee has little discretion with regard to when and how the job is completed. Standardization grew out of beliefs held by early organizational behaviorists who suggested that in order to make work more efficient, error should be reduced (Taylor, 1911). One way to do this was to standardize procedures to reduce errors and increase efficiency. As noted in Fig. 11-2, hierarchical and rational organizational cultures have high degrees of control usually through formalization and the standardization of procedures.

The degree of formalization can vary considerably within and between organizations (Robbins, 2005). Organizational charts depict different positions and/or units in an organization and formal lines of authority and decision-making. This is one type of formalization. Another type is related to performance of the work. Some pharmacies require all pharmacy personnel to punch a time clock at the beginning and ending of a shift; others do not have such a requirement. Positions that make up the organization can have very detailed job descriptions that inform employees what they can and cannot do, whereas other organizations are less formal and do not have written job descriptions. Or if they do, the descriptions are very vague. Individuals who are higher in the organization will have less formal job descriptions than those lower in the company. Some jobs also lend themselves to more or less formalization. The legal requirements of drug procurement and dispensing are highly formalized, but the individualized services that pharmaceutical care requires leave much discretion to the individual pharmacist.

Centralization

Centralization refers to the extent to which decision-making is concentrated at a single point in the organization. *Decision-making* and *authority* in this context refer to the rights inherent to the position that one holds in the organization. Usually the very top levels of management make most of the policy decisions in a centralized organization. More recently, the trend has been to decentralize decision-making and move it down in the organization to lower levels of management and/or even to staff-level employees. Problems with this approach arise when employees are responsible for achieving goals without the authority to make policies or gather the needed resources. Group and developmental organizational cultures have structures that allow for more flexibility in decision-making.

Centralization sometimes is confused with spatial differentiation. A hospital pharmacy that has satellite pharmacies located throughout the hospital is often referred to as being "decentralized." However, it is decentralized in location only if decision-making concerning the satellites still rests at one centralized point in the organization. Other organizational structure principles include division of labor, span of control, unity of command, and departmentalization.

Division of Labor

Division of labor divides work tasks into specific parts. This can be seen in pharmacy when there is a separation of pharmacists into those who only participate in dispensing functions and those who only participate in clinical functions. Even within clinical functions, pharmacists can specialize in a particular field (e.g., geriatrics, pediatrics, or disease states). This should result in more efficient use of the specialized skills of the individual. A negative consequence of the division of labor is that the professional may become very narrow in his or her abilities, and the job could become routine. Some suggest that enlarging rather than narrowing the scope of some jobs leads to greater productivity by using employees with interchangeable skills (Robbins, 2005). This can be seen in the health system setting, where pharmacists provide both traditional staffing functions on certain shifts and patient care (clinical) functions on others.

Unity of Command

Unity of command is the concept that an individual reports to only one supervisor, to whom he or she is responsible. As pharmacy organizations have tried to decentralize, employees may have more than one person to whom they are reporting. A structure that makes the most of this concept is called a *matrix organization.* A matrix organization integrates the activities of different specialists while maintaining specialized organizational departments (Tosi et al., 1994). Usually this takes the form of different specialists across several departments working in teams on specific projects. This type of structure works well in environments that are continually changing and in need of innovation. It also works well where project work is the norm, and people are required to get together in interdisciplinary terms (La Monica, 1994).

Pharmaceutical manufacturers and cross-disciplinary teams in health systems (e.g., nurses, physicians, pharmacists, and social workers) are particularly well suited for this endeavor. This allows for diversity of ideas and for the best possible solution to emerge. On the negative side, there is little evidence that employees prefer reporting to more than one supervisor, and confusion as to who is responsible for what can develop (Tosi et al., 1994).

Span of Control

Span of control refers to how many people a manager effectively controls. In pharmacies, we can see a wide variation in the number of individuals a pharmacist supervises. One pharmacist can supervise only one or two technicians in the pharmacy (in some states, there are legal regulations in this area), or the pharmacist can manage the entire store, including nonpharmacy personnel. Recently, there has been a push to increase the span of control of managers owing to a number of drawbacks to small spans of control: They are expensive because they add layers of management, complicate vertical communication by slowing down decision-making, and discourage employee autonomy because of the close supervision by management. It is also felt that highly trained employees do not need as much direct supervision (Robbins, 2005). Some individuals find it quite discomforting to have someone always looking over their shoulder, but others may prefer to have someone who can respond quickly to problems when they arise.

Departmentalization

Departmentalization refers to grouping individuals according to specific tasks. For example, persons responsible for purchasing, distributing, and managing drug products could constitute a department. One of the advantages of having departments is that the individuals in a department share a common vocabulary and training and expertise. This should increase efficiency and effectiveness of the unit. Given the increased complexities of health care and pharmacy in particular, some organizations are requiring that members work across departments so that a diversity of ideas and expertise is given to specific tasks. This team approach helps supplement the functioning of individual departments and allows for better communication between different areas.

Newer Approaches to Organizational Design

The idea that the best structure for an organization depends on the nature of the environment in which the organization operates is called the *contingency approach* to organizational design (Greenburg and Baron, 2003). In this approach, based on the work of Mintzberg (1983), there are five organizational forms: A *simple structure* is one in which a single person runs the entire organization. An independent community pharmacy would be an example of this structure. This type of organization is quite flexible and can respond to the environment quite quickly, but it is also quite risky because the success or failure of the business depends on one or two individuals. A *machine bureaucracy* is a highly complex formal environment with clear lines of authority. This type of organization is highly efficient in performing standardized tasks but may be dehumanizing and boring for employees. A chain or mail-order pharmacy may be like this depending on the degree of structure and formalization that exists in the organization. On the other hand, a *professional bureaucracy* is one in which much of the day-to-day decision-making is vested in the professionals who carry out most of the work. In this type of structure, there are many rules and regulations that may inhibit creativity. An example of this type of structure would be found in a health system pharmacy. The positive side of this structure is that it allows professionals to practice those skills for which they are best qualified. On the negative side, these professionals may become overly narrow, which may lead to errors and potential conflicts between employees as a result of not seeing the "big picture." A *divisional structure* is one that consists of a set of autonomous units coordinated by a central headquarters. In this design, divisional managers have a lot of control that allows upper-level management to focus on the "big picture." A negative side of this structure is high duplication of effort. A college or school of pharmacy that is structured around the various disciplines of the pharmaceutical sciences is an example of this structure. A fifth structure is called an "adhocracy." An "adhocracy" is very informal in nature. There is very little formalization and centralization. Most of the work is done in teams. An example of this structure may be found in the research and development department of a pharmaceutical company. This type of design fosters innovation but can be highly inefficient and has the greatest potential for disruptive conflict.

One of the newest forms of organizational structure is the *boundaryless organization.* In this type of organization, the chains of command are eliminated, the spans of control are unlimited, and departments are replaced by empowered teams (Greenburg and Baron, 2003). This type of organization is highly flexible and can respond quickly to the external environment. One form of the boundaryless organization is the virtual organization (Robbins, 2005). A virtual (also called *modular* or *networked*) *organization* is one that has a small core of individuals, and major organizational functions are outsourced to others. There are no departments in this type of organization, and all decisions are made centrally. An example of one aspect of this model in community pharmacy would be where all refill prescriptions are sent to a central location to be filled and then returned to the community pharmacy for distribution to patients or where technology is used to verify prescriptions while pharmacists are located at an off-site location.

Organizational Teams

As previously mentioned, one of the newest forms of organizational structure involves the establishment of teams. Teams in health care are not new, as we can think of teams of clinicians working together to provide care to patients in the hospital or clinic setting. We can also think of teams in terms of pharmacists and technicians working together at a community pharmacy on a particular shift. As health care becomes more specialized, there will be increasing need for team structures to coordinate the work of individual specialists (Fried et al., 2006).

A *team* is defined as small number of people who are committed to a common purpose, who possess complementary skills and who have agreed on specific performance goals for which team members hold themselves mutually accountable (Katzenbach and Smith, 1993). Teams differ from workgroups in that workgroups depend upon "individual bests" or the sum of individual performance for effectiveness. Workgroups usually do not want to risk conflict and to take collective action necessary to build a common purpose. Cohen and Bailey (1997) identified four types of teams: work teams, parallel teams, project teams and management teams.

Work teams are continuing work units responsible for producing goods or providing services. They are usually directed by managers who make most of the decisions on what is done, how it is done and who does it. An alternative form of the work team is the self-managing team that allows employees to decide how to carry out tasks, allocate work within the team, and make decisions. Many times the members of work teams are cross-trained in a variety of skills relevant to the tasks they perform.

Parallel teams draw members from different work units to perform functions that the regular organization is not equipped to perform well. These teams have limited authority and usually make recommendations to individuals higher up in the organizational hierarchy. A quality improvement team in a health system would be an example of a parallel team.

Project teams produce one-time outputs such as a new product or service. Product team members usually draw their members from different units so that specialized expertise can be applied to the project at hand. When the project is completed, the members either return to their functional unit or move on to the next project. A new drug development team that draws members from research and development, finance, marketing, and manufacturing would be an example of such a team.

Finally, *management teams* coordinate and provide direction to units under their authority. Management teams exist at the board of directors or trustee level, senior management level or at the departmental level.

While many individuals enjoy the interactions and synergies that come from working on teams, there is probably no other aspect of organizational life that causes as much ambivalence and cynicism (Fried et al., 2006). Many teams achieve far less than their potential because of coordination, communication, or motivation problems among group members (Steiner, 1972). Interprofessional rivalries and status differences are often played out in teams causing anger, dissatisfaction, lower productivity, and a sense that individual knowledge and skills are being underutilized.

A meta-analysis of 298 studies found pharmacists' to have positive effects on patient therapeutic and safety outcomes when participating in multidisciplinary teams that consist of physicians, nurses, and other health professionals (Chisholm-Burns, et al., 2010). Another study found that shared team learning occurred more often in teams in which members felt that "they were all in this together" rather than ones in which members felt they had to get others "on board" (Bunniss and Kelly, 2008).

A study of pharmacists' identity development within multidisciplinary primary health care teams found that it takes time to begin to feel like a contributing member of a team (Pottie et al., 2009). Pharmacists needed mentors outside of the team to whom they could share ideas and ask advice. The progression to team member was not always linear and many felt there were days when progress was made and other days when steps back were taken. Pharmacists also began to see their profession through the "eyes" of doctors or nurses. They began to develop empathy for their perspectives rather and complaining about how the other health professionals do not understand their roles.

So how can effective team performance be built? Biech as cited in Gordon (2002) identified ten characteristics of successful teams: (1) Clear goals—allows everyone to understand the function and purpose of the team; (2) defined roles—allows everyone to understand why they are on the team and enables them to form clear individual and team-based goals; (3) open and clear communication—is essential for team-building and is based on effective listening; (4) effective decision-making—the team must be in agreement with the decisions that are reached through a consensus-building process; (5) balanced participation—ensures that all members are fully engaged; (6) valued diversity—the team must recognize each member's expertise and value variety of knowledge, skills, and abilities; (7) managed conflict—all team members feel safe to freely state their points of view without fear of reprisal; (8) positive atmosphere—requires a climate of trust be developed that requires team members to spend significant amount of time with each other; (9) cooperative relationships—team members need to recognize that they need one another's knowledge and skill to complete the given tasks; and (10) participative leadership—need to have leaders who are willing to share responsibility and recognition with the team. Borkowski (2009) added one more to this list: reflection and appreciative inquiry—teams need to allocate time for reflection and debriefing on the results of their actions and decisions so they can develop a vision of what they want to accomplish in the future and build on what worked best to reach their goals.

Informal Organizational Structure

Alongside the formal organizational structure, an informal structure exists. The informal system has great influence in shaping individual behavior. Communication within the organization is one area that the informal structure affects. Formal communication patterns exist in the form of meetings, memos, and reports. Informal communication patterns ("the grapevine") can take the form of rumors, gossip, and speculation. The grapevine can be positive in that it allows formal communication to be translated into language that employees understand. In addition, it can provide feedback to the manager about pending problems in the organization. When employees feel frustrated at centralized decision-making and their level of input, the grapevine can be a useful source of information. Informal ways of influencing decision-making can also emerge through the formation of alliances and favoritism.

Organizational norms and accountability can be influenced by these informal means. *Norms* are explicit rules of conduct that govern such things as employee dress and punctuality in reporting for work. Informal norms can develop through peer-influence systems (i.e., if most pharmacists stay until all the prescription orders are processed, then someone who does not will be looked on unfavorably by peers). The *accountability* system considers ways to measure the achievement of organizational goals. This is usually accomplished through performance reviews (see Chapter 15).

Administrators and managers must monitor their treatment of employees continually to discern problems in the organization. Understanding and managing both the formal and informal structures of the organization are important for effective functioning and improved employee performance.

PROFESSIONALS IN BUREAUCRATIC ORGANIZATIONS

As noted previously, many organizations can be described as following the bureaucratic model of structure (characterized by control, hierarchy of authority, the presence of rules, and impersonality). While most pharmacists are employees of these organizations, they have been socialized through formal education and mentorship to value expertise, self-determination, and care to individual patients. This can be referred to as the *professional model*. Other aspects of this model include the use of professional associations as a major referent with regard to conduct and behavior, a sense of calling to the field (the dedication of the professional to work and the feeling that the practitioner would do the work even if few extrinsic reward were available), and autonomy (the feeling that the practitioner ought to be able to make decisions without external pressures from clients, those who are not members of the profession, or the employer) (Hall, 1968).

In recent years, the professional value system of health care has been challenged by escalating costs and the call for reform (Dye, 2000). Cost is particularly an issue for pharmacy because the cost of prescription drugs continues to escalate, and securing payment for nondispensing services (e.g., patient counseling and drug therapy monitoring) continues to be a struggle. One way in which health care organizations have responded to the need for change is to become more corporate or bureaucratic in values. The *corporate model* values the collective needs of its customers (not individual patients) both now and in the future and works to ensure institutional survival through measures of fiscal responsibility and operating efficiency (Stoeckle and Stanley, 1992). A professional values the care of individual patients and their present health needs, which leads to a focus on trust-building behaviors such as eliciting personal concerns and exercising technical competence. A professional responds to authority based on expertise, whereas the organization's authority is found in hierarchical positions. Allegiances of the professional outside the organization (professional associations) could conflict with organizational norms. The formalization and standardization found in organizations can stifle initiative and discourage creativity and risk taking. There are some positive aspects to the organizational model. A highly developed division of labor and technical competence should be related to a high degree of professionalism because professionals are considered experts. Accountability and responsibility are important to the professional as well as to the corporation.

While important, the focus on technical competence, expertise, accountability and responsibility has made it difficult for professionals to find meaning in their work (Cherniss, 1995). This focus encourages a critical, detached attitude toward the world that weakens the professional's ability to form a strong commitment to an ideology or a group. Frankl (1962) suggests that individuals can find meaning in activities done for the sake of a cause, a loved one, or a higher being. This research suggests that those individuals, who find meaning in their work, truly view their work as a "calling" to the field. These professionals are more likely to connect with clients, practice a set of ideals, and work in a community that shares and nurtures these ideals: a moral community.

How can we infuse pharmacy with a greater sense of moral relevance? One might envision pharmacy and the health care system as a moral community rather than a service delivery system (Cherniss, 1995). Moral communities are those that share ethical concerns, values pluralism and have a keen sense of social responsibility (Dharmasi, 2006). These communities are grounded in relationships with others (i.e., other pharmacists, health professionals, patients, and other stakeholders). The development of a moral community requires an interdisciplinary understanding of the moral and ethical situations that occur in the delivery of health care. Beginning a dialogue among these groups that address the multifaceted challenges that arise within each group could open new ways of thinking, inquiry, and methods of addressing these challenges (Austin, 2007). Students and pharmacists need to articulate their value system and search for employers that allow them to express this value system. Research suggests that the day-to-day experiences pharmacists have with their employing organization can influence how they view the entire profession of pharmacy (Gaither and Mason, 1992). Employers who exhibit a commitment to professional ideals and supportive management, in addition to their own organizational goals, are ones to consider. Organizations that allow pharmacists' expectations to be met find increased commitment to the organization (organizational commitment) (Gaither, 1999). Increased commitment to the profession also increases organizational commitment (Gaither, 1998a; Gaither and Mason, 1992; Gaither et al., 2008a). Support from management and administrators is positively related to organizational commitment for pharmacists working for pharmaceutical manufacturers (Kong et al., 1992). Employers who emphasize interpersonal relationships and those pharmacists and pharmacy technicians who experienced increased supervisor support felt increased commitment to both the profession and the employer (Desselle and Holmes, 2007; Gaither et al., 2008b; Kong, 1995). Pharmacists who believe that the call for pharmacy care would have a positive effect on pharmacy were more committed to their employer and to pharmacy as a career.

It can be concluded that pharmacists' responses to organizational demands can have important implications for their professional values and ability to find meaningful work. This behooves students and pharmacists alike to work for and with organizations that facilitate fulfillment of their expectations. If the values of the organization are not in line with the values of the health profession, negative personal and organizational behaviors will occur.

PHARMACISTS' ORGANIZATIONAL BEHAVIORS

Examining pharmacists' work-related attitudes and behaviors is important if an organization wants to improve the positive and decrease or minimize the negative actions of employees. Increased absenteeism, tardiness, and counterproductive behaviors such as not completing work in a timely manner or theft will decrease organizational productivity and performance significantly. This has the economic consequence of decreasing the profitability of the organization (Barnett and Kimberlin, 1984). An unhappy coworker also can make the work environment unpleasant for other workers. The entire day seems longer and more stressful. Negative organizational attitudes also can compromise patient care. An unhappy or dissatisfied pharmacist may be less motivated to keep skills and knowledge levels current. Job dissatisfaction also has been found to be associated with an increased risk of medication errors (Bond and Raehl, 2001). The physical and mental health of the pharmacist also can suffer, owing to the stress of working in an unappealing pharmacy environment with a heavy workload (Gaither et al., 2008b; Gidman et al., 2007; Kreling et al., 2006). Studies of pharmacists' organizational behaviors have focused on a variety of work-related attitudes and behaviors. The most common are job satisfaction, organizational commitment, job stress, and job turnover.

Job Satisfaction

Job satisfaction can be defined either as an emotional response (the pleasurable or positive emotional state resulting from the appraisal of one's job or job experiences) (Locke, 1976) or as a comparison between expectations and the perceived reality of the job as a whole (Bacharach et al., 1991). Each individual brings a set of expectations to a job. Research in pharmacy suggests that how closely the job meets expectations, performing more clinical or nondistributive work activities, higher levels of autonomy, recognition, ability utilization, good environmental conditions (i.e., better work schedules, less workload, control over work, good workplace teamwork and communication, and less stress), professional commitment, and working in an independent pharmacy environment are strong predictors of job satisfaction (Cox and Fitzpatrick, 1999; Gaither, 1999; Gaither et al., 2008a; Hardigan et al., 2001; Kuiper et al., 2011; Lerkiatbundit, 2000; Liu and White, 2011; Mott et al., 2004; Olsen and Lawson, 1996; Reuppell et al., 2003). Being younger, male, nonwhite, in a staff position, working full-time, high role stress (i.e., role ambiguity, role strain, or role overload), and negative interpersonal interactions with either coworkers, management, or patients (Ferguson et al., 2010; Gaither et al., 2008a; McHugh, 1999; Mott et al., 2004; Prince et al., 2003; Seston et al., 2009; Stewart and Smith, 1987) are factors associated with less satisfaction. In a study of physicians, an organizational emphasis on quality of care enhanced job satisfaction (Williams et al., 2002). The same should be true for pharmacists. Positive interactions with key stakeholders outside the pharmacy department were the largest drivers of job satisfaction for a group of health-system pharmacists (Lane et al., 2010).

Enhanced job satisfaction leads to more positive feelings toward the employing organization (organizational commitment) (Gaither et al., 2008a).

Organizational Commitment

Organizational commitment has been defined both as an emotional attachment (affective organizational commitment) (Allen and Meyer, 1990) and as accepting the organization's goals and values, putting forth effort, and wanting to maintain membership (Mowday et al., 1979). Organizational commitment is important because it is related to reduced job turnover intention for pharmacists (Gaither et al., 2008a; Kahaleh and Gaither, 2005). Organizational commitment is enhanced when health care professionals receive appropriate compensation and benefits (Gaither and Mason, 1992; Gaither et al., 2008a) and have access to important organizational information, resources to perform the job, opportunities for advancement within the organization, and organizational support (structural empowerment) (Kahaleh and Gaither, 2005). This enhancement holds true regardless of practice setting (Kahaleh and Gaither, 2007). Psychological empowerment (i.e., finding meaning, feeling competent, and having independence and influence in a job) positively influences commitment for independent community pharmacists (Kahaleh and Gaither, 2007). High job demands (stress) and unpleasant interpersonal interactions decrease affective organizational commitment for hospital pharmacists (Gaither and Nadkarni, 2011).

Job Stress

Role stress in the form of role conflict, role ambiguity, role overload, and work–home conflict increases job stress (Gaither, 1998b; Gaither et al., 2008a). Job dissatisfaction is also associated with increased job stress (Wolfgang and Wolfgang, 1992). Role expansion in the form of increased expectations to provide medication use reviews and other nondispensing services without the supporting infrastructure or support of other health care professionals has led to increased job stress, decreased job satisfaction, and increased intentions to leave the profession (Eden et al., 2009; McCann et al., 2009; Rothmann and Malan, 2007). Stress that continues to be ignored can lead to a phenomenon known as burnout. Burnout is thought to develop through a series of stages, and if caught at anytime, it can be reversed.

Traditionally, burnout has been conceptualized as a problem confined to the individual (i.e., flaws in a person's character, behavior, or productivity). However, growing evidence suggests that burnout is tied to the social environment of the workplace (Maslach and Leiter, 1997). The structure and functioning of the workplace shape how people interact and carry out tasks. Failure to recognize the human side of work increases the risk of burnout. Engagement with work requires a person's full participation in the social environment. Support, recognition and collaboration help people focus their energy more effectively, justify their involvement and extend their achievements. Consequently this leads to a more robust organization and lessens burnout (Maslach and Leiter, 1997). More information on how to manage job stress and burnout is found in Chapter 10.

Job Turnover

Job turnover is one of most pressing concerns of organizations. The decreased productivity from voluntary turnover is very costly to an organization because less experienced workers must be used to replace the more experienced workers who leave. Advertising, recruiting, and training a replacement employee for someone who has left can be costly not only in monetary terms but also in terms of lost productivity owing to the time spent bringing the new employee up to speed. In a time of shortage of available employees, it is important to retain existing employees. Actual job turnover rates of pharmacists have been estimated to be between 14 and 23 percent per year (Gaither, 1998a; Paavola, 1990; Stewart et al., 1987). In an interview of chain pharmacists who recently left their employers, the main reasons pharmacists gave for leaving were related to working conditions: inflexible and long working hours and inadequate support personnel (Schulz and Baldwin, 1990). Other reasons for leaving an organization relate to job dissatisfaction, role stress, and culture and climate factors (Gaither, 1998a; Gaither et al., 2007,

2008a; Mott, 2000). Personal variables such as number of children (more), race (whites less), age (older more or less), education (e.g., having an advanced degree), and having a major life event (e.g., getting married, getting divorced, or death in family) also can result in job turnover intention (Gaither et al., 2007; McHugh, 1999). Market conditions such as the number of jobs available are important because this may make it easier to leave one job for another.

As with burnout, job turnover is viewed as a process in which an individual will first think about leaving, search for job alternatives, form an intention to leave, and then actually leave. Therefore, it can be influenced at various stages. Managers may not be able to control all the factors related to job turnover (e.g., major life events or market conditions), but they can be very influential as mentioned earlier and should be on the lookout for ways in which the organization can foster commitment, improve job satisfaction, and decrease role stress. A place to start would be with the structure of the organization. Looking for problems in the amount of decision-making ability given to pharmacists, the tasks/workload assigned, the reward structure, and communication between management and staff is a good way to determine areas that need improvement. Another factor that may be particularly important for professional employees such as pharmacists is organizational identification.

Organizational identification is defined as the perception of oneness with or belongingness to a group/organization (Ashforth and Mael, 1989). To identify with an organization implies that one sees oneself as a personal representative of the organization and feels that the organization's successes and failures are one's own. Fostering organizational identification may be a very important way to shape health professionals' organizational behavior because outside influences (e.g., professional associations, colleagues, or patients) are important in the formation and maintenance of professional behavior (Dukerich et al., 2002).

The more strongly employees identify with an organization, the more likely they are to engage in citizenship behaviors related specifically to the organization (e.g., courtesy, conscientiousness, sportsmanship, civic virtue, and altruism) (Konovsky and Pugh, 1994). These behaviors are actions that typically are not captured in the normal reward structure of the organization. A recent study of community pharmacists found that participation in pharmaceutical care activities was associated with greater organizational identification (O'Neill and Gaither, 2007). Higher levels of organizational identification were related to lower job turnover intention. In addition, the way in which an employee believes the organization is viewed by outsiders has a direct impact on both organizational identification and job turnover intention; the more positive the image, the greater is identification. Joe Smart may want to ask some of the patients and even the doctors and nurses who come into the ambulatory care pharmacy how they view the pharmacy and the services it provides. If these "outsiders" have a negative view of the pharmacy, it may be contributing to the tense atmosphere in the pharmacy. This brings us to an emerging area in pharmacists' organizational behaviors: emotions.

Emotions

Emotions are intense feelings that are directed at someone or something (Greenburg and Baron, 2003). Emotions are sometimes confused with moods, which are pervasive emotions not directed at any particular person or object (Fiske and Taylor, 1991). Moods have been shown to be related to withdrawal behaviors such as absenteeism and turnover (Pelled et al., 1999). Health care organizations put more emotional demands on employees and patients than many other organizations, yet very little is known about what these demands are and the strategies people use to deal with their emotions (Ovretveit, 2001). One study in pharmacy found that the emotional expression of anger, defensiveness, or disgust is related to job dissatisfaction and depression, whereas the expression of resentfulness and disappointment is related to emotional exhaustion, a major component of job burnout (Abunassar and Gaither, 2000).

Health care demands both the suppression and expression of emotion and skills to know and manage feelings appropriately (Ovretveit, 2001). Emotional regulation in the workplace has been termed *emotional labor* and is particularly important to health care professionals. Emotional labor is defined as expressing organizationally desired emotions during service transactions (Hochschild, 1983). The difference between the emotions that an individual expresses and those he or she actually feels can be the basis of emotional exhaustion.

Individuals who have the ability to take another's perspective or to know what another is feeling (empathic concern) or who generally express or feel positive emotions (positive affect) will have less of a need to expend emotional labor (Zammuner and Galli, 2005). It is also suggested that persons who are more emotionally mature (or possess greater emotional intelligence) will experience greater job satisfaction than those who do not. The pharmacists in the scenario's ambulatory care pharmacy may be expending high levels of emotional labor. The pharmacy director may want to explore training for pharmacists to enhance their empathic behaviors, which also may decrease their emotional labor and possibly enhance emotional intelligence. The concept of emotional intelligence has also been linked to another important influence on the organizational behavior of employees: the leadership abilities of those in management or administrative positions.

LEADERSHIP BEHAVIOR

In an era of increasing corporatization of health care, securing the welfare of patients requires that health professionals participate in the creation of optimal frameworks to deliver care (Stoeckle and Stanley, 1992). No longer should the individual pharmacist say, "I am not the manager or administrator, so I have no role in determining how the pharmacy is structured or organized." Without highly competent and aggressive leadership, the provision of pharmaceutical care and other new roles advocated by the pharmacy profession could be usurped by other health professionals, corporate entities, or technologies (O'Neil, 2002). This will require the development of leadership abilities in all pharmacists.

Management versus Leadership

Leadership can be thought of as getting a group of people to move toward a particular vision or ideal. Leadership is concerned with change and with motivating employees to move toward a shared vision. *Management,* on the other hand, is concerned with handling the complexities involved in running an organization (i.e., planning, control, evaluation, and financial analysis) (Kotter, 1990). Given this distinction, a manager or an administrator may not necessarily be a leader. She may be more concerned with the day-to-day functioning of the organization. The manager may give little thought to the overall goals of the organization and how her department/pharmacy fits into the overall scheme. In addition, managers may not give much thought to the future and to developing a shared vision with employees as to where the organization should be moving. A good manager should also be a leader because one needs to be concerned with the present situation but have an eye on the future. The future should include not only the tasks and activities in which the organization engages but also the development of motivation and future leadership in the staff. This motivation and energy are essential to facilitate the transformation of pharmacy from drug procurement and dispensing into the provision of pharmaceutical care.

THEORIES OF LEADERSHIP

Trait Theories

Much of the early research on leadership focused on identifying personality traits that could distinguish leaders from nonleaders. Intelligence, self-confidence, a high energy level, and technical knowledge about the task at hand are positively correlated with leadership abilities (Robbins, 2005). The problem with the search for traits of leaders is that it implies that leaders are born and not made. Individuals without these traits could never be leaders. It also ignores the influence and needs of the employees one is trying to lead. Trait theories focus more on leaders and less on followers. Research findings in this area have been inconsistent. Some studies found that one trait was related to leadership ability, whereas another study found that it was not related (Stodgill, 1948; Yukl, 1989).

Recent research suggests that traits do make a difference when categorized into five basic personality characteristics (Judge et al., 2002): *extroversion*—one's comfort level with relationships; *agreeableness*—an individual's propensity to defer to others; *conscientiousness*—how reliable a person is; *emotional stability*—a person's ability to withstand stress; and *openness to experience*—an individual's range of interests and fascination with novelty (Robbins, 2005). High energy and self-confidence can be categorized under extroversion and emotional stability. The other main drawback with the trait approach is that it does a better job of predicting who may emerge as a leader than determining what constitutes effective leadership. This has led contemporary researchers to take a behavioral approach to leadership and to focus on the preferred behavioral styles that good leaders demonstrate.

Behavioral Theories

Researchers have observed three very basic leadership styles: autocratic, democratic, and laissez-faire. *Autocratic leaders* make all the decisions and allow for no or very little input from the employees. *Democratic leaders* consult with their subordinates and allow them some input in the decision-making process. *Laissez-faire leaders* allow employees complete autonomy. In such an approach, employees set their own goals and work toward them with no direction from management. Let's say a pharmacy manager would like to implement a disease management program in the pharmacy. An autocratic leader would just inform the employees of the change in approach and then assign the tasks necessary to implement the program. A democratic leader would present the idea to the employees and ask for their input about the appropriateness of the idea and take into consideration their ideas on how to implement the program. Finally, a laissez-faire leader would not mention the idea unless the employees came to him with it. The leader then would allow the employees to develop the entire program and implement the plan. It has been found that all three styles of leadership behavior can be appropriate depending on the situation (La Monica, 1994). These findings led researchers to begin examining the components of leadership behavior and the determination of appropriate behavior for the specific situation.

Situational or Contingency-Based Theories

Hersey's Situational Leadership® model is a leadership theory based on three basic dimensions: task and relationship orientation behavior and follower readiness (Hersey and Blanchard, 1988). *Task orientation behavior* refers to the extent to which a leader engages in one-way communication by defining the roles of individuals and members of the group by explaining (telling or showing or both) what each subordinate is to do, as well as when, where, how much, and by when specific tasks are to be accomplished. This dimension also includes the extent to which the leader defines the structure of the organization (i.e., chain of command, channels of communication, etc.) and specifies ways of getting jobs accomplished. *Relationship orientation* behavior refers to the extent to which the leader engages in two-way communication, provides socio-emotional support, and uses facilitative versus directive efforts of bringing about group change. This component takes into account the establishment of effective interpersonal relationships between the leader and the group based on trust. The third component consists of *follower readiness or maturity*. In this case, maturity readiness is related the group's or individual's willingness or ability to accept responsibility for a task and whether they are currently performing the task at a sustained and acceptable level. Certainly, the possession of the necessary training or experience to perform the task impacts on their ability to perform but what matters most in assessing readiness is whether they are doing the task now rather than what they are potentially capable of doing. As in the example given earlier, a group of pharmacists may be quite willing to develop a disease management program but may be inexperienced at implementing such a program.

Each of these dimensions can be located on a continuum that is divided into four quadrants (Waller, Smith, and Warnock, 1989). Fig. 8-4 illustrates these quadrants.

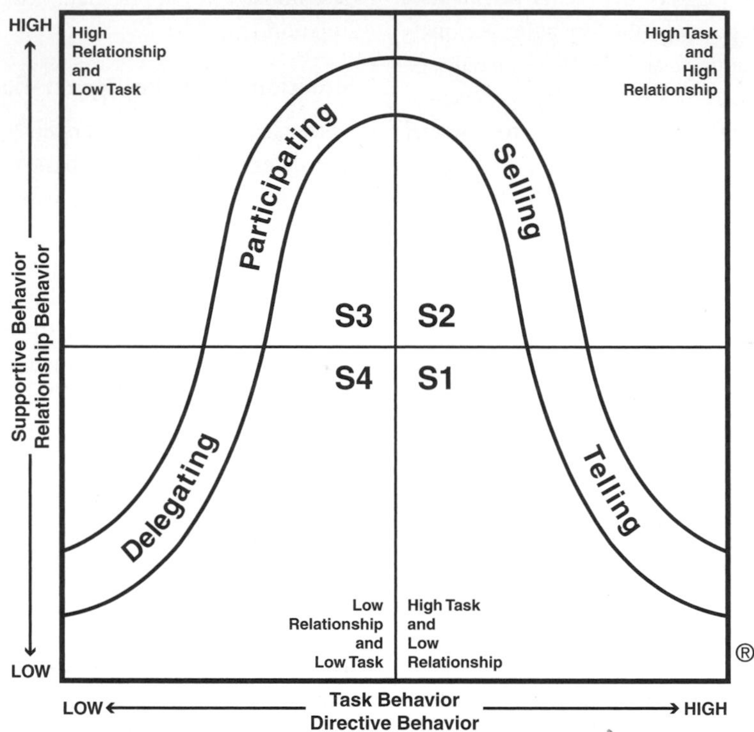

Performance Readiness®

HIGH	MODERATE		LOW
R4	**R3**	**R2**	**R1**
Able and Confident and Willing	Able but Insecure or Unwilling	Unable but Confident or Willing	Unable and Insecure or Unwilling

Figure 11-4. Situational leadership theory. (*Adapted with permission from Hersey and Blanchard, 1988.*)

1. *High task/low relationship.* The leader determines the roles and goals of the group and closely supervises the task. Communication is one way and usually flows from the leader to the followers. This style, also known as *telling* (S1), is most appropriate when followers are unable/unwilling or insecure (R1).
2. *High task/high relationship.* The leader still closely supervises the task but will also explain why decisions are made. The leader may alter the plan given the followers' reactions. This style, also known as *selling* (S2), is most appropriate when followers' are unable but more willing or secure (R2).

3. *High relationship/low task.* In this case the leader is more concerned about process and how the group works together to accomplish the task rather than the task itself. In this style, also called participative or *supportive* (S3), the leader still may define the problem but supports the group's efforts at accomplishing the task. Followers in this case are able but unwilling or insecure (R3).
4. *Low task/low relationship.* The leader turns over all decisions and responsibility for task accomplishment, goal attainment, and implementation to followers. The leader may be available for consultation but usually maintains a low profile. In this case, also called *delegation* (S4), followers are very able, willing, and secure (R4).

It is the leader's job to determine the performance readiness of the group and then apply the appropriate leadership style to the situation.

A final component of this model is *leader effectiveness* (La Monica, 1994). A leader's influence over an individual or group can be either successful or unsuccessful. When a leader's behavior fails to influence an individual or group to achieve a specified goal, then the leader must reevaluate what occurred and redesign a strategy for goal accomplishment. Even when a goal is accomplished, a leader's influence still can range from very effective to ineffective depending on how followers feel about the leader's behavior. If a leader knows the personal strengths of her followers and assigns goals or tasks with them in mind, this can make goal accomplishment quite rewarding for the followers. On the other hand, if the followers feel coerced to accomplish by a leader who uses positional power, close supervision, and rewards and punishments, the followers may be very unhappy and carry negative feelings toward the leader. Leadership effectiveness is very important because effective leadership will lead to followers who are motivated and goal oriented even when the leader is not present. Ineffective leadership will lead to followers who often will relax the drive to accomplish when the leader is absent.

A study of pharmacists who worked in community settings or for national and state pharmacy associations found that the most common leadership style was selling (high task/high relationship), and the next most common was participation (low task/high relationship) (Ibrahim et al., 1997; Ibrahim and Wertherimer, 1998). About 26 percent of the pharmacists did not have a dominant style. Not surprisingly, most pharmacists scored in the low- (community pharmacists) to-moderate (association executives) range in their ability to adapt their style to the needs of their subordinates (leadership effectiveness). These results suggest that while pharmacists possess a dominant leadership style, there is room for improvement in terms of learning to respond and modify their style to best fit the needs and motivational levels of their staff.

Leader–Member Exchange Theory

Another theory related to the leader–follower relationship is the leader–member exchange (LMX) theory (Green and Uhl-Bien, 1995). This theory suggests that leaders establish special relationships with a small group of followers early on in the tenure of the leader. These individuals make up the leader's in-group, whereas others are considered part of the out-group. It is unclear how these relationships form, but most likely they result from the followers either having similar personality characteristics to the leader or exceptional abilities to perform the job. The in-group gets special attention from the leader and tends to have higher job satisfaction and lower job turnover intention than members of the out-group (Robbins, 2005). These findings suggest that leaders need to pay attention to the nature of their relationships with followers because these relationships can greatly affect employee morale (Greenberg and Baron, 2003).

Leader-Participation Model

One of the more recent additions to contingency-based leadership theories relates leadership behavior and participation in decision-making (Vroom and Yetton, 1973). This model assumes five behaviors that may be feasible given a particular situation. These behaviors are (1) you solve the problem yourself using the information you have available at the time; (2) you obtain the necessary information from subordinates and then decide on a solution yourself; (3) you share the problem with relevant subordinates individually, getting their ideas and suggestions without bringing them together as a group, and then you make the decision; (4) you share the problem with your subordinates as a group and collectively obtain their ideas and suggestions, and then you make the decision that may or may not reflect your subordinates' influence; and (5) you share the problem with the group and together you generate and evaluate alternatives and attempt to reach consensus on a solution. The leader-participation model then uses a series of eight yes–no questions to determine how much participation should be used. Questions include:

- Do I have enough information to make a high-quality decision?
- If the decision were accepted, would it make a difference which course of action was adopted?
- Do subordinates have sufficient additional information to result in a high-quality decision?
- Do I know exactly what information is needed, who possesses it, and how to collect it?
- Is acceptance of the decision by subordinates critical to effective implementation?
- If I were to make the decision by myself, is it certain that my subordinates would accept it?
- Can subordinates be trusted to base solutions on organizational considerations?
- Is conflict among subordinates likely in the preferred solution?

These questions allow the leader to determine which of the five behaviors is most appropriate. Results from research on this model suggest that leaders should consider the use of participatory methods when the quality of the decision is important, when it is crucial that subordinates accept the decision and it is unlikely that they will if they do not take part in it, and when subordinates can be trusted to pay attention to the goals of the group rather than simply their own preferences (Robbins, 2005). A more recent update of this model adds several more yes–no questions to consider regarding time constraints that limit subordinate participation, costs of bringing subordinates together, minimizing the time needed to make the decision, and the importance of developing subordinates' decision-making skills (Vroom and Jago, 1988).

This approach may be fruitful in pharmacy because new leadership models of organizing health care have been proposed. Governance models that focus on shared decision-making between management and health care professions offer a way to combine both professional and organizational concerns (Young, 2002). The management style of leaders in an era of change is one that has a high regard for people and production and emphasizes shared responsibility, involvement, commitment, and mutual support (Williams, 1986). The most productive and motivated staff members are those who have strong relationships with others with whom or for whom they work (Abramowitz, 2001).

Transactional versus Transformational Leadership

Most of the theories presented in this chapter are considered transactional in nature. In other words, they are largely oriented toward accomplishing the task at hand and maintaining good relations with those working with the leader by exchanging promises of rewards for performance (Dessler, 1998). A newer approach to leadership takes a transformational approach. Transformational leaders make subordinates more conscious of the importance and value of their task outcomes and provide followers with a vision and motivation to go beyond self-interest for the good of the organization (Osland et al., 2001). This focus on task outcomes is a major shift in the health care arena because much of the focus of health care has been on the process of care (DeYoung, 2005). It is suggested that health care organizations need both transactional (for control and efficiency) and transformational (for innovation) leadership. A recent survey of health system pharmacists indicated that pharmacists did possess both transactional and transformational characteristics, but few were interested in becoming the director of pharmacy (Abraham, 2006). This suggests that more research is needed as to why this type of leadership is unattractive to pharmacists and what can be done to remedy this situation. More information on leadership theories can be found in Chapter 16.

There is always the question of whether leadership is really necessary. As mentioned earlier, advocating for patients and the fulfillment of new roles for pharmacists will require that all pharmacists demonstrate leadership behaviors. Such factors as ability, intrinsic motivation, the nature of technology, and the structure of the organization can affect the performance and satisfaction of its members. Upon graduation, pharmacists possess the basic task knowledge to practice pharmacy. Pharmacists may also try to maintain good working relationships with patients and management because of professional values. These factors can substitute for effective leadership. Goals will be met regardless of what the leader or manager does or does not do. But managers and leaders need to recognize that by no means will motivated pharmacists continue to be motivated and energized in working environments that are negative and highly stressful. It is important for leaders to develop a shared vision with individual units in their organizations and support and empower employees to move toward that vision an effective leader conducts self-diagnoses and is aware of his or her blind spots, seeks ways to address them, and also surrounds himself or herself with people having complementary strengths.

One final note regards the increasing diversity in health care organizations regarding not only the type of personnel working together (i.e., physicians, nurses, pharmacists, technicians, and assistants) but also in the demographic characteristics of these workers (i.e., gender, race/ethnicity, and age). Leaders must be able to effectively manage this diversity to maximize individual performance. An approach that links diversity to the actual work performed and values it for what it adds to the organization leads to an environment in which the benefits of diversity can be maximized (Ely and Thomas, 2001).

REVISITING THE SCENARIO

Joe Smart knew that something was wrong with the internal environment of the ambulatory care pharmacy. What he probably noticed was a lack of leadership on the part of the pharmacy director and how the pharmacists were very task oriented in their behavior and seemed not to find their work meaningful. It may be that the employees of the pharmacy do not feel like a part of the health system organizational team and are feeling frustrated by a lack of recognition by others. It seems as though not a lot of time has been spent building relationships within or outside the department. Since Joe is the newest employee of the pharmacy, he is a bit hesitant to get involved, but he may be the perfect person to inquire about the values and goals of the ambulatory care pharmacy and how the pharmacy is structured to meet these goals. This would be a perfect time to examine the climate in the pharmacy to find out why the employees are dissatisfied. Although Joe does not have a leadership position in the organization, he should think about what he could do to improve the environment of the pharmacy. It is everyone's responsibility to make sure that health care is being delivered in the best manner possible, and unhappy staff members probably are not doing their best. Joe also could work on building relationships with others on the staff. This may help the employees talk about what is going on at the pharmacy. Improved dialogue within the pharmacy and with other stakeholders outside the pharmacy department could enhance the sense of community among the employees. With the help of more experienced employees, Joe could bring these matters to the attention of the pharmacy director. By taking a proactive stance, Joe is developing leadership skills that will serve him throughout his career.

CONCLUSION

An understanding of organizational behavior is needed by pharmacists to function productively in an organizational environment. Looking for employers who facilitate professional goals is necessary for the continued development of new roles for pharmacists. Employers must constantly monitor the work environment for signs of job dissatisfaction, job stress, and burnout in their employees. It is important that health care professionals do not stay away from participating in organizational governance. It is a part of their professional responsibility to ensure that health care is delivered appropriately to patients. Leadership ability can greatly influence pharmacists' attitudes and behaviors. Without a clear and shared vision between management and staff, innovative practices will be difficult to implement.

QUESTIONS FOR FURTHER DISCUSSION

1. Why did the focus of organizational behavior change over time?
2. Given that organizations are trying to empower employees at all levels, are organizational charts still necessary? Why or why not?
3. How important is division of labor, span of control, unity of command, departmentalization, and other structural aspects in pharmacy today? Do you see more or less of these structures in pharmacy organizations? What new organizational forms do you see developing in the future?
4. What are some ways in which professionals respond to organizational demands? Are these appropriate? What are other ways of responding?
5. What role do values play in an organization?
6. How might pharmacists find meaningful work in their organizations?
7. Why is it important for pharmacists and employing organizations to monitor organizational behaviors?
8. How can organizations assist pharmacists in expanding their role without inadvertently increasing their workload to unmanageable levels?
9. What role does emotion have in a health care organization? How might we better understand its importance?
10. What are some key features of leadership? Is it important for pharmacists to develop leadership skills? How will you develop your leadership abilities?

REFERENCES

Abraham D. 2006. Pharmacy leadership crisis: Is it the people or the job? Paper presented at American Society of Health-System Pharmacists Midyear Clinical Meeting, Anaheim, CA.

Abramowitz PW. 2001. Nurturing relationships: An essential ingredient of leadership. *Am J Health Syst Pharm* 58:479.

Abunassar SM, Gaither CA. 2000. The effects of cognitive appraisals and coping strategies on job satisfaction, commitment and burnout levels in hospital pharmacists. Paper presented at the 147th Annual Meeting of the American Pharmaceutical Association, Washington, DC.

Allen NJ, Meyer JP. 1990. The measurement and antecedents of affective, continuance and normative commitment to the organization. *J Occup Psychol* 63:1.

Ashforth BE, Mael FA. 1989. Social identity theory and the organization. *Acad Manage Rev* 14:20.

Austin W. 2007. The ethics of everyday practice: Healthcare environments as moral communities. *ANS Adv Nurs Sci* 30:81.

Bacharach SB, Bamberger P, Conley S. 1991. Work-home conflict among nurses and engineers: Mediating the impact of role stress on burnout and satisfaction at work. *J Org Behav* 12:39.

Barnett CW, Kimberlin CL. 1984. Job and career satisfaction in pharmacy. *J Soc Admin Pharm* 2:1.

Bond CA, Raehl CL. 2001. Pharmacists' assessment of dispensing errors: Risk factors, practice sites, professional functions and satisfaction. *Pharmacotherapy* 21: 614.

Borkowski N. 2009. Teams and team building. In Borkowski N (ed.) *Organizational Behavior, Theory, and Design in Health Care.* Sudbury, MA: Jones and Bartlett.

Boyle TA, Mahaffey T, Mackinnon NJ, Diehl H, Hallstrom LK, Morgan H. 2011. Determinants of medication incident reporting, recovery, and learning in community pharmacies: A conceptual model. *Res Soc Adm Pharm* 7:93.

Bunnies S, Kelly DR. 2008. 'The unknown becomes the known': Collective learning and change in primary care teams. *Med Educ* 42:1185.

Bush J, Langley CA, Wilson KA. 2009. The corporatization of community pharmacy: Implications for service provision, the public health function, and pharmacy's claim to professional status in the United Kingdom. *Res Soc Adm Pharm* 5:305.

Cameron KS, Freeman S. 1991. Culture, congruence, strength and type: Relationship to effectiveness. *Res Organ Change Dev* 5:23.

Cherniss C. 1995. *Beyond Burnout.* New York: Routledge.

Chisholm-Burns MA, Lee JK, Spivey CA, et al. 2010. US pharmacists' effect as team members on patient care: Systematic review and meta-analysis. *Med Care* 48:923.

Clark BE, Mount JM. 2006. Pharmacy Service Orientation: A measure of organizational culture in pharmacy practice sites. *Res Soc Adm Pharm* 2:110.

Cohen SG, Bailey DE. 1997. What makes team work: Group effectiveness research from the shop floor to the executive suite. *J Manage* 23:239.

Cox ER, Fitzpatrick V. 1999. Pharmacists' job satisfaction and perceived utilization of skills. *Am J Health Syst Pharm* 56:1733.

Dessler G. 1998. *Management: Leading People and Organizations in the 21st Century,* 1st edn. Upper Saddle River, NJ: Prentice-Hall.

Desselle SP, Holmes ER. 2007. A structural model of CPhTs' job satisfaction and career commitment. *J Am Pharm Assoc* 47:58.

Desselle SP, Skomo ML. 2010. Factors related to pharmacists' care of migraineurs. *Res Social Adm Pharm* 6:232–245.

DeYoung R. 2005. Contemporary leadership theories. In Borkowski N (ed.) *Organizational Behavior in Health Care.* Sudbury, MA: Jones and Bartlett.

Dharamsi S. 2006. Building moral communities? First, do no harm. *J Dent Educ* 70:1235.

Dukerich JM, Golden BR, Shortell SM. 2002. Beauty is in the eye of the beholder: The impact of organizational identification, identity, and image on the cooperative behaviors of physicians. *Admin Sci Q* 47:507.

Dye CF. 2000. *Leadership in Healthcare*: Values at the Top. Chicago: Health Administration Press.

Eden M, Schafheutle EI, Hassell K. 2009. Workload pressure among recently qualified pharmacists: An exploratory study of intentions to leave the profession. *Int J Pharm Pract* 17:181.

Ely RJ, Thomas DA. 2001. Cultural diversity at work: The effects of diversity perspectives on work group processes and outcomes. *Admin Sci Q* 46:229.

Feletto E, Wilson LK, Roberts AS, Benrimoj SI. 2010. Building capacity to implement cognitive pharmaceutical services. *Res Social Adm Pharm* 6:163–173.

Ferguson J, Ashcroft D, Hassell K. 2010. Qualitative insights into job satisfaction and dissatisfaction with management among community and hospital pharmacists. *Res Soc Admin Pharm.*

Fiske ST, Taylor SE. 1991. *Social Cognition.* New York: McGraw-Hill.

Fjortoft N. 2006. Identifying caring behaviors of pharmacists through observations and interviews. *J Am Pharm Assoc* 46:582.

Frankl VE. 1962. *Man's Search for Meaning.* New York: Clarion.

Freidson E. 1970. *Profession of Medicine: A Study of the Sociology* of Applied Knowledge. New York: Dodd, Mead, p. 73.

Fried BJ, Topping S, Edmondson AC. 2006. Groups and teams. In Shortell SM, *Kaluzny AD (eds.) Health Care Management: Organization Design and Behavior,* 5th edn. Clifton Park, NY: Thomson Delmar Learning.

Gaither CA. 1998a. The predictive validity of work/career-related attitudes and intentions on pharmacists' turnover behavior. *J Pharm Mark Manage* 12:3.

Gaither CA. 1998b. An investigation of pharmacists' role stress and the work/non-work interface. *J Soc Admin Pharm* 15:92.

Gaither CA. 1999. Career commitment: A mediator of the effects of job stress on pharmacists' work-related attitudes. *J Am Pharm Assoc* 39:353.

Gaither CA, Kahaleh AA, Doucette WR, et al. 2008a. A modified model of pharmacists' job stress: The role of organizational, extra-role and individual factors on work-related outcomes. *Res Soc Admin Pharm* 4:231.

Gaither CA, Mason HL. 1992. A model of pharmacists' career commitment, organizational commitment and career and job withdrawal intentions. *J Soc Admin Pharm* 9:75.

Gaither CA, Nadkarni A. 2011. Interpersonal interactions, job demands and work-related outcomes in pharmacy. *Int J Pharm Pract*: 165-173.

Gaither CA, Nadkarni A, Mott DA, et al. 2007. Should I stay or should I go? The influence of individual and organizational factors on pharmacists' future work plans. *J Am Pharm Assoc* 47:165.

Gibb JR. 1978. *Trust: A New View of Personal and Organizational Development.* Los Angeles: Guild of Tutors Press.

Gidman WK, Hassell K, Day J, et al. 2007. The impact of increasing workloads and role expansion on female community pharmacists in the United Kingdom. *Res Soc Adm Pharm* 3:285.

Gordon J. 2002. A perspective on team building. *J Am Acad Bus* 2:185.

Green GB, Uhl-Bien M. 1995. Relationship-based approach to leadership: Development of leader-member exchange (LMX) theory of leadership over 25 years: Applying a multi-domain perspective. *Leadership Q* 6:219.

qualified candidates from distant areas would be reimbursed for travel for the interview. Another consideration is targeting an appropriate demographic. For example, if an organization is seeking a pharmacist with considerable years of experience for a management position, it need not advertise in a newspaper or magazine that targets teenagers. On the other hand, if an organization consistently recruits for a large number of positions, it should be conscious about trying to reach populations diverse in age, gender, and race/ethnicity.

After choosing the advertising medium, an advertisement is written. When writing any advertisement, it is important to keep it simple. It should not make false promises and should not use hyperbolic rhetoric or technical jargon. It should only capture the eye of qualified candidates and persuade them to contact the pharmacy.

Placement

Placement refers to candidate application, screening, interviewing, selection, and hiring processes. In many organizations, pharmacists are assisted in this process by corporate personnel offices. Personnel offices offer valuable assistance in advertising positions, managing applications and paperwork, screening candidates, advising about legal and policy questions, checking references, and extending job offers. They free pharmacy personnel to develop criteria for selecting employees, to interview qualified candidates, and to make the final choice.

It is important to emphasize, however, that pharmacists need to monitor and influence the personnel office's performance in the placement process. One reason is that personnel employees do not understand as well as pharmacists the requirements of pharmacy practice. They may emphasize different knowledge and capabilities than pharmacists. A second reason is that the personnel office does not have to suffer as much from the consequences of a bad employee choice. Pharmacy personnel will bear the brunt of a bad employee hire. Therefore, it is incumbent on pharmacists to maintain as much control over the process as necessary to ensure a good choice.

Application

One of the first steps in hiring is for a candidate to fill out a job application. Job applications serve two purposes. The first is to help screen unqualified candidates. Applications can identify whether candidates have the necessary training, degrees, and experience for the job. The second purpose of applications is to provide background about the candidate for the interview.

Screening

Once they have submitted an application, applicants are screened to see if they meet the requirements of the job. Screening is a process that attempts to weed out unqualified applicants from the pool of potential candidates. Common screening criteria include lack of job qualifications (e.g., license, degree, residency, or experience), poorly completed applications (e.g., misspelling, missing information, or sloppy writing), and negative applicant history (e.g., felony conviction, lying on the application, or frequent changes in employment).

Screening criteria are developed from job analyses. Job analyses are systematic reviews of the requirements of a job (Donnelly et al., 1995). Job analyses attempt to identify some of the following aspects of a job:

- Behaviors, tasks, and outcomes required of the employee on the job
- Skills, capabilities, and knowledge required
- Physical requirements
- Required information, technology, and resources
- Expected interpersonal relationships
- Budget and managerial responsibilities

The job analysis provides useful information for both employees and managers. For managers, information from the job analysis is used in writing job descriptions, interviewing job candidates, screening candidates, and setting performance criteria. For employees, information from the job analysis tells employees how work is to be done and the outcomes expected.

Interviewing

When qualified candidates are identified, interviews are scheduled. Qualified candidates normally are ranked according to desirability, with the top-ranked

Table 12-2. Sample Job Description and Performance Standards for a Hospital Pharmacist

Description

Responsible for safe distribution and drug administration for patient care, supervising technicians, order entry, drug monitoring, and providing drug information to nurses and physicians

Qualifications

Bachelor's degree (5-year program) or advanced pharmacy degree (Pharm.D. or M.S.) from an accredited college of pharmacy, hospital pharmacy experience preferred, licensure or eligibility for licensure

Performance Standards

Dispensing	Dispenses medications in accordance to all state and federal laws
Clinical skills and professional judgment	Integrates clinical, procedural, and distributive judgments using acceptable standards of practice to achieve positive patient outcomes
Productivity	Prioritizes work to ensure that all tasks are completed in a timely manner
Service	Fosters favorable relations between hospital personnel, patients, coworkers, families, visitors, and physicians. Accepts chain of command, supervision, and constructive criticism
Written documentation and communication	Follows all state and federal laws, regulatory agency rules, and hospital policies and procedures regarding written documentation. Consistently, clearly, and concisely communicates oral and written information to all hospital personnel, physicians, and patients
Technical supervision	Provides oversight and feedback to pharmacy technicians that ensures quality care and adherence to departmental policies and procedures
Attendance and punctuality	Meets all hospital policies regarding attendance and punctuality

candidates receiving initial invitations to interview. If a candidate is not chosen from the first round of applicant interviews, a second round is scheduled, drawing from the remaining pool of applicants.

Preparation for an interview is as important for the interviewer as it is for the candidate. The following is a suggested list of interview preparation steps:

- *Send information about the position to the candidate.* It is helpful to provide candidates with specific information about the job description and standards for performance to help them prepare for the interview.
- *Identify interview objectives.* It is important to ask yourself what you want to achieve with the interviews. For example, if you have acute, immediate needs, you may only consider candidates who are available immediately. However, if your interest is long term, you may be willing to wait for an excellent candidate to graduate from pharmacy school or complete a commitment made to another employer.
- *Review the position description and performance standards.* The position description and performance standards will form the basis of your interview questions. Examples of a position description and performance standards are provided in Table 12-2.
- *Develop a list of interview questions.* Pay particular attention to assessing the requirements of the job specified in the performance standards.
- *Study the applications and résumés.* Look for accomplishments and credentials on which you want the candidate to expand. Also note frequent job changes, gaps in employment, demotions, inconsistencies in history, or incomplete information on references about which you want to learn more.

- *Schedule a quiet, uninterrupted interview.* It shows disrespect to the candidate if you permit interruptions and distractions from giving your full attention to the interview.
- Alert coworkers whom you want the candidate to meet so that they can schedule a time to meet.

Most interviews follow a relatively predictable number of steps. The first step consists of introductory small talk designed to put the candidate at ease. Rather than jumping immediately into the questioning, a few minutes may be spent developing some rapport with the candidate. After the small talk, interview questions are posed of the candidate. When the questioning phase is finished, the interviewer describes and promotes the job to the candidate. At this point, candidates typically ask questions of the interviewer about the job. At the end of the interview, applicants either meet with other interviewers or are given a tour of the facilities.

Interviews can be conducted in several different ways. The *traditional interview* attempts to engage candidates in a general discussion about themselves. A common question from a traditional interview might be, "Tell me a little about yourself" or "What are your strengths and weaknesses?" *Situation* (or *role-play*) *interviews* direct applicants to describe how they would handle a difficult imaginary situation. For example, "You are the pharmacy manager, and one of your employees has just told you that another worker is stealing merchandise. What would you do?" Situation interviews assess candidates' problem-solving capabilities and communication. *Stress interviews* attempt to replace the polite conversation seen in traditional interviews with a deliberate attempt by the interviewer to unnerve the candidate with blunt questions (e.g., "Why would a person with your background want to work here?"), interruptions, and persistent pursuit of a subject. It attempts to discern candidate preparation and ability to handle stress. *Behavioral interviews* try to evaluate an applicant's past behavior, experience, and initiative by asking for specifics about past events and the candidate's role in those events. Classic behavioral questions start with "Give me an example when you . . . " or "Describe your worst . . . " Behavioral interviewing is based on the assumption that past behavior best predicts future behavior. In many cases, interviewers employ more than one style in an interview.

Other tools used by some employers to select candidates are standardized personality and skills tests. Their use stems from a belief that persons with certain personality traits (e.g., one who employs a particular leadership style) may be best suited for a position or may fit best within a company's culture. Similarly, a person may have to demonstrate one or more particular abilities on a skills test to minimally qualify for a job.

The use of standardized tests has limitations, and thus such tests may not be used to a great extent in health care. One limitation is that they may not validly differentiate potential success in employee candidates. For instance, personality is difficult to accurately assess in humans and its relationship with employee success may not be clear or actionable. Other limitations include potential bias toward minorities and nonnative speakers, inability to apply standardized tests for nonstandardized jobs, the potential to game the exams, and the negative message the tests might send to potential candidates.

Most interviewers have limited experience and are prone to common interview mistakes (Umiker, 1998). One is lack of preparation. Managers who are very busy with immediate problems may be tempted to skimp on interview preparation. However, that savings of time is not a bargain if it leads to a bad hire. Another typical mistake occurs when the interviewer does most of the talking and does not give the candidate an opportunity to speak. It is hard to learn much about a candidate when the interviewer is talking. In other situations, interviewers treat the interview as an inquisition designed to squeeze the candidate into revealing his or her flaws. Although this may reveal some insights about the candidate, it is also likely to drive the candidate to another employer. Finally, some interviewers assume that the candidate wants the position, so no attempt is made to sell its benefits. Any of these mistakes can result in

Table 12-3. Interview Mistakes That May Immediately Exclude a Job Candidate from Consideration

- Inappropriate dress or body adornment
- Lack of knowledge about the position and hiring organization
- Tardiness
- Being unengaged in the interview
- Responding badly to predictable questions
- Poor body language
- Unclear or irritating speech patterns
- Focusing on self interest over that of the hiring organization
- Showing under-confidence or over-confidence

either losing a desirable candidate or choosing the wrong one.

Selecting Candidates

During the interview process, it is important to keep good notes about each candidate. This is essential for keeping details about candidates organized and for documenting the selection process in case any claims of discrimination should occur. It is better to save note taking until immediately after the interview to avoid distracting the candidate during the interview. It is also helpful to develop an interview checklist to structure interview notes. Table 12-3 lists several interview mistakes candidates make frequently that can exclude them immediately from further consideration.

The final choice of the interviewer often comes down to how well a candidate can address the following questions:

- *Can this person perform the basic job?* This addresses the ability of the candidate to contribute to the organization's performance. For instance, a good clinical pharmacist who has little dispensing experience may not be chosen for a position in a community pharmacy setting. Although good clinical skills may be helpful in a community position, basic dispensing capabilities are essential.
- *How well do the candidate's skills and capabilities mesh with the organization's needs?* Sometimes the best employee for a position does not have the greatest credentials or the most talent. In many circumstances, the best employee is the one who can fill skill deficiencies in the organization and complement the talents of other employees.
- *Will the candidate make my job easier?* Everyone has some self-interest in the selection of a candidate. Successful applicants often highlight how they will be able to solve problems of individuals and the organization.
- *Would I want to work with this person?* This question deals with the rapport between the applicant and the interviewer. If the rapport is good, the chances of selection are enhanced significantly.

Hiring

In most cases, a candidate cannot be hired until the personnel department completes a reference check. If everything is found to be acceptable, a compensation package is put together, and an offer is extended. Once again, it is important that the pharmacy department be involved in the process to ensure that an offer is not mishandled. For example, if an uncompetitive compensation package is put together for the candidate, pharmacy personnel may need to argue for a better one. Once an applicant accepts a position, the hard part of HRM begins.

Hiring is just the first step in the HRM process. Once hired, employees must be given the training and feedback necessary to do their jobs. There are many reasons why employees may not perform their tasks as they should. Table 12-4 gives a list of them (Fournies, 1999). A quick scan of the list indicates that employees either do not know (1) what they are supposed to do or (2) how to do it and/or (3) they benefit from not doing it. Managers must communicate to employees what is expected of them, train them to do it, and provide feedback about how well they are doing and how they might improve. The remainder of this chapter addresses how employees can achieve these goals.

Table 12-4. Reasons Why Employees Do Not Always Do What They Are Supposed to Do

- They don't know what they are supposed to do.
- They don't know why they should do it.
- They don't know how to do it.
- They think something else is more important.
- There are no positive consequences for them doing it.
- There are no negative consequences for them not doing it.
- They are rewarded for not doing it.
- They are punished for doing what they are supposed to do.
- They are not and will never be capable to perform as desired.
- They have personal problems that get in the way.

Source: Fournies, 1999.

TRAINING AND DEVELOPMENT

Training

A manager's job is to help staff members succeed at their jobs. One key task in employee success is training. The purpose of training is to help employees meet the changing demands of their jobs. Training benefits both the organization and the employee. For the organization, it improves the quality and quantity of work provided by each employee. For the employee, it can make the job more interesting and meaningful and lead to greater morale and sense of accomplishment (Holdford, 2003). Excellent pharmacy service organizations invest in the training and development of their employees.

Training and development serve different purposes. *Training* is meant to improve employee performance with current tasks and jobs, whereas *development* prepares employees for new responsibilities and positions. Therefore, training is essential for meeting current needs, and development is an investment in future needs.

Training comes in two primary forms: orientation and job training. The purpose of *orientation training* is to welcome new employees, present a positive first impression, provide information that will permit them to settle into their new responsibilities, and establish early expectations of performance and behavior (Umiker, 1998). It also involves familiarizing new hires with the company's/department's mission, goals, cultural norms, and expectations. Examples of things covered in orientation training include coworker introductions, a tour of the facilities, discussion of employee benefits, review of departmental policies and procedures, discussion of performance objectives for the job, description of behavioral expectations, demonstration of the computer system, and special organizational training (e.g., HIPAA, sexual harassment, and discrimination). It is a good idea to develop a checklist that covers all orientation topics to ensure that nothing is overlooked.

Job training helps current employees learn new information and skills to do their jobs and refresh capabilities that may have diminished over time. Although pharmacists are highly trained professionals, the changing nature of medical and business practice requires continual training throughout their careers. Job training is a responsibility of both the individual and the organization. For example, a pharmacist might attend a continuing-education program offered by a pharmacy school to fill a perceived gap in knowledge about a disease state and its treatment. Alternatively, a pharmacist may be asked by an employer to receive on-the-job training in customer service methods to fulfill a perceived employer need. Job training can be used to develop habits (e.g., time management), knowledge (e.g., new drug treatments), skills (e.g., blood pressure monitoring), procedures (e.g., handling drug insurance claims), and policies (e.g., sexual harassment).

Pharmacy organizations formally or informally may employ a type of training called *job rotation* (also known as *cross-training*). Job rotation is designed to give an individual broad experience through exposure to different areas of the organization. In a hospital pharmacy, for example, newly hired technicians can be trained in filling carts, outpatient dispensing, intravenous admixture preparation, inventory management, billing and crediting, and working in one or more satellite pharmacy units. Such training would diversify technicians' skills, allowing them to work in any number of areas should one be short staffed, and may help improve their self-esteem and sense of contribution to the organization.

Development

Development requires a long term focus by preparing for future needs of the individual or organization. Professional development typically consists of answering the following questions: (1) What is my present situation? (2) Where do I want to be? (3) What skills, knowledge, and training do I need to get where I want to be?

Development differs from training in that it requires a greater intensity of education and instruction. Whereas job training might be met sufficiently with continuing-education programs, on-the-job instruction, and short courses, professional development may require formal education and structured experiences such as college courses, multiday seminars and certificate programs, residencies, or fellowships.

PERFORMANCE FEEDBACK

Types of Performance Feedback

While training and development prepare employees for current and future jobs, performance feedback communicates how well they are doing in their jobs and how they can improve. Managers commonly provide employee feedback in three ways. The first and most important is the *day-to-day feedback* provided on the job. This refers to the verbal and visual messages provided daily to employees through conversations, body language, and behaviors. Daily communication is the most effective performance feedback because it is immediate and often. Other forms of managerial feedback are provided less frequently and often long after the behavior occurred. The following is a list of suggestions for providing useful daily feedback to employees:

- *Practice management-by-walking-around (MBWA).* This management approach consists of getting out the office or from behind the desk and interacting with employees. It is hard to provide feedback to individuals without frequent personal contact.
- *When practicing MBWA,* listen more than talk. The purpose of MBWA is to learn what is happening within the organization and to solicit input and advice from others. That information is then acted on to improve the organization and the work of employees.
- *Focus on the positive.* Encourage people by catching them doing something right, not catching them doing something wrong. Employees get enough negative feedback. Surprise them with positive comments specific to an action that you want them to continue doing, for example, "I liked how you went out of your way to listen to the concerns of that patient and find exactly the right solution for her needs."
- *Take notes.* When people make suggestions or you make promises, write them down. Provide a deadline for getting back to them about any documented issue. Then keep your promise to get back to them by that deadline.
- *Make individuals see your presence as helpful.* Try not to waste peoples' time, interrupt their work, nitpick, complicate things, or do anything that makes their day-to-day job more difficult. The purpose of MBWA is to assist and support employees, not to criticize and inspect their work.

A second form of feedback comes through the employees' *annual* (or *semiannual*) *performance reviews.* Annual performance reviews act as long-term planning sessions where managers help employees review their previous progress, identify successes and areas that need improvement, and establish goals and objectives for the next year (Umiker, 1998). Annual performance reviews augment and summarize feedback provided by managers on a day-to-day basis. Annual performance reviews are discussed in greater detail in Chapter 14.

The final form of managerial feedback comes from reviews scheduled ad hoc in response to certain particularly good or bad performances. Good *ad hoc performance reviews* are designed to provide recognition for outstanding performance and may be accompanied by some award or gift. Bad ad hoc reviews are designed to address unacceptable employee behavior or performance immediately. These negative ad hoc reviews are part of a process called *progressive discipline.*

Progressive Discipline

Progressive discipline is defined as a series of acts taken by management in response to unacceptable performance by employees. The role of progressive discipline is to escalate the consequences of poor employee performance incrementally with a goal of improving that behavior. Responses by management to undesirable behavior become progressively severe until the employee either improves, resigns, or is terminated from the position. Although punitive in nature, the purpose of progressive discipline is not to punish. Rather, the aim is to make explicit to an employee the consequences of unsatisfactory behavior in order to encourage improved behavior. Indeed, improved behavior is always the preferred outcome, never the loss of an employee through resignation or termination. Progressive discipline may be initiated in response to employee behaviors such as discourtesy to customers or coworkers, tardiness, absenteeism, unsatisfactory work performance, and violation of departmental policies. Progressive discipline usually consists of the following steps: verbal warning, written warning, suspension, and termination.

Verbal Warning

A verbal warning is a formal oral reprimand about the consequences of failing to perform as expected. A manager might verbally warn a technician that she is performing below expectations in regard to tardiness and that if performance is not improved, further disciplinary action may be warranted. Verbal warnings are relatively common and often the only action needed to correct unacceptable employee performance.

Written Warning

If an employee does not respond to a verbal warning, a more formal written warning is issued. A *written warning* is the first formal step in progressive discipline that may result in eventual discharge of the employee. It differs from verbal warnings, which are relatively informal acts that only require the manager to note the time and place of the reprimand and what was discussed. A written warning is a legal document that can end up as evidence in a court case. If an employee is discharged and any disciplinary step is handled inappropriately, the employer can be sued successfully for financial damages by the employee. Therefore, written warnings should be crafted carefully with help from superiors and the human resources department.

The written warning should describe the unacceptable behavior clearly, previous warnings, specific expectations of future behavior to be achieved by a precise deadline, and the consequences of not meeting expectations. For example, "You were verbally warned about tardiness on January 16 of this year. You have continued to be tardy at a rate above that specified in your performance standards. If you are late for work more than twice within the next month, you will be suspended for one day without pay." As shown by this example, it is essential for a manager to keep good records of previous warnings because they will be used as the basis for potential written warnings.

Suspension

Suspensions are punitive actions meant to demonstrate the seriousness of a situation. Sometimes written warnings do not result in improved employee performance and need to be backed up by actions. Suspensions are meant to act as a final warning that current behavior is unacceptable. Like written warnings, they must be crafted carefully to include previous warnings, requirements for future actions, and consequences for not improving behavior (e.g., termination).

TERMINATION OF EMPLOYEES

Some managers are hesitant to terminate employees because it can be a difficult circumstance for all involved. For the terminated employee, it can have a tremendous impact on self-esteem, reputation, and personal finances. For the manager, it can be an emotionally charged event that results in an unpleasant confrontation. It also can lead to legal action for the business and individual manager. Therefore, some managers avoid dealing with such situations by insisting wrongly that laws and rules make it impossible to fire anyone.

However, if employees are provided clear performance standards and the procedures for progressive discipline are observed, firing bad employees usually is not difficult procedurally. This means that every step leading up to the termination must be appropriate and documented.

Procedures for terminating employees differ depending on the circumstances. For newly hired employees who are on probation (i.e., a trial period for assessing new employees), the process of progressive discipline ordinarily does not need to be followed. The employee can be terminated at any time during the probationary period if it is clear that the employee will not succeed in the job. The steps of verbal warning, written warning, and suspension are not necessary before termination. The same is true for employees who commit acts that can lead to immediate termination, such as fighting on the job, drug or alcohol use at work, stealing, vandalism, or periods of absence without notice.

For employees who do not fall into the preceding categories, termination should not come as a surprise. Following progressive discipline procedures should give employees explicit expectations of what is going to occur when performance is not improved. Many employees will resign before being terminated. Employees who do not resign are asked to attend a termination meeting.

Prior to the termination meeting, the manager must be certain that all the following statements are true:

- The employee is not being terminated for anything but poor job performance or breaking major rules (e.g., theft or fighting).
- The reason for termination can be stated in measurable, factual terms.
- The employee has been given specific feedback regarding the performance deficiency in measurable, factual terms.
- The organization's policies and procedures regarding discipline have been observed and actions documented.
- The employee has been given ample opportunity to correct the poor performance.
- Employee treatment is consistent with similar situations of employee performance.
- The personnel department has been kept informed throughout the disciplinary process and is currently aware of plans to terminate the employee. If there is no personnel department with whom to confer, a lawyer should be consulted.

Most businesses have a procedure for terminating employees, so the manager simply follows that procedure. Most termination procedures require that a witness be present during the meeting to verify conversations and actions.

The primary goal of the termination meeting is to terminate the employee compassionately and in a manner that maintains the employee's dignity and self-respect. This is better achieved by being direct and to the point by stating something such as, "You have not achieved the performance objectives specified in our last meeting, so we have decided to terminate you from your position."

The employee may respond in multiple ways (e.g., anger, tears), but the manager's response should be neutral. The manager should not argue with or criticize the employee or engage in any negotiations. It is essential to state that the decision is final. Let the employee vent any frustrations, but do not permit abusive or violent behavior. Be ready to discuss a severance package or direct the person to the human resources department, and then end the meeting.

Since an employee may be upset and not thinking very clearly after termination, it is useful to offer recommendations on what he or she should do next. For instance, the employer may tell the employee that he does not need to complete his shift and that his belongings will be packed and left for him to pick up the following day at some designated place.

After termination, several final steps need to be concluded. Documentation of final actions should be completed and filed. All people involved should be reminded about the confidentiality of discussions and actions. Finally, the manager should reflect on how the process went and what changes may be necessary to prevent further terminations.

REVISITING THE SCENARIO—TACKLING HUMAN RELATIONS

Scot Phinney's problems in the scenario revolve around HRM. There appear to be three related problems: (1) There are three pharmacist position vacancies that need to be filled, (2) employee morale is low, and (3) current employee productivity and behavior are unacceptable. Scot has identified several specific employee behaviors that hinder the performance of the pharmacy, including frequent arguments, excessive complaints, pharmacists not supervising technicians, and rude behavior and poor service to nursing. He has decided to focus on these problems first.

Scot's first step should be to examine the current job and performance descriptions of the employees to see if they address the problem behaviors described. If they do, then he can use them to illustrate that specific behaviors are documented as unacceptable. If job descriptions and performance standards do not address problem behaviors, then they need to be updated. With clearly defined duties and performance standards for all employees, Scot can start a dialogue with employees about expected behavior using specific examples. For instance, if a pharmacist states that it is not her job to supervise technicians, Scot can review the performance standards that relate to her supervisory duties. Scot needs to communicate clear expectations of employees and provide feedback in day-to-day discussions, annual reviews, and disciplinary actions.

Scot should realize that changing entrenched employees is a long process, so he should be patient and persistent. Some employees may not accept his efforts immediately and may refuse to alter their conduct. Scot will have to apply pressure through progressive discipline to encourage them to change or find a new employer. If he is consistent and fair, most employees will go along with and even embrace the changes. With successful change, employee morale should also increase and the turnover rate slow down.

CONCLUSION

Good HRM is an important requirement for providing excellent pharmacy services. Pharmacy personnel who are well managed are more likely to be satisfied in their jobs, effective, and productive. Good HRM in health care fields enhances the likelihood that patients will be better served and achieve better health outcomes. Any pharmacist who is serious about serving patients and the profession needs to be committed to good HRM.

QUESTIONS FOR FURTHER DISCUSSION

1. What are the potential advantages and limitations of affirmative action to a pharmacy organization?
2. What knowledge and skills are employers looking for in pharmacists?
3. What questions might an interviewer ask of a candidate for the job described in Table 12-2?
4. Which interview method do you think is most effective? Least effective? Why?
5. When should the job search process for pharmacist jobs start for pharmacy students? What actions should be taken?
6. How effective would you be at terminating an employee for poor job performance? Why or why not?
7. Think about your last job search and employment. Rate your employer's performance in the areas of
    a. Recruitment and selection
    b. Interviewing
    c. Orientation and training
    d. Performance feedback
8. What type of performance feedback have you received from previous employers? Describe a specific example in which an employer did a particularly good or bad job of providing feedback.

REFERENCES

American Society of Health-Systems Pharmacists. 2011. Cost of pharmacist turnover (practice managers resource). Available at www.ashp.org/s_ashp/docs/files/turnovercost.pdf; accessed on June 3, 2011.

CNN/Money. 2011. Top 100 companies to work for. Available at money.cnn.com/magazines/fortune/bestcompanies/2011/index.html; accessed on June 3, 2011.

Donnelly JH, Gibson JL, Ivancevich JM. 1995. Human resource management. In *Fundamentals of Management*, Vol 13. Chicago: Irwin, p. 444.

Fournies FF. 1999. *Why Employees Don't Do What They're Supposed to Do and What to Do About It.* New York: McGraw-Hill.

Holdford DA. 2003. *Marketing for Pharmacists.* Washington, DC: American Pharmaceutical Association.

Occupational Safety & Health Administration (OSHA), U.S. Department of Labor. 2007. Available at www.osha.gov/; accessed on August 15, 2007.

Umiker W. 1998. *Management Skills for the New Health Care Superviser.* Gaithersburg, MD: Aspen Publishers.

Waldman JD, Kelly F, Arora S, Smith HL. 2004. The shocking cost of turnover in health care. *Health Care Manage Rev* 29(1):2–7.

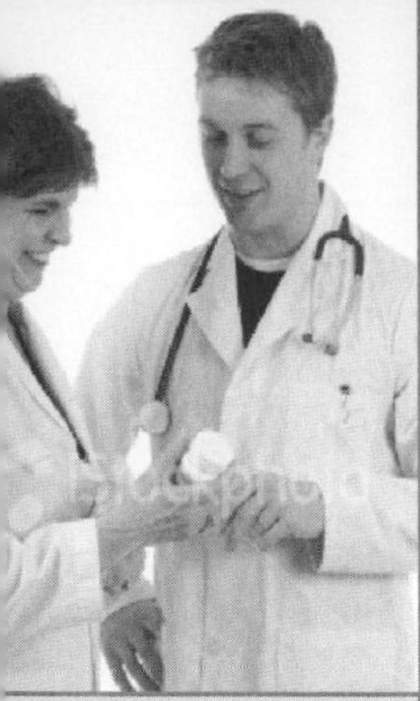

13

CUSTOMER SERVICE

Erin R. Holmes and Leigh Ann Bynum

About the Authors: Dr. Holmes is an assistant professor with the School of Pharmacy and research assistant professor of the Research Institute for Pharmaceutical Sciences, both at the University of Mississippi. Dr. Holmes received a Pharm.D. degree and MS in pharmacy administration from Duquesne University and a Ph.D. in pharmacy administration from the University of Mississippi. She teaches courses in pharmacy management, pharmacy law, personal finance and health care policy. Her research focuses on organizational behavior, human resource management and operations management in community pharmacy practice. Dr. Holmes is codeveloper of RxSync Service, an adherence management program for community pharmacies.

Dr. Bynum is an assistant professor with the Belmont School of Pharmacy. Dr. Bynum received a BA degree in psychology and M.S. in wellness from the University of Mississippi and a Ph.D. in pharmacy administration from the University of Mississippi. Her professional experience includes human resource training and development and directing market services for health services groups. She teaches courses in pharmacy management and communications. Dr. Bynum's research focuses on human resource management and organizational behavior issues such as psychological contracts, equity sensitivity, and organization citizenship behaviors.

LEARNING OBJECTIVES

After completing this chapter, readers will be able to

1. List the principles for ensuring good customer service.
2. Provide ways of meeting each standard that patients and customers use to evaluate services.
3. Define and describe the significance and implications of service failure, service recovery, service recovery paradox, and zone of tolerance.
4. Choose service recovery efforts for low-, mid-, and high-criticality service failures.

5. Explain the four perspectives of customer satisfaction assessment.
6. Identify ways to develop pharmacy staff members to provide good customer service.
7. Describe how an employee's work life can affect customer service.
8. Recommend steps for dealing with "difficult" patients and customers.

SCENARIO

Sarah Laird, a 60-year-old woman, walked into the retail chain pharmacy in the morning with a prescription for promethazine 25-mg tablets. After suffering a back injury on an assembly line job at her workplace last week, she had been taking a pain medication as prescribed for a couple of days. While her pain has significantly reduced, the nausea from the pain medication has been difficult to deal with.

Upon presenting the prescription directly to the pharmacy manager and telling him that it should be covered by her workman's compensation insurance, he returned to her a clearly puzzled look. The look was not judgmental—just puzzled. He knew that promethazine is not a drug that is usually covered by workman's compensation insurance and that a prior authorization from the physician would be needed. She did not take his look as a puzzled one; rather, she took it as a judgmental one. "Um, ma'am, this promethazine is not a drug typically covered by your workman's comp. I need to get a prior authorization from your doctor. You'll have to come back tomorrow for it." The pharmacist said this to her pretty hastily, as he had quickly moved from his puzzled look to her on toward gazing at the computer to fill the next prescription. This morning was one of the busiest mornings that he could remember in a long time. Confused and still not quite sure what was going on, she left the pharmacy.

Sarah returned to the pharmacy later in the afternoon to pick up her prescription, but it still was not ready. She was steamed. On top of feeling bad from the nausea, now the pharmacist just will not fill the prescription. To be honest, she really believed that the pharmacist was discriminating against her because of the workman's compensation insurance. "You just don't want to fill my prescription, do you?" she angrily told him. Now, the pharmacy manager is agitated by and frustrated with Sarah because all he hears is, "What is taking so long?" "How many times have I heard *that* one," he thought to himself. "Didn't I tell you this morning that your prescription wasn't going to be ready until tomorrow?" he said in an impatient and very angry tone.

Sarah went home and immediately called the pharmacy back, asking the pharmacy manager for *his* manager. Not wanting to bring this to the attention of the pharmacy district manager, he forwarded the call to the general store manager. "I don't know why that pharmacist doesn't want to fill my prescription" she said. Sarah's daughter, a nurse, who was also on the line, repeated the question. "I want you to explain it to me," she said. Not knowing about the situation, the general manager took down Sarah's phone number and assured her that he would look into the situation and call her back within the next hour. He spoke with the pharmacy manager about the situation and called her back within 15 minutes. "It's not that he doesn't want to fill the prescription," the general manager told Sarah in a very slow and calming tone. "It's just that this is a medication that isn't usually covered by workman's comp. The pharmacist needs to call your doctor for a prior authorization. A prior authorization is a special permission for you to get the drug paid for by workman's comp. The doctor needs to fill out some paperwork and send it to the pharmacist, so that's why it is taking so long. The pharmacist wasn't trying to be mean or not want to fill your prescription. He was just confused about the promethazine being covered on workman's comp, and then had to go through some special procedures to get it covered for you." "Oh, well, is that all?" she asked. Well then, that's just fine!" The general manager assured Sarah he would call her in the morning when the prescription was ready so that she could come pick it up. He took no further action on the matter. After receiving the general manager's phone call the next morning Sarah returned to the pharmacy and picked up her prescription without any additional problems.

■ CHAPTER QUESTIONS

1. Why is the provision of service particularly challenging in the pharmacy setting?
2. What standards do patients and customers use to evaluate the quality of services?
3. What should pharmacy managers do when customer service goes wrong?
4. How does an employee's quality of work life affect the quality of service they provide?
5. What are the potential outcomes of both good and bad customer service?

■ INTRODUCTION

While there is no one universal definition of "good" or "bad" customer service, most of us have probably experienced some of each and most likely can distinctly remember the feelings that ensued from these experiences. Maybe a customer service agent went well above and beyond the call of duty to resolve a problem. Their efforts greatly surpassed your expectations, and you felt a huge sense of relief and gratitude after your experience. You left that interaction with a very positive impression of that company. You may also have encountered a store clerk with an "I couldn't care less" attitude and wondered; how could that person have so little regard for their job and for other people? Maybe the encounter left you feeling offended, invisible, angry, and with a bad taste in your mouth about the company.

Regardless of the pharmacy setting, there is no question that providing good customer service is intricately tied to patient care and gives an organization or business a competitive advantage. Providing good customer service, however, is sometimes easier said than done, especially in a very busy pharmacy. Think of a time you have worked in a pharmacy. Did you give your patients and customers your complete attention and use eye contact and avoid other activities like working on the computer when having a conversation with them? Did you sincerely apologize to a patient or customer if a mistake was made by you or the pharmacy? When speaking to a patient or customer over the phone, did you use inflection in your voice to convey interest and concern (Leland and Bailey, 2006)? How would you rate your customer service skills based on these questions? How would you rate the customer service skills of other employees with whom you have worked? How would you rate the pharmacist presented in the scenario?

There is no question that unique characteristics of the pharmacy profession make the provision of good customer service challenging. First, the medications dispensed are typically viewed as "negative goods," which means that patients purchase them because they *have* to, not because they *want* to (Kolassa, 1997). Additionally, customers may already come in with negative perceptions of the price of medicines, other health care professionals, or their insurance plan, which can sometimes be transferred (either intentionally or unintentionally) to the pharmacy staff. Pharmacy customers may be symptomatic and not feeling well. At the same time, they likely have high expectations for pharmacy service given the very serious consequences of potential medication errors. Moreover, work in the pharmacy can be very hectic at times, making the provision of customer service especially challenging. In the scenario presented at the beginning of the chapter, Sarah was not feeling well, and the pharmacy manager was busy. The combination of these factors likely contributed to the misunderstanding and the resultant service failure.

With these unique characteristics of the pharmacy profession in mind, this chapter begins by providing ways that pharmacy managers can ensure good customer service and provides strategies for addressing service failures that can occur in the pharmacy setting. Then, satisfaction and other outcomes of a patient's or customer's experience in the pharmacy are discussed. Next, how employees' work life, as well as how the management of pharmacy employees affects the provision of customer service in a pharmacy will be addressed. Later, methods for collecting patients', customers' and employees' feedback about customer service will be discussed. Finally, techniques for dealing with "difficult" customers and customer complaints will be explored.

First, a few clarifications of terminology are warranted. Although the primary topic of this chapter is *customer* service, there is significant debate as to whether the term "patient," "client," "consumer," or "customer" is the most appropriate term to describe those who are served by pharmacists, especially in the community pharmacy setting. While often used interchangeably, these terms have different meanings. In fact, one study described the characteristics and needs of patients, clients, consumers, and customers of community pharmacies and outlined the best ways pharmacists can the meet the needs of each of these groups that they serve (Austin et al., 2006). For example, the authors describe a *patient* as being more reliant on a pharmacist than a *customer*, who tends to be more autonomous. It follows, then, that a pharmacist may appropriately treat and communicate with a *patient* who is inquiring about the side effects of her infertility treatment differently than a *customer* who approaches the pharmacy counter to purchase pseudoephedrine for a cold. Regardless, both patients and customers are entitled to high-quality service in a pharmacy. Therefore, both the terms "customer" and "patient" will be used when appropriate in this chapter. In a final note of clarification, while many concepts of customer service in this chapter are presented in the context of the community pharmacy setting, the concepts also are intended to apply to other pharmacy practice settings.

PRINCIPLES FOR ENSURING GOOD CUSTOMER SERVICE

Whether perusing the Internet, reading business publications, or evaluating research studies, there appears to be a consistent set of principles to which pharmacy managers can (and should) adhere to in providing good customer service. Table 13-1 provides a summary of these principles. This list of principles can be captured into an easy-to-remember concept known as the "golden ule of customer service." That is, treating your customers as you would want to be treated (Obarski, 2010).

Table 13-1. Principles for Ensuring Good Customer Service

Anticipate patients' and customers' needs and wants
Solve patient–customer problems without hassle
Solve patient and customer problems promptly
Treat patients and customers with dignity, empathy and respect
Correct mistakes when they are made
Apologize for mistakes when they are made
Underpromise and overdeliver
Do work right the first time
Actively listen to patients and customers
Make patients and customers feel important and appreciated
Help patients and customers understand how your pharmacy works
Always look for ways to help patients and customers

Sources: Friedman (2010); Tipton (2009); Umiker (1998).

STANDARDS PATIENTS AND CUSTOMERS USE TO EVALUATE SERVICES

While abiding by this list can be challenging, it is worth remembering that patients and customers keep an "invisible report card" in their head, and they grade you on the basic needs (standards) that they require. They are not going to overtly ask for those standards. They are not going to approach the pharmacist and say, "Here is my prescription to be filled. Can you please make sure

Table 13-2. **Description of Standards that Patients and Customers Use to Evaluate Services**

Standard	Description	How Standard Can Be Met
Reliability Parasuraman et al. (1988)	Receiving the promised service dependably and accurately	Accurate prescription filling and patient counseling
Responsiveness Parasuraman et al. (1988)	Receiving help and prompt service	Staff who are eager to help patients and customers any way they can
Assurance Parasuraman et al. (1988)	Knowledgeable and courteous employees who convey trust and confidence	Staff who are knowledgeable about the location of products in the store and help customers find products
Empathy Leland and Bailey (2006); Parasuraman et al. (1988)	Caring, individualized attention; appreciating a patient's or customer's circumstances and feelings without criticism or judgment	Acknowledging that patients may be sick, scared, confused, worried, and responding to their feelings
Tangibles Parasuraman et al. (1988)	The appearance of physical facilities, equipment, personnel, and communication materials	Using spare minutes in the day to wipe shelves or counters (Kneeland, 2009); providing medication information that is easy to understand and read
Friendliness Leland and Bailey (2006)	Polite and courteous treatment	Friendly and upbeat staff; calling patients by their name; having packages ready as patients and customers walk to the counter
Fairness Leland and Bailey (2006)	Fair treatment from service providers	Helping patients and customers in order of their arrival at the pharmacy
Control Leland and Bailey (2006)	The patient's or customer's need to have an impact on the way things turn out	Letting patients know that the remainder of a partial fill will not be available for two days
Options Leland and Bailey (2006)	The patients or customer's need to feel that other options are available	Ordering products for patients and customers when necessary
Information Leland and Bailey (2006)	The patient's or customer's need to be educated and informed about products, policies, and procedures	Patient counseling and patient information to take home

that you fill it accurately and treat me with empathy and fairness?" However, they are going to evaluate you for accuracy, empathy, and fairness (Leland and Bailey, 2006). The literature suggests ten standards that patients and customers use to evaluate services: (1) reliability, (2) responsiveness, (3) assurance, (4) empathy, (5) tangibles, (6) friendliness, (7) fairness, (8) control, (9) options, and (10) alternatives (Leland and Bailey, 2006; Parasuraman et al., 1988). Table 13-2 provides a description of each standard and an example of how each standard can be met in the pharmacy setting.

It should be noted here that the "responsiveness" standard should be interpreted with caution. There is no question that some patients who come to the pharmacy are in a hurry. And, indeed, pharmacies have recently advertised "15-minute prescription guarantees" for prescription fills (Gamble, 2011) (although these guarantees have exceptions for calling a prescriber or third party, orders, professional services, or before or during lunch break). Prescriptions cannot always be processed quickly. Sometimes the prescriber needs to be called for a drug-related problem or reauthorization. Sometimes the pharmacy benefits manager (PBM) needs to be called for a problem or prior authorization. Patient education takes time. Hastily filled prescriptions can result in service failure that is much worse than waiting on a prescription—one that potentially can be very detrimental to the patient. However, it is not necessarily a long wait that is perceived as a service failure; but rather, it is a wait that was longer than *expected* or *promised*. So, pharmacists must provide honest and realistic expectations about the time needed to fill a prescription or provide other services. The pharmacist must clearly explain why there will be a delay (this also meets the standard of "control" in Table 13-2). If the pharmacist in the scenario at the beginning of the chapter clearly communicated in simple language the reason for delay, the ensuing confusion and inconvenience may have been avoided. Because this can be challenging in a busy pharmacy, it might be best to overestimate sparingly the time required to fill a prescription when communicating with a patient. As noted in Table 13-1, underpromise and overdeliver exceeding a patient's or customer's expectations can result in their satisfaction, or even delight, with the pharmacy.

PHARMACY ISSUES THAT ARE IMPORTANT TO PATIENTS

Providing quality customer service in a pharmacy requires understanding what aspects of pharmacy services are most important to patients, and subsequently focusing on improving those aspects. A 2010 survey of over 34,000 pharmacy customers identified issues most important to them. Not surprisingly, filling prescriptions accurately and efficiently was the most important factor for pharmacy customers, followed in order by overall convenience, prescription pricing, pharmacy staff, printed health information, and additional medical services (Boehringer Ingelheim, 2011).

WHEN CUSTOMER SERVICE GOES WRONG

Even the best efforts to ensure customer service can result in failure to meet the expectations of a patient or customer. Failing to meet the expectations of a patient or customer is called *service failure*. Examples of service failures include patients and customers not getting what they expected or were promised; having to wait longer than they expected or were promised; rude, patronizing, or indifferent treatment from a pharmacy staff member; and a "can't do" attitude or a "sorry, it's our policy" response from a pharmacy staff member (Umiker, 1998). A widespread example of service failures in pharmacies occurred with the implementation of the Medicare Part D program on January 1, 2006. Pharmacists struggled to dispense medications under the new drug benefit and required more time to sort out the new rules and regulations. Data suggest that overall satisfaction with pharmacies decreased during that time but has since recovered (Boehringer Ingelheim, 2008).

By their very nature, service failures in the pharmacy can range from the inconvenient (a long wait for a prescription, or a partial fill due to limited stock), to the very serious (giving a patient the wrong drug or wrong dose). *Service criticality* refers to the magnitude of the consequences of a potential service failure to the patient or customer (Webster and Sundaram, 1998). For example, a car dealer forgetting to wash your car as promised during servicing has a low service criticality while a serious car accident due to fixing your brakes incorrectly during that servicing has a high service criticality. Obviously, the higher the service criticality, the more seriously the patient or customer will perceive the service failure, and the more important it is for the pharmacy to address the failure. Service criticality is important; it has been shown that with increasing service failure criticality, satisfaction with, trust in, and commitment to the business by the customer is more likely to decrease, and negative word of mouth can become that much more problematic (Weun et al., 2004). It is important to keep in mind that patients and customers will have varying perceptions of the severity of a failure. Just because the provider of the service may perceive a service failure as insignificant does not mean that the patient or customer will perceive it, likewise.

RIGHTING THE WRONG

Given the negative consequences of service failures on patients and businesses, the way in which a service provider responds to a failure is critical. While it is well understood that service failures are sometimes inevitable, this does not mean that dissatisfied patients and customers are inevitable (Hart et al., 1990). That is the premise of service recovery. *Service recovery* is the attempt to correct the service failure and make things right for the patient or customer (Tipton, 2000). Service recovery has been formally defined as an effort to "alter the negative perceptions of dissatisfied customers and to ultimately maintain a business relationship with these customers" (Schweikhart et al., 1993, p. 3). Service recovery requires more than correcting the error and making things right, but requires going above and beyond to satisfy the patient or customer (Bell and Zemke, 1987). The way in which a provider responds to service errors can dictate patients' and customers' satisfaction and dissatisfaction (Bitner et al., 1990) and whether they will continue to patronize the pharmacy (Hoffman et al., 1995).

RECOVERING FROM LOW- AND MID-CRITICALITY SERVICE FAILURES IN THE PHARMACY

As previously mentioned, low-criticality service failures in the pharmacy can include a longer than expected wait for a prescription, a partial fill, and rude treatment from pharmacy staff, among others. Mid-criticality failures can include drug errors that are easily reversible or have resulted in little or no patient harm such as mislabeling a prescription bottle and providing the wrong dose to a patient, among others. Ideally these types of errors in the pharmacy are minimal; however, they do occur. In pharmacy, an estimated 51.5 million errors occur during the filling of 3 billion prescriptions each year (Flynn et al., 2003). Readers are referred to Chapters 8, 27, and 29 for a more detailed discussion about medication errors. For low- and midcriticality service failures, similar recovery efforts can be applied. Suggested recovery efforts for these types of failures are provided in Table 13-3.

In one pharmacy service failure study, pharmacy students were asked to indicate the best way a pharmacist can handle the following hypothetical situation (Tipton, 2000, p. 75):

> Having picked up your prescription, you do not notice that it is incorrect and take the medication for several days. This results in headaches and several days missed at work. You fully recover, and there are not permanent damages. You return to the pharmacy to discuss this situation with the pharmacist.

The most commonly mentioned "best way" that pharmacy students thought the pharmacist should respond to the situation was an apology, followed by compensation for financial losses, assurance about the system, explanation about how the mistake was made, and expression of sincerity and genuine concern (Table 13-3). Other qualitative studies of consumers' perceptions of pharmacy service failures have lent less credence to an apology by the pharmacist (Bunniran et al., 2010). This contradiction in findings may be a result of pharmacy students being more empathetic than a consumer with a pharmacist's mistake. Additionally, the latter study also examined low-criticality service failures. It has been suggested that in low-criticality situations, an apology might be perceived as more trivial to a patient then actual correction of the problem (Tipton, 2000). That being said, regardless of the criticality of the failure, an apology is called for in addition

Table 13-3. Suggested Recovery Efforts for Low- and Midcriticality Service Failures

Bell and Zemke (1987)	• Apology • Urgent reinstatement • Empathy • Symbolic atonement • Follow-up
Johnston (1995)	• Provide information about the problem • Provide information about what is being done • Action in response to customer (but preferably without being asked) • Staff appearing to go out of their way to help • Involving the customer in decision making
Kelley et al. (1993)	• Discount • Correction • Manager/employee intervention • Correction plus • Replacement • Apology • Refund
Tipton (2000)	• Apology • Compensation for substantial financial losses • Assurance system is either not defective and this was a unique situation, or that system is defective and will be corrected • Explanation of how the mistake was made • Expression of sincerity and genuine concern

to correcting the problem and compensating the patient when necessary.

The importance of recovering from a service failure in a pharmacy is clear. It has been found that reducing customer loss by 5% can increase profits from 25% to 85% (Reichheld and Sasser, 1990). Additionally, it is estimated to cost up to five times more to recruit a new patient or customer than it does to keep a current customer happy (Hart et al., 1990). The good news is that effective recovery from a service failure can potentially result in a more satisfied patient than if no service failure ever happened. This phenomenon is known as the *service recovery paradox* (Smith and Bolton, 1998).

Readers should be warned, however, that some research suggests that the service recovery paradox does not always occur, especially if the service failure is one of high criticality. It has been found that after a severe service failure, a customer may remain dissatisfied and engage in negative word of mouth about the pharmacy, even if the service recovery appears strong (Weun et al., 2004). A study of service failure and service recovery in community pharmacy also was unable to demonstrate that a service recovery paradox exists (Bunniran, 2010). It has been suggested that after a mistake in health care, it may be impossible to return to an "error-free state in the patient's mind" and that it may be "better not to fail than to have a great recovery from a service failure" (Bunniran, 2010, p. 86). *These findings, however, are not meant to imply that service recovery efforts should not be taken for every service failure, regardless of the level of criticality.* Even if a patient's or customer's satisfaction does not exceed the prefailure state after a service recovery, they still can potentially return to a level of satisfaction that exceeds postfailure levels. A study of service failure and service recovery in pharmacy suggests that assurance of correction of the problem and a $25 gift card can result in satisfaction ratings that are higher after the recovery than after the failure (Bunniran, 2010).

Although she may feel differently, we can assume that the service failure that Sarah experienced in the scenario was one of low criticality, and one that probably happens quite often in pharmacies. The general manager attempted to recover from the failure by explaining how the mistake was made. For Sarah, that was all that was needed. If this was not enough to remedy the situation, the manager could have used additional techniques to recover from the service failure, such as providing her with store credit. Not all service recovery techniques are going to be effective for all patients and customers. Blanket policies for service recovery are not recommended. Rather, a variety of recovery efforts should be made available and staff empowered to utilize them as needed.

RECOVERING FROM HIGH-CRITICALITY SERVICE FAILURES IN THE PHARMACY

It should not be surprising that methods to recover from a high-criticality service failure in the pharmacy are different from recovering from low- and midcriticality service failures. High-criticality service failures (also known as catastrophic prescription errors) in the pharmacy include those causing severe harm that is irreversible (Tipton et al., 2003). Relative to low- and midcriticality service failures, high-criticality service failures are emotionally disturbing in addition to being potentially or actually life-threatening. The implications of a catastrophic error are without question, significant. Implications can include loss of trust in the pharmacist and/or pharmacy, and injured public image, spread of negative-word-mouth may spread, legal action, board of pharmacy action, as well as loss of customers and profit. Not only are patients and their families affected, but so are a variety of other stakeholders such as employees, management, other patients, regulators, competitors, media, suppliers, accrediting bodies, the legal system, and stockholders/investors; making service recovery infinitely more complex (Pearson and Mitroff, 1993).

To the extent possible, victims of catastrophic medication errors are due just and equitable compensation for their suffering Tipton (2009) outlines recommendations for response to a victim and his or her family after a catastrophic event:

1. *Tell the truth* about what happened.
2. Attempt to compensate for *emotional costs* with an apology.
3. Attempt to compensate for *psychological costs* with assurances the system will be fixed.
4. Attempt to compensate for costs related to *time, money,* and *inconvenience* through financial settlements.

Managing media relations after a catastrophic event requires thoughtful consideration due to audiences and stakeholders with different interests. For example, the general public will want to be informed because they are asking the question, "what if I went or had to go there?" They demand openness and forthrightness. Another group of stakeholders who have financial or other interests in the organization may be concerned about how their interests are affected and demand circumspection (Tipton et al., 2003). Six options have been detailed for dealing with the media including (1) saying nothing at all, (2) denying or repudiating the charge, (3) claiming no responsibility for the event, (4) minimizing the impact of the event, (5) admitting the mistake and asking for forgiveness, and (6) any combination of the above (Benoit and Brinson, 1994).

It has been suggested that one way to deal with the media is to say nothing, slowly. However, the recommended approach is to be honest and open immediately while emphasizing the good your organization has done because this helps disarm the media. Doing the former puts you on the defensive and may further tarnish the organization's reputation (Tipton, 2009). Then there is the question of whether to apologize.

While apologies are good for the conscience, it is argued that apologies may lead to legal consequences (American Academy of Family Physicians, 2005). Some recommend ambiguity in announcements rather than an outright apology (Sellnow and Ulmer, 1995). For example, Jack in the Box in 1993 following reported deaths due to *Escherichia coli*–contaminated burgers stated: "Although it is unclear as to the source of an illness lined to undercooked beef, Jack in the Box announced today that it has taken measure to ensure [that] all menu items are prepared in accordance with an advisory issued yesterday by the Washington State Department of Health" (Sellnow and Ulmer, 1995, p. 142).

When it comes to consequences of a catastrophic service failure, there are four things to be considered; (1) a price cannot be put on human life, (2) no one can adequately compensate for the suffering that a catastrophic service failure causes, (3) no one can really understand the impact of the failure on the practitioners, and (4) the event cannot be undone (Tipton, 2009). However, Tipton (2009 p. 194) best summarizes what can (and should) be done as health care professionals:

> The response can be open, caring, concerned, empathetic, and ethical. It is a test of character. The choice, ultimately, is between taking the high road or taking the expedient path of self-interest. As practitioners involved in the higher moral activity of health care as opposed to pure commerce, is an obligation. The high road also will be good for business.

OUTCOMES OF SERVICE FAILURE AND SERVICE RECOVERY

It should be no surprise that service failures can result in negative consequences for the pharmacy if not adequately addressed after they occur. Service failures and how well pharmacies recover from them have serious implications not only for patients and customers, but for the future of the business. The implications can be permanent. While many outcomes of service failure and recovery have been studied, including word of mouth communications (positive and negative), relationship quality, attitude toward the service provider, loyalty, repurchase intentions, service provide switching behaviors, and complaining behaviors; this section of the chapter focuses on satisfaction, word of mouth, trust, and customer retention.

Satisfaction

Satisfaction can be defined as the extent to which patients' and customers' needs and wants are met (Chui, 2009) or as meeting the expectations of the patient's or consumer's anticipation of how a service encounter should occur (Bunniran, 2010).[1] In a study of hotel service failures, it was found that a strong recovery can have a positive influence on satisfaction. However, satisfaction still remains negative after recovery if a more severe service failure occurs (Weun et al., 2004).

There are four perspectives of customer service including performance evaluation, affect-based assessment, equity-based assessment, and disconfirmation of expectations. *Performance evaluation* refers to determining satisfaction with characteristics of a particular service such as the physical environment of the pharmacy (e.g.convenient location, availability of parking, safety, cleanliness). *Affect-based assessment* refers to emotional reaction that a patient or customer experiences as a result of the service (e.g., "I am delighted with this service"). *Equity-based assessment* refers to a

[1] A discussion of ***patient satisfaction***, or the "degree to which a consumer perceives a healthcare good or service (or delivery of said good or service) to be valuable, beneficial, useful, appropriate, and effective" (von Waldner and Abel, 2011) is beyond the scope of this chapter. In the context of the economic, clinical, and humanistic outcomes (ECHO) model, patient satisfaction is a humanistic outcome (see chapter 9 for a more detailed discussion of evaluating the outcomes of pharmacy services). As a humanistic outcome, patient satisfaction is becoming an increasingly salient measure of pharmacy quality. However, patient satisfaction should be kept in mind during this discussion of customer service, as customer service is integral to patient satisfaction.

patient's or customer's perceptions of fairness in the provision of service based on inputs and outputs and other individuals' service experiences (Schommer et al., 2002; von Waldner and Abel, 2011).

When assessing satisfaction, one of the most prevalent approaches is *disconfirmation of expectations* (Oliver, 1980; Spreng et al., 1996). With this approach, patients and customers evaluate the gap between their expectations and perceptions of a service. If a patient or customer perceives that a service outperforms their expectations, they will be satisfied (or delighted, if their expectations are significantly outperformed) with the service. Conversely, if the service does not meet their expectations, they will be dissatisfied. Their expectations may come from their own experiences with that particular service, other services like it, or the experiences of others (Oliver, 1980). The challenge from the service provider's perspective is that the expectations are dynamic—they can differ among patients and customers and change constantly (Tipton, 2009). For example, if a patient enters the pharmacy with the expectation that their prescription will be filled in 20 minutes, and it is filled in 10 minutes, they will be satisfied (perhaps even delighted). However, if it takes 45 minutes to fill because the prescriber needs to be called about a problem, they may be dissatisfied. This is not unlike having one's satisfaction with a movie being governed to a large extent by the expectations of the movie they had before seeing it.

A similar theory, the *perceptions–expectations gap* conceptualization, suggests that patients and customers also evaluate the gap between their expectations and perceptions of service *quality* (Parasuraman et al., 1985). An extension of this theory is the *zone of tolerance* (Zeithaml et al., 1993). This suggests that for patients and customers, there is a level of service that is *desired* and a level of service that is *adequate*. For example, at the airport, a desired level of service would include on-time arrivals and departures, graciously helpful staff, and luggage that is never damaged or lost. Realistically, an adequate level of service might include 15-minute delays, staff that helps when asked, and the occasional lost bag (Tipton, 2009). The zone of tolerance includes any level of service between desired and adequate. Pharmacy managers should keep in mind that the zone of tolerance may be narrow or wide depending on the particular element of service. For example, the zone of tolerance for accurate prescription filling is likely narrow, and the zone of tolerance for pharmacy appearance may be wide (Tipton, 2009). Pharmacy managers also should be cognizant of the fact that patients and customers can vary in their tolerance for service failure. In other words, some patients and customers are less affected by, or more tolerant to service failures than others.

Word of Mouth

Word of mouth occurs when patients and customers provide each other with information about products or services in a noncommercial way (Arndt, 1967). Word of mouth can be positive or negative. It has been suggested that unhappy customers may tell up to 20 people about a bad service experience (Mattila, 2001). The recent growth of web-based social networking through media such as Facebook and Twitter can result in an exponential dissemination of word of mouth by making it possible for one person to communicate their experience to hundreds, even thousands of people (Mangold and Faulds, 2009). Data suggests that negative word of mouth can be hard to mitigate even with strong service recovery. In a study of hotel service failures, it has been found that perceived severity of a service failure can increase negative word of mouth and negative effect on satisfaction. In cases of a severe service failure, even strong recovery efforts might not be enough to stop negative word of mouth (Weun et al., 2004).

Trust

Just as with negative word of mouth, it similarly has been found that trust in the organization can be hard to regain even with strong recovery efforts in the event of severe service failures (Weun et al., 2004). In contrast, an encouraging finding was made with regard to service failures and service recovery in pharmacy. In the pharmacy setting, it appears that trust in the pharmacy and pharmacist remains relatively high, regardless of how severe a patient condition is (symptomatic cough or severe infection) or how serious the service failure is (partial fill or medication error); even before the service recovery is initiated (Bunniran, 2010).

Customer Retention

A single service failure is one of the primary reasons customers switch service providers (Keaveney, 1995). This is significant considering the aforementioned cost to recruit a new customer (Hart et al., 1990). Although previously cited research suggests that the *service recovery paradox* (exceeding pre-service failure satisfaction levels after a service recovery) may not exist, evidence suggests that service recovery efforts can be effective in retaining 75% of customers who experience service failures (Hoffman et al., 1995). It should be noted here that the service recovery paradox does not necessarily have to exist to retain a customer. If a service recovery does not result in a service recovery paradox, it can likely result in satisfaction levels that exceed postfailure satisfaction. Consistent with other earlier findings (Hoffman et al., 1995; Weun et al., 2004), Bunniran (2010) found that in the case of more serious service failures, it is generally more difficult to execute an effective recovery.

COLLECTING FEEDBACK AND SATISFACTION RATINGS

Pharmacy satisfaction studies suggest that patients and customers continue to raise the bar on their expectations, demanding higher levels of service and convenience. The good news is that pharmacies appear to be meeting or exceeding patients' and customers' expectations (Boehringer Ingelheim, 2008). Measuring patient and customer satisfaction and feedback with the service they receive at the pharmacy requires time and effort, but is important for two reasons. First, it helps identify any gaps or deficits in service provision. Second, the pharmacy manager can implement strategies to improve customer service (von Waldner and Abel, 2006). However, one should not measure *only* patient or customer satisfaction feedback. It is a good idea also to survey or interview staff to get their feedback about customer service in the pharmacy. They may see problems that the manager does not see, and they may even provide effective solutions (which, of course, boosts their own morale). When surveying patients, a variety of methods can be used, such as web-based surveys, written questionnaires, telephone surveys, focus groups, or face-to-face interviews. The best method chosen depends on the type of patients or customers being surveyed (young, elderly, low literacy, etc.) and the type of information, or data needed. A combination of methods might be required (Leland and Bailey, 2006).

THE EMPLOYEE'S PERSPECTIVE

If you have ever wondered why a service associate in a retail establishment seems to care so little about their job, there may be good reason why they do not. Ideally, pharmacy employees should be enthusiastic and passionate about what they do. There is no question that employees who are passionate about what they do will take great care of patients and customers; however, not all employees are going to display such enthusiasm. Table 13-4 outlines ten items that are critical for pharmacy managers to remember when wanting to create a climate for the provision of good customer service to patients and customers by their employees. One of the most important points of the information in Table 13-4 is the idea of ensuring employees' quality of work life and job satisfaction. Researchers in customer service consistently have found that employee satisfaction and customer satisfaction are positively correlated (Harter et al., 2002; Wangenheim et al., 2007). The stressful environments of pharmacies have been found to be related to decreased job satisfaction in pharmacy technicians (Desselle and Holmes, 2007). That being said, job stress can be mitigated by supervisor support, which, along with employer support is related positively to job satisfaction (Desselle and Holmes, 2007). These findings lend credence to pharmacy managers providing a supportive and quality work environment

Table 13-4. Developing a Staff That Provides Good Customer Service

Recommendation
1. Hire employees with a caring attitude
2. Reinforce customer service in employee training and orientation
3. Monitor employees' customer service and coach deficiencies
4. Empower employees to solve patient and customer problems
5. Reward employees who make special efforts to please patients customers
6. Get feedback from employees
7. Make customer satisfaction a condition of satisfactory employee performance
8. Model good customer service as a manager
9. Ensure employees' quality of work life and job satisfaction
10. Treat employees fairly

Sources: Bowen et al., (1999); Umiker (1998); Wangenheim et al. (2007).

for their employees for not only the provision of customer service, but for the good of their employees.

Another phenomenon that employees experience (and pharmacy managers should be aware of) is emotional labor. *Emotional labor* describes the process of modifying the emotions you *feel* or the emotions you *express* to meet the goals of your organization (Grandey, 2000). For example, a customer lashing out at a gate agent in an airport over a cancelled flight may induce an emotional response in the agent (such as yelling back at or insulting the customer). Because this would not be a desired response for her or her airline (and may result in disciplinary action or termination of the agent) the agent may choose to regulate her emotions (Holmes, 2008). There are two types of emotional labor. If the gate agent modifies the emotions she *feels* about the situation (e.g., feels empathy for the customer and the inconvenience the cancelled flight has caused) she is undergoing *deep acting*. If the gate agent does not really change her feelings about the situation, but rather, puts on a "mask" to simply change her expression, this is known as *surface acting* (Hochschild, 1983). The pharmacist in the chapter scenario is a good example of someone *not* undergoing emotional labor. He was agitated, frustrated, and angry. He did not modify what he felt or what he expressed to respond to Sarah more appropriately, and it certainly escalated the situation.

The phenomenon of emotional labor has been studied in pharmacists and pharmacy technicians, and a number of things have been observed. First, pharmacists and pharmacy technicians' perception that they have role overload (feeling that there is too much needed to accomplish at work), appears positively related to emotional labor (particularly, surface acting) (Holmes et al., 2009a; Holmes and Bunniran, 2011). Additionally, surface acting appears to be related to negative outcomes in pharmacists, such as reduced job satisfaction, intentions to leave their pharmacy, and emotional exhaustion (in technicians, surface acting has been shown to predict all but intentions to leave their job) (Holmes et al., 2009b; Holmes and Bunniran, 2011). In these same studies, pharmacists and technicians did not seem to undergo deep acting, nor did deep acting seem to be related to other work variables. This is not surprising, as pharmacists may feel that deep acting requires more effort than surface acting and therefore not use it as much (Holmes, 2008).

There are important considerations for managers with regard to emotional labor. First, despite the seemingly negative consequences of emotional labor, it is not likely to go away and it most likely should not. While some employees will a have very high tolerance for difficult customers and never have to undergo emotional labor, not everyone does, and there always will be "difficult" patients and customers. It is not acceptable to pharmacy organizations, or to the profession of pharmacy to act out negative feelings toward patients and customers like the pharmacist did in the scenario. What can pharmacy managers do about the negative consequences? It has been demonstrated that coworker social support (Abraham, 1998) and perceived organizational support (Duke et al., 2009) can mitigate the negative effect of emotional labor on job satisfaction (although, organizational support has not been shown to do this for pharmacy technicians [Holmes and Bunniran, 2011]). Pharmacy chain managers and administrators are encouraged to implement various support mechanisms to mitigate the negative effects of emotional labor (Holmes et al., 2009b).

How far can the way in which you manage your employees and ensure their quality of work life go when it comes to good customer service? Some companies' extraordinary reputations are a result of the legendary customer service they provide as a function of their employees. Probably the most prominent example is Southwest Airlines. Southwest is well known for keeping fares low, getting passengers and their baggage to their destinations on time, and ensuring that passengers enjoy their flight (and even have fun!) (Freiberg and Freiberg, 1996). How do they do it? It is Southwest's policy that employees are first, and customers are second. Their philosophy is that customers will always be treated well because employees are treated well and fairly. They hire only employees who are passionate about people and who fit Southwest's mission. They do their best to ensure that employees' quality of life is exceptional. They give employees the authority to solve customer problems on their own, thus resolving problems faster and providing those employees with a greater sense of autonomy (Freiberg and Freiberg, 1996).

Another company that is legendary for its customer service as a result of employee management is Nordstrom. Nordstrom has been described as having a cult-like culture among its employees (Collins and Porras, 1994). Employees emphatically claim that is the best job they have ever had. At Nordstrom, employee empowerment (see recommendation 4 in Table 13-4) is job number one. Nordstrom one rule for employees is to "use your good judgment in all situations." There are no other rules for employees. As a result, employees at Nordstrom ("Nordies", as they are called) are said to have (Collins and Porras, 1994):

- Ironed a new-bought shirt for a customer who needed it for a meeting that afternoon
- Cheerfully wrapped gifts a customer bought at Macy's
- Warmed customer's cars in the winter while they finished shopping
- Personally knitted a shawl for an elderly customer to be of a length that did not get caught in her wheel chair
- Delivered party clothes at the last minute to a frantic hostess
- Refunded money for a set of tire chains (which aren't sold at Nordstrom's)

Granted, the highly regulated nature of the pharmacy profession and its associated risk makes the Southwest Airlines and Nordstrom examples somewhat extreme and not necessarily appropriate for the pharmacy profession. However, it does speak to the influence employee treatment and development can have on the provision of customer service.

DEALING WITH PATIENT–CUSTOMER COMPLAINTS

Customer complaints are a natural part of the service industry no matter how hard managers and employees try to ensure good customer service. Some patients and customers will never complain no matter how poor the service they receive, while others will do nothing *but* complain. Regardless, few things irritate customers more than not having a venue to lodge complaints, or concerns (Leland and Bailey, 2006). Most likely they will find another venue for their complaints (like Facebook and Twitter) if they cannot use their pharmacy as a venue. While stressful and challenging, complaints should not be perceived negatively but rather as a way to improve the service the pharmacy provides (Leland and Bailey, 2006). It is important not to take a defensive approach to complaining patients and customers, as this may hinder employees' and managers' ability to hear what they are saying and think about ways to improve the provision of service in the pharmacy. Leland and Bailey (2006, p. 250) suggest that complaints can "prove to be a great source of information, innovation, and inspiration." That is because you can discover problems you did not know existed (which may be frustrating other customers) or get ideas for new products or services. Thus, the complaints ultimately help retain current customers, recover customers thought to have been lost, or even gain new ones (Leland and Bailey, 2006).

Leland and Bailey (2006) provide eight principles for constructively dealing with customer complaints.

1. View complaints as gifts.
2. Make it easy for customers to complain.
3. Identify the elements of the complaint.
4. Thank customers for complaining.
5. Sincerely apologize.
6. Fix the problem.
7. Practice prevention.
8. Follow up.

DEALING WITH "DIFFICULT" PATIENTS AND CUSTOMERS

Working in a pharmacy or other service environment can present challenges, including having to deal with "difficult" patients and customers. But rather than think of these patients and customers as "difficult," it is more important to keep in mind *why* patients and customers may be unhappy. As noted in the beginning of the chapter, (1) patients likely view their medications as "negative goods" (Kolassa, 1997), (2) patients may already come in with negative perceptions of the price of medicines, their other healthcare professionals, or their insurance plan, which can sometimes be translated to the pharmacy and to pharmacists, and (3) patients may be symptomatic and not feeling well. It is also important to reinforce that patients and customers will have varying perceptions of the severity of a failure, which may not coincide at all with employees' own perceptions of the severity of failure. Moreover, even after employing the principles of good customer service and ensuring that standards for customer service are met, there can still be the occasional patient or customer who is not happy. While it is very rare, some patients or customers may even become threatening or violent. If a patient's or customer's behavior appears to be escalating out of control, staff in your pharmacy should be trained to call security or dial 911. Such behavior can result in serious consequences and should never be tolerated in the pharmacy setting. For the rest of the dissatisfied patients and customers, Leland and Bailey (2006) suggest a six-step process.

Step 1: Let the customer vent. When patients and customers are upset, their priorities are to vent (not necessarily to the person who is at fault), and to solve their problem. Service providers are encouraged to let the patient or customer express his or her feelings without interruption. Trying to calm them down can anger them further.

Step 2: Avoid getting trapped in a negative filter. This occurs when employees' negative thoughts about a patient or customer bleed into their conversation with them. For example, a patient may come in for a refill not realizing that they do not have a refill authorization left. When a pharmacist informs the patient that he or she will need to call the doctor to get the refill authorization, they may respond with frustration toward the pharmacist because of the delay. A negative filter (perceptions that the patient for customer is being unreasonable) may result in a response by the pharmacist such as, "Look, you are the one who came in with no refills left." Leland and Bailey (2006) suggest replacing this "negative filter" with a "service filter." Pharmacy employees should ask themselves, "What does this customer need, and how can I provide it?" This will change an employee's focus from anger and frustration (and a possible argument) to that of problem solving.

Step 3: Express empathy to the customer. Expressing empathy allows employees to recognize and appreciate a patient's or customer's feelings. But, employees should not sympathize, or overidentify with the patient's or customer's feelings.

Step 4: Begin active problem solving. Once the patient or customer has aired their grievances, employees can begin active problem solving by gathering additional information and double-checking the facts of the situation.

Step 5: Mutually agree on the solution. In this stage, employees should work with the customer to come up with an acceptable solution to the problem. By doing this, employees are meeting the patient's or customer's requirement for control (see Table 13-2).

Step 6: Follow up. Following up to make sure that the solution worked can go a long way with patients and customers. If the solution did not work, this is the employee's opportunity to try again.

Looking back at the scenario at the beginning of the chapter, how did the general manager approach Steps 1–6? How did the pharmacist approach Steps 1–3?

PREVENTING PATIENT AND CUSTOMER CONFLICT AND COMPLAINTS

When it comes to dealing with "difficult" patients and customers, sometimes prevention is the best medicine. Avoid using phrases and language that make patient or customer feel like an adversary or that express disinterest on your part. For example, phrases such as "I don't know," "no," "that's not my job," "you're right; this stinks," "that's not my fault," "you need to talk to my manager," "you want it by when?," "calm down," "I'm busy right now," and "call me back," can demonstrate to patient and customers that you are not willing to help, and can sometimes be a catalyst to conflict (Leland and Bailey, 2006). However, phrases such as "I'll find out," "what I can do is . . . ," "this is who can help you," "I understand your frustration," "let's see what we can do about this," "I can help you," "I'll try my best," "I'm sorry," "I'll be with you in just a moment," and "I will call you back," can demonstrate to the patient or customer that you are willing to go the extra mile, and create a positive image in the mind of the patient or customer (Leland and Bailey, 2006).

In addition to avoiding certain phrases and language, also important, if not more important, is avoiding body language, tone of voice, and other nonverbal behaviors that can express similar negativity. Body language and tone of voice can say a lot, even if nothing is said at all. In fact, it has been shown that 55% of what is learned from others comes from body language, 33% comes from tone of voice, and 7% comes from actual spoken words (Leland and Bailey, 2006). For example, in a restaurant a customer might request from the server that their hamburger come without mayo or onion, with extra pickle, and no salt on the fries. The server might roll her eyes in exasperation. She is connoting that the customer has annoyed her with his request. Ways in which eye contact, facial expressions, nodding, hand gestures, and personal space are used can drastically affect the patient or customer encounter and communicate to them whether an employee is engaged in helping him or her, is uninterested in helping or sees them as an adversary (Leland and Bailey, 2006).

Body language might have played a significant role in the scenario presented at the beginning of the chapter. The pharmacy manager's look toward the patient was a puzzling one. He was simply confused and perplexed. However, Sarah did not interpret it that way. She interpreted his look to be judgmental. Additionally, the pharmacy manager did not look at her directly while explaining the situation. This may have sent the message that he did not care about her situation, even if he did (Leland and Bailey, 2006).

Tone of voice also can send a message to the customer. A flat, monotone voice suggests boredom or disinterest in the patient or customer; a slow speed and low pitch suggests that an employee wants to be left alone; a high-pitched emphatic voice suggests enthusiasm; an abrupt speed and loud tone suggests an employee is too busy for the patient or customer; and, high pitch and drawn out speed expresses disbelief in what the customer is saying. Additionally, inflection (wave-like movement of highs and lows in the pitch of your voice), stress on words, breathing, volume, and pacing can influence communication to the patient or customer (Leland and Bailey, 2006).

REVISITING THE SCENARIO

Sarah's experience at the pharmacy is probably not an unusual one. Pharmacies get hectic, and misunderstandings occur and escalate due to a patient's fragile state and the communication methods of the staff. The concepts from this chapter, such as the principles for ensuring good customer service, standards that customer use to evaluate services, how to help and motivate employees to provide good customer service, and how to prevent customer conflict are worth remembering. Despite a provider's best efforts, service failures likely will still occur. After they do, every effort should be made to genuinely compensate for a patient's loss, however big or small. Sarah seemed satisfied with the information provided to her by the general manager. Will she return to the pharmacy? Will she still trust the pharmacist? Will she tell her friends about what happened? In the end, the high road will be good for business.

QUESTIONS FOR FURTHER DISCUSSION

1. Describe a time when you, as a customer, received great customer service, and bad customer service. Why was it great or bad, and how did it make you feel?
2. What kind of impact has social media like Facebook and Twitter had on the provision and evaluation of customer service?
3. How do Leland and Bailey's (2006) Steps 1–3 in dealing with difficult customers compare and contrast to the concept of emotional labor?

REFERENCES

Abraham R. 1998. Emotional dissonance in organizations: antecedents, consequents, and moderators. *Genet Soc and Gen Psych Mono* 124(2):229–46.

American Academy of Family Physicians. 2005 Liability: doctor apologies. Available at http://www.aafp.org/online/etc/medialib/aafp_org/documents/policy/state/liability-apologies.Par.0001.File.tmp/stateadvocacy_Liability_Doctor%20Apologies.pdf; accessed on August 21, 2011.

Arndt J. 1967. Role of product-related conversations in the diffusion of a new product. *J Market Res* 4:291–95.

Austin Z, Gregory PAM, Martin JC. 2006. Characterizing the professional relationships of community pharmacists. *Res Soc Admin Pharm* 2:533–46.

Bell CR, Zemke RE. 1987. Service breakdown, the road to recovery. *Manag Rev* 76(10):32–35.

Benoit W, Brinson S. 1994. Apologies are not enough. *Commun Q* 42(1):75–88.

Bitner MJ, Booms BH, Tetreault MS. 1990. The service encounter: diagnosing favorable and unfavorable events. *J Mark* 54:71–84.

Boehringer Ingelheim. 2008. Pharmacy Satisfaction Digest (on-line). Available at http://www.rx-edge.com/research%20pdfs/PharmacySatisfactionDigest_2008.pdf; accessed on July 20, 2011.

Boehringer Ingelheim. 2011. Topline Data Report (on-line). Available at http://www.pharmacysatisfaction.com/pharmacy-data.jsp; accessed on December 15, 2011.

Bowen DE, Gilliland SW, Folger R. 1999. HRM and service fairness: How being fair with employees spills over to customers. *Organ Dyn* 27(3):7–23

Bunniran S. 2010. *Patient Service Experiences in Community Pharmacy: an Examination of Health Criticality in Service Failures and Service Recovery Incidents and Its Influence on Trust, Satisfaction, Repurchase Intentions and Word-of-Mouth [doctoral dissertation].* Oxford: The University of Mississippi.

Bunniran S, McCaffrey DJ, Bentley JP. 2010. Service failure and service recovery incidents in community pharmacy. *American Pharmacists Association Annual Meeting.*

Chui MA. 2009. Evaluating the outcomes of value-added pharmacy services. In Desselle S, Zgarrick D (eds.) *Pharmacy Management.* New York: McGraw-Hill, p. 475.

Collins J, Porras J. 1994. *Built to Last.* New York: HarperBusiness, pp. 115–21

Desselle SP, Holmes ER. 2007. Structural model of certified pharmacy technicians' job satisfaction. *J Am Pharm Assoc* 47:58–72.

Duke A, Goodman J, Treadway D, Breland J. 2009. Perceived organizational support as a moderator of emotional labor-outcomes relationships. *J Appl Soc Psychol* 39:1013–34.

Flynn EA, Barker KN, Carnahan BJ. 2003. National observational study of prescription dispensing accuracy and safety in 50 pharmacies. *J Am Pharm Assoc* 43(2):191–200.

Freiberg K, Freiberg J. 1996. *Nuts! Southwest Airlines' Crazy Recipe for Business and Personal Success.* New York: Broadway Books, pp. 282–95.

Friedman S. 2010. Customer Service Manager. At your service: the ten commandments of customer service.

Available at http://www.customerservicemanager.com/at-your-service-the-ten-commandments-of-great-customer-service.htm; accessed on July 12, 2011.

Gamble KH. 2011. Pharmacy Times. Do speedy prescription guarantees compromise safety? Available at http://www.pharmacytimes.com/web-exclusives/Do-Speedy-Prescription-Guarantees-Compromise-Safety; accessed: July 21, 2011.

Grandey A. 2000. Emotion regulation in the workplace: A new way to conceptualize emotional labor. *J Occup Health Psychol* 5:95–110.

Hart CWL, Heskett JL, Sasser WE. 1990. The profitable art of service recovery. *Harv Bus Rev* 68:148–56.

Harter JK, Schmidt FL, Hayes TL. 2002. Business-unit-level relationship between employee satisfaction, employee engagement, and business outcomes: a meta-analysis. *J Appl Psychol* 87(2):268–79.

Hochschild A. 1983. *The Managed Heart: Commercialization of Human Feeling.* Berkley, CA: University of California Press, pp. 48–49.

Hoffman KD, Kelley SW, Rotalsky HM. 1995. Tracking service failures and employee recovery efforts. *J Serv Market* 9(2):49–61.

Holmes E. 2008. *The Role of Emotional Dissonance as an Affective State on the Emotional Labor Process of Retail Chain Pharmacists [doctoral dissertation].* Oxford: The University of Mississippi.

Holmes E, Bentley, Bouldin A, Garner D. 2009a. The role of affective emotional dissonance as an affective state on the emotional labor process of retail chain pharmacists. *American Pharmacists Association Annual Meeting.*

Holmes E, Bentley, Bouldin A, Garner D. 2009b. The impact of emotional labor on retail chain pharmacists work life outcomes. *American Pharmacists Association Annual Meeting*.

Holmes E, Bunniran S. 2011. Community pharmacy technicians' emotional labor and resultant work life outcomes. *American Pharmacists Association Annual Meeting.*

Johnston R. 1995. Service failure and recovery: impact, attributes, and process. *Adv Ser Mark Manage* 4:211–28.

Keaveney S. 1995. Customer switching behavior in service industries: an exploratory study. *J Mark* 59:71–82.

Kelley SW, Hoffman KD, Davis MA. 1993. A typology of retail failures and recoveries. *J Retail* 69(4):429–52.

Kneeland B. 2009. Delivering the WOW. *Am Pharm* 28–31.

Kolassa EM. 1997. Pricing, politics, and problems-a pricing philosophy. In Kolassa EM (ed.) *Elements of Pharmaceutical Pricing.* Binghamton, NY: Pharmaceutical Products Press, p. 22.

Leland K, Bailey K. 2006. *Customer Service for Dummies.* Hoboken, NJ: Wiley Publishing, Inc.

Mangold W, Faulds D. 2009. Social media: the new hybrid element of the promotion mix. *Bus Horiz* 52: 357–65.

Mattila A. 2001. The effectiveness of service recovery in a multi-industry setting. *J Serv Mark* 15:583–96.

Obarski AM. 2010 Customer Service Manager. Customers are us! The golden rule of customer service. Available at http://www.customerservicemanager.com/customers-are-us-the-golden-rule-of-customer-service.htm; accessed on July 12, 2011.

Oliver R. 1980. A cognitive model of the antecedents and consequences of satisfaction decisions. *J Mark Res* 17(4):460–69.

Parasuraman A, Zeithaml VA, Berry LL. 1985. A conceptual model of service quality and its implications for future research. *J Mark* 49:41–50.

Parasuraman A, Zeithaml VA, Berry LL. 1988. SERVQUAL: A multiple-item scale for measuring consumer perceptions of service quality. *J Retail* 64(1):12–40.

Pearson CM, Mitroff II. 1993. From crisis prone to crisis prepared: a framework for crisis management. *Acad Manage Exec* 7(1):48–59.

Reichheld FF, Sasser WE. 1990. Zero defections: Quality comes to services. *Harv Bus Rev* 68:105–11.

Schommer JC, Wenzel RG, Kucukarslan SN. 2002. Evaluation of of pharmacists services for hospital inpatients. *Am J Health Syst Pharm* 59:1632–637.

Schweikhart SB, Strasser S, Kennedy MR. 1993. Service recovery in health service organizations. *Hosp Health Serv Admin* 38(1):3–21

Sellnow T, Ulmer R. 1995. Ambiguous argument as advocacy in organizational crisis communication. *Arg Advoc* 31:138–50.

Smith A, Bolton R. 1998. An experimental investigation of customer reactions to service failure and recovery encounters: paradox or peril. *J Serv Res* 1(1):65–81.

Spreng R, MacKenzie S, Olshavsky R. 1996. A reexamination of the determinants of consumer satisfaction. *J Mark* 60:15–32.

Tipton DJ. 2000. Service recovery in pharmacies. *J Pharm Mark Manage* 13(3):71–83.

Tipton DJ. 2009. Customer service. In Desselle S, Zgarrick D (eds.) *Pharmacy Management.* New York: McGraw-Hill.

Tipton DJ, Giannetti VJ, Kristofik JM. 2003. Managing the aftermath of medication errors: managed care's role. *J Am Pharm Assoc* 43:662–29.

Umiker W. 1998. *Management Skills for the New Health Care Supervisor.* Gaithersburg, MD: Aspen Publishers, Inc.

von Waldner TK, Abel SR. 2011. Achieving and measuring patient satisfaction. In Chisholm-Burns M, Vaillancourt A, Shepherd M (eds.) *Pharmacy Management, Leadership, Marketing, and Finance.* Sudbury, MA: Jones and Bartlett.

Wangenheim F, Evanschitzky H, Wunderlich M. 2007. Does the employee-customer satisfaction link hold for all employee groups? *J Bus Res* 60:690–97.

Webster C, Sundaram DS. 1998. Service consumption criticality in failure recovery. *J Bus Res* 41:153–59.

Weun S, Beatty SE, Jones MA. 2004. The impact of service failure severity on service recovery evaluations and post-recovery relationships. *J Serv Market* 18(2): 133–46.

Zeithaml VA, Berry LL, Parasuraman A. 1993. The nature and determinants of customer expectations of service. *J Acad Market Sci* 21(1):1–12.

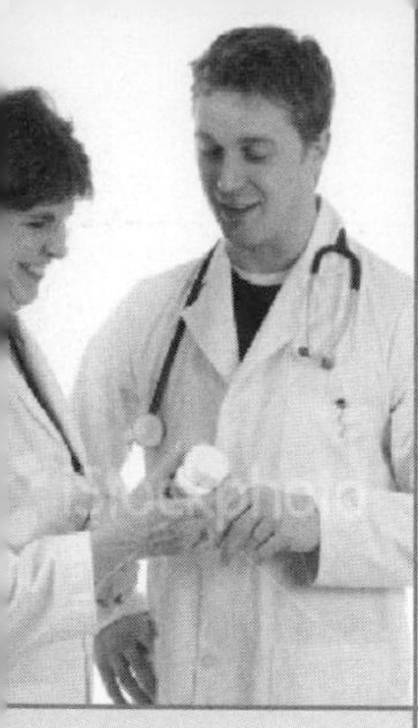

14

MANAGING THE WORKPLACE TO PROTECT THE ORGANIZATION AND IMPROVE EMPLOYEE QUALITY OF WORKLIFE

Alan R. Spies

About the Author: Dr. Spies is an associate professor at the University of Oklahoma College of Pharmacy. He completed a B.S. in Pharmacy at Southwestern Oklahoma State University, an M.B.A. and J.D. at the University of Oklahoma and a Ph.D. in Pharmacy Administration at the University of Mississippi School of Pharmacy. At the University of Oklahoma, Dr. Spies teaches professional students about pharmacy law/ethics, leadership, and management. His current research interests focus on professionalism, generational differences, psychological contract violations, and the role of exercise in pharmacy students' well-being.

LEARNING OBJECTIVES

After completing this chapter, readers should be able to

1. Compare and contrast the role various federal employment laws play in the pharmacy workplace.
2. Describe what is meant by "sexual harassment" and how employers and employees can resolve issues of quid pro quo and hostile work environments.
3. Discuss the concept of drug testing and why it is necessary in the pharmacy workplace.
4. Determine the appropriate steps in preventing a successful false imprisonment lawsuit.
5. Identify the best ways to resolve pharmacy robbery, burglary, theft and shoplifting incidents.
6. Describe fundamental issues in occupational safety.
7. Identify and discuss methods to maximize employee productivity and minimize turnover, such as career planning and use of employee assistance programs.
8. Discuss potential workplace issues associated with intergenerational dynamics and other aspects of managing an increasingly diverse workforce.

SCENARIO

Michael Davis is a brand new pharmacy school graduate, and after receiving his pharmacist license, is immediately made store manager at Sooner Drug and Apothecary, a large chain pharmacy located in the Midwest and Southern United States. Michael is excited about his managerial position. There are two clerks, three pharmacy technicians and one other pharmacist at Michael's store, all women employees except for the other pharmacist. After a couple months, one of the pharmacy technicians approaches Michael and tells him that Mark, the other pharmacist, has been making rather suggestive comments to her and that it makes her feel uncomfortable. Michael regularly plays golf with Mark and really likes him, as they have similar interests. Michael tells the technician not to worry about it, as he cannot imagine Mark saying anything close to what the technician is telling him.

A couple of weeks later, this same technician tells Michael she noticed another technician taking some hydrocodone 10-mg tablets and placing them in her purse. After conducting an informal inventory of the hydrocodone in stock and noticing a shortage of 20 tablets, Michael calls both technicians into the break room and confronts the suspected employee. The employee adamantly denies this, but Michael is convinced she committed theft. He tells the suspected employee to wait in the break room while he and the technician making the complaint exit the room. Michael then locks the door to the break room and calls the police. The police arrive 15 minutes later and after questioning the technician, determine that she, in fact, stole the hydrocodone.

After terminating the technician's employment, Michael decides to hire a new technician, a recent high school graduate. As a millennial, she is the youngest employee in the pharmacy. Michael is very happy with his new hire but is concerned when she begins texting and Tweeting when no patients are in the pharmacy. This behavior has caused friction especially with one of the pharmacy's clerks, a baby boomer, and 20-year employee of Sooner Drug and Apothecary. This senior clerk believes there is no reason to surf the Internet or use a cell phone while at work and to do so is unprofessional. A couple days later, Michael notices that one of the other technicians has started using her cell phone at work, occasionally when patients are in the pharmacy.

CHAPTER QUESTIONS

1. What are some of the principal workplace issues that involve federal employment laws?
2. What are some of the skills and abilities managers must possess in order to ensure a safe and healthy working environment?
3. What are the potential legal issues associated with drug testing in the workplace? Should employers require drug testing of job applicants and employees?
4. What are the main sources of conflict in the workplace?
5. What role, if any, do generational differences play in the workplace?
6. What are the benefits for managers providing professional and career development opportunities for their employees? What are some reasonable approaches to developing employees?

FEDERAL EMPLOYMENT LAWS

There are numerous federal laws that impact the pharmacy workplace. Chapter 12 describes several laws that help govern how pharmacist employers recruit, interview, select, hire, discipline, and terminate employees. The principles illustrated in that chapter are critical for pharmacists to understand and apply. This chapter will examine, in more detail, a few select federal employment laws in the context of discrimination and sexual harassment. Though a thorough discussion is beyond the scope of this chapter, specific provisions for discrimination and sexual harassment will be examined, supplemented with specific examples from various areas of pharmacy practice.

Title VII of the Civil Rights Act of 1964 (Title VII) prohibits discrimination on the basis of race, color, national origin, religion, or sex. Discrimination in the workplace can occur in other ways, too, in addition to the five areas listed earlier. For instance, individuals may bring a claim of discrimination based on age, pregnancy, compensation, or disability. As such, other federal employment laws were enacted, such as the Age Discrimination in Employment Act, the Equal Pay Act, and the Americans with Disabilities Act. To protect pregnant individuals, Title VII was amended to include the Pregnancy Discrimination Act. At first glance, it may appear overwhelming to comply with these federal laws. However, the next few sections hopefully will illustrate methods pharmacists can adopt to create, develop, and maintain a workplace free from discrimination. The majority of information for this section comes directly from the U.S. Equal Employment Opportunity Commission Web site (http://www.eeoc.gov/).

Title VII of the Civil Rights Act of 1964

Race Discrimination

Discrimination on the basis of an immutable characteristic associated with race, such as skin color, hair texture, or certain facial features violates Title VII, even though not all members of the race share the same characteristic. Title VII also prohibits discrimination on the basis of a condition that predominantly affects one race unless the practice is job related and consistent with business necessity. For example, since sickle cell anemia predominantly occurs in African Americans, a policy that excludes individuals with sickle cell anemia is discriminatory unless the policy is job related and consistent with business necessity. Similarly, a "no-beard" employment policy may discriminate against African American men who have a predisposition to pseudofolliculitis barbae (severe shaving bumps) unless the policy is job related and consistent with business necessity.

In a race discrimination lawsuit, the courts will examine whether a particular policy is related to the conditions of employment and consistent with business necessity. This evaluation is conducted on a case-by-case basis but some factors the courts examine include

- Education
- Employment testing
- Conviction and arrest records

In the profession of pharmacy, pharmacists are required by law to be licensed by their respective licensing board (e.g., state board of pharmacy). So, a nonpharmacist (regardless of race) will not prevail in a race discrimination lawsuit against an employer advertising specifically for a pharmacist position, assuming that the job qualifications require a licensed pharmacist. As illustrated in the example below, a situation could arise regarding education involving a pharmacy technician.

Case 1

Samantha, a 22-year-old white female, is the head pharmacy technician at Drugs R' Us. She took the job right after college and now is departing after 3 years to go to pharmacy school. The employer was thrilled with Samantha's work, and when he receives notice that she is leaving, he sets out to find a replacement. Sylvia, an African American, applies for the job. Sylvia is a successful graduate of the local technical institute, and has spent the last 5 years working as a pharmacy technician for another pharmacy, being promoted a year ago to become the head pharmacy technician in one of the largest pharmacies in the city. The employer rejects Sylvia's application because she is not a college graduate, which triggers the lawsuit. Statistical evidence shows that in the local labor market African Americans and Hispanics in the pool of pharmacy technicians are significantly less likely to have college degrees than whites. The employer defends its education requirement by attributing Samantha's success to the fact that she was college educated, noting that the head pharmacy technician position involves not only traditional technician work, but also more complex responsibilities such as preparing reports, and training and supervising other technicians and clerks. The investigation reveals, however, that none of the pharmacy's prior successful head pharmacy technicians had college degrees, and it is not the industry standard. Most importantly, the employer presents no evidence that a college degree is more predictive of, or correlated with, job performance than a degree from a technical institute plus significant relevant experience (e.g., Sylvia's qualifications), or other credentials and experiences that would render a person qualified for the job. The evidence establishes that the employer has violated Title VII because the college-degree requirement screens out African Americans and Hispanics to a significant degree but it has not been demonstrated to be job related and consistent with business necessity.

An employer, to show an employment decision was made related to the conditions of employment and consistent with business necessity, may use conviction and arrest records. Unlike many other places of employment, pharmacists are required by federal (and some state) law to receive a waiver for any employee with a controlled substance-related felony. If a waiver is not obtained for the employee prior to the beginning of employment, the pharmacy will be in violation of the law. So, it is imperative for any pharmacy that dispenses controlled substances to make sure all of its employees have undergone criminal background checks. It is also important to note that these policies of conducting background checks must be applied to all employees. Failure to do so could result in a successful discrimination lawsuit.

Color Discrimination

Title VII prohibits employment discrimination because of "color" as a basis separately listed in the statute. The statute does not define "color." The courts and the Equal Employment Opportunity Commission (EEOC) read "color" to have its commonly understood meaning—pigmentation, complexion, or skin shade or tone. Thus, color discrimination occurs when a person is discriminated against based on the lightness, darkness, or other color characteristic of the person. Even though race and color clearly overlap, they are not synonymous. Thus, color discrimination can occur between persons of different races or ethnicities, or between persons of the same race or ethnicity. It is important to note that discrimination can occur when the victim and the person who inflicted the discrimination are the same race or color.

National Origin Discrimination

Whether an employee or job applicant's ancestry is Mexican, Ukrainian, Filipino, Arab, American Indian, or any other nationality, he or she is entitled to the same employment opportunities as anyone else. EEOC enforces the federal prohibition against national origin discrimination (in addition to race, color, sex, and religion) in employment under Title VII that covers employers with fifteen or more employees.

It is unlawful to discriminate against any employee or applicant because of the individual's national origin. No one can be denied equal employment opportunity because of birthplace, ancestry, culture, and linguistic characteristics common to a specific ethnic group, or accent. Equal employment opportunity cannot be denied because of marriage or association with persons of a national origin group; membership or association with specific ethnic promotion groups; attendance or participation in schools, churches, temples or mosques generally associated with a national origin group; or a surname associated with a national origin group. Title VII prohibits offensive conduct, such as ethnic slurs, that creates a hostile work environment based on national origin.

In addition, the following items are important for employers to keep in mind:

- *Accent discrimination.* An employer may not base a decision on an employee's foreign accent unless the accent materially interferes with job performance.
- *English fluency.* A fluency requirement is only permissible if required for the effective performance of the position for which it is imposed.
- *English-only rules.* English-only rules must be adopted for nondiscriminatory reasons. An English-only rule may be used if it is needed to promote the safe or efficient operation of the employer's business.
- *Coverage of foreign nationals.* Title VII and the other antidiscrimination laws prohibit discrimination against individuals employed in the United States, regardless of citizenship. However, relief may

be limited if an individual does not have work authorization. The Immigration Reform and Control Act of 1986 (IRCA) requires employers to prove all employees hired after November 6, 1986, are legally authorized to work in the United States. IRCA also prohibits discrimination based on national origin or citizenship.

Case 2

Luis, a Mexican citizen and licensed pharmacist in the United States, files a charge with the EEOC alleging that he was not promoted from his staff pharmacist position to a pharmacy store manager position by XYZ Pharmacy because of his Mexican national origin. The investigation reveals that XYZ has many Mexican Americans employed as pharmacists, but has a policy requiring that all of its higher-paid store and district pharmacy managers be US citizens. In addition, Hispanic applicants for pharmacy intern, technician, and pharmacist jobs are rejected at a much higher rate than non-Hispanic applicants, even accounting for differences in qualifications and/or experience. Hispanic employees also are generally given less favorable work assignments and paid less than non-Hispanic employees who are performing similar work. Under the circumstances, the evidence establishes that the citizenship requirement is part of a wider scheme of unlawful national origin discrimination and was adopted for unlawful discriminatory reasons.

Religion Discrimination

Title VII prohibits employers from discriminating against individuals because of their religion in hiring, firing, and other terms and conditions of employment. The Act also requires employers to reasonably accommodate the religious practices of an employee or prospective employee, unless to do so would create an undue hardship upon the employer. A reasonable religious accommodation is any adjustment to the work environment that will allow the employee to practice his religion. Flexible scheduling, voluntary substitutions or swaps, job reassignments, and lateral transfers are examples of accommodating an employee's religious beliefs.

Employers generally should not schedule examinations or other selection activities in conflict with a current or prospective employee's religious needs, inquire about an applicant's future availability at certain times, maintain a restrictive dress code, or refuse to allow observance of a Sabbath or religious holiday, unless the employer can show that not doing so would cause an undue hardship.

An employer can claim undue hardship when asked to accommodate an applicant's or employee's religious practices if allowing such practices requires more than ordinary administrative costs, diminishes efficiency in other jobs, infringes on other employees' job rights or benefits, impairs workplace safety, causes coworkers to carry the accommodated employee's share of potentially hazardous or burdensome work, or if the proposed accommodation conflicts with another law or regulation. Undue hardship also may be shown if the request for an accommodation violates the terms of a collective bargaining agreement or job rights established through a seniority system.

It should be noted that what appears as an undue hardship for one pharmacy may not appear as an undue hardship for another pharmacy. As such, there is no definitive standard that determines undue hardship. An accommodation would pose an undue hardship if it would cause more than diminish cost on the operation of the employer's business. Factors relevant to undue hardship may include the type of workplace, the nature of the employee's duties, the identifiable cost of the accommodation in relation to the size and operating costs of the employer, and the number of employees who will need a particular accommodation.

Costs to be considered include not only direct monetary costs but also the burden on the conduct of the employer's business. To prove undue hardship, the employer will need to demonstrate how much cost or disruption a proposed accommodation would involve. An employer cannot rely on potential or hypothetical hardship when faced with a religious obligation that conflicts with scheduled work, but rather should rely on objective information. A mere assumption that many more people with the same religious practices as the individual being accommodated may also seek accommodation is not evidence of undue hardship.

For example, many pharmacies are open on Sunday, a day traditionally reserved for attending church services. However, what does a pharmacy employer do if all its employees do not want to work on Sunday? The typical attorney answer is "it depends."

One way to resolve this potential issue it to address it prior to hiring an employee. Though an employer is prohibited from asking an applicant questions regarding his/her religious beliefs, the employer is allowed to ask the following question: "Are you able to perform all the essential qualifications for the position, qualifications that include working on Sunday?" If the applicant responds "yes," the employer is then allowed to require the employee to work on Sunday. It should be noted, though, that it could appear discriminatory if the same employee (or select employees) are always required to work on Sunday, while other employees (assuming same seniority or less) are not required to work Sunday.

Pregnancy Discrimination

As mentioned earlier, Title VII was amended to prohibit pregnancy discrimination. Pregnancy discrimination involves treating a woman (an applicant or employee) unfavorably because of pregnancy, childbirth, or a medical condition related to pregnancy or childbirth. An employer may not single out pregnancy-related conditions for special procedures to determine an employee's ability to work. However, if an employer requires its employees to submit a doctor's statement concerning their inability to work before granting leave or paying sick benefits, the employer may require employees affected by pregnancy-related conditions to submit such statements.

If an employee is temporarily unable to perform her job because of her pregnancy, the employer must treat her the same as any other temporarily disabled employee. For example, if the employer allows temporarily disabled employees to modify tasks, perform alternative assignments, or take disability leave or leave without pay, the employer also must allow an employee who is temporarily disabled because of pregnancy to do the same.

Pregnant employees must be permitted to work as long as they are able to perform their jobs. If an employee has been absent from work as a result of a pregnancy-related condition and recovers, her employer may not require her to remain on leave until the baby's birth.

Further, under the Family and Medical Leave Act (FMLA) of 1993, a new parent (including foster and adoptive parents) may be eligible for 12 weeks of leave (unpaid or paid, if the employee has earned or accrued it) that may be used for care of the new child. To be eligible, the employee must have worked for the employer for 12 months prior to taking the leave and the employer must have 50 or more employees.

Sex Discrimination

Sex discrimination involves treating someone (an applicant or employee) unfavorably because of that person's sex. For example, a pharmacy manager only wants to hire a male pharmacist because he does not believe women should be in the profession of pharmacy. So, he hires only male pharmacists at his store, even though he receives both qualified male and female pharmacist employment applications. Sex discrimination also can involve treating someone less favorably because of his or her connection with an organization or group that is generally associated with people of a certain sex.

Sexual harassment is also a form of sex discrimination under Title VII. There are two types of sexual harassment: quid pro quo and hostile work environment. Unfortunately, many cases of sexual harassment are never reported. As pharmacy interns and pharmacists, it is important to identify cases when they occur. The information (and subsequent case) below provides an overview of sexual harassment.

Unwelcome sexual advances, requests for sexual favors, and other verbal or physical conduct of a sexual nature constitute sexual harassment when this conduct explicitly or implicitly affects an individual's employment (quid pro quo), unreasonably interferes with an individual's work performance, or creates an intimidating, hostile, or offensive work environment (hostile work environment). Sexual harassment can occur in a variety of circumstances, including but not limited to the following:

- The victim as well as the harasser may be a woman or a man. The victim does not have to be of the opposite sex.
- The harasser can be the victim's supervisor, an agent of the employer, a supervisor in another area, a coworker, or a nonemployee (pharmacy patient).
- The victim does not have to be the person harassed but could be anyone affected by the offensive conduct.
- Unlawful sexual harassment may occur without economic injury to or discharge of the victim.
- The harasser's conduct must be unwelcome.

It is helpful for the victim to inform the harasser directly that the conduct is unwelcome and must stop. The victim should use any employer complaint mechanism or grievance system available.

When investigating allegations of sexual harassment, EEOC looks at the whole record: the circumstances, such as the nature of the sexual advances, and the context in which the alleged incidents occurred. A determination on the allegations is made from the facts on a case-by-case basis.

Prevention is the best tool to eliminate sexual harassment in the workplace. Employers are encouraged to take steps necessary to prevent sexual harassment from occurring. They should clearly communicate to employees that sexual harassment will not be tolerated. They can do so by providing sexual harassment training to their employees and by establishing an effective complaint or grievance process and taking immediate and appropriate action when an employee complains. In the scenario, Michael's response to complaints of potential sexual harassment is probably not the most prudent of actions. At the very least, Michael should investigate the matter further, carefully listening to the technician and also speaking with Mark about the alleged remarks. Whether Mark admits to making the sexually suggestive remarks, responsibility falls onto Michael to remind all employees (either himself, or someone trained in the laws/ethics of such) of what constitutes proper behavior in the workplace and that the organization will not tolerate sexual harassment. Any further actions against Mark will be dictated by the response, situation, and any future behaviors by all parties involved.

It is also unlawful to retaliate against an individual for opposing employment practices that discriminate on the basis of sex or for filing a discrimination charge, testifying, or participating in any way in an investigation, proceeding, or litigation under Title VII.

Case 3

CT, a male pharmacist, has recently been promoted to pharmacy manager and transferred to XYZ Drugs, a large pharmacy chain, at its location on Harvard and Main Street, to replace the current pharmacy manager who recently retired. AH, a female pharmacy technician, has been working at XYZ Drugs for just over one year and is described by others as an "exemplary employee." CT's first 3 months as pharmacy manager go very smoothly, and everyone is pleased with their new manager, including AH. In fact, it is not uncommon for all the pharmacy employees to go to dinner together after work on Friday evenings. One Friday evening during dinner at a local restaurant, CT asks AH if she has a boyfriend. AH awkwardly replies, "no." Nothing else is said. A couple of weeks later, CT compliments AH by saying, "you look really nice today." AH does not respond. The following day, CT hears AH telling the other pharmacy technician that her neck is really sore from working out. CT comes up to AH and begins giving her a neck massage. Again, AH does not say anything and allows CT to give her the massage. Two days later, CT asks AH if she would like to go to a concert with him. AH declines. Assume you are CT's pharmacy district manager and that AH has just filed a grievance with you, alleging CT sexually harassed her. As the district manager, it is imperative to investigate this matter immediately. The investigation is not implying CT has violated Title VII, but an investigation must be commenced to resolve the situation. That being said, the district manager must individually meet with and interview all parties involved. Once the facts are known, the district manager must take appropriate steps (and discipline, if needed) to make sure the workplace is free from sexual harassment. Failure to do so may place XYZ Drugs and the district manager at risk for legal action, as well.

Age Discrimination in Employment Act

Age discrimination involves treating someone (an applicant or employee) less favorably because of his or her age. The Age Discrimination in Employment Act (ADEA) forbids age discrimination only against people who are age 40 or older. It does not protect workers under the age of 40, although some states do have laws that protect younger workers from age discrimination. It is not illegal for an employer or other covered entity to favor an older worker over a younger one, even if both workers are age 40 or older. Discrimination can occur when the victim and the person who inflicted the discrimination are both over 40. It is also important to note that an employment policy or practice that applies to everyone, regardless of age, can be illegal if it has a negative impact on applicants or employees age 40 or older and is not based on a reasonable factor other than age.

Based on this information, must a pharmacy manager promote a pharmacist over the age of 40 rather than promote a pharmacist who is 30 years of age? The answer is no, provided age was not a factor in the decision. The ADEA is not automatically violated if a pharmacy employee over the age of 40 is not promoted. There are several factors the employer may use in its decision-making process so as to protect the pharmacy (and the pharmacy management/owner) from an ADEA claim. These factors include

- Output
- Productivity
- Education
- Experience (Robinson et al., 2002).

Regarding the previous example, the pharmacy employer must demonstrate that in promoting the 30-year-old pharmacist over the 40-year-old pharmacist, the younger pharmacist performed his job more efficiently, possessed greater education, had more experience as a pharmacist and/or had a greater number of years with the organization. The presence of these factors is no guarantee the employer will win a possible ADEA lawsuit but they do provide a stronger defense. It should be noted that the employer must have documentation to support its claim, chiefly performance evaluations (see Chapter 12).

The Equal Pay Act

The Equal Pay Act (EPA) requires that men and women in the same workplace be given equal pay for equal work. The jobs need not be identical, but they must be substantially equal. Job content (not job titles) determines whether jobs are substantially equal. All forms of pay are covered by this law, including salary, overtime pay, bonuses, stock options, profit sharing and bonus plans, life insurance, vacation and holiday pay, cleaning or gasoline allowances, hotel accommodations, reimbursement for travel expenses, and benefits. If there is an inequality in wages between men and women, employers may not reduce the wages of either sex to equalize their pay.

An individual alleging a violation of the EPA may go directly to court and is not required to file an EEOC charge beforehand. The time limit for filing an EPA charge with the EEOC and the time limit for going to court are the same: within 2 years of the alleged unlawful compensation practice or, in the case of a willful violation, within 3 years. The filing of an EEOC charge under the EPA does not extend the time frame for going to court.

Title VII also makes it illegal to discriminate based on sex in pay and benefits. Therefore, someone who has an Equal Pay Act claim may also have a claim under Title VII.

Title VII, the ADEA, and the Americans with Disabilities Act (covered in next section) prohibit compensation discrimination on the basis of race, color, religion, sex, national origin, age, or disability. Unlike the EPA, there is no requirement under Title VII, the ADEA, or the ADA that the jobs must be substantially equal.

At first glance, it may appear that all pharmacy technicians and all pharmacists must be respectively compensated the same amount for working the same hours at the same pharmacy. This, however, is not the case. If the employer can demonstrate that the pharmacists at Pharmacy XYZ, for example, differed in job performance, seniority, or an incentive system (e.g., generic utilization percentage), then pay differentials are allowed. As mentioned earlier, it is imperative these factors have empirical data to support these claims.

Case 4

TW, a licensed pharmacist, claims that Memorial Hospital violated the EPA by offering her a lower starting salary than it offered a male licensed pharmacist. Memorial Hospital proves that it offered a higher salary to the male because he had very favorable job references based on his productivity and successful track record in starting new clinical pharmacy services; he received other job offers at the higher salary; he relied on those job offers as a bargaining tool for negotiating the higher salary. Memorial Hospital began salary discussions with TW with the same opening offer as given to the male, and indicated it was "willing to go higher if necessary." But TW did not bargain as assertively as her male counterpart, and ended up with a lower starting salary. There is no evidence that Memorial Hospital treated TW any differently than the male in salary negotiations. Memorial Hospital has proved that the compensation disparity is based on a factor other than sex, and therefore no EPA violation is found.

The Americans with Disabilities Act

Title I of the Americans with Disabilities Act of 1990 (ADA) prohibits private employers, state and local governments, employment agencies and labor unions from discriminating against qualified individuals with disabilities in job application procedures, hiring, firing, advancement, compensation, job training, and other terms, conditions, and privileges of employment. The ADA covers employers with 15 or more employees, including state and local governments. It also applies to employment agencies and to labor organizations.

An individual with a disability is a person who

- Has a physical or mental impairment that substantially limits one or more major life activities;
- Has a record of such an impairment; or
- Is regarded as having such an impairment.

A qualified employee or applicant with a disability is an individual who, with or without reasonable accommodation, can perform the essential functions of the job in question.

Reasonable accommodation may include, but is not limited to

- Making existing facilities used by employees readily accessible to and usable by persons with disabilities
- Job restructuring, modifying work schedules, reassignment to a vacant position
- Acquiring or modifying equipment or devices, adjusting or modifying examinations, training materials, or policies, and providing qualified readers or interpreters

An employer is required to make a reasonable accommodation to the known disability of a qualified applicant or employee if it would not impose an "undue hardship" on the operation of the employer's business. Reasonable accommodations are adjustments or modifications provided by an employer to enable people with disabilities to enjoy equal employment opportunities. Accommodations vary depending upon the needs of the individual applicant or employee. Not all people with disabilities (or even all people with the same disability) will require the same accommodation.

For example:

- A deaf applicant may need a sign language interpreter during the job interview.
- An employee with diabetes may need regularly scheduled breaks during the workday to eat properly and monitor blood sugar and insulin levels.
- An employee with cancer may need leave to have radiation or chemotherapy treatments.

An employer does not have to provide a reasonable accommodation if it imposes an "undue hardship."

Undue hardship is defined as an action requiring significant difficulty or expense when considered in light of factors such as an employer's size, financial resources, and the nature and structure of its operation. An employer is not required to lower quality or production standards to make an accommodation; nor is an employer obligated to provide personal use items such as glasses or hearing aids.

An employer generally does not have to provide a reasonable accommodation unless an individual with a disability has asked for one. If an employer believes that a medical condition is causing a performance or conduct problem, it may ask the employee how to solve the problem and if the employee needs a reasonable accommodation. Once a reasonable accommodation is requested, the employer and the individual should discuss the individual's needs and identify the appropriate reasonable accommodation. Where more than one accommodation would work, the employer may choose the one that is less costly or that is easier to provide.

Title I of the ADA also covers:

- *Medical examinations and inquiries.* Employers may not ask job applicants about the existence, nature, or severity of a disability. Applicants may be asked about their ability to perform specific job functions. A job offer may be conditioned on the results of a medical examination, but only if the examination is required for all entering employees in similar jobs. Medical examinations of employees must be job related and consistent with the employer's business needs. Medical records are confidential. The basic rule is that with limited exceptions, employers must keep confidential any medical information they learn about an applicant or employee. Information can be confidential even if it contains no medical diagnosis or treatment course and even if it is not generated by a health care professional. For example, an employee's request for a reasonable accommodation would be considered medical information subject to the ADA's confidentiality requirements.
- *Drug and alcohol abuse.* Employees and applicants currently engaging in the illegal use of drugs are not covered by the ADA when an employer acts on the basis of such use. Tests for illegal drugs are not subject to the ADA's restrictions on medical examinations. Employers may hold illegal drug users and alcoholics to the same performance standards as other employees. The subject of drug testing will be covered in the next section.

Case 5

A qualified candidate for a pharmacist's position is required to have a medical exam after he has been extended a job offer. During the exam, he reveals that he has had diabetes for five years. He also tells the doctor that since he started using an insulin pump 2 years ago, his blood sugar levels have been under control. The candidate also mentions that in his 6 years as a pharmacist working for another pharmacy, he never had an incident related to his diabetes. Because there appears to be no reason why the candidate could not safely perform the duties of a pharmacist, it would be unlawful for the employer to withdraw the job offer.

One final note is worth mentioning here. Recently, the ADA was amended to make it easier for an individual seeking protection under the ADA to establish that he or she has a disability within the meaning of the Act. Specifically, the Act

- expands the definition of "major life activities" by including two nonexhaustive lists:
    - The first list includes many activities that the EEOC has recognized (e.g., walking) as well as activities that EEOC has not specifically recognized (e.g., reading, bending, and communicating)
    - The second list includes major bodily functions (e.g., "functions of the immune system, normal cell growth, digestive, bowel, bladder, neurological, brain, respiratory, circulatory, endocrine, and reproductive functions")
- states that mitigating measures other than "ordinary eyeglasses or contact lenses" shall not be considered in assessing whether an individual has a disability;
- clarifies that an impairment that is episodic or in remission is a disability if it would substantially limit a major life activity when active.

Table 14-1. Summary of Federal Employment Laws

	Summary	Type of Employer Covered by Act
Title VII of the Civil Rights Act of 1964	Prohibits discrimination in the conditions and privileges of employment based on an individual's race, color, sex, religion or national origin	An employer having 15 or more employees[a]
The Age Discrimination in Employment Act	Prohibits discrimination in the conditions of employment based on an individual's age (persons 40 years of age or older)	An employer having 20 or more employees[a]
The Equal Pay Act	Prohibits differentials in wages and benefits based on an employee's sex	Virtually all employers[a] (no minimum number of employees required)
The Americans with Disabilities Act	Prohibits discrimination in the conditions of employment based on an individual's physical or mental disability provided the individual is qualified for the position, or could be qualified through reasonable accommodation	An employer having 15 or more employees[a]

[a]There are exceptions to these rules so it is important for each employer to determine whether or not these federal laws cover the organization.

Before the recent amendments to the ADA, an employee with well-managed diabetes might not be considered as having a disability. Under the new law, all individuals with diabetes (whether controlled or not) or a similar chronic condition limiting a major life activity are covered. Table 14-1 provides a summary of the federal employment laws covered in this section.

DRUG TESTING IN THE WORKPLACE

There are a number of Constitutional concerns associated with drug testing in the workplace. The Fourth Amendment to the United States Constitution protects citizens against unreasonable searches and seizures. In providing a drug (blood) or urine sample, many individuals claim this is an intrusive search and seizure. Furthermore, plaintiffs bringing a lawsuit alleging their Fourth Amendment rights have been violated often assert their right of privacy. It is important to note that pharmacists, as health care professionals and members of a highly regulated industry, have a lessened expectation of (and therefore less right to) privacy. Here, the reasoning is that these workers have voluntarily subjected themselves to licensing and regulation, and this could include drug testing. As such, pharmacists can expect drug testing in the workplace, provided certain conditions exist.

Employers are allowed to conduct drug testing in the workplace. Failure to do so could place the employer at risk for subsequent litigation, especially if the employer was aware one of its employees had a drug/alcohol problem and did nothing to try and resolve the issue, possibly endangering patients. This being said, employers are still not allowed carte blanche discretion when it comes to drug testing its current and future employees.

The Drug-Free Workplace Act provides significant protection for employers by requiring holders of government contracts as well as federal grant recipients in excess of $100,000 to implement programs reasonably expected to reduce and eliminate employee drug use (Robinson et al., 2002). If a pharmacy receives reimbursement from the government (e.g., Medicare claims) in excess of $100,000, it is required to comply with this federal law. However, private sector employers may also (and should) initiate drug-testing programs provided the testing is applied uniformly to all job applicants and employees. Employers who "select" individuals for drug testing solely on the basis of race, color, sex, religion, national origin and/or the basis of a disability run a significant risk of losing a discrimination lawsuit. Random screening is allowed, provided all employees are eligible for the screenings and that the screenings do not result in only certain protected classes (groups protected in Title VII and ADA) undergoing testing.

There is a situation where random screening is not required. Drug testing may be implemented in circumstances where the employer has a reasonable basis for suspecting that an employee is under the influence of drugs during work hours and when an employer has a legitimate business interest in having the work performed by employees who are not impaired by drugs or alcohol use (*Kraslawsky v Upper Deck Co*).

Case 6

TC, the pharmacist who normally works the graveyard shift at the local hospital, slips on some ice at home, breaking his leg. As a result, a part-time relief pharmacist, BW, is called to come to the hospital late in the evening to cover TC's shift. When BW arrives, a pharmacy technician notices that his speech appears slightly impaired and believes she smells alcohol on his breath. She calls the Director of Pharmacy who requires that the pharmacist submit to a blood alcohol test. The alcohol test, as well as any resulting discipline for violation of a uniformly applied conduct rule, is permissible under the ADA.

Since the results of the actual drug test can ultimately result in tarnishing an employee's work record or perhaps even cause the employee's termination of employment, it is imperative to have accurate and valid test results. There are times when a false positive test may be reported. Before making any employment decision, it is crucial to verify the results. In fact, many states require more than one test be performed if a positive test result is reported (Gianutsos, 2011). For pharmacists, pharmacy technicians and pharmacy students who test positive, there are a variety of state pharmacy organizations that can provide valuable assistance and support in overcoming addiction.

FALSE IMPRISONMENT

False imprisonment is a claim brought by an individual who has, in essence, been held against his/her will. Essentially, false imprisonment or false arrest is detaining someone without a legal reason, using either force or a threat of force. In a chapter describing various workplace issues, why would a section be devoted to false imprisonment? The following case example will hopefully shed additional light as to the need for pharmacists to be aware of this potential legal pitfall.

Case 7

LG, one of the pharmacy's technicians, notices two men acting very suspicious around the prescription department, moving to the front of the store and back several times. On more than one occasion, LG asks the two men if they need help with anything. They respond "no" each time and appear to be scoping out the pharmacy. A few minutes later, one man begins asking LG several random questions. Out of the corner of his eye, LG notices the other man placing some batteries in his overcoat. LG cannot tell exactly how many packages he conceals but when he makes eye contact with him, he turns and heads for the front door. LG, a former high school all-State defensive lineman, takes off after the man and catches him before he exits the store. LG then grabs the man's overcoat, pulls out three packages of batteries and drags him to the back where the pharmacist in charge is waiting. They both begin to interrogate the man, telling him that if he tries to leave, the pharmacist will stop him using the baseball bat he is holding. Furthermore, LG is standing directly between the man and the front door, the only available exit from the store. Several minutes later, the police arrives and promptly arrests the man as his accomplice fled the scene. The man who was arrested later files a false imprisonment lawsuit against the pharmacist and the pharmacy technician.

ROBBERY, BURGLARY, AND THEFT

Pharmacies make an attractive target for robberies, burglaries, and theft, as pharmacies carry not only cash, but medications, some of which have the potential to be abused or use for self-manufacture of dangerous and addictive substances. Crimes against pharmacies have become very prevalent and problematic, particularly in some areas of the United States. As such, it is imperative pharmacists do everything they can to try and make the pharmacy a less appealing and more difficult target.

It is important to differentiate the terms robbery, burglary, and theft. The reason is that there is not a "one size fits all" approach to preventing and handling these crimes. However, pharmacy employees and employers who possess an awareness of the issues surrounding these crimes will be better equipped to resolve any difficulties that might arise. Rather than go through an extensive legal comparison of these crimes, suggested methods of dealing with these situations will be presented so that readers will gain practical tips to apply in the workplace (Pharmacists Mutual Insurance Company, 2011).

Robbery

Robbery is "the illegal taking of property from the person of another, or in the person's presence, by violence or intimidation." (*Black's Law Dictionary* 1996). Armed robbery involves the use of a gun or other weapon that can do bodily harm, such as a knife or club.

One key point to make initially is the health and safety of employees and patients is of utmost importance. So, it is imperative for managers and employees to comply with the individual's demands. Considering the fact that many robberies involve individuals who are impaired and/or "drug seeking," the first goal should focus on having the individual spend as little time as possible inside the pharmacy. An armed robbery is no time for an employer or employee to be a hero in resisting the individual's demands. Controlled substances, money, and merchandise can be replaced; individual lives cannot.

There is no way to guarantee a robbery will never take place in the pharmacy. However, the following tips may help prevent a robbery from occurring:

- Arrange stock shelves so that the most targeted drugs are not visible from the sales floor.
- Rearrange stock shelves periodically so that the most targeted drugs are not always in the same location.
- If feasible, place a short, "working" supply of the most targeted drugs in one location on the shelves, and keep the bulk of your supply of those drugs under lock and key or in another location on the shelves. A robber may accept that short supply as being all that is on hand.
- Pharmacy personnel should not discuss these inventory controls to even other store personnel that do not have a "need to know," and certainly not within earshot of patients.
- Install a surveillance system. Make the cameras or camera housings obvious. Even "dummy" cameras can be effective deterrents. Hide and make secure the recording devices.
- Install an alarm system connected to the local law enforcement center or to a central station alarm company. Include strategically placed "panic buttons."
- Place any controls or circuit panels for the alarm or surveillance systems away from areas that can be accessed by the public, such as restrooms or the corridor leading to a back exit.
- Place signs and placards such as "Protected by ABC Alarm Systems" conspicuously throughout the store and on exterior doors; these will normally be available from the alarm system vendor.
- Train the sales floor staff to be alert, observant and to offer assistance to patients regularly and often (Pharmacists Mutual Insurance Company, 2011)

Preventing a robbery from occurring is the first step but once a robbery occurs, it is important to stay

Table 14-2. What to Do during a Robbery

Remember, the objective is to get the robber out of the store as quickly as possible.

- Try to stay calm. Say to yourself – "stay calm".
- *Do exactly as you are told.* No more, no less.
- *Using caution, being careful is not cowardice.*
- Alert the robber to any event or action you know is going to happen that may startle or upset the robber. (e.g., someone is due to arrive soon).
- Be observant, make a conscious effort to get a description of the robber, *but* avoid making direct eye contact. (The perception is that eye contact promotes recognition.)
- Do not make any sudden or quick movements.
- When it is necessary to move or reach to comply with demands, tell the robber what you are going to do and why.
- Listen carefully. Not only in order to obey commands but perhaps to hear a name used or something else said that could be used in the investigation.
- *Do not resist!* Take a step back. Place your hands in front of you with palms held outward.
- Passively try to keep any note or written instructions the robber may have given you. If you can, turn this over to the police later.
- Activate "panic button" or "toe kick" alarms only when you do it secretly. Take no chances!
- Give the robber adequate time to leave. Avoid the urge to give chase! Note the direction of travel when he/she leaves.
- Try to get a description of any vehicle used in the getaway *if* you can do so without compromising your personal safety. Make, model, color, license number, distinguishing features (decals, dents, bumper stickers, hubcaps, etc.).

Source: Pharmacists Mutual Insurance Company, 2011.

calm and comply with the individual's requests. Refer to Table 14-2 for tips on what to do during a robbery.

Burglary

Burglary is "the offense of breaking and entering into a structure for the intent of committing a felony" (*Black's Law Dictionary* 1996). No great force is needed (pushing open a door or slipping through an open window is sufficient) if the entry is unauthorized. In the context of burglary of a pharmacy, force is almost always involved. Unlike robbery, burglary does not involve the threat or use of force against an individual. The most common example of a pharmacy burglary would be a pharmacy that is broken into during the middle of the night, resulting in the loss of medications, money and/or merchandise. Preventing a burglary is similar to preventing a robbery so those same tips are very applicable here.

Case 8

JD, a community pharmacy owner, is sound asleep at home when he gets a call on his cell phone. JD looks at the clock and notices it is 2 a.m. He notices on his caller identification that the call is from his security alarm company. Once he answers the call, JD is told the pharmacy's alarm system was triggered 5 minutes earlier. JD gets dressed and arrives at the pharmacy a few minutes later. JD, with ball bat in hand, begins to search the exterior of the pharmacy. He notices the back door was kicked in and that there appears to be

Table 14-3. What to Do upon Discovering a Burglary

- **Call the police**—even if the alarm has been triggered.
- **Lock the doors. Prevent anyone from entering!** Preserve the crime scene for the law enforcement investigators. Don't touch anything the burglar may have touched and block off any areas the burglar(s) was to protect evidence they may have left behind.
- Post signs at entries that the store opening will be delayed! If there has been damage to the property, call a contractor to **make repairs as soon as possible.**
- Protect property still on the premises from further damages or loss.
- When law enforcement arrives, greet them and assist in assessing whether or not the premises are secure. At this point, turn the matter over to the law enforcement officials. **Cooperate fully!**
- Refer any inquiries from outsiders (media, etc.) to the responding law enforcement agency.
- Do not discuss items or amounts taken with anyone other than law enforcement.
- Management—**call the alarm company** vendor to reset or repair the alarm system!
- Management—**call a third-party/independent source to assess** the effectiveness of your alarm system. What can and should be done to enhance the system?
- Management—call insurance provider to **open a claim file** and get instructions on the claims process.
- Management—fill out internal burglary report.

Source: Pharmacists Mutual Insurance Company, 2011.
Note: If controlled substances are discovered missing, it is imperative to also notify the DEA, the State Board of Pharmacy (depending on the state) and fill out a DEA Form 106.

some broken items in the pharmacy. JD makes a quick inspection and notices several prescription stock bottles are on the floor, indicating someone had been there earlier. Assume you are JD, what should you do? Would you have done anything differently? See Table 14-3 for more information.

Theft

Theft (larceny) is "the unlawful taking and carrying away of someone else's personal property with the intent to deprive the owner of it permanently" (*Black's Law Dictionary*, 1996). Though robbery and burglary are types of theft, each is categorized as a different criminal act. The two types of theft that are more commonly seen in the workplace will be addressed in these sections: Shoplifting and Employee Theft.

Shoplifting

Prevention also is key to preventing this type of theft. In fact, training pharmacy employees to detect shoplifters is very important. The following tips are important in trying to prevent shoplifting from occurring:

1. Watch for suspicious behavior(s) from customers:
   a. Is (are) the customer(s) wearing heavy bulky clothing even though the weather is good?
   b. Is the customer constantly looking behind, left or right, or above as if to see if anyone, or anything, is watching?
   c. Is a group of customers acting in a boisterous manner as if to call attention to themselves?
   d. Is a customer spending an inordinate amount of time looking at the same relatively high-priced merchandise?
   e. Is a customer seemingly resentful or uneasy when a sales associate asks if they can assist?

   Make mental and/or written notes, including descriptions, of any of the conditions noted earlier. Report any of the preceding conditions to store management. (Pharmacists Mutual Insurance Company, 2011)

As demonstrated in an earlier section on false arrest (imprisonment), there are potentially very serious legal ramifications for pharmacy personnel who either inappropriately detain a shoplifter (as seen in Case 7) or who falsely identify shoplifting suspects (unlike the example in Case 7). Though identification and subsequent prosecution are key methods to deter larceny, it is important to be very diligent before accusing a suspect. According to Pharmacists Mutual, there are six universally accepted steps managers and employees should follow when suspecting shoplifting is taking place. See Table 14-4 for more information.

Employee Theft

Employee theft can range from an employee simply eating a candy bar without paying for it to stealing hydrocodone tablets. As mentioned earlier, it is important to prosecute all types of theft in a timely and legally sound manner. Furthermore, it is critical for employers to convey to all employees the expectations of employment, expectations that include zero tolerance for theft. It may appear harsh, at first glance, to tell your employees this information. However, what may appear as "common sense" information to an employer (or even an employee) may not be viewed the same way

Table 14-4. What to Do if Shoplifting Is Taking Place

To prevent false arrest claims and establish probable cause for detaining a suspected shoplifter, there are **six universally accepted steps** a manager or employee should follow:

1. You must see the shoplifter approach your merchandise or enter your store without any merchandise in their hand(s). This prevents the scenario of falsely detaining a customer who carried an item to be returned or exchanged into your store.
2. You must see the customer select your merchandise. If you can say without doubt that you saw the customer pick up your merchandise before putting it into a pocket or otherwise concealing it, you again protect yourself from that false arrest claim as in #1.
3. You must see the shoplifter conceal, carry away, or convert the merchandise in question. Concealment can be in pockets, in shopping bags, in a child's stroller. It can even be accomplished in full view as in when tags are removed from articles of clothing. A good example of conversion is a shoplifter eating food before paying for it. In some, *but not all,* states, this step is enough to constitute shoplifting.
4. In most states, at this point, you must maintain continuous surveillance of the suspect. You must comply with this step in the strictest sense.
5. You must see the shoplifter fail to pay for the stolen merchandise. Sometimes the thief will walk directly out of the store, but sometimes they will pay for some items but not the concealed one. It is important to see that the concealed item is not retrieved and paid for. There are all sorts of pitfalls for the merchant in this step. Examples--the person concealing or converting a candy bar pays for it along with other items at checkout, the person pays for batteries or a newspaper at the cashier and then picks up the item between the cashier stand and the door on his/her way out. As a double check, ask the cashier if the specific item(s) has/have been paid for.
6. You must see the shoplifter leave the store. Your approach to the thief should be outside the store. This eliminates all arguments that the shoplifter intended to pay for the item(s).

Source: Pharmacists Mutual Insurance Company, 2011.
Note: These steps may vary from state to state so please make sure the pharmacy adheres to the particular laws of its state.

by a fellow employee. Thus, in order to protect itself, employers should have a clear company policy for employee theft. Often times, this information is contained in an employee handbook or manual.

The following are some examples of employee theft:

- Taking merchandise without paying for it.
- Forgery. Signing company checks or endorsing a customer's check for personal use.
- Pilfering office supplies and converting them to personal use outside the store.
- Embezzlement. Conversion of company funds for personal use. Can range from using petty cash for personal use to complicated purchasing/billing/payables.
- Short-changing customers or the register and pocketing the cash.
- Abusing the company's sick leave policies to obtain personal time off while not ill or injured.
- Abusing the company's time clock policies by having someone clock in or out for you.
- Overbilling expense accounts.
- Charging personal expenses on company credit cards. (Pharmacists Mutual Insurance Company, 2011)

Case 9

Dave's Drugs, a small retail pharmacy chain of five stores, operates a snack bar in all its pharmacies. As part of the snack bar, there is a soda fountain. Dave's Drugs has a policy whereby all employees receive a discount on food and drinks purchased at the snack bar. Dave's also has a policy where there are no free refills on fountain drinks. This policy applies to everyone, including employees. Every Wednesday afternoon, Dave hires a relief pharmacist to come work for him so that he can run errands or go fishing. The relief pharmacist comes after lunch, so he never eats lunch at the snack bar. However, the pharmacist loves diet soda. He never goes anywhere without his 64 ounce cup. CD, a pharmacy technician, often notices the pharmacist filling up his cup from home with a diet soda from the fountain. To the best of CD's knowledge, the pharmacist has never paid for a beverage. What should CD do? In a professional manner, CD should remind the pharmacist about the store's policy. This should be done in private so as to not draw any unnecessary attention to the situation. Hopefully, this has been merely an oversight on the part of the pharmacist.

There are numerous opportunities for employee theft. Though not mentioned in this section, fraud has become a major issue in health care. In fact, third-party providers and pharmacy benefit managers have increased the frequency of pharmacy audits. Thus, it is imperative for pharmacy managers and employees to conduct and operate a workplace free from dishonesty.

WORK SAFETY ISSUES

Robbery, burglary, and theft are among a number of issues affecting the safety of your employees; however, there are others, as well. The Occupational Safety and Health Act created the Occupational Safety and Health Administration (OSHA) and established the federal government's role in promulgating and enforcing safety and health standards for places of employment that engage in interstate commerce. It is the responsibility of every employer to provide a work environment that is free from recognized hazards. Employees have a right to have an inspection of the workplace performed, have dangerous or hazardous substances or situations identified, be properly informed of hazards, have accurate records kept regarding exposure to hazards, and have violations posted at the workplace (Occupational Safety and Health Administration, 2011). Failure to comply with rules and regulations can result in severe fines and other penalties from OSHA.

The National Institute for Occupational Safety and Health (NIOSH) conducts research on criteria for specific functions and occupations. NIOSH publishes numerous safety and health standards related to workplace hazards. There is an entire section of standards devoted to the safety of health care workers. Of particular interest are standards regarding blood-borne pathogens and chemical hazards. These standards require employers to develop exposure plans and implement specific control methods for individual positions, to develop postexposure follow-up plans, and to develop procedures for evaluating situations in which employees have been exposed (National Institute of Occupational Safety and Health, 2011). As with all other workplace issues, simply complying with relevant government regulations is a minimalist approach. Job hazard analysis and periodic safety awareness programs are essential for ensuring a safe workplace. It is essential that managers in large organizations interact regularly with safety staff and risk managers or consultants to ensure the well-being of their employees. Managers of smaller organizations must be familiar with the necessary rules and regulations to ensure compliance with the law and a safe, productive workforce.

INTERGENERATIONAL DYNAMICS AND THE WORKPLACE

In addition to knowledge of applicable laws and regulations governing human resources management policies and actions, the pharmacy manager also must be adept at applying knowledge in an ever-changing contemporary workplace. One issue with which the manager must be increasingly aware involves intergenerational dynamics and how differences in generations can either enhance or limit the workplace. Given the potential of having four different generational employees working at the same pharmacy, it is imperative to examine the strengths and weaknesses each generation brings to the workplace.

The Evolution of the Pharmacy Workplace

The profession of pharmacy has undergone tremendous change during the past century including many that involve technology.

This is relevant in that the majority of pharmacists will remember and even prefer practicing pharmacy in various ways, including even prior to the advent of computers. Today's pharmacy school graduates may find it almost impossible to comprehend working in the pharmacy without a computer. This difference, by itself, can create perspective differences in the pharmacy workplace. Differences, if not handled appropriately, can lead to unhealthy conflict.

The Four Generations in Today's Pharmacy Workplace

For the most part, generations are typically time periods of 15 to 20 years in duration. The specific starting and ending dates are not critical for purposes of this section. Rather, it is important to focus on the significant events and characteristics of each generation. Generational characteristics are a tool for helping individuals understand each other, whether in personal or professional relationships. As previously discussed, stereotyping is never appropriate in the workplace, whether the stereotype involves an individual's race or generation. Furthermore, there are many other influences (e.g., family, friends) that help shape an individual's attitudes and behaviors, influences that are beyond the discussion of this section.

The four generations representative of today's pharmacy workforce include

- The Silent Generation
- The Baby Boomers
- Generation X
- The Millennials.

For an overview of the four generations, see Table 14-5.

As demonstrated from Table 14-5, there are many, notable differences and with these differences, there is potential for conflict. It should be noted that not all conflict is treated the same. For instance, constructive conflict can be healthy to the growth of the individual and organization. It is important to have varying and differing points of view in the pharmacy. However, if a healthy resolution is not achieved, everyone suffers. So, what are some ways to effective resolve conflict? Before answering that question, consider the following case.

Case 10

AS, a 25-year-old recent pharmacy school graduate and licensed pharmacist begins work at Rogers County Hospital as a clinical pharmacist. AS is enthusiastic, as

Table 14-5. An Overview of the Four Generations in the Pharmacy Workplace

	The Silent Generation	The Baby Boomers	Generation X	The Millennials
Years	1925–1945	1946–1964	1965–1979	1980–2000
Events	Great Depression The New Deal World War II Korean War Labor Unions	Civil Rights Movement Assassinations (MLK, JFK, RFK) Walking on Moon Watergate	Challenger Tragedy Iran-Contra AIDS Video Games Rise of Computers	OKC Bombing 9/11 Persian Gulf War Columbine Enron, WorldCom Rise of Internet
Characteristics	Conservative Fiscally prudent Employer loyalty Conformity Respect authority Duty before pleasure	Free-spirited Questioning Working longer, Retiring later If unhappy in a relationship, exit it Organize life around work	Independent ("latch-key" children) Immediate, ongoing feedback Loyalty to work, Team and boss but not necessarily organization Value expertise Need accountability and flexibility Less hierarchy More fun	Most child-centered generation (told they are "special") Entitlement Self-confident Celebrate diversity Multitaskers Respect titles and positions Group/team players Technologically savvy Big concern for personal safety

she has numerous innovative ideas for improving the delivery and quality of pharmacy services at the hospital. In fact, AS completed two advanced pharmacy practice experiences at the hospital during her fourth year of pharmacy school, so she saw first hand how things could be improved. DR, the hospital pharmacy director, is 58 years old and has worked at the hospital for nearly 30 years, the past 15 years as director. When AS interviewed for her current position, she shared several ideas for the creation of a new clinical pharmacy service supported with the latest technology. Her ideas seemed to be well received, and given the fact she was offered the highly competitive position, AS had every reason to believe her ideas would be quickly implemented. Every couple of weeks, AS would stop by DR's office to share her ideas for improving the pharmacy. DR would always tell AS the same thing, "you need to be patient . . . Rome was not built in a day." After hearing this line for the tenth time, AS responded, "if you are not going to take my suggestions, I will go work for someone who cares about patients!" Needless to say, DR was not pleased with this comment. When AS arrived for work the next day, she noticed she had been switched to working the nightshift with little time for patient interaction. She stomped down to DR's office and demanded an explanation. DR told AS "she should be glad she has a job and that if she 'pays her dues,' there is a good chance she will eventually get to work the day shift again."

Resolving conflict in the workplace can be a daunting challenge. In fact, there are entire books devoted to the subject. There are many reasons why conflict exists but this section will only examine intergenerational dynamics and how generational differences can lead to conflict in the workplace. As noted in the preceding case example, conflict can exist when employers and employees do not see eye to eye about job expectations. This can be due, in part, to generational differences. In the case example, DR is a baby boomer and AS is a millennial. DR may approach the concept of "change" very differently than AS. Furthermore, AS suggesting the use of the newest technology may make DR uncomfortable, especially if he cannot see the need to replace the existing system. These are but a couple of the many generational differences that could be the source of conflict between AS and DR.

The following responses to multigenerational challenges could assist DR and Rogers County Hospital:

1. Accommodate generational differences
2. Create choices by allowing workplace to shape itself around the work being done
3. Operate from a sophisticated management style
4. Respect competence and initiative by assuming the best of your people
5. Nourish retention (Howell et al., 2005).

It is important to note that AS also has a responsibility in this example. AS needs to develop emotional intelligence skills. Emotional intelligence "means managing feelings so that they are expressed appropriately and effectively, enabling people to work together smoothly toward their common goals" (Goleman, 1998). In fact, emotional intelligence has been described as the single, biggest predictor of performance in the workplace (Bradberry and Greaves, 2009). AS needs to work on appropriately expressing her frustration to DR if she wishes to be successful at the hospital.

Given that conflict is inevitable in the pharmacy workplace, employers must develop timely and effective methods for resolving conflict. One of the biggest sources of intergenerational conflict involves differences (or perceived differences) in work ethic. For example, a Silent Generation pharmacy owner may have an expectation that all pharmacists should work 9 a.m. to 6 p.m. (Monday to Friday) with an hour lunch break, no exceptions. The millennial pharmacist, on the other hand, may view the workweek as being flexible so that if he is able to work 4, 10-hour shifts in the pharmacy and/or have the ability to work on developing new pharmacy services outside the physical pharmacy location (e.g., at home, coffee shop), that would be more appealing. Other sources of conflict could include, but not be limited to, communication styles and the expectations of what constitutes an appropriate work/life balance. This statement is not meant to imply that some generations are not interested in spending time with their families but rather, to demonstrate that for some generations, spending time with friends and family is a top priority, a factor that plays a major role in job selection.

When conflict does arise in the pharmacy workplace, the following steps are helpful in resolving the conflict:

1. Focusing on the issue
2. Emphasizing key points
3. Be specific about what you think or want
4. Acknowledge the other person's point of view
5. Avoid "hot button" language (e.g., "back in my day") (Gravett and Throckmorton, 2007).

It should be noted that resolving conflict may appear more complicated than simply following these five steps. And, the techniques that work for one employee may not work well for another. These steps, however, provide a solid foundation for resolving conflict. Furthermore, it is imperative for pharmacy managers to keep their eye on the "big picture" and not allow petty, personal differences to interfere in helping meet the pharmacy's mission and vision. There are many ways to improve the quality of services provided to patients. And, it is likely that no two employees would handle the situation the exact same way. That being said, each person's point of view must be heard. It is only then that the best solution can be reached. And though this section has examined generational conflict, these steps can be applied to other sources of conflict as well.

Though differences exist among the four generations, these differences are extremely valuable to the pharmacy and to the pharmacy's patients. Oftentimes, differences are viewed as negative and/or divisive to the organization's mission. However, if valued and developed, differences make the workplace more diverse with the potential to accomplish more than having employees who all think and act the same way. Thus, the challenge for any pharmacy manager is how to capitalize on each employee's strengths while motivating the employee to continually strive for improvement.

MANAGING A DIVERSE WORKFORCE

Intergenerational dynamics is critically important, yet only one component of an increasingly diverse workforce. As previously mentioned, managing diverse individuals requires creating a workplace environment of equality of opportunity and respect. In its simplest form, equal opportunity and managing a diverse workforce involve the basic ethical imperatives of a commitment to fairness and justice and respect for the basic dignity of all persons.

Ideally, managers will develop ongoing interventions to orient organizational culture to respect diversity and equality. Compliance with the various laws to ensure equal opportunity in the workplace is a necessary but not sufficient condition for managing diversity in organizations. Training programs that increase awareness of and respect for cultural pluralism and that educate people regarding practices that involve negative stereotyping and negative impact on minorities should be ongoing and institutionalized. Counseling and intervention are necessary when stereotyping and potential discriminatory practices take place. For example, training sessions can identify "flag" words that can be demeaning to certain groups, explain why these words may be offensive, and remove the words from discourse within the organization. Simple choice of language such as addressing grown women as "girls" or telling ethnic jokes that ridicule certain groups can create hostile environments. An organizational culture that has a high degree of awareness of cultural pluralism and provides clear guidelines with managerial monitoring will be able to fully use the diverse talents of all its employees and also avoid the stress and negative publicity of possible regulatory and legal action.

There are a number of benefits to having a diverse workforce, such as a larger talent pool, greater knowledge of broader and diverse markets, and better organizational agility. The ability to recruit and retain a diverse workforce allows organizations to draw on varying perspectives, thus escaping the tunnel vision that often accompanies operating under only one set of cultural assumptions. Second, organizations that are more diverse have a greater probability of addressing the unique needs, preferences, and values of a diverse customer base. Finally, when diverse views and minority viewpoints are present, problem solving and creativity are enhanced by overcoming the problems of "groupthink" in organizations (Carnevale and Stone, 1995).

OTHER ISSUES PROMOTING PRODUCTIVITY AND QUALITY OF WORKLIFE

Career Planning

In addition to providing a stable, hospitable, and safe working environment, managers can help promote quality of work life and minimizing conflict by assisting employees with their careers, preferably within the organizations in which they are currently employed. Career progression can be a source of fulfillment or frustration as employees pursue job pathways. Employee retention and productivity can be enhanced with proper career planning by managers. Companies have an interest in identifying, mentoring, developing, and retaining their employees who hold promise for significant contributions to the organization. However, each individual needs to view his or her career as an important source of both financial and personal rewards and take responsibility for the optimal development of that career.

There are a number of models for organizing and understanding career development and progression. Career development goals vary with general stages of adult development beginning with early-adult transition to the late-adult era. The developmental tasks of establishing an identity, stable value systems, and relationships are correlated with career progression (Levinson, 1978).

Transition into adulthood usually is characterized by advanced education and exploration of occupation through course work and practical experiences. Early adulthood involves experimenting with different job settings and deciding on specific lifestyles and roles, including stabilizing relationships and possibly starting a family. The adult continues through various transitional phases, refocusing efforts and emphases on career, family, and lifestyle.

A career-anchor approach can facilitate the organization of talents, motives, and values into "anchors" that allow the individual to pursue a career pathway that is consistent with both his or her aspirations and capabilities. These career anchors are technical/functional, managerial, security oriented, autonomy oriented, and creativity oriented (Schein, 1975). Persons with a technical/functional anchor tend to enjoy the detail of the work itself and avoid responsibilities that take them away from the day-to-day performance of specific tasks that produce the product or service. In contrast, persons with a management anchor tend to like analyzing and problem solving, seek influence through interpersonal communication, and are emotionally and intellectually able to take responsibility and exercise power. Individuals, who value security in work, seek jobs and organizations that offer long-term work stability and retirement benefits with clear and predictable career pathways and will sacrifice other opportunities to have security. Autonomy seekers are most concerned with freedom in decision making and a minimum of constraints, whereas individuals who value creativity seek innovation and invention as the primary motivation in work.

These anchors can be used as guides in managing career pathways in pharmacy. For example, a pharmacist who prefers the technical and functional anchor may seek employment focused on the dispensing and compounding aspects of pharmacy practice in initial career choice and move into nuclear pharmacy, where more technical aspects of pharmacy can be realized. By contrast, pharmacists who seek management careers would develop competency with advanced management degrees while seeking increased responsibility for management across a variety of settings before settling in on a specific organization, such as a pharmaceutical company or managed-care organization to gain specific skills in an industry of interest. Security-oriented individuals may look to government positions such as the U.S. Public Health Service or the military, which offer predicable and stable career progression.

That being said, while much of career planning rests with the individual, managers play a key role. Employees need to know that there is a potential future for them with the organization. They also need to know that their current skills/talents are valued, and what additional training might be required to stay with, prosper, and even move up in an organization. If management can create an environment for employees to achieve fulfillment, then productivity is likely to increase and interpersonal conflict is likely to decrease. Moreover, it should be noted that some turnover and change is inevitable. The best managers are those looking to identify and groom persons to fill higher positions in the organization, even if those positions are not currently vacant.

Case 11

LG, a recent pharmacy school graduate, has demonstrated tremendous leadership skills during his 3 years working at The Prescription Shoppe. LG's immediate pharmacy supervisor, BH, senses real potential in LG. Though BH would like to mentor LG, BH is swamped and can barely fulfill his administrative responsibilities, as his pharmacy is one of the busiest in the city. From time to time, LG approaches BH and asks him about opportunities for advancement and whether pursing an MBA degree would be beneficial. BH repeatedly replies, "sure . . . what's your hurry?" A few months later, LG asks BH if they can talk. As they sit down to chat, LG shares with BH that he has accepted a job with a rival pharmacy across town, a job that carries with it a promotion to pharmacy manager, plus the opportunity to enroll in a part-time MBA program. BH is stunned and cannot believe he is losing his best staff pharmacist. BH is surprised that LG would leave The Prescription Shoppe after nearly 4 good years of employment.

Employee Assistance

Even in well-managed organizations, individual employees will face any number of professional or personal problems that can impact them, others in the workplace, and the organization, as a whole. One resource many organizations have for such issues are confidential employee assistance programs (EAPs) that refer employees for counseling and that train managers in early identification and referral (Smith, 1992). EAPs can be established by contract with independent behavioral health providers. Through a confidential intake, professionals and supervisors can identify employees with problems, and costs can be stabilized by early identification and referral. In addition, employees who are valuable to a company often can benefit from brief interventions and return to work more productive and committed to the organization.

Referral to a company-sponsored EAP program normally is voluntary; however, managers can suggest a referral based on a history of poor work performance or other work-related problems. Managers can use work performance as a vehicle for discussion of employee problems that are affecting the workplace. EAP professionals are licensed and regard the information on assessment and treatment as confidential and subject to Health Insurance Portability and Accountability Act (HIPAA) regulations. Employees can sign releases to share limited information with employers, especially if there is a clear relationship between the personal problem and work performance.

Drug and alcohol problems are personal problems that can affect work performance significantly. Many states have mandatory reporting requirements for pharmacists who have substance abuse problems so that interventions and referrals for treatment and follow-up may be made. Pharmacists and managers have special responsibilities and obligations not to "enable" another's substance abuse through lack of intervention because of the potential harm posed to the public health from an impaired pharmacist. Pharmacists can be at special risk for substance abuse problems because they have universal access to drugs and may have a false sense of invulnerability owing to their extensive education regarding the mechanisms and effects of drugs. In addition, the tendency to self-medicate among some pharmacists can cause serious difficulty when applied to addictive medications.

The general procedures for managing impaired pharmacists are summarized as follows:

1. Mandatory state board reporting requirements for pharmacists who have substance abuse problems but are not receiving treatment
2. Intervention by an organization usually working with the state board
3. Professional assessment
4. Treatment recommendations
5. After-care counseling and monitoring usually involving Alcoholics Anonymous or Narcotics Anonymous, as well as random drug testing for a defined period
6. Reinstatement to practice contingent on successful completion of treatment

For the program to be effective, all employees should be educated about the issue of substance abuse, with special attention paid to early identification, intervention, and responsibilities of management in ensuring intervention and referral for treatment.

■ REVISITING THE SCENARIO

Michael Davis has a variety of issues facing him as the new pharmacy manager. They include (1) a claim by an employee of sexual harassment, (2) possible theft by one of his pharmacy technicians, and (3) potentially disruptive employee behavior during working hours in the pharmacy. As evidenced from the scenario at the beginning of this chapter, Michael did not handle these issues well, possibly leading to costly litigation against him and the pharmacy. This section will examine each of these issues separately, suggesting other more appropriate courses of action.

The first issue of concern was the way Michael handled his pharmacy technician's claim of sexual harassment. Any manager should treat a claim of sexual harassment very seriously, immediately investigating the claim to determine its validity. Here, Michael simply dismissed the claim because Mark was his friend and that Michael could not believe Mark would say such things. Properly resolving a claim of sexual harassment is not whether or not a manager could imagine such an event (or events) taking place, but rather, the results of an unbiased and thorough investigation. In this example, the technician's claim could be false but Michael must investigate before making that determination.

The second issue, a very serious and unfortunately, very common issue, is employee theft of hydrocodone tablets. Once again, Michael did not handle the situation well. Though he did attempt to resolve the issue quickly, he should not have locked the accused technician in the break room. As such, he set himself up for a possible false arrest (imprisonment) lawsuit. Here, the technician was found guilty of stealing the hydrocodone but this does not excuse Michael's inappropriate handling of the situation. It is a good idea to have a witness (not the other technician, though) present for interviewing a suspected employee but locking a suspect in a break room opens the employer up to potentially costly litigation.

The final issue is one involving workplace behavior and appears to be intergenerational in nature. Here, a millennial employee is texting and Tweeting at work. From the facts of the scenario, it is not clear whether Sooner Drug and Apothecary has a workplace policy prohibiting this type of behavior. If so, it is imperative for Michael to inform the technician that her behavior is unacceptable and should cease. If there is no policy prohibiting texting, then Michael must determine whether to allow the behavior or not. As noted from the scenario, another technician has adopted the behavior, potentially decreasing the pharmacy's quality of patient care services. And, the technician's behavior has created conflict with Michael's baby boomer employee. If Michael avoids the conflict, it will only become worse. Therefore, Michael must address it in a timely manner.

CONCLUSION

It is important to develop a workplace free from discrimination, where employees from all generations are allowed to contribute to the organization's mission and vision and where diverse opinions are valued. Furthermore, it is important to encourage discussion while resolving conflict in a timely and appropriate manner. Employers who are able to address and resolve potential issues before they occur will maintain a tremendous advantage in avoiding legal pitfalls. Though no workplace is guaranteed to be "litigation free," applying these principles will go a long way in helping protect the pharmacist and pharmacy from damaging lawsuits while striving to make patients' needs their top priority.

QUESTIONS FOR FURTHER DISCUSSION

1. Must a pharmacy manager hire an individual from a "protected class" if there are other individuals from nonprotected classes that apply for a pharmacist position?
2. What are the similarities and differences between the two main types of sexual harassment? How should an employer handle each type?
3. What are some examples of "reasonable accommodations" for a small chain pharmacy? For a large hospital pharmacy? Are they the same? Why or why not?
4. Would you recommend pharmacy employers conduct a drug screen test on its job applicants? Its employees? Give reasons why you would or would not recommend this.

5. What is the best way to "detain" a suspected shoplifter? Suspected theft by an employee?
6. Should a pharmacist chase down a shoplifter? An armed robber? Why or why not?
7. What do intergenerational dynamics have to do with working in a pharmacy?
8. How does emotional intelligence impact performance?

REFERENCES

Black's Law Dictionary. 1996. St Paul, MN: West Publishing Company.

Bradberry T, Greaves J. 2009. *Emotional Intelligence 2.0.* San Diego, CA: TalentSmart.

Carnevale AP, Stone SC. 1995. *The American Mosaic.* New York: McGraw-Hill.

Fink JL. 2009. Is a contractual covenant not to compete enforceable? *Pharm Times* 2009.

Gianutsos G. 2011. *Pharmacy Law: Workplace Testing.* Continuing Education Seminar. Temple University. Available at http://secure.pharmacytimes.com/lessons/html/workplace_testing.htm; accessed on July 4, 2011.

Goleman D. 1998. *Working with Emotional Intelligence.* New York, NY: Bantam Dell.

Gravett L, Throckmorton R. 2007. *Bridging the Generation Gap.* Franklin Lakes, NJ: Career Press.

Howell LP, Servis G, Bonham A. 2005. Multigenerational challenges in academic medicine: UCDavis's response. *Acad Med* 80(6):527–32.

Kraslawsky v Upper Deck Co., 65 Cal.Rptr.2d 297 (Cal. App. 1997).

Levison DJ. 1978. *The Seasons of a Man's Life.* New York: Knopf.

National Institute of Occupational Safety and Health. 2003. Available at www.cdc.gov/niosh; accessed on July 5, 2011.

Occupational Safety and Health Administration. 2011. Available at www.osha.gov; accessed on July 5, 2011.

Payne v Western & Atlantic Railroad Co., 81 Tenn. 507, 518 (1884).

Pharmacists Mutual Insurance Companies. 2011. Model Policy and Procedure Templates (Burglary, Robbery, Shoplifting and Employee Dishonesty Policies). Available at http://www.phmic.com/phmc/services/RM/rmlcs/Pages/ModelPolicyProceduresTemplates.aspx; accessed on July 4, 2011.

Robinson RK, Franklin GM, Wayland R. 2002. *The Regulatory Environment of Human Resource Management.* Fort Worth, TX: Harcourt College Publishers.

Schein EH. 1975. *Career Dynamics.* Reading, MA: Addison-Wesley.

Smith J. 1992. EAPs evolve into health plan gatekeeper. *Employee Benefit Plan Rev* 46:18.

The United States Equal Employment Opportunity Commission. Available at www.eeoc.gov; accessed on July 4, 2011.

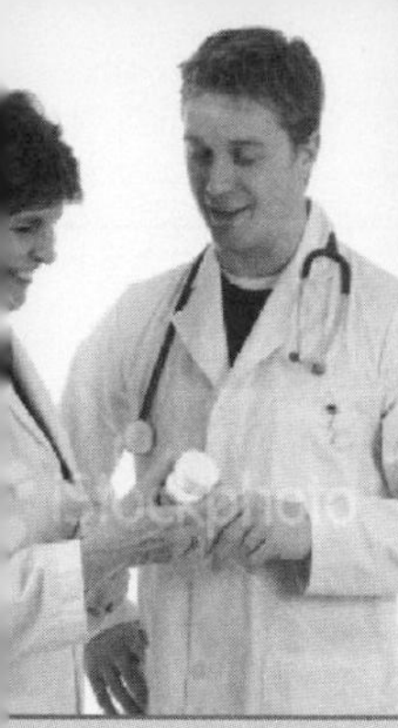

15

PERFORMANCE APPRAISAL SYSTEMS

Shane P. Desselle

About the Author: Dr. Desselle is Dean and professor at the California Northstate University, College of Pharmacy. He received a B.S. degree in pharmacy and a Ph.D. in pharmacy administration from the University of Louisiana at Monroe. He has practice experience in both community and hospital pharmacy settings. He teaches courses in American health care systems, health care economics, social and behavioral aspects of pharmacy practice, and research methods. His research interests include performance appraisal systems in pharmacy, quality of work life among pharmacy technicians, direct-to-consumer prescription drug advertising, Web-based pharmacy services, and pharmacy benefit design. Dr. Desselle won the Duquesne University School of Pharmacy's President's Award for Teaching and President's Award for Scholarship and was recognized for his contributions to pharmacy by being named a Fellow of the American Pharmacists Association in 2006.

■ LEARNING OBJECTIVES

After completing this chapter, readers will be able to

1. Discuss the rationale behind the implementation of a systematic performance appraisal system.
2. Discuss the difficulties in implementing a performance appraisal system within a pharmacy organization.
3. Identify various types of performance appraisal processes, and evaluate the strengths and weaknesses of each type.
4. Discuss issues of reliability and validity within the context of evaluating a performance appraisal system.
5. Describe how to conduct a performance appraisal interview and how to handle disagreements that may arise during or subsequent to the interview.
6. Discuss the linkage of performance appraisal results with the proper allocation of organizational rewards.

7. Discuss the importance of formal and informal feedback and describe best practices for providing informal feedback and praise to employees to maximize their work satisfaction, commitment, and productivity.

SCENARIO

"What?" asked Marcus Green, emphatically. "You've got to be kidding! That's just not fair. I've been here for $3^1/_2$ years, and I've received only one raise—and that may as well have been nothing. Why did she get another raise? She's probably making more money than I am, and she's only been here for a little more than 1 year." With a look of consternation, Marcus lowers his voice and asks his colleagues at the lunch table, "Where did you hear this from, anyway? Ah, never mind. I don't want to discuss it any further," Marcus chimed as he finished scarfing up the remainder of his lunch and left the table in a huff.

Marcus's fellow pharmacy technicians at Community Hospital were equally upset that Susan Klecko allegedly had received another raise, but they were not sure that they had done the right thing by telling Marcus about it. Marcus, having worked at Community Hospital for nearly 4 years, generally was regarded as the "best tech" in the pharmacy. He filled orders twice as fast as anyone else, always showed up on time, and came to work on short notice when others called in sick, even though he was perhaps a bit more prone to making a dispensing error and was well known for being a "hothead." Susan Bostik, on the other hand, seemed to be the "boss's pet." Indeed, she was regarded as a very pleasant person who got along with everyone, especially the director, Cynthia Broedl, with whom she shared an appreciation for poetry and theater.

Marcus continued to stew over his plight throughout the afternoon. He didn't really *feel* like looking for another job, making phone calls, filling out forms, and going on interviews. But he also did not understand why other technicians seemed to be rewarded at Community Hospital pharmacy more frequently with raises than he did. He wondered just what about his performance was not up to par. He did not recall being formally evaluated in over 2 years, when he and Ms. Broedl had a few words on his suggestion that he often had to "pick up the slack" for pharmacists "not doing their jobs." Meanwhile, Terrence Whitfield, the assistant director, appeared in Cynthia's office to discuss his relief that the apparent exodus of staff occurring during the previous few months appeared to be over.

CHAPTER QUESTIONS

1. What is a performance appraisal system? What does formal appraisal have to do with employee motivation, productivity, and turnover?
2. What is the difference between absolute, relative, and goal-oriented systems for appraising employee performance?
3. What kinds of appraisals typically are performed in pharmacy environments? How might these appraisal systems be improved?
4. How are formal performance appraisal mechanisms implemented? What are some strategies to maximize the effectiveness of the appraisal interview?
5. How should performance appraisals be linked to the allocation of organizational rewards? What are some innovative reward strategies that can be used to optimize employee satisfaction and productivity?
6. What is the difference between formal and informal performance feedback? Why is frequent and regular informal feedback so important? What are some methods to provide informal feedback?

WHAT ARE PERFORMANCE APPRAISALS?

Virtually every practitioner and many students reading this text have either participated in or know of a discussion similar to the one taking place at the beginning of the scenario. Pharmacists and pharmacy support staff typically are hardworking, honest people who want the best for their patients and their organizations. However, they are made of the same fabric as everyone else and desire equitable treatment and fair compensation for their work.

The scenario begs the question of precisely what qualities signify a "good" pharmacy technician. Are promptness, dedication, and hard work the attributes most revered by administrators, or are collegiality and amicability? What is more important—the quantity or the quality of the work performed? The scenario raises some additional concerns. Do some employees get preferential treatment because they have things in common with those in administrative positions? How do other employees in the pharmacy feel about the way they are being treated and compensated by their employer? Why have so many employees left the pharmacy department at Community Hospital of late? Do the director and assistant director know how Marcus feels and that he is contemplating quitting as well? What do the pharmacists at Community Hospital think about the situation?

As humans, we are concerned primarily for the interests of ourselves, our families, and our closest loved ones. Each person's concern for self, manifesting within the cornucopia of personalities that exist among us, practically ensures occasional discontent among employees. And discontent, coupled with the consistency of life changes (e.g., birth of a new family member, sickness, death, or new opportunities) guarantees some level of turnover within all organizations that is beyond the control of management. The lack of a well-planned, well-executed, and equitable performance appraisal system can be a major source of discontent among employees of any pharmacy operation. However, putting such a system in place is well within management's control.

Strictly defined, a *performance appraisal* is a formal assessment of how well employees are performing their jobs, but it is much more than that. It is a way of formally communicating the organization's mission and goals, a foundation on which to establish informal channels of communication, a method on which to base organizational rewards, and a tool to improve the performance of each and every employee within the organization. Unfortunately, performance appraisal is a frequently neglected function. Managers have cited performance appraisals (also known as *performance reviews*) as their least favorite activity (Campbell and Barron, 1982). Constructing, implementing, and monitoring a performance appraisal system presents many formidable challenges.

THE RATIONALE FOR A FORMAL PERFORMANCE APPRAISAL SYSTEM

As Chapters 11 and 12 pointed out, human resources are among a pharmacy's most valuable assets. Employee wages are the greatest operating or overhead expense for almost all pharmacies (see Chapter 17). Employees, however, should not be viewed simply as an expense, but as an essential asset for organizational success. The ramifications of executing a good performance appraisal system extend to most human resources decisions. In fact, evidence suggests that the quality of poor performance appraisal systems results in employees' lower job satisfaction, lower organizational commitment, and higher quit intentions (Brown et al., 2010). The scenario depicting Marcus Greene's plight is not at all uncommon. Employees need to feel that their contributions to the organization are valued and appreciated, and if they feel otherwise, lower job satisfaction is only the beginning of a possible cascade of negative consequences. Table 15-1 summarizes some important points about the need for performance appraisals.

Legal

Performance appraisals are necessary to document employees' progress toward achieving goals and heeding the advice of administrators on how to improve performance. Documentation is necessary to demonstrate fairness in promotion and termination (discharge) practices. Title VII of the Civil Service Reform Act ushered in heightened concern regarding appraisal

Table 15-1. Rationale for Implementing Effective Performance Appraisals

Legal
- Title VII of the Civil Service Reform Act
- Age Discrimination in Employment Act

Communicative
- Ensures understanding of performance expectations by managers and staff
- Provides a formal means for employees to voice concerns and make suggestions for system improvement
- Indicates management's commitment to open dialogue and fairness

Productivity of labor
- Provides direction to employees on how to improve
- Establishes an environment conducive to self-motivation
- Assists employees with career planning
- Promotes satisfaction and elicits commitment of employees
- Mitigates turnover

Equity in rewards
- Provides a means for accurate and equitable distribution of organizational rewards
- Provides recognition for past service
- Helps to establish support for terminating "problem" or underachieving employees

Other managerial functions
- Supplies evidence to review organizational and systems problems
- Provides data on recruitment and selection procedures
- Identifies deficiencies in orientation and training programs

Financial position
- Assists in reducing operating costs
- Avoids costly litigation
- Reduces replacements costs

issues (Martin and Bartol, 1991). Title VII is a federal statute that applies to and sets forth constitutionally protected classes as they pertain to employment, including religion, national origin, race or color, and gender (Blackwell et al., 1996). An employee can initiate a Title VII claim based on disparate treatment, disparate impact, or retaliation (see Chapter 14). As such, the claimant would have to demonstrate that a hiring, promotion, or discharge had a significant adverse impact on a member of a protected class. Should a pharmacy be accused of any one of these, there are a limited number of defenses, most notably the bona fide occupational qualification (BFOQ). With the BFOQ, the pharmacy must demonstrate that the employee claimant could not perform essential job duties safely and effectively. Having implemented a formal performance appraisal system, the pharmacy possesses critical documentation that an employee's performance was lacking and that the employee was provided adequate warning that failure to improve would result in certain consequences (termination/discharge, failure to obtain a promotion or pay increase, etc.).

Communicative

An employee typically will come to know what is expected of him during the performance appraisal process. These expectations may or may not have been communicated adequately during the hiring, training, or informal feedback processes. The performance appraisal process affords managers the opportunity to inform employees of the importance of their roles and responsibilities to the organization and how their performance will be measured, thus mitigating the possibility of *role stress* among employees (Eulburg et al., 1988). Role stress typically is viewed as having two components: role ambiguity and role conflict. *Role ambiguity* exists when an employee is unsure about his responsibilities. *Role conflict* is the simultaneous occurrence of two or more role expectations (Kong et al., 1992). The prevalence of role conflict and role ambiguity have been widely studied in pharmacy (Desselle and Tipton, 2001; Kong, 1995; Smith et al., 1985). It is not difficult to envision their occurrence. In hospital pharmacies, technicians often experience stress over who maintains responsibility for cleaning the laminar flow hood, delivering medications to the floors, and filling stat orders. In community pharmacies, conflicting roles for pharmacists may involve demands from administrators to increase prescription volume while spending more time performing clinical functions like patient education and medication therapy management.

If it becomes apparent to an administrator that productivity among their staff is suffering, information can be gathered during the performance appraisal process that can lead to constructive changes in nonpersonnel aspects of the business (e.g., workflow design). In any event, the dialogue emanating from the appraisal process provides data *for* administrators, as well as data to employees *from* administrators.

Performance appraisals have been increasingly used to communicate and inculcate an organization's values to employees. An appraisal system can be designed to reflect a company's mission by incorporating performance criteria deemed important to the organization (Park and Huber, 2007). These criteria may be written as specific competencies among employees needed to transform an organization's entire approach to its business (Kalb et al., 2006). Many pharmacy organizations stress a need to improve the medication use process and increase medication safety as part of their culture. As such, they are incorporating these values into their performance appraisal systems (Schneider, 1999). Community Hospital had not reviewed Marcus' performance with him in over 2 years, so if the organization had decided to put more weight on activities related to medication safety in employees' evaluations, this had not yet been communicated, at least not to Marcus Greene.

Productivity of Labor

A principal reason for conducting appraisals is to enhance performance. During the appraisal process, employees should be provided feedback on their strengths and areas of performance that requirement improvement. Suggestions for improvement may be in reference to general areas of competence or to very specific roles or functions. This feedback, coupled with other components of the appraisal (equitable distribution in rewards and career planning), provides specific goals that an employee may strive to attain in the future. It is said that managers cannot motivate employees, but rather can establish an environment conducive to self-motivation (McConnell, 2010, p. 207). Thus, a supervisor cannot force or trick employees into being good performers. A well-planned performance appraisal can make employees aware of what they have to do to be judged as good performers and leaves it up to them to strive and achieve these goals.

The feedback and open dialogue present in performance appraisals are valuable to the career planning process. Career planning helps employees formulate personal goals and evaluate strategies for integrating their goals with the goals of the organization. This is important because very few people work in the same jobs their entire career, often changing jobs within one organization and/or changing organizations. When these changes are poorly conceived, both the individual and the organization suffer (Griffin, 1996, p. 403). Career planning informs employees that they are valued enough by their organizations to be considered in their long-range plans. Career planning increasingly has been suggested for use among pharmacy technicians (Desselle and Holmes, 2007) and pharmacists (Gaither et al., 2007). Chapter 14 provides additional detail on career planning.

Employees are more likely to be satisfied with their jobs if they have directed feedback and specific goals for which to aim. It has been shown that satisfaction with the performance appraisal process itself is closely linked to overall job satisfaction (Blau, 1999), which precedes commitment to the employer (Gaither and Mason, 1992a), and averts costly turnover (Gaither and Mason, 1992b). A high level of turnover often leaves an organization temporarily short staffed, which creates even more stress for current employees. It also results in administrators having to invest inordinate amounts of time in recruiting, selecting, and training new employees rather than engaging in activities more productive to the organization. If Community Hospital were to lose Marcus Greene, it would take a hit in productivity that might not be so easily remedied. Marcus may have his drawbacks and limitations, as all employees do. However, the performance appraisal process can assist employees in working through those limitations, even leveraging them into strengths with the proper feedback and job structuring. This could create a "win-win" for Community Hospital and for Marcus.

Equity in Rewards

One of the key factors in providing an environment conducive to self-motivation is to distribute rewards equitably. The allocation of rewards (e.g., promotions and salary increases) cannot be arbitrary or even be perceived as arbitrary by staff, as might be the case with Marcus Green in the scenario. Evidence suggests that employees in service organizations, such as pharmacies, who have equitable performance appraisal and reward systems treat customers more fairly (Bowen et al., 1999).

Many performance appraisal systems allow the manager to either rate employees on a given set of attributes, or provide them feedback on how they might compare to benchmarks or work standards created by the department or organization. The quantification of performance into a score or ranking creates a foundation from which to base rewards. The culmination of a series of performance appraisals taken over several years can be used as support for recognizing top performers with extraordinary rewards (such as a gift, plaque, or reimbursement for travel to a conference) that exceed annual merit increases.

OTHER HUMAN RESOURCE MANAGEMENT (HRM) FUNCTIONS

The performance appraisal process inherently generates a considerable amount of data for administrators. Poor performance of a group or an entire unit of personnel may be indicative of poor direction from an immediate supervisor or a lack of adequate resources for employees to perform their jobs. If not stemming from an organizational or systems problem, deficiencies among a significant number of employees could indicate that management has been ineffective in recruiting and selecting employees or perhaps in orientation and training, particularly if the underachieving employees are new hires (see Chapter 12).

Financial Position

Enhanced productivity translates into efficiency and the reduction of labor costs. For example, Community Pharmacy A may be able to dispense 200 prescriptions per day on average with 10 fewer employee hours worked per week than Community Pharmacy B without any excess stress or burden. The 10 fewer hours is less costly to Pharmacy A and thus enhances profitability. In addition, having well-constructed performance appraisals can save an organization a significant amount of money by avoiding damage awards from litigation brought on by employees in the types of wrongful termination suits described previously. Finally, if the performance appraisal system is effective in holding turnover to a minimum, this saves the organization money that would have been dedicated to recruiting and training new employees.

TYPES OF PERFORMANCE APPRAISALS

A variety of performance appraisal systems are in use. These systems are summarized in Table 15-2. Performance appraisal methods typically are categorized into three broad types: absolute, relative, and outcome oriented (Segal, 1992).

Absolute Systems

Absolute systems require the rater to indicate whether or not the employee is meeting a set of predetermined criteria for performance. This usually involves the use of a scale or index. Absolute systems are the most commonly employed of the three types of performance appraisal methods (Byars and Rue, 2000, p. 277). The main advantage that absolute systems have over other types of appraisal methods is the feedback that is derived inherently from the process. Allowing employees to see how they are evaluated among criteria deemed important by their organization enables them to learn

Table 15-2. Performance Appraisals and Their Advantages and Disadvantages

System	Brief Description	Advantages	Disadvantages
Absolute			
Essay	Rater prepares a written statement describing the employee's strengths and weaknesses	May provide rich data	Differences across raters, lack of objectivity
Critical incident	Rater maintains a record of incidents indicative of both positive and negative behaviors of the employee	Derived from documented data	Burdensome and subject to interpretation
Checklist	Rater answers with a yes or a no aseries of questions about the employee's behavior	Easy to complete, indicative of specific behaviors	Less precision
Graphic rating	Rater indicates various employee traits and behaviors on a scale	Often based on trait measures	Leniency, central tendency, use of traits
Behaviorally anchored rating scales	Rater employs highly descriptive scales to indicate employee's tendency to demonstrate desirable behaviors	Quantitative, conducive to supplying feedback	Central tendency, burdensome
360° feedback	Employees rate themselves, and comparisons are made with ratings by various stakeholders	Multiple points of view, facilitates reflection	Very time consuming, subject to role conflict
Forced choice	Rater ranks a set of statements describing the employee's performance	Mitigates bias	Irksome to raters, feedback is challenging
Relative			
Alternation ranking	Rater selects most and least valued employee from remaining pools of employees	Eliminates leniency and central tendency	Limited feedback, perceptions of bias
Paired comparisons	Each employee is compared with every other employee one at a time on each criterion	May appear to be less subjective than alternation ranking	Limited feedback
Forced distribution	Rater categorizes employees into one of three groups according to how well they meet expectations tendency	Eliminates leniency and central tendency	Limited feedback, skewing
Outcome-Oriented			
Management by objectives	Rater establishes goals for the employee to achieve during the next period, and employee is evaluated on his/her success	Highly participatory and incentive driven	Employees evaluated by different standards
Work standards approach	Rater sets a standard or an expected level of output and compares each employee's performance to the standard	Evaluation is more standardized	Standards may be viewed as unfair

about their strengths and areas that may require improvement.

There are two types of absolute systems that do *not* employ any sort of scaling procedure. One is the *essay method,* in which the rater responds to a series of brief open-ended questions concerning the employee's performance, such as, "What are the employee's strengths?" and "How does this employee get along with coworkers?" By allowing the rater to include what she thinks is most valuable, the data can be richer than those obtained from the use of scales. However, it is more difficult to translate these data into numeric quantities for the purpose of allocating rewards and communicating organizational goals. In addition, differences among raters in their detail and writing abilities can subject the process to charges of bias. A second method, the *critical-incident appraisal,* may mitigate some concerns over subjectivity because it requires that the rater keep a written record of significant incidents (both positive and negative) as they occur. These incidents provide a basis for the evaluation. The data are still subject to interpretation, however, and maintaining such detailed records can be cumbersome. Employees who do a "steady" job may complain that this type of evaluation fails to capture their strongest suit.

The *checklist* is one of three types of summated rating scale methods. In a summated rating scale, a rater indicates the employee's level of performance along a list of criteria. The ratings assigned to each criterion are then summed to provide a total score for the employee. With the checklist, the rater simply answers a set of yes/no questions concerning whether or not the employee exhibited certain characteristics. The employee receives a point when the rater assigns an affirmative response to a desirable characteristic or a negative response to an undesirable characteristic. While indicative of specific behaviors and easy for the rater to complete, the checklist ignores levels of performance along each performance criterion. Thus, it is less precise and does not generate as much feedback as other summated scale methods.

The *graphic rating* appraisal, on the other hand, has the rater assess the employee's level of performance on a scale, usually from one to five or one to seven. Some graphic rating scales may include written descriptions along with the numerical ranges. An example of such is given in Table 15-3.

Although it has the advantage of lending greater precision and feedback, the graphic rating appraisal, like many absolute systems, is prone to rater biases. One is *central tendency,* which occurs when the rater appraises everyone at or near the median of the scale or rates everyone similarly for fear of causing angst or feelings of injustice among employees. With *leniency,* the rater not only judges each employee similarly but also rates each on the high end of the performance scale. Leniency is common in many appraisal systems. Raters might inflate their ratings more for low performers than for others because they believe this will help achieve harmony and boost morale. The primary reasons identified were under the auspices of achieving harmony and boosting motivation. However, this can backfire. If better performers believe that they are not being recognized accordingly for their efforts, then the result can be more disharmony. This might be a component of what is going on with the case of Marcus Greene.

Some graphic rating appraisals may consist mostly of traits as criteria rather than particular performance indicants. While traits may manifest into certain behaviors, they are innately part of every person's character. To this end, managers should avoid evaluating an employee on characteristics such as appearance, knowledge, or friendliness without specifying how this translates into actual performance. The *halo effect* occurs when a rater allows a single prominent characteristic of an employee to influence her judgment on each separate item in the appraisal. For example, a pharmacy technician who is very friendly may be rated more highly on performance than someone not as outwardly amicable, despite the latter outperforming the technician on other aspects of the job. While the halo effect can be problematic for any type of appraisal system, it can be especially problematic when traits are used in a graphic rating scale. In the scenario, Susan Bostik might not being favored overtly; however, she could be the beneficiary of some halo effect originating from her pleasant demeanor.

Table 15-3. Sample Items on a Graphic Rating Scale Evaluation Form

Quantity of work—the amount of work an employee does in a workday				
Does not meet minimum requirements	Does just enough to get by	Volume of work is satisfactory	Very industrious, does more than is required	Has a superior work production record
Dependability—the ability to do required jobs well with a minimum of supervision				
Requires close supervision; is unreliable	Sometimes requires prompting	Usually completes necessary tasks with reasonable promptness	Requires little supervision; is reliable	Requires absolute minimum of supervision
Job knowledge—information an employee sbould have on work duties for satisfactory job performance				
Is poorly informed about work duties	Lacks knowledge of some phases of job	Is moderately informed; can answer most questions about the job	Understands all phases of job	Has complete mastery of all phases of job
Attendance—faithfulness in coming to work daily and conforming to work hours				
Is often absent without good excuse or frequently reports for work late, or both	Is lax in attendance, or reporting for work on time, or both	Is usually present and on time	Is very prompt, regular in attendance	Is always regular and prompt; volunteers for overtime when needed
Accuracy—the correctness of work duties performed				
Makes frequent errors	Careless, often makes errors	Usually accurate, makes only average number of mistakes	Requires little supervision; is exact and precise most of the time	Requires absolute minimum of supervision; is almost always accurate

Source: Byars and Rue, 2000, p. 283; reprinted with permission.

Table 15-4. Example of a Behaviorally Anchored Rating Scale for "Providing Customer Service" in a Community Pharmacy

Scale	Values	Anchors
1	Poor	Does not interact well with customers, who frequently complain about the employee; employee instigates conflict with customers
2	Below Average	Courtesy is inconsistent; is not responsive to customer needs
3	Average	Is polite and friendly with customers but lacks creativity in meeting customer needs
4	Above average	Is polite, friendly, and professional in dealing with customers; is adept at meeting customer needs and strives to improve in this area
5	Excellent	Has managed to develop a bond with customers, who anticipate coming to the pharmacy and interacting with this employee; is innovative in creating ways to satisfy customers

The *behavior-anchored rating scale* (BARS) method of performance appraisal is designed more specifically to assess behaviors necessary for successful performance. Most BARS methods use the term *job dimension* to mean those broad categories of duties and responsibilities that make up a job, requiring development of unique scales for each dimension. Managers often develop BARS in collaboration with employees well versed in the responsibilities that comprise the dimensions of job performance. An example of how a BARS may look for a community pharmacy technician in dealing with customers is illustrated in Table 15-4. The BARS system lends itself to providing quality feedback, particularly if supplemented with qualitative comments on how to improve. A drawback is the time and effort required to develop an effective BARS appraisal.

More common to larger organizations than retail or institutional pharmacies, *360-degree feedback,* also known as *multirater assessment,* involves the use of a summated rating scale or brief closed-ended questions requiring the employee to rate himself and compare these ratings with those afforded to him by supervisors, peers, customers, suppliers, and/or colleagues on a similar instrument. This mitigates an employee's concern that one particular rater may be biased against him, and engenders a degree of reflection by any employee who receives feedback from so many points of view. Moreover, supervisors are relieved from being the exclusive "heavies" in evaluating performance, as they learn from other evaluators in the process (Anonymous, 2001). Aside from the time it takes to gather and collate all of the data used in 360-degree feedback, another disadvantage from the employee's point of view is the role conflict that may arise owing to differing demands placed by various stakeholders in the process. This problem is further exacerbated when there is a lack of inter-rater reliability among evaluators, as is often the case in many organizations (Valle and Bozeman, 2002).

Another type of absolute method that seeks to mitigate bias or perceptions of bias is *forced-choice rating.* Forced-choice rating is used more often in larger organizations with formal human resources departments. With this method, the rater is presented with a set of statements that describe potentially how the employee might be performing on the job and ranks each statement on how well it describes that employee's behavior. The weights and scoring, known and performed by the human resources department, are unknown to the rater. An example is given in Table 15-5.

Relative Systems

Rather than requiring the rater to evaluate employees on a predetermined set of characteristics or standards, relative systems require the manager to make

Table 15-5. Sample Set of Statements in a Forced-Choice Rating Scale

Instructions: Rank the following statements according to how they describe the manner in which this employee carries out duties and responsibilities. Rank 1 should be given to the most descriptive and rank 5 to the least descriptive. No ties are allowed.

Rank	Description
____	Is easy to get acquainted with
____	Places great emphasis on people
____	Refuses to accept criticism
____	Thinks generally in terms of money
____	Makes decisions quickly

Source: Byars and Rue, 2000; reprinted with permission.

comparisons among employees. Relative systems have an advantage over absolute systems in that central tendency and leniency effects are minimized. The likelihood of the halo effect occurring also is reduced. The fact that employees are pitted against one another, so to speak, makes it easier to base organizational rewards on merit. Moreover, social comparison theory implies that it may be more efficacious for raters to compare an employee to other employees rather than use absolute rating standards, and some research suggests that certain types of relative systems showed greater validity and precision over absolute systems (Goffin et al., 2009). It has been shown that relative measures induce raters to consider social comparison information and behavioral information when making their responses more than absolute measures, which might be problematic, but yet shows higher correlations of accuracy with relevant criteria (Olson et al., 2007).

Relative systems have a significant drawback in that they are not conducive to generating substantive feedback to employees. If, for example, an employee is rated below two-thirds of her colleagues on overall performance, what does this mean to the employee? What behaviors are being demonstrated that resulted in this ranking? What behaviors could be demonstrated that would result in improved performance and a higher ranking during the next evaluation? This adds to the manager's challenge of establishing an environment for employee self-motivation. An employee may be performing well but still ranked below a majority of colleagues, and vice versa. These are among the reasons that types of performance evaluations are undergoing scrutiny and various mutations. While relative systems inform employees where they stand in comparison to the whole of their colleagues in a department or in an organization, it should be kept in mind that generally the rankings of each employee are not made public. Rather, each employee is made aware of their performance in comparison to a selected group, as a whole, on certain indicators or benchmarks.

Three types of relative performance appraisal systems are used. One is called *alternation ranking,* a method in which the rater chooses the most and least valuable persons from a list of employees with similar jobs. Both names are crossed off, and then the procedure is repeated until every employee on the list has been ranked. With its ability to eliminate central tendency and leniency and with its ease of implementation, alternation ranking may appear appealing. However, aside from its failure to generate feedback, the halo effect could come into play. Moreover, employees may be concerned with the potential for bias and inaccuracy by the evaluator, especially when criteria for performance have not been delineated clearly.

The method of *paired comparisons* has the rater comparing each employee against every other employee, one by one, on either specific aspects of performance or on overall performance. During each comparison, the rater places a checkmark by the name of the employee who was considered to have performed better. The employee with the most checkmarks is considered to be the best performer. While more precise and perhaps seemingly less ambiguous to employees, paired comparisons still may fail to generate substantive feedback and is more burdensome to implement than other relative systems.

The *forced distribution* method requires the rater to compare the performance of employees and place a certain percentage of them into various groupings. It assumes that the performance level in a group of employees will be distributed according to a bell-shaped or normal distribution curve. While lending itself well to the allocation of organizational rewards, levels of actual performance may be skewed by forcing their distribution into a bell-shaped curve, ignoring the possibility that perhaps most or all employees are performing well or performing poorly. Forced distribution, as well as other relative systems, may fail to demonstrate system deficiencies that can be improved by management.

As previously mentioned, absolute systems have strengths, but also limitations. The lack of feedback was discussed, but there are additional drawbacks. While the exact rankings of employees are not (at least should not be) publicly aired, some employees might still come under the impression that they are being pitted against one another. Some "healthy competition" might be good for an organization. However, if managed poorly, this could result in downwardly spiraling morale and even behaviors indicative of poor cooperation and citizenship among employees supposedly working toward the same goal.

Outcome-Oriented Systems

Where absolute and relative systems focus on behaviors, outcome-oriented systems are concerned with evaluating end results. These systems involve setting quantifiable goals for the succeeding period, to be followed with a performance review at its conclusion. Outcome-oriented systems can be used to generate feedback, but equity issues arise because rewards are allocated according to how well goals are met, and employees with similar jobs may receive substantially different sets of goals and expectations for performance. Because these systems are used more frequently for persons in autonomous positions (e.g., attorneys, college professors, clinical pharmacists), flexibility has to be built in to allow for contingencies that resulted in an employee changing his goals or not being able to meet them. On the other hand, an employee can always come up with excuses as to why certain goals were not met.

The most commonly employed type of outcome-oriented system is *management by objectives* (MBO), also known as *results management, performance management,* and *work planning and review.* The MBO process typically consists of six steps (Byars and Rue, 2000, p. 277):

1. Establishing clear and precisely defined statements of objectives for the work to be done by an employee.
2. Developing an action plan indicating how these objectives will be accomplished.
3. Allowing the employee to implement the action plan.
4. Measuring objective achievement.
5. Taking corrective action when necessary.
6. Establishing new objectives for the future.

The establishment of objectives is critical to the success of MBO. The objectives must be challenging but attainable. They should be expressed in terms that are objective and measurable and should be written in clear, concise, unambiguous language. Table 15-6 presents examples of how some poorly stated objectives for pharmacists might be better stated. It is important that the objectives be derived through collaboration and consent of the employee. In this respect, the objectives and action plan can serve as a basis for regular discussions between the manager and the employee.

A concern of MBO is the potential incongruence among the goals and objectives of employees with similar jobs, especially when it comes to allocating organizational rewards. One study confirmed that when using such an approach, persons with higher accountability come under more intense scrutiny during performance evaluations (Roch and McNall, 2007). Other research shows the importance of feedback, and attribution of the feedback to factors within the employee's control to improve self-efficacy, which in turn can assist her with creating more accurate, yet cautiously ambitious goals (Tolli and Schmidt, 2008).

While shortcomings of an MBO system can be overcome to some degree by basing the rewards on the outcomes themselves, use of another method, the *work standards approach,* can further mitigate the problem. The work standards approach is a form of goal setting

Table 15-6. Examples of How to Improve Work Objectives in Pharmacy

Poor:	To maximize the number of prescriptions dispensed
Better:	To increase the average daily prescription volume by 10 percent at the end of the year
Poor:	To make as few dispensing errors as possible
Better:	To commit no dispensing errors that result in an untoward event during the next 6 months
Poor:	To get all medications up to the floors more quickly
Better:	To get unit dose medications to the floors within 30 minutes after the order arrives to the pharmacy
Poor:	To make sure that nurses are happy with the clinical services you provide
Better:	To achieve a mean score of at least 80 out of 100 on a survey measuring nurses' satisfaction with the clinical services provided

in which each employee is compared with some sort of standard or an expected level of output. In other words, the objectives are the same or similar for each employee in the group. Without as much input from each employee, however, the standards established may be viewed as unfair, and employees may not have as much incentive to strive to attain them.

SPECIAL CONSIDERATIONS FOR APPRAISAL SYSTEMS IN PHARMACY

A community pharmacy is typically a for-profit organization that must be concerned with its financial position to remain solvent over the long term. Community pharmacies also must conduct their business in an ethical manner. Moreover, it can hardly be argued that pharmacists and support personnel must practice altruism, putting patients ahead of personal motives (Wolfgang, 1989). Like any organization, a pharmacy will be more likely to achieve its goals when its employees derive gratification from performing their jobs (Etzioni, 1964). The pharmacy profession has experienced numerous environmental changes that affect the work experiences of pharmacy personnel. These include higher prescription volumes, greater complexity in third-party reimbursement, increasing professional emphasis on patient care, and implementation of automated dispensing technologies (Alvarez, 1997). These trends behoove pharmacy managers to take special care in developing effective performance appraisal systems. One first has to determine whether a similar performance appraisal should exist among technicians and pharmacists working within the same organization. Certain similarities in the jobs of pharmacists and support personnel exist. In addition, there are certain values (e.g., dependability, dedication, altruism) that the organization may want to assess in all its employees regardless of their position or status. There are, however, certain aspects of pharmacists' jobs and those of support personnel that may call for alternative systems or at least different components of a similar system. Most notable of these is the level of autonomy and responsibility they share.

Considerations for Support Personnel

A pharmacy organization's effectiveness often is linked to the productivity of its technicians and other support personnel. Pharmacy technicians, for example, are now beginning to take responsibility for more functions, including drug preparation, order entry, and managing technology (Collins, 1999). The profession has recognized the need for thorough job descriptions, training manuals, equitable pay, and productivity-monitoring systems among pharmacy support personnel, (Desselle, 2005) yet the literature offers little in the way of performance appraisal systems devised specifically for pharmacy technicians. One study found that relatively few community pharmacies engage in routine performance monitoring of support personnel (Desselle et al., 2002). In the same study, a method predicated on a study of the "scope of pharmacy practice" (Muenzen et al., 1999) was suggested. It involved the use of 20 practice functions each with a different weight (for importance) combined with a BARS-type scale to produce a highly quantitative measure. The 20 practice functions and weights are provided in Table 15-7. A similar method can be used to derive a performance appraisal system for technicians working in alternative settings.

Considerations for Pharmacists

Evaluating pharmacist performance may be more challenging than evaluating technician performance because of pharmacists' greater levels of autonomy and responsibility. This may be further compounded by the presence of disparate roles various pharmacists may play within an organization. It may be fruitful to gather information from customers, including patients and other health care professionals, when evaluating pharmacists for the services they provide. This may be accomplished through informal feedback, surveys, or even through critical incidents appraisal previously described. While it is beyond the scope of this chapter to describe them in detail, a few types of performance appraisal systems have been suggested for pharmacists, particularly those whose responsibilities are more clinical in nature (Schumock et al., 1990; Segal, 1992).

Other Types of Bias to Consider

The discussion of different types of appraisal systems described various biases that could be introduced into the process, such as leniency, central tendency, and the tendency to expect more from potential high performers and set goals that are too high. As previously mentioned, a focus on traits and/or aspects of personality not affiliated with specific work behaviors can introduce bias and even make your organization more subject to litigation. As described in Chapter 14, there are laws and moral codes that govern organizations and protect certain populations. In addition to discrepancies that could arise due to race/ethnicity and gender, intergenerational dynamics also come into play. While each individual is unique, certain values emanating from major events occurring during development years permeate each generation, and thus become the source of conflict, or rater bias. The rater must be culturally competent and trained in various facets of conducting performance evaluations. The chapter scenario does not provide the ages of those employed; however, there could very well be intergenerational or other dynamics at play when considering the different values placed by employees on different aspects, or components of performance. Unless the organization communicates what it values most, there will be misconceptions and battle lines drawn between employees with competing values.

THE FUTURE OF PERFORMANCE APPRAISAL SYSTEMS

While the debate between the advantages and disadvantages of various systems will likely continue for some time, there are some trends worth noting. While not necessarily employing a full 360-degree feedback mechanism, more organizations are seeking a wider array of input to make more accurate assessments of employee performance and provide more ample feedback. Technology will be useful in advancing various performance appraisal systems. Employees reported being more informed and sensed greater interpersonal justice in the organization when an electronic performance monitoring system was used (McNall and Roch, 2009). Overall, employees have expressed favorability toward systems with high differentiation of rewards, frequent feedback, and large comparison groups (Blume et al., 2009). Using an absolute system, anonymity is all but lost as the comparison groups grow smaller. When rater teams are used, and they are required to reach a consensus, greater accuracy is manifest in part from rater motivations being negated (Roch, 2007).

Another issue widely agreed upon is the need for specific and additional training for raters, or those evaluating and motivating the performance of others. One study demonstrated that even in the presence of less behaviorally oriented or more vague job dimensions performance measures, raters can overcome bias and

Table 15-7. Community Pharmacy Technicians' Practice Functions and Corresponding Weights

1.	Maintaining inventory II (receiving goods) 3.79
2.	Maintaining inventory II (receiving goods) 2.25
3.	Maintaining inventory III (other, such as stock appearance and inventory analysis) 3.36
4.	Collecting productivity information 1.63
5.	Participating in quality assurance and quality improvement activities 4.00
6.	Solving problems (of prescribers, customers, and colleagues) 3.80
7.	Billing and accounting 2.00
8.	Customer service activities 4.88
9.	Training other staff members 2.70
10.	Maintaining a positive image 3.93
11.	Being a team player 4.00
12.	Exhibiting a positive attitude 4.75
13.	Maintaining cleanliness 3.00
14.	Receiving and interviewing patients 4.88
15.	Communicating with prescribers 3.72
16.	Assessing prescription orders for completeness and accuracy 3.00
17.	Processing prescription orders 4.00
18.	Filling prescription orders 4.25
19.	Compounding prescription orders 1.00
20.	Appropriately concluding a patient's visit 4.73

Source: American Pharmacists Association. 2002;42(8):774; reprinted with permission.

subjectivity with the proper training (Roch et al., 2009). There is additional evidence to suggest that at least some personality-related cues and traits can be evaluated more precisely with the proper training (Powell and Goffin, 2009). Also important in this process is training rates, as organizations continue to identify means of enhancing both rater and rate reactions to the appraisal system (MacDonald and Sulsky, 2009). Organizations are continually seeking ways to improve the process, and one method currently being evaluated and implemented in some organizations is a reflection component by the employee shortly after the formal review process (Anseel et al., 2009). A more direct form of training for raters is frame-of-reference training, which separates what is considered good organizational citizenship behaviors by employees from more specific behaviors to be evaluated. Frame-of-reference training also provides effectiveness levels of alternative behaviors in comparison to those most desired and thus increases accuracy in evaluations (Uggerslev and Sulsky, 2008).

It should be noted that the trends in performance appraisal systems are finally catching up with other aspects of management. For example, many are advocating a quality improvement (QI) model of performance appraisal system rather than a quality assessment (QA) system (Edwards, 2009). In the traditional QA model, performance was judged to be effective or ineffective, and either remediation or punishment is offered to poor performers. In the QI model, the performance appraisal system is viewed as one tool to shift the curve of performance for an entire department or organization upward. This concept is commensurate with the aforementioned goals in frame-of-reference training and with the ideals of continuous quality improvement in operations management described in Chapter 8.

THE PERFORMANCE APPRAISAL INTERVIEW

Regardless of the type of system selected, the written appraisal should be accompanied by a formal interview of the employee. It is during the interview that the results of the written appraisal are discussed. The success of the performance appraisal hinges significantly on the interview. If the supervisor is mindful of taking a few precautionary steps and follows some helpful guidelines, most appraisal interviews will come off without a hitch.

Preparing the Employee for the Interview

An appointment should be made with the employee well in advance, at least 3 to 4 weeks. The employee should be provided with a copy of the position description and corresponding performance standards, a copy of the evaluation form used in the appraisal process, a copy of the report of the previous formal review, departmental/organizational objectives for the current and subsequent year, and instructions on how to prepare for the meeting. The employee may be instructed to prepare comments on how well objectives set during the last review were met and to prepare a list of new objectives. The employee also may be asked to discuss what she considers her most valuable contribution to the organization to be since the last review, barriers to her achieving current goals, and what the organization or supervisor can do to facilitate her progress (McConnell, 2010, p. 229). In some organizations, employees are asked to complete a self-evaluation on an instrument similar to the one used by the employer. This may help identify gaps in perceptions of effectiveness in certain areas and reinforce strengths and limitations in others.

Planning for the Interview

The supervisor should enter the interview well informed of prior appraisals and be intimately familiar with the responsibilities of the employee's job. The supervisor also should have appropriate documentation and evidence to support claims of the employee's performance, particularly in areas of deficiency but also in areas of strength. To prepare for the interview, the supervisor should have answered the following questions (Byars and Rue, 2000, p. 286):

1. What results should the interview achieve?
2. What good contributions is the employee making?
3. Is the employee working up to his potential?
4. Is the employee clear about the organization's performance expectations?

5. What strengths does the employee have that can be built on or improved?
6. Is there any additional training available that can help the employee improve?

Conducting the Interview

The interview should be conducted in the following sequence: (1) review and update the position description and performance standards, (2) discuss the performance ratings assigned to the employee using the prescribed appraisal form, (3) highlight strengths and accomplishments since the previous appraisal, (4) discuss objectives that were not reached since the previous review, and (5) discuss future performance and assist with career planning.

Supervisors should establish a comfortable, professional atmosphere and maintain a positive tone when conducting the interview. They should be careful not to stereotype or prejudge employees. There may be occasions in which the rater simply does not like the person whom she is evaluating but must be careful to remain focused on the relevant behaviors and performance. Nonetheless, circumstances will arise in which the supervisor has to address performance deficiencies with an employee. Some suggestions for addressing these situations are as follows (McConnell, 2010, p. 233):

- Limit criticism to one or two major problems. Do not search for significant problem areas when none exist.
- Reserve critical remarks until after some of the positives have been accentuated.
- Maintain open dialogue with the employee. Offer the employee a chance for self-criticism. Allow the employee to offer reasons why performance was below standard. Allow the employee to suggest ways and an appropriate time frame to expect significant improvement.
- Avoid the use of terms that potentially could be misconstrued, such as *attitude, work ethic, professionalism,* and *weakness.*

Remain firm but supportive. Use assertiveness skills by reinforcing points of agreement, handling disagreements diplomatically, and avoiding defensiveness.

The interview should be concluded with an expression of confidence that the employee will be able to meet the new objectives. The supervisor also should thank the employee for her time spent in the interview and for her contributions to the organization.

ENSURING VALID RESULTS FROM THE PERFORMANCE APPRAISAL SYSTEM

A pharmacy manager must carefully consider the advantages and drawbacks of each type of appraisal system. Aside from those specifically designed for pharmacy organizations described in this chapter, the prevailing consensus among employers is that summated rating scales, particularly derivations of BARS methods, are the best systems to employ. Regardless of the type of system selected, managers must be mindful of ensuring that the system is reliable and valid and is helping the organization to achieve its objectives. *Reliability* is another word for consistency, inferring that the system produces similar results in multiple iterations. For example, given a certain employee's level of performance, any rater should view the performance similarly. If a system is unreliable, then it cannot be valid. *Validity* implies that the system is measuring what it purports to measure.

Implementing the System

A primary consideration when implementing a system is how frequently to conduct the formal appraisal. Rating periods usually are annual, either on the employee's anniversary of hire date or during a rating period in which all employees are evaluated, the latter of which is easier to implement (Mohrman et al., 1989). Evidence suggests, however, that better results are obtained from more frequent evaluations, such as semiannually or quarterly (Martin and Bartol, 1998). Everyone in the organization should be well informed about the role each person plays in the appraisal process and how the appraisal results are used (Latham and Wexley, 1994).

Monitoring the System

The effectiveness of the appraisal system itself should be monitored. Certain indicators can be helpful, including the quality of performance standards, effective use of appraisal results, tracking of the raters, and elimination of adverse impact. *Quality of performance standards* refers to the standards being specific, challenging, realistic, dynamic, understandable, and consistent with organizational goals. *Use of performance appraisal results* refers to how well these results are tied with rewards and recognition and to what extent the appraisal process has contributed to improved performance among all employees. Tracking the raters consists of reviewing the ratings awarded by individual raters and giving them feedback concerning the quality of their ratings, which may be overly stringent, lenient, or biased in some way in comparison with other raters. *Adverse impact* refers to a performance appraisal system whose use results in significantly lower ratings for members of any protected group described previously.

PERFORMANCE AND ORGANIZATIONAL REWARDS

Organizational rewards consist of both intrinsic rewards (those internal to the individual and derived from involvement in the job, such as achievement, feelings of accomplishment, informal recognition, satisfaction, and status) and extrinsic rewards (those controlled and distributed by the organization, such as formal recognition, incentive pay, fringe benefits, and promotions). Proper allocation of both is critical for varied reasons. Recent evidence rejects a popular view that satisfaction leads to performance (Byars and Rue, 2000, p. 303). It does suggest, however, that (1) rewards based on current performance enhance subsequent performance and (2) job dissatisfaction leads to turnover, absenteeism, tardiness, accidents, grievances, and strikes. Research also supports the notion that while extrinsic rewards do not in and of themselves cause satisfaction, perceived deficiencies or inequities can result in dissatisfaction among employees (Barnett and Kimberlin, 1988). A study of pharmacists suggested that perceptions of inadequate pay were predictive of their intentions to withdraw from a current job (Gaither and Mason, 1992b).

In addressing employees' base and merit pay, managers must consider internal, external, and individual equity. Internal equity concerns what an employee is being paid for doing a job compared with what other employees in the same organization are being paid to do their jobs. External equity concerns what employees in an organization are being paid compared with employees in other organizations performing similar jobs. Individual equity addresses the rewarding of individual contributions and is related closely to linking pay with performance. Internal and external equity are factors considered more in determining base wage and fringe benefits, or those rewards are based merely on employment and seniority with an organization. Pharmacy managers must ensure that pharmacist and support staff salaries and benefits (e.g., vacation, paid holidays, health insurance, child care, and pension plans) are competitive with those offered in similar pharmacy settings and even other types of pharmacy settings in the region.

Managers also must address individual equity and allocate certain rewards (pay increases, promotions, and formal recognition) in a manner that corresponds with the right types of behaviors. Such behaviors include but are not limited to working extra hours when required, volunteering for unenviable tasks or assignments, substituting for others willingly, and pleasing customers. More specifically, rewarding behaviors listed and evaluated in the performance appraisal system eliminates ambiguity about what constitutes good performance. Other suggestions for allocating rewards are as follows (Byars and Rue, 2000. pp. 360–361):

- *Consider the presence of performance constraints.* The employee's performance should not be hampered by things beyond his control.
- *Provide a clear distinction between cost-of-living, seniority, and merit pay increases.*
- *Enlist trust among employees.* Similarly, employees should not be misled into thinking that their rewards were based on merit, only to find out later

that the increases were across the board. This could result in distrust and dissatisfaction.

- *Make merit pay substantial.* While operating within the organization's budget, merit pay has to be worthwhile. Employees will not appreciate being evaluated very highly and praised only to see very small pay increases as a result.
- *Be flexible in scheduling rewards.* It is easier to establish a credible pay-for-performance plan if all employees do not receive pay adjustments on the same date.
- *Effectively communicate merit and total pay policy to employees.* In addition, do not prohibit employees from discussing pay because this may be a violation of the National Labor Relations Act.

There are detractors to using performance appraisals as a means to allocate rewards. It has been suggested that appraisals used in this way create "winners" and "losers," ultimately, a zero-sum game for an organization, which should not use systems to make miniscule distinctions in pay adjustments (Kennedy and Dresser, 2001). Monetary rewards are said to work best when completely unanticipated by the employee, rather than based upon the appraisal feedback. Moreover, while managers' ability to reward with pay is limited, there are no such constraints on other forms of recognition.

MOTIVATION AND OTHER REWARDS NOT TIED TO BASE PAY

Chapters 11, 12, and 16 discuss motivation of employees through leadership and support. Support by the supervisor goes a long way toward keeping employees satisfied. In fact, supervisor and organizational support has proved to be an effective deterrent to pharmacists' uncertainty about their future in an organization (Desselle and Tipton, 2001) and a buffer against the stress that accompanies work (Kong and Wertheimer, 1994; Lahoz and Mason, 1991). Pharmacy managers should also keep this in mind when dealing with support personnel. Managers may believe that support personnel do not value intrinsic rewards, but this is certainly not true. Managers should be cognizant of the desire for autonomy and personal growth by all employees.

Informal Feedback: Providing Consistent, Constructive Criticism and Giving Praise

Support from supervisors need not be confined to the formal appraisal period. Informal feedback should be rendered on a consistent basis. Not only is feedback helpful in improving performance, employees have several motives for seeking feedback, including reduction of uncertainty, goal achievement, protection of ego, self-esteem, and desire to be responsive (Anseel et al., 2007). Employees should be instructed immediately when they demonstrate behaviors detrimental to the organization or if they are not performing to standards, as long as it is done in a professional manner. For example, the supervisor should never criticize an employee in the presence of others. Offering praise to an employee for a job well done should be done in public, however, as long as the employee truly deserves such praise, the praise is not overdone, and it is not overly repetitive (Rosendahl, 1993). Supervisors also should consider following up praise with an official memo and boasting of the employee to colleagues so that it may get back to her indirectly. Other suggestions include complimenting the employee as soon as possible after the behavior, address the person by name when giving praise, compliment a specific action, and explaining why the action being praised was important to you and the organization (Byers, 2010).

Supervisors should avail themselves of opportunities to provide performance feedback whenever possible. Seldom should either laudatory or critical comments during the formal appraisal process come as much of a surprise to employees. Supervisors can seek training on how to provide consistent and continuous feedback without giving employees the impression that they are losing autonomy. When the supervisor handles these situations deftly and develops a positive relationship with the employee, the latter will have a positive reaction toward any type of feedback and are more likely to believe that the organization is promoting fairness among its employees (Feys et al., 2008).

Other Benefits

Pharmacy managers may consider the use of other strategies to recognize and reward good performers:

- Offer to pay for attendance at local continuing education programs.
- Provide funding for attendance at national conferences.
- Offer to offset the cost of professional recognition and certification processes for pharmacists and technicians.
- Fund membership in a professional association.
- Buy lunch.
- Allow someone to represent you at an important meeting.
- Assign tasks with greater levels of responsibility if the employee is ready to handle them.

REVISITING THE SCENARIO

Administrators may consider the fact that Marcus has made more errors than other technicians to be of greater consequence than his promptness and vigorous effort. Marcus may contend that a greater frequency of errors is bound to occur as a result of him filling a greater number of medication orders. The technicians may not be clear on who is responsible for certain tasks. Pharmacy staff may be concerned that management plays favorites among the employees. Overall, it would appear as though Community Hospital does not even have a formal system of evaluation in place, or at least is not abiding by it. This is problematic for all the reasons discussed throughout the chapter.

Marcus is confused and frustrated for having seldom been evaluated formally. Has management avoided subsequent appraisals because the last one did not run so smoothly? Has this been the case with other employees as well? None of these questions is necessarily an indictment of management at Community Hospital pharmacy because there is much information not known in the scenario. However, it is certain that all employees at the pharmacy must be evaluated formally at least once a year, informed of behaviors that are viewed as desirable, instructed on how they may improve performance, and shown how various aspects of performance translate into the allocation of organizational rewards.

CONCLUSION

Supervisors often view performance appraisals as an undesirable task, but careful planning and implementation should make them less onerous. Performance appraisals are closely linked to employee motivation, performance, commitment, and turnover. Numerous systems are available, each of which has its strengths and drawbacks. The formal appraisal must be accompanied by frequent and substantive informal feedback. The appraisal interview is key to the success of the appraisal system. The allocation of organizational rewards must be linked closely to the results of the appraisal process.

QUESTIONS FOR FURTHER DISCUSSION

1. What types of skills do you think are necessary for selecting and implementing a performance appraisal system? What about for conducting an appraisal interview?
2. How would you feel about having responsibility for determining whether or not an employee will receive merit pay?
3. Has your performance ever been assessed formally at a job? How was that experience? What do you think the supervisor could have done better when assessing your performance?
4. How would you react if you were told that your performance was not measuring up to the expectations of an organization?
5. Does everyone with similar jobs in a pharmacy deserve the same level of pay raises, or should they be based more on performance?
6. Do you know anyone who has left a job because, in part, of the kinds of issues raised in the chapter scenario?

REFERENCES

Alvarez NA. 1997. Searching for utopia. *J Am Pharm Assoc* 37:632.

Anonymous. 2001. Conducting effective performance appraisals. *Clin Leadersh Manag Rev* 15:348.

Anseel F, Lieens F, Levy PE. 2007. A self-motives perspective on feedback-seeking behavior: Linking organizational behavior and social psychology research. *Intl J Manage Reviews* 9:211.

Anseel F, Lievens F, Schollaert E. 2009. Reflection as a strategy to enhance task performance after feedback. *Org Behav Hum Decision Processes* 110:35.

Barnett CW, Kimberlin CL. 1988. Levels of satisfaction among Florida pharmacists. *J Pharm Mark Manage* 2:23.

Blackwell S, Szeinbach S, Garner D, Smith M. 1996. Legal issues in personnel management. *Drug Top* 140:74.

Blau G. 1999. Testing the longitudinal impact of work variables and performance appraisal satisfaction on subsequent overall job satisfaction. *Hum Relat* 52:1099.

Blume BD, Baldwin TT, Rubin RS. 2009. Reactions to different types of forced distribution performance evaluation systems. *J Bus Psychol* 24:91.

Bowen D, Gilliland SW, Folger R. 1999. HRM and service fairness: How being fair with employees spills over to customers. *Organ Dynam* 27:7.

Brown M, Hyatt D, Benson J. 2010. Consequences of the performance appraisal system. *Pers Rev* 39:396.

Byars LL, Rue L. 2000. *Human Resource Management*, 6th edn. New York: McGraw-Hill.

Byers M. 2010. Nicely done! The power of genuine compliments. *J Mich Dental Assoc* 92:26.

Campbell B, Barron C. 1982. How extensively are human resource management practices being utilized by practitioners? *Person Admin* 27:67.

Collins PM. 1999. Pharmacy technician: Valuable asset in today's pharmacy. *Wash Pharm* 41:38.

Desselle SP. 2005. Job turnover intentions among certified pharmacy technicians. *J Am Pharm Assoc* 45:676.

Desselle SP, Holmes ER. 2007. A structural model of CPhTs' job satisfaction and career commitment. *J Am Pharm Assoc* 47:58.

Desselle SP, Tipton DJ. 2001. Factors contributing to the satisfaction and performance ability of community pharmacists: A path model analysis. *J Soc Admin Pharm* 18:15.

Desselle SP, Vaughan M, Faria T. 2002. Creating a performance appraisal template for pharmacy technicians using the method of equal-appearing intervals. *J Am Pharm Assoc* 42:768.

Edwards MT. 2009. Measuring clinical performance. *Physician Exec* 35:40.

Etzioni A. 1964. *Modern Organizations.* Englewood Cliffs, NJ: Prentice-Hall.

Eulburg JR, Weekley J, Bhahat RS. 1988. Models of stress in organizational research: A meta-theoretical perspective. *Hum Relat* 41:331.

Feys M, Libbrecht N, Anseel F, Lievens F. 2008. A closer look at the relationship between justice perceptions and feedback reactions: The role of the quality of the relationship with the supervisor. *Psychol Belg* 48:156.

Gaither CA, Mason HL. 1992a. Commitment to the employer: Do pharmacists have it? *Am Pharm* NS32:41.

Gaither CA, Mason HL. 1992b. A model of pharmacists' career commitment, organizational commitment and job withdrawal intentions. *J Soc Admin Pharm* 9:75.

Gaither CA, Nadkarni A, Mott DA, et al. 2007. Should I stay or should I go? The influence of individual and organizational factors on pharmacists' future work plans. *J Am Pharm Assoc* 47:165.

Goffin RD, Jelley RB, Powell DM, Johnston NG. 2009. Taking advantage of social comparisons in performance appraisal: The relative percentile method. *Hum Resour Manage* 48:268.

Griffin RW. 1996. *Management*, 5th edn. Boston: Houghton-Mifflin.

Kalb KB, Cherry NM, Kauzloric J, et al. 2006. A competency-based approach to public health nursing performance appraisal. *Public Health Nurs* 23:115.

Kennedy PW, Dresser SG. 2001. Appraising and paying for performance: Another look at an age-old problem. *Empl Benefits J* 26:8.

Kong SX. 1995. Predictors of organizational and career commitment among Illinois pharmacists. *Am J Health Syst Pharm* 52:2005.

Kong SX, Wertheimer AI. 1994. Social support: Concepts, theories, and implications for pharmacy research. *J Pharm Mark Manage* 9:63.

Kong SX, Wertheimer AI, McGhan WF. 1992. Role stress, organizational commitment and turnover intention among pharmaceutical scientists: A multivariate analysis. *J Soc Admin Pharm* 9:159.

Lahoz MR, Mason HL. 1991. Reducing pharmacists' stress. *Am Drug* 200:38.

Latham GP, Wexley KM. 1994. *Increasing Productivity Through Performance Appraisal*, 2d edn. Reading, MA: Addison- Wesley.

MacDonald HA, Sulsky LM. 2009. Rating formats and rater training redux: A context-specific approach for enhancing the effectiveness of performance management. *Can J Behav Sci Revue* 41:240.

Martin DC, Bartol KM. 1991. The legal ramifications of performance appraisal: An update. *Employee Relat Law J* 17:257.

Martin DC, Bartol KM. 1998. Performance appraisal: Maintaining system effectiveness. *Public Person Manag* 27:223.

McConnell CR. 2010. *Umiker's Management Skills for the New Health Care Supervisor.* Sudbury, MA: Jones and Bartlett.

McNall LA, Roch SG. 2009. A social exchange model of employee reactions to electronic performance monitoring. *Hum Perform* 22:224.

Mohrman AM, Resnick-West SM, Lawler EE III. 1989. *Designing Performance Appraisal Systems.* San Francisco: Josey-Bass.

Muenzen PM, Greenberg S, Murer MM. 1999. PTCB task analysis identifies role of certified pharmacy technicians in pharmaceutical care. *J Am Pharm Assoc* 39: 857.

Olson JM, Goffin RD, Haynes GA. 2007. Relative versus absolute measures of explicit attitudes: Implications for predicting diverse attitude-relevant criteria. *J Personal Soc Psychol* 93:926.

Park EJ, Huber DL. 2007. Balanced scorecards for performance management. *J Nurs Adm* 37:14.

Powell DM, Goffin RD. 2009. Assessing personality in the employment interview: The impact of training on rater accuracy. *Hum Perform* 22:465.

Roch SG. 2007. Why convene rater teams: An investigation of the benefits of anticipated discussion, consensus, and rater motivation. *Org Behav Hum Decision Processes* 104:29.

Roch SG, McNall LA. 2007. An investigation of factors influencing accountability and performance ratings. *J Psychol* 141:523.

Roch SG, Paquin AR, Littlejohn TW. 2009. Do raters agree more on observable items? *Hum Perform* 22:409.

Rosendahl I. 1993. Keeping them happy. *Drug Top* 137:50.

Schneider PJ. 1999. Creating an environment for improving the medication-use process. *Am J Health Syst Pharm* 56:1769.

Schumock GT, Leister KA, Edwards D, et al. 1990. Method for evaluating performance of clinical pharmacists. *Am J Hosp Pharm* 47:127.

Segal R. 1992. A framework for evaluating the work of pharmacists. *Top Hosp Pharm Manag* 12:130.

Smith HA, Branecker J, Pence BS. 1985. Role orientation, conflict and satisfaction among pharmacists and students. *J Soc Admin Pharm* 3:19.

Tolli AP, Schmidt AM. 2008. The role of feedback, causal attributions, and self-efficacy in goal revision. *J Appl Psychol* 93:692.

Uggerslev KL, Sulsky LM. 2008. Using frame-of-reference training to understand the implications of raer idiosyncrasy for rating accuracy. *J Appl Psychol* 93:719.

Valle M, Bozeman DP. 2002. Interrater agreement on employees' job performance: Review and directions. *Psychol Rep* 90:975.

Wolfgang AP. 1989. Challenging students to consider pharmacy's professional status. *Am J Pharm Educ* 53:177.

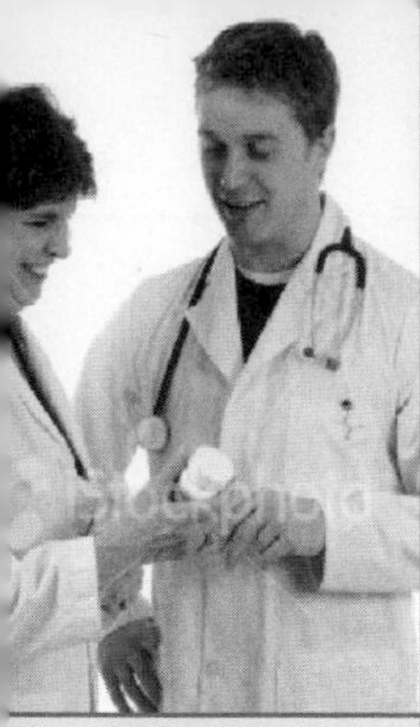

16

LEADERSHIP THEORY AND APPLICATION

Virginia (Ginger) G. Scott

About the Author: Dr. Scott is professor and director of Continuing Education in the Department of Pharmaceutical Systems and Policy at West Virginia University School of Pharmacy. She received a B.S. in pharmacy from the University of Kentucky, an M.S. in pharmacy administration from Purdue University, and a Ph.D. in social and administrative pharmacy from the University of Minnesota. Her teaching interests include patient health education, outcomes and quality improvement, pharmacoeconomics, and patient-reported outcomes. Her research interests include health services and health outcomes research, specifically patient-reported outcomes and cost-effectiveness of patient care services and drug therapy; educational research on continuing professional development; and examining the relationship between educational programming and the implementation of pharmacy services. She has been involved actively in pharmacy professional organizations, has served in numerous leadership positions on the state and national levels since 1977, and was selected as an academic leadership fellow for the American Association of Colleges of Pharmacy in 2004.

LEARNING OBJECTIVES

After completing this chapter, readers will be able to

1. Define leadership and identify qualities needed to be an effective leader.
2. Discuss the integration of organizational culture into leadership models and theories.
3. Explain how leadership theories and models can be used as a guide to promote change within an organization.
4. Identify ways to develop leadership skills in others, such as delegation and the use of leadership evaluative tools.
5. Discuss how to leverage personal strengths to advance an organization.
6. Describe leadership roles within the profession and community for students and pharmacists.

SCENARIO

Jennifer Leader is a fourth-year pharmacy student who is involved in several student pharmacy organizations at her college of pharmacy. Recently, she was recognized by her peers and inducted into Phi Lambda Sigma, a pharmacy organization that fosters and recognizes student pharmacist leaders. Jennifer's long-term goal is to become a director of pharmacy or a regional manager or to own her own store. Other goals are to be actively involved in local, state, and national pharmacy organizations and to have a leadership position in one of the pharmacy organizations on both the state and national levels. Based on her leadership class in pharmacy school, Jennifer feels that she has a broad understanding of the concepts of leadership and leadership theories. During her rotations to date, she has encountered several leaders who do not exhibit the leadership styles and skills that she was taught in pharmacy school. Thus, she is thinking that she may need additional leadership development to further self-awareness of her strengths and leadership skills as well as to gain a better understanding on how to interpret the leadership style of others.

CHAPTER QUESTIONS

1. How is leadership defined? What sorts of things distinguish leading from other seemingly interchangeable terms like supervising or managing?
2. How can leadership theories and models be applied to promote change within an organization?
3. If a person wants to become a leader within the organization or profession, how could they assess or enhance their leadership ability and skills?
4. How are one's personal strengths leveraged to advance the organization and profession?
5. What qualities are needed for effective leadership?
6. How are employees developed to be future leaders of the organization?
7. What leadership styles are important in pharmacy?
8. What types of leadership roles should pharmacists and/or pharmacy students assume?

LEADERSHIP

The hallmarks of effective leadership are important from both a personal and an organizational perspective, and the concepts of leadership have intrigued individuals for centuries. A wealth of literature exists related to the meaning of leadership, qualities of an effective leader, leadership styles, leadership theories, the development of a leader, and other dimensions of leadership.

This chapter builds on the leadership theories related to organizational behavior discussed in Chapter 11. Specifically, this chapter will promote a greater understanding of the definitions and concepts of leadership; qualities of an effective leader; leadership theories and styles; how leadership theories and styles incorporate the organizational culture; how leadership theories are used to make changes within the organization; how to use one's personal strengths to enhance leadership abilities, developing leadership in others, including the pros and cons of delegation; evaluative tools to identify personal leadership style; and leadership roles within the profession and community for students and pharmacists.

WHAT IS LEADERSHIP?

Leadership has been described in many ways by many persons, but there exists no universally accepted definition. Carson Dye (2000) confirmed this when he stated, "After all these years ... no one is able to articulate a comprehensive, absolute definition of leadership." Common to many leadership definitions are the following dimensions: Leadership is a learned skill (Dye, 2000; Giuliani, 2002; Maxwell, 2003), adapting principles to circumstances (Axelrod, 1999), a process that focuses on making organizational changes (Kotter, 1990), not controlling people (Autry, 2001), a blend of characteristics and talents that individuals can use to develop into a leader (Lombardi, 2001), and attracting the voluntary commitment of followers to reach for common goals (Kreiter and Kinicki, 1997; Nanus, 1992; Tichy, 1997).

Even though there are many leadership definitions, Komvies et al. (1998) noted several basic assumptions about leadership that are incorporated into the preceding definitions. These assumptions are that leadership is a learned behavior, is teachable, occurs at all levels of the organization, does not require a charismatic personality, is a relational process, is culturally influenced, requires followership, involves purposeful change that satisfies collective needs and aspirations, includes the components of effectiveness and ethics, and develops over life.

Leadership is an important concept that transcends all health care professions. The acceptance of this role by all health care professionals is vital to the invention of new technologies and dosage forms, changes in the delivery of health care, enhancement of patient outcomes and quality of life, and success of their specific health care organization. The opportunities for pharmacists to be leaders in their practice setting, the pharmacy profession, and the community are plentiful. Leadership is a critical component for positive change within pharmacy organizations and the profession.

LEADERSHIP THEORIES AND STYLES

Leadership theories help us to understand the leadership style of your immediate supervisor and other administrators. Understanding leadership theory and leadership styles enables us to identify the personal values and vision that guide the organization's management team. It also provides insight into employers' expectations of their employees.

The leadership theories discussed in Chapter 11 were trait, behavioral (i.e., autocratic, democratic, and laissez fare), situational or contingency based, transactional, and transformational. The majority of these theories are transactional in nature; however, transformational leadership is used more often to implement innovation and change within the profession and achievement of organizational goals (Bass, 1985). Building on Chapter 11, leadership theories and phases that incorporate an organization's culture into leadership models and theories are emerging in the health care industry and other organizations to address the implementation of change in a dynamic and competitive environment. Some leadership theories focus on the individual, such as servant and strengths-based leadership, and the value of these related to the organization's leadership team. On the contrary, the four-frame model for reframing organizations emphasizes the importance of using the abilities and skills of all members of the leadership team to overcome deficits in an individual's abilities and skills to accomplish the organization's vision and mission.

Organizational Culture

Leadership models and theories that incorporate organizational culture are becoming increasingly important (Ledlow and Coppala, 2011). To understand this phenomenon, it is important to understand the definition of culture. Schein's (1992) definition of culture is more formal. He states that culture is "a pattern of shared basic assumptions that a group learned as it solved its problems of external adaptation and integration, that has worked well enough to be considered valid and therefore be taught to new members as the correct way to perceive, think, and feel in relation to those problems." Less formal definitions of culture are "a set of important understandings (often unstated) that members of a community share in common" (Sathe, 1985) or "as the way we do things around here" (Deal and Kennedy, 1982).

Bolman and Deal (2003) noted that there are still controversies as to the relationship between culture and leadership. Some areas of disagreement include "Do leaders shape culture or are they shaped by it?" "Do organizations with strong cultures outperform those relying on policies and rules?" and "Does success breed a cohesive culture or does culture breed success?" (Bolman and Deal, 2003). Where Ledlow and Coppola (2011) emphasize the importance of incorporating organizational culture into leadership theories and models. They noted that these models "require leaders to determine, develop, and maintain an organizational culture that best meet the expectations—if not thrive—in the external environment." After all, culture of an organization also includes its language/communication, citizenship behaviors, power structure, the way things get accomplished, mores, esprit de corps, and many other components. Nonetheless, there are strong links between leadership and culture. Even though several leadership phases or models are emerging that incorporate organizational culture and leadership, only two of these will be discussed in this chapter. These are the culture creation contingency leadership (CCCL) phase and the dynamic culture leadership (DCL) model.

Culture Creation Contingency Leadership

CCCL is defined by Ledlow and Coppala (2011) as a phase "which combines situational or contingency leadership with organizational culture creation, refinement and enhancement." In this phase, leaders of the organization predefine the organization's culture based on the needs of the external environment for the purpose of achieving success within the organization. In contrast to situational leadership described in Chapter 11, leaders are more proactive than reactive, since they predetermine the organizational culture.

Dynamic Culture Leadership Model

The DCL model (Ledlow and Coppala, 2011) incorporates the organizational culture's development process with transformational and transactional leadership theories discussed in Chapter 11. The DCL model is robust in the fact that the leadership team and management team are aligned to ensure that the knowledge, skills, and abilities of all individuals are utilized while maintaining an appropriate organizational culture (Ledlow and Coppala, 2011). The DCL model processes consist of six constructs: communication improvement; strategic planning; decision-making alignment; employee enhancement; knowledge management and organizational learning; and evaluating, reflecting, and retooling. The theory behind the model is that with process repetition and consistency, the organizational culture will align with the leadership's vision and respond to dynamic changes in the environment. An example of this is the strategic plan of ABC pharmacy to include the addition of disease management programs. After conducting a needs assessment to determine the disease state(s) on which to focus, the pharmacy owner/manager identifies diabetes as being the most prevalent in the pharmacy's patient population. Prior to implementation of the program, all pharmacists are sent to a diabetes certificate program. After the program is implemented and established, the pharmacy implements other patient care programs such as smoking cessation or asthma so that their pharmacy will remain competitive in the marketplace.

A model used to respond to change by many organizations is Kotter's (1996) eight-step process for leading change. This process is based on the premises that change does not occur within the organizations due to barriers or errors created by the leadership. These barriers are allowing too much complacency, failing to create a sufficiently powerful guiding coalition, underestimating the power of vision, undercommunicating the vision by a factor of 10 (or 100 or even 1,000), permitting obstacles to block the new vision, failing to create short-term wins, declaring victory too soon, and neglecting to anchor changes firmly in the corporate culture (Kotter, 1996). Any or all of these errors can have a negative effect on the success of the organization in a dynamic and competitive environment. Heller (1999) emphasizes the importance on addressing changes within the organization in a systematic way. Kotter's eight-step processes are listed in Table 16-1 and offer a systematic way to implementing change in the organization and addresses how to avoid the errors noted earlier. Prior to implementing a change, administrators must know how the change is going to affect them, their team, and organization and be able to relate the change to the vision and mission of the organization. Osborne (2008) echoes the importance of making this connection so that individuals understand their role and conflict is avoided (Bolman and Deal, 2003). When staff understand their role, they are also more likely to commit to the change (Osborne, 2008). Based on the above example, the addition of a diabetes management program is a big change for the employees in ABC pharmacy. To gain acceptance for the change, the administrator must communicate to all employees the importance of the diabetes management

Table 16-1. The Eight-Stage Process of Creating Major Change

1. Establish a sense of urgency
   - Examine the market and competitive realities
   - Identify and discuss crises, potential crises, or major opportunities
2. Create the guiding coalition
   - Put together a group with enough power to lead the change
   - Get the group to work together like a team
3. Develop a vision and strategy
   - Create a vision to help direct the change effort
   - Develop strategies for achieving that vision
4. Communicate the change vision
   - Use every vehicle possible to constantly communicate the new vision and strategies
   - Have the guiding coalition role model the behavior expected of employees
5. Empower broad-based action
   - Get rid of obstacles
   - Change systems or structures that undermine the change vision
   - Encourage risk taking and nontraditional ideas, activities and action
6. Generate short-term wins
   - Plan for visible improvement in performance, or "wins"
   - Create those wins
   - Visibly recognize and reward people who made the wins possible
7. Consolidate gains and produce more change
   - Use increased credibility to change all systems, structures, and policies that do not fit together and do not fit the transformation vision
   - Hire, promote, and develop people who can implement the change vision
   - Reinvigorate the process with new projects, themes, and change agents
8. Anchor new approaches in the culture
   - Create better performance through customer- and productivity-oriented behavior, more and better leadership, and more effective management
   - Articulate the connections between new behaviors and organizational success
   - Develop means to ensure leadership development and succession

Source: Used with permission from Kotter JP. 1996. Leading Change. Harvard Business School Press: Boston, MA.

program to the organization and the patients it serves, the employees' role in the implementation and success of the program, and how the program relates to the vision and mission of the organization.

Servant Leadership

Servant leadership is a term coined by Robert Greenleaf in 1970, and it has been studied and expanded on by other authors, such as Covey et al. (1998), Autry (2001), and Martin (2002). It is based on the philosophy that an individual's first desire is to serve. Later, the individual makes a conscious decision to lead (Greenleaf, 2002). Authors have identified many characteristics that are important in the development of servant leaders. Larry Spear, chief executive officer (CEO) of the Greenleaf Center, identified ten principles of servant leadership (*10 Principles of Servant Leadership,* 2010) based on Greenleaf's original writings. These characteristics are listening, empathy, healing, persuasion, awareness, conceptualization, foresight, stewardship, commitment to the growth of people, and building community (Spears, 2003). Autry (2001) noted that servant leaders have a deeper connection to their work, and the connection transcends power and money. In his writings, he discusses several other characteristics of a servant leader. These are to be authentic (i.e., the same person in every circumstance), vulnerable (i.e., to realize that you are not in total control but depend on others), accepting (i.e., to focus on ideas presented, not on the person), present (i.e., available, centered, and grounded), and useful (i.e., caring, useful, and creating a meaningful workplace). An example of a pharmacist exhibiting servant leadership is one who establishes a health care program including medication management to the homeless or underserved population. The program was established from their passion and desire to serve this population of people. By establishing the program, the individual emerged as a leader in this area, since communities relied on this individual to establish similar programs within the state.

Strengths-Based Leadership

Strengths-based leadership is based on the theory of positive psychology. The theory implies that individuals are more effective leaders when they become aware of and understand their unique talents and capitalize on these strengths (Hendricks, 2001). Talents, knowledge, and skills of the individual are the basis for strength-based leadership. Talents are naturally unique to each individual and can be maximized by knowledge and skill development (Buckingham, 2005; Buckingham and Clinton, 2001; Coffman and Gonzalez-Molins, 2002). Research in this area has been conducted by Gallup University (2011) using interviews of great leaders and a Web-based assessment tool to determine the importance of using strength-based leadership in the workplace. An evaluative tool (StrengthsFinder Profile, 2011) to assess an individual's strength and the importance of identifying their strengths is discussed later in the chapter (see Section "Leadership Evaluative Tools").

REFRAMING LEADERSHIP

Bolman and Deal (2003) present another concept of leadership style that incorporates the use of *frames* to maximize the success of the organization. Frames are defined as "windows on the world of leadership and management. A good frame makes it easier to know what you are up against and what you can do about it." These authors further noted that "frames [are] like maps; frames are both windows on a territory and tools for navigation. Every tool has distinctive strengths and limitations. The right tool makes the job easier, but the wrong one just gets in the way" (Bolman and Deal, 2003). These frames are an essential part of the leadership process and are labeled *structural, human resources, political,* and *symbolic.* Most leaders will not exhibit strengths in all four frames. The key is for the leader of an organization to surround himself or herself with individuals who have strengths in the other frames to maximize the success of their organization.

Structural leaders do homework; rethink the relationship of structure, strategy, and environment; and focus on implementation. On the contrary, human resources leaders believe in people and communicate their beliefs. They are visible, accessible, empower others, and refer to employees as partners or associates. Political leaders clarify what they want and what they can get. They persuade first, negotiate second, and coerce only if necessary. Symbolic leaders lead by example, offer plausible interpretations of experience, communicate a vision, tell stories, and respect and use history. Reframing leadership is a leadership style that will be valuable in assisting future leaders to create new opportunities within their environments. For example, the CEO of ABC Pharmacy may have strengths related to the human resources frame (e.g., communication, relator, and connectedness) but is weak in skills related to the political frame such as negotiation and competitiveness. As the CEO, he or she would want another pharmacist on their administrative staff who has these skills. The CEO should then assign all tasks involving negotiations to this individual. By supplementing the administrative staff with individuals who supplement your own strengths, the organization is more likely to be successful.

QUALITIES OF EFFECTIVE LEADERS

Recent authors (Ahoy, 2007; Buckingham, 2005, Maxwell, 1995) have identified five hallmark characteristics of effective leaders. These are modeling, mentoring, motivating, monitoring, and multiplying successes (i.e., reproducing future leaders). Leaders must be role models within the organization because employees will model the role they exhibit. They are also mentors by teaching other employees on the workings of the organizations and guiding their employee development. Administrators with good leadership abilities motivate employees to be responsible for their performance within the organization. Responsible employees assist leaders in helping the organization grow and succeed. The administrator must monitor the operations of the organization on a daily basis to ensure that the organization remains efficient and effective. *Multiplying success* refers to the fact when individuals are given greater responsibility for and control of their own work; they are more likely to work toward improving the organization. Ahoy (2007) noted that other characteristics, such as empowering, guiding, and coaching others while delegating responsibility, are also important characteristics of leadership. The W. K. Kellogg Foundation Report (2000) indicated that collaboration between administrators and employees, shared purpose, respect, and an enhanced learning environment are also important to the success of organizations.

Additional qualities frequently mentioned include vision (Ahoy, 2007; Bolman and Deal, 2003), integrity (Maxwell, 1995), communicating a vision effectively (Clifford and Cavanaugh, 1985; Kouzes and Posner, 1987), commitment (Bolman and Deal, 2003; Clifford and Cavanaugh, 1985; Collins, 2001; W. K. Kellogg Foundation Report, 2000), positive attitude (Maxwell, 1995), confidence (Maxwell, 1995), character (Maxwell, 1995), passion (Bolman and Deal, 2003; Clifford and Cavanaugh, 1985; Collins, 2001), (Bolman and Deal, 2003; Kotter, 1990; Kouzes and Posner, 1987; Nanus, 1992), honesty (Bolman and Deal, 2003), relationship building (Coleman, 2002; Kotter, 1990; Kouzes and Posner, 1987; Nanus, 1992), charisma (Denny, 2002), team spirit (Barnes et al., 2002), creativity (Dave, 2002), being ethical (Kcim, 2002), courage (Haverson, 2002), networking (Malinchak, 2002), self-knowledge (W. K. Kellogg Foundation Report, 2000), authenticity/integrity (W. K. Kellogg Foundation Report, 2000), empathy/understanding of others (W. K. Kellogg Foundation Report, 2000), and competence (W. K. Kellogg Foundation Report, 2000).

After decades of research and thousands of interviews with great leaders, Gallup University research discovered seven challenges, referred to as the "seven demands of leadership" that leaders must meet to maximize their leadership impact on an organizations and critical to their leadership success (Conchie, 2004). These challenges are visioning, mentoring, knowing self, making sense of experience, maximizing values, building a constituency, and challenging experience.

LEADERSHIP DEVELOPMENT

A prevailing myth about leadership is that it is innate or, in other words, something with which you are born. In the definitions of leadership above, many great leaders stated that leadership is a learned behavior (Dye, 2000; Giuliani, 2002; Maxwell, 2003). Maxwell (2003) classified four levels of leadership based on the concept that leadership is a learned behavior. These are the *leading leader,* the *learned leader,* the *latent leader,* and the *limited leader.* Each category is based on the individual's level of leadership and desire to become a leader. The classifications vary along a continuum from being born with leadership qualities (the leading leader) to the leader who has had little or no exposure to leadership (the limited leader). Other characteristics used to classify an individual into a specific category depend on whether the individual has seen leadership modeled, has had leadership training, and has the desire to be a leader. In all four classifications, the only characteristic not acquired is "born with leadership qualities." Thus, any individual with the desire to be a leader can develop his or her leadership skills. Mason and Wetherbee (2004) noted two assumptions of leadership development. The first emphasizes the preceding point that leaders can be developed through education and training. The second is that management differs from leadership and that managers can be transformed into leaders.

Dye (2000) identified four stages in the growth of leadership. Individuals in Stage 1 do not think that leadership is their job, and they resist leadership development (unconscious incompetence). Stage 2 refers to individuals being consciously incompetent or who have the desire to grow and improve but may not realize it until they lose their job. Stage 3 is conscious competence, where individuals are competent but are not seen as strong leaders. They need the opportunity to practice skills and continue learning. Stage 4 refers to unconscious competence and is the ultimate stage of leadership. In this stage, an individual's leadership skills are smooth and happen without hesitation.

A different concept to enhancing leadership effectiveness was presented by Jim Collins (2001) in his book, *Good to Great.* He encouraged the development of a "stop doing" list by business leaders. Collins's rationale for this concept is that leaders lead busy lives with many "to do" lists. By developing a "stop doing" list, leaders can channel their resources into a few focused areas.

Maxwell (2003) developed a workbook to correspond to the material presented in his book, *The 21 Irrefutable Laws of Leadership,* to aid in the development of leaders. The workbook provides multiple instruments that individuals can employ for the purpose of identifying strengths related to leadership skills, such as vision, relationship building, coaching, and connectivity. This is a good place to begin to identify your strengths as a leader. The results can be used in the development of a more elaborate leadership development plan. Reliable and valid instruments have been developed to identify an individual's personality style and skills related to the resolutions of conflicts, critical thinking, motivation, and personal strengths.

Strengths-based development at the individual level is a more recent model for leadership development. There are three steps in the development process. First, an individual's talents are identified, and the person is made aware of these talents. Second, the individual begins to integrate these into his or her daily routines, shares with other members of the organization, and identifies ways to maximize his or her strengths. Last, a behavior change occurs as the individual is able to tie his or her successes to his or her themes of talent (Clifton and Harter, 2003). Being cognizant of your own strengths and leadership skills enhances your ability to develop leadership in others.

Developing Leadership in Others

Stanley (2003) stated, "Sometimes it really is easier and less time-consuming to do things yourself than to train someone else." But leadership is not always about getting things done "right." Leadership is about getting things done through other people. In Covey's (1989) *The 7 Habits of Highly Effective People,* he notes that transferring responsibility or delegation results in growth for both the individual and the organization.

Delegating responsibilities and tasks to other individual(s) or team(s) within the organization not only develops staff (Heller, 1999) but also increases time for meeting your own responsibilities (Heller, 1999), allowing for better time management (Heller, 1999; Yaverbaum and Sherman, 2008). Delegation also empowers the staff to take responsibility for obtaining the organization's goals (Yaverbaum and Sherman, 2008). This contribution by the individual to the organization gives him or her a greater sense of self-worth, confidence in their leadership ability, and commitment to the success of the overall organization.

Even though a leader delegates responsibilities and tasks to other individuals or teams, many administrators still tend to micromanage (Heller, 1999; Yaverbaum and Sherman, 2008) by retaining overall responsibility for the task or project. Administrators must find a balance between micromanaging a project and task and outlining their expectations and outcomes (Yaverbaum and Sherman, 2008). This is important for leaders to remember; otherwise, they increase the risk of stifling the creativity (DeCoske et al., 2011) of individuals within the organization.

As an administrator, you also have the responsibility to develop future leaders to ensure the continual success of your organization. Conger (1992) and Conger and Benjamin (1999) identified four types of leadership development used in corporations. These are skills building training (e.g., practice exercises for skills, simulations, lectures, and video case studies), intensive feedback programs (e.g., observational exercises, survey and verbal feedback, and fellow colleagues), conceptual approaches (e.g., written and video case studies, lectures on conceptual models, and discussion groups), and personal growth approaches (e.g., teamwork, risk taking, and personal values exploration). Other types of leadership development used are mentoring, coaching, and profile evaluative instruments.

LEADERSHIP EVALUATIVE TOOLS

Numerous leadership evaluative tools help individuals increase self-awareness, recognize interpersonal communication skills, and identify thinking skills. Some of the most commonly used evaluative tools are the Myers–Briggs Type Indicator (MBTI) (Myers and Briggs, 1988), the Strength Deployment Inventory (SDI) (Scudder, 1996), the Watson–Glaser Critical Thinking Appraisal (WGCTA) (Watson and Glaser, 2000), the Thomas Kilmann Conflict Mode Instrument (TKI) (Kilmann and Kilmann, 1972), StrengthsFinder Profile (Buckingham and Clifton, 2001), 360-Degree Feedback (2011), and Q12.

Myers–Briggs Type Indicator

The Myers–Briggs Type Indicator (MBTI) personality inventory was developed in the 1940s by Isabel Myers and Katherine Briggs. The instrument was based on Carl Jung's theory of psychological types introduced in 1920. Jung's theory indicates that random behavior variation is due to differences in the way individuals prefer to use their perception and judgment. The instrument identifies an individual's preference for the four dichotomies specified in Jung's theory. These are favorite world (i.e., extroversion or introversion), information (i.e., sensing or intuition), decisions (i.e., thinking or feeling), and structure (i.e., judging or perceiving). Your answers to questions comprising the inventory are used to place you into 1 of 16 personality types. It is assumed that none of the personality types is "better" or "superior" to others. As such, the purpose of the feedback is to help you to understand and appreciate differences between people (Myers and Briggs, 1988).

Currently, there are two MBTI forms, MBTI Step I and MBTI Step II. MBTI Step I (Form M) consists of 93 questions and is based on preferences, whereas MBTI Step II (Form Q) consists of 144 questions. Feedback from this form provides a broader picture related to communication, decision making, and ability to deal with change and conflict. The MBTI, after more than 70 years, continues to be the most popular personality measure for understanding individual differences and helping a person to uncover different methods to use when interacting with other people (Myers and Briggs, 1988). Identification of your personality style is important in interacting with other members of your organization. Feedback from this tool provides tips on interacting with individuals who exhibit a different personality style. By knowing how to interact with individuals with different personality styles, the organization can grow, and conflicts can be avoided.

The Strength Deployment Inventory

The Strength Deployment Inventory (SDI) is based on relationship awareness theory. This theory implies that individual relationships can be improved and/or transformed by a better understanding not only of themselves but also of others through the creation of shared meanings (Noce, 1999; Porter, 1996). The SDI differs from other instruments assessing an individual's behavior in that an individual's motivation value system is also assessed. Values are assessed when things are going well for an individual, as well as when the person faces conflict. The questions are self-scored and worded to measure behaviors and the motivations and values that underlie those behaviors. Some applications of the SDI are conflict management, enhanced awareness of self and others, development of communication and negotiation skills, team building, and leadership development. It also includes instructions for drawing a visual representation of an individual's SDI results (Jones, 1976). This information is important because leaders must build relationships within the organization for the organization to grow and succeed.

The Watson–Glaser Critical Thinking Appraisal

The Watson–Glaser Critical Thinking Appraisal (WGCTA) is the most commonly used tool in business today to assess critical thinking skills. It assesses inference, recognition of assumptions, deduction, interpretation, and evaluation of arguments skills (Watson and Glaser, 2000). The WGCTA has been used extensively in business settings to determine hiring, promotion, and development of individuals for succession planning of a company. It is believed that high-potential performers with good critical thinking skills use sound decision making (Watson and Glaser, 2000).

Individuals being assessed are asked to evaluate reading passages that include statements, problems, arguments, and interpretations. When completed, a single score is determined for each individual. The score and information related to interpretation of the score are then provided to the individual. Since critical thinking skills are important in all organizations, individuals need to have critical thinking skills or develop this skill to be an effective leader. As the pharmacy profession requires pharmacists to use critical thinking skills daily, the WGCTA is an excellent tool to assess an employee's skill in this area.

The Thomas Kilmann Conflict Mode Instrument

The Thomas Kilmann Conflict Mode Instrument (TKI) was developed to assess an individual's preferred mode of five conflict-handling styles. These are avoiding, accommodating, competing, compromising, and collaborating. Individuals completing the instrument are forced to choose between two possible statements that describe their most likely behavior in a given situation. Responses then are transferred to a scoring sheet, and scores are totaled for each of the five modes of conflict resolution. Feedback allows individuals to determine their primary mode of conflict resolution and to identify situations when other modes of conflict resolution might be more effective. This is important in an organizational setting because leaders may be faced with a variety of conflicts that need to be resolved by different techniques.

The StrengthsFinder Profile

The StrengthsFinder Profile was developed by the Gallup Organization (Buckingham and Clifton, 2001) to identify the strengths that an individual possesses. The profile actually measures an individual's themes of talents. Since strengths are a result of talents, knowledge, and skills, a profile of various talent themes can be developed for an individual (Buckingham and Clifton, 2001). The profile consists of a pair of statements. The responses are then sorted. The feedback lists your five most dominant patterns of behavior. These are referred to as your signature theme. Research by Gallup University has identified 34 themes.

The book "*Now, Discover Your Strengths*" by Buckingham and Clifton (2001) discusses development of the profile and describes each of the signature themes in depth. A second version of the StrengthsFinder Profile was released in the fall of 2007. Version 2 can be accessed by using the personal identification code in the back jacket of the book "*Now, Discover Your Strengths: StrengthsFinder Profile 2.0*" (Rath, 2007). By knowing their strengths and the strengths of their employees, leaders can assign individuals' responsibilities based on their strengths, resulting in a more effective and successful organization.

360-Degree Feedback

This is a performance appraisal tool focusing on leadership effectiveness, planning, and teamwork (Edwards and Even, 1996). The system or process ultimately helps individuals to be more effective managers and/or leaders by better understanding their overall strengths and weaknesses (Chapter 15). There is a self-evaluation and a peer evaluation. Employees (i.e., managers, peers, and staff) provide their perceptions on a broad range of workplace competencies. Participants use a rating scale to respond to the questions in addition to providing written comments. Afterwards, responses for each category of employees (e.g., peers) are collated to ensure anonymity. Feedback is provided on the difference between the self-evaluation and peer evaluation in relation to leadership skills such as listening, goal setting, and planning. The feedback is provided in a format such that the individual can create a development plan. An advantage of the 360-Degree Feedback is that it can also be used as a development tool for nonmanagers (DeBare, 1997). Even though nonmanagers have no staff reporting directly to them, feedback from coworkers can be useful in helping them to be more effective in their current position. Second, it serves as a development tool for individuals aspiring to move into an administrative position. By identifying their strengths and areas for improvement, they can adjust their behaviors or develop new skills to be effective leaders within the organization and excel in their jobs.

Q12

The Q12 was developed by the Gallup Organization (Gallup Organization, 1999; Coffman and Gonzalez-Molins, 2002) to determine the level of employees' engagement within the organization. The Q12 assesses 12 key dimensions that describe a great workplace (Gallup Organization, 1999). The report from the Q12 instrument identifies how the leader's management style influences the perception of team members and engagement of employees. This information is important to leaders within the organization because disengaged employees are often not productive, which eventually may lead to a decline in the success of the organization.

LEADERSHIP ROLES FOR PHARMACY STUDENTS AND PHARMACISTS

Pharmacists and pharmacy students have unlimited opportunities to become leaders within their individual practice settings; pharmacy professional organizations on the local, state, and national levels; the overall health care profession; and their communities. Leaders will make changes within their practice setting prior to other pharmacists within their immediate vicinity, such as implementing medication therapy management (MTM) services or providing a new pharmacy service in the hospital. Other professional leadership opportunities include being an officer in local, state, and/or national pharmacy organizations. Community leadership roles involve community organizations such as the Lion's Club and Rotary Club, public health initiatives, and political involvement. Students can be leaders in their student pharmacy organizations by providing services to local community organizations and providing disease management services such as blood pressure, cholesterol, and glucose screening to the citizens within their local communities and state. Leadership in each of these areas is important to provide effective patient care, to enhance the quality of life of patients, to advance the profession of pharmacy, to make for a healthier community, and to advance your own self-worth and actualization.

REVISITING THE SCENARIO

Jennifer Leader is a month away from graduation. On her last two rotations, her preceptors have modeled the qualities of an effective leader that Jennifer learned about in pharmacy school. She has talked extensively to both individuals about serving as a mentor when she graduates from pharmacy school. Her preceptors suggested that she be willing to accept a supervisory position in her selected practice setting on graduation. Several types of leadership development were recommended to enhance Jennifer's leadership skills. These include exploring the opportunities to attend a leadership development program with her future employer; becoming active in her local, state, and national organizations for the purpose of networking and building relationships with other pharmacists; identifying who administers the different leadership evaluative tools such as StrengthsFinder and Myers–Briggs; and attending a pharmacy leadership program such as the American College of Clinical Pharmacy (ACCP) Academy Leadership and Management Certificate Program (2011), American Society of Health-System Pharmacists (ASHP) Conference for Leaders in Health-System Pharmacists (2011), ASHP Leadership Institute, experiential programs in association management and leadership (such as with the American Pharmacists Association), and/or other pharmacy leadership programs. The results from the leadership evaluative instruments will help Jennifer to develop a plan to enhance her leadership skills. This will also be the beginning of a process to realize her goal of becoming a pharmacy leader within her practice setting and in professional pharmacy associations on the state and national levels.

CONCLUSION

Pharmacists have assumed administrative and leadership roles in their practice settings, profession, and communities. However, opportunities for pharmacists to demonstrate leadership have never been greater or more needed. This is occurring as a result of changes in the provision of health care such as MTM and the invention of new technologies. Employers will be seeking pharmacists who can be leaders in this changing environment so that patients will receive the best quality of care. Leadership resources are plentiful, and many tools are available to assist individuals in developing their leadership skills. Resources are available in both print- and Web-based format. Other resources include leadership development programs and evaluative tools. Recent evaluative instruments provide feedback on a pharmacist's strengths. Once an individual knows his or her strengths, the information can be used to maximize his or her strengths, resulting in greater successes. Pharmacists are encouraged to use these resources not only for their own leadership development but also to develop leadership skills in others.

QUESTIONS FOR FURTHER DISCUSSION

1. What are the challenges to becoming a leader? What characteristics of an effective leader mentioned in this chapter do you currently possess? How might you acquire or improve on some others?
2. What is the importance of developing insight into your personal leadership style?
3. Which of the evaluative tools mentioned in this chapter do you feel might be of most benefit to you? Why?
4. As a leader, how do you help to promote change within the profession and in your practice setting?
5. How comfortable are you with delegating things to others? What are some factors that might keep you from delegating certain responsibilities? How might this be improved?

REFERENCES

About StrengthsFinder 2.0. 2011. Available at http://strengths.gallup.com/110440/About-StrengthsFinder-2.aspx; accessed on August 27, 2011.

ACCP Academy Leadership and Management Certificate Program. 2011. Available at www.accp.com/academy/leadershipandmanagement.aspx; accessed on August 27, 2011.

Ahoy CK. 2007. *Leadership in Educational Facilities Administration.* Alexandria, VA: Association of Higher Education Facilities Officers.

ASHP Conference for Leaders in Health-System Pharmacy. 2011. Available at www.ashp.org/menu/Meetings/Leadership-Conference; accessed on August 27, 2011.

Autry JA. 2001. *Servant Leadership.* Roseville, CA: Prima Publishing, pp. 20–21.

Axelrod A. 1999. *Patton on Leadership.* Paramus, NJ: Prentice-Hall, p. 31.

Barnes R, Coleman D, Cureton D, et al. 2002. *Let Your Leadership Speak: How to Lead and Be Heard.* Paxton, MA: The Future is Yours to Create! Company.

Bass B. 1985. *Leadership and Performance Beyond Expectations.* New York: Free Press.

Bennis W. 1989. *On Becoming a Leader.* Reading, MA: Addison-Wesley.

Bolman LG, Deal TE. 2003. *Reframing Organizations: Artistry, Choice, and Leadership,* 3rd edn. San Francisco, CA: Jossey-Bass.

Buckingham M. 2005. *The One Thing You Need to Know: About Great Managing, Great Leading, and Sustained Individual Success.* New York: Free Press.

Buckingham M, Clifton DO. 2001. *Now, Discover Your Strengths.* New York: Free Press.

Clifford DK, Cavanagh RE. 1985. *The Winning Performance: How America's High Growth Midsize Companies Succeed.* New York: Bantam Books.

Clifton DO, Harter JK. 2003. Strengths investment. In Cameron KS, Dutton JE, Quinn RE (eds.) *Positive Organizational Scholarship.* San Francisco, CA: Berrett-Koehler.

Coffman C, Gonzalez-Molina G. 2002. *Follow This Path.* New York: Warner Books.

Coleman DD. 2002. On relationships. In Barnes R, Coleman D, Cureton D, et al. (eds.) *Let Your Leadership Speak: How to Lead and Be Heard.* Paxton, MA: The Future is Yours to Create! Company.

Collins J. 2001. *Good to Great.* New York: Harper Collins, pp. 139–140.

Conchie B. 2004. The seven demands of leadership: What separates good leaders from all the rest? *Gallup Manag J,* May 13.

Conger JA. 1992. *Learning to Lead: The Art of Transforming Managers into Leaders.* San Francisco, CA: Jossey-Bass.

Conger JA, Benjamin B. 1999. *Building Leaders: How Successful Companies Develop the Next Generation.* San Francisco, CA: Jossey-Bass.

Covey SR. 1989. *The 7 Habits of Highly Effective People.* New York: Simon and Schuster, p. 171.

Covey SR, Merrill RA, Jones D. 1998. *The Nature of Leadership.* Salt Lake City, UT: Franklin Covey Co.

Dave L. 2002. On creativity. In Barnes R, Coleman D, Cureton D, et al. (eds.) *Let Your Leadership Speak: How to Lead and Be Heard.* Paxton, MA: The Future Is Yours to Create! Company.

Deal TE, Kennedy AA. 1982. *Corporate Cultures.* Reading, MA: Addison-Wesley.

DeBare I. 1997. 360 Degrees of evaluation: More companies turning to full circle job reviews. *San Francisco Chronicle,* May 5.

DeCoske MA, Tryon JE, White SJ. 2011. *The Pharmacy Leadership Field Guide: Cases and Advice for Everyday Situations.* Bethesda, MD: American Society of Health-System Pharmacists.

Denny NH. 2002. On leading with charisma. In Barnes R, Coleman D, Cureton D, et al. (eds.) *Let Your Leadership Speak: How to Lead and Be Heard.* Paxton, MA: The Future is Yours to Create! Company.

Dye CF. 2000. *Leadership in Healthcare.* Chicago, IL: Health Administration Press, pp. 12, 15.

Edwards MR, Even AJ. 1996. *360-Degree Feedback: The Powerful New Model for Employee Assessment and Performance Improvement.* New York: American Management Association.

Gallup Organization. 1999. What is a great workplace? The twelve key dimensions that describe a great workplace (part 1). *Gallup Manag J,* March 15.

Gallup University. 2011. *Great Manager's Program.* Available at www.gallup.com/university/1399/gallup-university; accessed on August 27, 2011.

Giuliani RW. 2002. *Leadership.* New York: Hyperion, p. xii.

Greenleaf RK. 2002. *Servant Leadership.* New York: Paulist Press.

Haverson R. 2002. On leading with courage. In Barnes R, Coleman D, Cureton D, et al. (eds.) *Let Your Leadership Speak: How to Lead and Be Heard.* Paxton, MA: The Future is Yours to Create! Company.

Hedricks M. 2001. Play to your strengths: Skills testing and evaluation. *Entrepreneur,* May.

Heller R. 1999. *Learning to Lead.* New York, NY: DK Publishing, Inc.

Jones JE. 1976. A review of E. H. Porter's Strength Deployment Inventory. *Group Organ Manag* 1:121–123.

Keim WS. 2002. On becoming an ethical leader. In Barnes R, Coleman D, Cureton D, et al. (eds.) *Let Your Leadership Speak: How to Lead and Be Heard.* Paxton, MA: The Future is Yours to Create! Company.

Kilmann T, Kilmann RH. 1972. *Thomas Kilmann Conflict Mode Instrument.* Palo Alto, CA: CPP, Inc.

Komives SR, Lucas N, McMahon TR. 1998. *Exploring Leadership: For College Students Who Want to Make a Difference.* San Francisco, CA: Jossey-Bass.

Kotter J. 1990. *Leadership Theories: A Force for Change—How Leadership Differs from Management.* New York: Free Press.

Kotter JP. 1996. *Leading Change.* Boston, MA: Harvard Business School Press.

Kouzes JM, Posner BZ. 1987. *The Leadership Challenge.* San Francisco, CA: Jossey-Bass, p. 48.

Kreiter R, Kinicki A. 1997. *Organizational Behavior.* New York: Irwin.

Ledlow GR, Coppola MN. 2011. *Leadership for Health Professionals Theory, Skills, and Applications.* Sudbury, MA: Jones and Barlett Learning.

Lombardi V Jr. 2001. *What It Takes to Be #1: Vincent Lombardi on Leadership.* New York: McGraw-Hill, p. 2.

Malinchak J. 2002. On masterful networking. In Barnes R, Coleman D, Cureton D, et al. (eds.) *Let Your Leadership Speak How to Lead and Be Heard.* Paxton, MA: The Future Is Yours to Create! Company.

Martin J. 2002. On leading by serving. In Barnes R, Coleman D, Cureton D, et al. (eds.) Let Your Leadership Speak: How to Lead and Be Heard. Paxton, MA: The Future Is Yours to Create! Company.

Mason FM, Wetherbee LV. 2004. Learning to lead: An analysis of current training programs for library leadership. *Library Trends* 53:187–217.

Maxwell JC. 1995. *Developing the Leaders Around You in Three Books in One Volume.* Nashville, TN: Nelson Business.

Maxwell JC. 2003. *Developing the Leader within You.* Nashville, TN: Nelson Business.

Myers I, Briggs K. 1988. *Myers–Briggs Type Indicator.* Mountain View, CA: CPP, Inc.

Nanus B. 1992. *Visionary Leadership.* San Francisco, CA: Jossey-Bass, p. 10.

Noce DJD. 1999. Seeing theory in practice: An analysis of empathy in mediation. *Negotiation J* 15:277.

Osborne C. 2008. *Leadership.* New York, NY: DK Publishing, Inc.

Porter E. 1996. *Relationship Awareness Theory.* Carlsbad, CA: Personal Strengths Publishing.

Rath T. 2007. *Now, Discover Your Strengths: StrengthsFinder 2.0.* New York: Gallup Press.

Sathe V. 1985. *Culture and Related Corporate Realities: Text, Cases, and Reading on Organizational Entry, Establishment, and Change.* Homewood, IL: Irwin, p. 6.

Schein EH. 1992. *Organizational Culture and Leadership,* 2nd edn. San Francisco, CA: Jossey-Bass, p. 12.

Scudder T. 1996. *Strength Deployment Inventory.* Carlsbad, CA: Personal Strengths Publishing.

Spears L. 2003. Introduction: Understanding the growing impact of servant leadership. In Beazley H, Beggs J, Spears C (eds.) *The Servant-Leader Within: A Transformative Path.* Mahwah, NJ: Paulist Press.

Stanley A. 2003. *The Next Generation Leader.* Sisters, OR: Multnomah Publishers.

10 Principles of Servant Leadership. 2011. Available at www.butler.edu/volunteer/resources/principles-of-servant leadership; accessed on August 27, 2011.

Tichy N. 1997. *The Leadership Engine.* New York: Harper Collins, p. 42.

Watson G, Glaser E. 2000. Watson–Glaser Critical Thinking Appraisal. San Antonia, TX: Harcourt Brace & Co.

What is 360-Degree Feedback. 2011. Available at www.custominsight.com/360-degree-feedback/what-is-360-degree-feedback.asp; accessed on August 27, 2011.

W. K. Kellogg Foundation Report. 2000. *Leadership Reconsidered: Engaging in Higher Education in Social Change.* Battle Creek, MI: W. K. Kellogg Foundation.

Yaverbaum E, Sherman E. 2008. *The Everything Leadership Book,* 2nd edn. Avon, MA: Adams Media.

SECTION IV

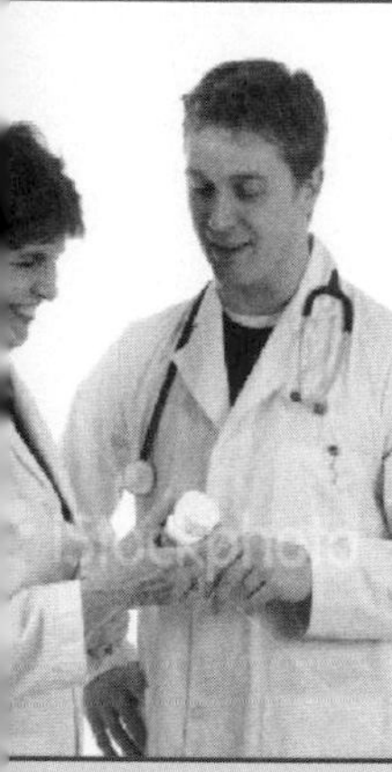

MANAGING MONEY

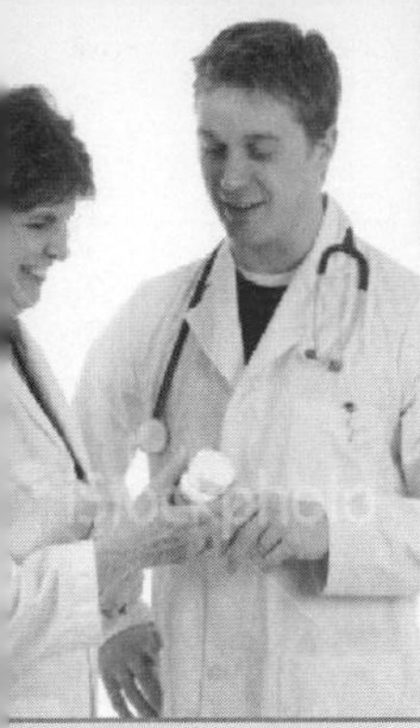

17

FINANCIAL REPORTS

Rashid Mosavin

About the Author: Dr. Mosavin is associate dean of academic affairs and associate professor in the Department of Pharmacotherapy and Outcomes Science at Loma Linda University's School of Pharmacy. He received a B.S. in Pharmacy from the University of Kansas, a Ph.D. in Pharmaceutical Sciences from the University of Wisconsin–Madison, and an MBA from the University of Chicago. He has experience in pharmaceutical industry, hospital pharmacy, and ambulatory care pharmacy settings. His research interests encompass economic evaluation of health care delivery systems and the role of pharmacists in these systems (especially as it relates to management of chronic diseases by pharmacists). Another key area of his research is analysis of economic gains achieved by health information technology implementation in ambulatory care pharmacy practice.

LEARNING OBJECTIVES

After completing this chapter, readers should be able to

1. Compare and contrast the fundamental objectives of a balance sheet and an income statement.
2. Demonstrate the relationship between a balance sheet and an income statement for a given fiscal year.
3. Describe the utility of financial ratios and interpret basic financial ratios used in community pharmacy practice.
4. Describe and integrate the financial information depicted in a balance sheet and an income statement in community pharmacy practice.
5. Define the flow of funds involved in community pharmacy practice, including expenses, prescription adjudication, receipt of payment, and revenue generation.
6. Describe the basic financial and productivity reports used in hospital pharmacy practice.

SCENARIO

It was a beautiful summer day when Marco and Diana met at a coffee shop near where they had gone to pharmacy school. It had been just a couple of years since they had graduated, but they had a lot to catch up on. Marco had always wanted to own a community pharmacy but was currently working in a chain community pharmacy to gain experience and save money. Diana had recently finished a cardiology fellowship and had accepted a clinical faculty position at a large teaching hospital. Diana was interested in hospital pharmacy management and was hoping eventually to be given some administrative and leadership responsibilities in the pharmacy department.

Over the past 2 years, Marco and Diana had begun to gain an appreciation for the need to track the use of money. On a personal level, Marco was beginning to pay off his student loans. Not only was he successfully paying off his loans, he was actually beginning to save some money for his future. While Diana was able to defer payment on her loans during her residency and fellowship, she had to learn to manage her own money wisely, given that she earned substantially less during the past 2 years than many of her friends who took pharmacist positions immediately on graduation. Both were beginning to understand that to become a successful hospital pharmacy administrator or independent pharmacy owner, one needs to also understand how money moves through an organization. Just as Marco and Diana have had to carefully track their own finances to meet their personal financial goals, tracking the uses and flows of money is an essential element in operating any type of pharmacy. They hoped that if they could understand the flows of money in personal finance, they would be able to learn the financial management principles necessary to succeed as pharmacy administrators.

Marco and Diana decided to meet once a month for the next 3 months. Over the course of these meetings, they planned to learn more about accounting, financial reports, and their uses in pharmacies.

CHAPTER QUESTIONS

1. Why is it essential for pharmacy students to understand the fundamentals of financial accounting?
2. Even though they may not be responsible for the organization's financial performance, why is it important for pharmacists to have a basic understanding of the financial reports in their workplace?
3. How do financial reports in hospital pharmacy practice differ in the type and scope of information they contain from the financial reports of a community pharmacy?
4. How would mastering financial reports make a pharmacist a more effective manager?

INTRODUCTION

As mathematics is the language of the physical sciences, accounting is the language of business. The American Institute of Certified Public Accountants (AICPA) defines *accounting* as "a service activity, whose function is to provide quantitative information, primarily financial in nature, about economic entities that is intended to be useful in making economic decisions." Although society may perceive accounting as a mundane task involving the endless juggling of numbers, the truth is that accounting provides the framework for critical decision-making processes essential for the success of any organization. Accounting is the dynamic process by which corporations, small businesses, and even individuals determine and report how they finance their activities and use their money. A major use of accounting is to track the flow of money (cash or credit) between financing and investing activities. Understanding financial reports is essential to understand the flow of money. Financial reports are prepared based on standard accounting principles. Determining profitability, future growth, and tax liability are examples of the vital functions accounting plays in the day-to-day operations of any type of organization or even at the personal level.

Let us use a simple example to define a few terms fundamental to our understanding of an organization's financial health. If your goal is to operate a taxicab, you need to obtain a car. The car is an *asset.* By definition, assets are things that a business owns that can be used to generate income (e.g., driving paying passengers to their destinations in your cab). Obtaining the money needed to acquire an asset requires *financing.* Financing for the taxi may come from a combination of personal savings, gifts, a bank loan, or even money borrowed from friends and relatives. These sources of financing can be further classified as *liabilities* (money owed to others) and *owner's equity* (the owner's own funds). Whatever the total amount invested in an asset, it always must equal the amount financed for its acquisition. If you paid $25,000 for the car, the value of your asset is recorded as $25,000. Now let us say that you financed this asset by putting up $10,000 of your own money and getting a $15,000 from your bank. In accounting language, this *investment* in the *asset* ($25,000 for the car) is financed by *owner's equity* (your $10,000) and a *liability* (the $15,000 you owe the bank).

This brings us to the most important rule in accounting, often referred to as the *accounting equation:*

$$\text{Assets} = \text{owner's equity} + \text{liabilities}$$

This rule always holds, whether you own a small community pharmacy or a major multinational corporation. Mastering this relatively simple equation will help you to better understand even the most complex financial concepts that arise over the course of your professional career!

REVIEW OF ACCOUNTING PRINCIPLES

Accounting principles are essential tools that can be applied in all areas of pharmacy practice (Stickney et al., 2010). This is so because any pharmacy, just as any other type of organization, engages in three fundamental activities:

- Obtaining financing
- Making investments
- Conducting a profitable operation

Obtaining Financing

To start a business, one needs to acquire assets. Financing activities to acquire assets involve obtaining funds from owners as well as creditors (i.e., banks). When owners fund the activities of a corporation, they become shareholders of the corporation. Shareholders have a claim on the company's assets, and their investments in the company are rewarded by either regular distributions from the company to the owners (also known as *dividends*) or by an increase in the value of company's total assets owing to profitable operations.

Creditors, on the other hand, provide funds to the company but do not receive dividends. They require the company to repay the funds with interest over a specified period of time. This period of time can range from days from vendors that supply companies with inventory or raw materials, to years from banks that grant long-term loans. There are many other types of financing, the discussion of which is beyond the scope of this chapter. Interested readers can learn more by reading *Investments* (6th edition) by Bodie et al. (2010) and *Principles of Corporate Finance* (6th edition) by Brealy and Myers (2007).

Making Investments

The types of investments a company makes depend largely on the type of business it is conducting. In pharmacy settings, funds are invested in acquisition of inventory, equipment and supplies, information systems, dispensing systems, buildings, and land. Acquiring the resources necessary to employ the appropriate number of pharmacists, pharmacy technicians, and other staff also can be viewed as an investment activity.

Conducting a Profitable Operation

We started this cycle by obtaining financing for our business. We invested those funds to acquire needed assets. Our final step is to engage in operations. In general, the operating activities of pharmacy settings include purchasing, distribution (i.e., prescription-filling activities), clinical activities, and administration. In many pharmacies, marketing is also a significant operation activity, in that it is required so that others can learn of the goods and services that the pharmacy offers (see Chapters 21 and 22).

THREE ESSENTIAL FINANCIAL STATEMENTS

Most organizations use a number of different financial statements. However, there are three types of financial statements that are essential to the operations of any organization. Before learning about these essential financial statements, though, it is important to define the term *fiscal year.* A fiscal year is a unit of time—a year as the term implies—that businesses use to record their financial interactions. A fiscal year can start on January 1 and end on December 31, or it can start on any other date and end 1 year later. Businesses (such as retail department stores) that experience heavy sales during the month of December usually begin their fiscal years in March or April. Businesses have to pay their taxes to the Internal Revenue Service (IRS) based on dates set by IRS rules regardless of the calendar dates of their fiscal year. IRS rules on corporate taxes are beyond the scope of this discussion, but readers can learn more by visiting the IRS Web site at www.irs.gov (United States Department of the Treasury, 2011). Search the site for Publication 538, Accounting Periods and Methods.

The three financial reports that are essential to the operation of any organization are the *balance sheet,* the *income statement,* and the *statement of cash flows* (Table 17-1). Please note that several other types of financial reports are also generated by organizations that are not discussed in this chapter. A publicly traded organization, that is an organization whose shares are traded on the stock market, is required to file a number of other financial reports with the Securities and Exchange Commission (SEC). One of these reports is Form 10-Q, which describes the organization's quarterly financial performance. The methodology used to prepare these and other financial reports is established by the Financial Accounting Standards Board (FASB) (2007), a nongovernmental agency dedicated to establishing standards in accounting practice.

Table 17-1. Three Main Types of Financial Statements

Type	Use
Balance sheet	Snapshot of the firm's investments (assets) and how they are financed (liabilities and owner's equity)
Income statement	Connects the beginning and ending balance sheets in any given period by providing the details of operating activities (such as sales and expenses)
Statement of cash flow	Connects the beginning and ending balance sheets by indicating the impact of the company's investments, financing, and operations on cash flows

For investor protection, Congress passed the Securities Act of 1933 and the Securities Exchange Act of 1934. These acts provided government oversight on US capital markets to prevent the kind of fraud that had resulted in the 1929 stock market crash. In 1934, Congress established the SEC to enforce the new laws and to provide stability for US capital markets (United States Securities and Exchange Commission, 2011).

The Balance Sheet

Table 17-2 shows the balance sheet for Whole Health Partners Pharmacies (WHP). The *balance sheet* provides a snapshot of an organization's assets, liabilities, and shareholder equity at any particular point in time. While organizations generally prepare a balance sheet at the end of a fiscal year, they may prepare this statement at any point in time (e.g., at the end of a month or a quarter). In holding with the accounting equation described earlier, the balance sheet's total assets must equal the total liabilities plus shareholders' equity at all times.

As of November 1, Year 0, WHP had not yet started operations. However, WHP had acquired all the

Table 17-2. **Whole Health Partners Balance Sheet**

November 1	Year 0 ($)	Year 1 ($)
Assets		
Current assets		
Cash	50,000	100,000
Accounts receivable	0	50,000
Inventories	200,000	300,000
Noncurrent assets		
Building	300,000	300,000
Equipment	50,000	50,000
Total assets	**600,000**	**800,000**
Liabilities		
Current liabilities		
Accounts payable to wholesalers	200,000	170,000
Salaries payable to employees	0	30,000
Noncurrent liabilities		
Bonds payable	100,000	100,000
Total liabilities	**300,000**	**300,000**
Shareholders' equity		
Common stock	300,000	300,000
Retained earnings	0	200,000
Total shareholders' equity	300,000	500,000
Total liabilities and shareholders' equity	**600,000**	**800,000**

assets it needed to begin operations. When we examine WHP's balance sheet after 1 year of operations (Year 1), we notice changes in assets, liabilities, and shareholders' equity. WHP's goal, like that of most businesses, is to increase its assets through profitable operations throughout the fiscal year. Assuming that WHP is able to keep its liabilities unchanged, an increase in assets would result in an increase in shareholders' equity, and that will make for one happy pharmacist owner! Remember that owner's equity represent the funds that an owner puts up to start the business. WHP's balance sheet indicates that the owners started with $300,000 of their own money. At the end of Year 1, the owners have increased this amount by $200,000 to $500,000 owing to profitable operations during Year 1. The owners could leave this extra $200,000 of profit to be used in the business (known as *retained earnings*), or they could take some or all of the money to pay themselves (known as *dividends*).

The Income Statement

The balance sheet in Table 17-2 shows the values of assets, liabilities, and shareholders' equity, but because it is only a snapshot, it does not reveal much about what caused these values to change over the course of the year. The balance sheet also does not tell us how income was generated and what types of expenses were incurred during the accounting period.

The *income statement* is a dynamic document that provides information about money coming into an organization (*income*) and money necessary to obtain that income (*expenses*). The difference between income and expenses is commonly referred to as *net income, net profit,* or *earnings.* The income statement tells the

Table 17-3. Whole Health Partners Income Statement for Year 1 ($)

Revenue	
Sales—prescription	2,000,000
Sales—nonprescription	500,000
Total revenue	**2,500,000**
Expenses	
Cost of goods sold	1,800,000
Administrative expenses	350,000
Income tax expense	50,000
Total expenses	**2,200,000**
Net income	**300,000**

reader what happens to an organization over a period of time. While organizations generally create income statements that span their fiscal year, they often create income statements that describe revenues, expenses, and net income over shorter periods of time, such as quarters, months, weeks, or even over a single day.

Table 17-3 shows WHP's income statement for Year 1. The income statement shows all the operating activities that resulted in either revenues or expenses. It also shows the net income for Year 1. It is important to understand that the terms *net income* and *earnings* are used interchangeably in financial reports. You will note that the net income for Year 1 is $300,000. The balance sheet (Table 17-2) shows retained earnings of $200,000. This is the portion of the net income that the owners have reinvested in the business. Where did the rest ($100,000) of the net income go? It was redistributed among owners as dividends (as depicted in Table 17-4). The connection between the net income value from the income statement and retained earnings from the balance sheet is an example of how these two reports are linked. In this particular example, the details of this linkage can be examined by the statement of retained earnings (Table 17-4).

Table 17-4. Whole Health Partners Statement of Retained Earnings for Year 1 ($)

Retained earnings Year 0	0
Net income Year 1	300,000
Dividends distributed to shareholders	100,000
Retained earnings Year 1	200,000

The Statement of Cash Flows

Throughout the fiscal year, the inflows and outflows of cash are recorded in the *statement of cash flows.* These recorded values generally fall into three categories: operating, investing, and financing. Table 17-5 shows WHP's statement of cash flows. It is customary in accounting to represent negative values (i.e., cash outflows) in parentheses. By the end of Year 1, WHP has increased its cash by $50,000. The last line in the statement of cash flows, indicating the amount of cash available at the end of a fiscal year, is always the same as the amount of cash recorded on the balance sheet for the beginning of the following fiscal year. Once again, you should note the fluid nature of these reports and the degree to which they are linked.

Table 17-5. Whole Health Partners Statement of Cash Flows for Year 1 ($)

Operating	
Revenues providing cash	2,300,000
Expenses using cash	2,150,000
Cash flow from operating	150,000
Investing	
Acquisition of noncurrent assets	0
Sales of noncurrent assets	0
Cash from investing	0
Financing	
Issue of bond	0
Dividends	(100,000)
Cash from financing	(100,000)
Change in cash	50,000
Cash—end of Year 0	50,000
Cash—end of Year 1	100,000

FINANCIAL RATIOS

Organizations, investors, creditors, and even individuals use financial ratios to examine an organization's financial performance. Some financial ratios, such as net income/average total assets, provide useful information on the profitability of the organization. Other ratios can be calculated that provide insight into the liquidity of the organization (how much cash is available to pay the bills) or how well the organization is converting its accounts receivable to cash. Data are taken from the balance sheet and income statement for calculating most ratios. Although financial ratios can be used to quantify many aspects of an organization, they should not be used in isolation from other financial reports. In general, financial ratios allow users of financial information to make comparisons between:

- A single organization and the entire industry average
- Differences within an organization over time (e.g., months, quarters, years)
- Two or more units within a single organization (e.g., pharmacies within the same chain)
- Two or more organizations with each other (e.g., comparisons between chain pharmacy corporations)

Financial ratios should be compared to a reference point (such as historical values of the same company). Financial ratio analysis is only as valid as the financial information on which it is based. If the information provided in the financial statements has not been independently verified (audited), the results of a financial ratio analysis are not likely to give the reader an accurate assessment of the financial performance of that organization. While financial ratio analysis can provide valuable insight to the performance of any organization, it is important that the users of financial ratios are also mindful of their limitations.

When calculating financial ratios for terms shorter than 1 year (i.e., day, week, month, quarter), keep in mind seasonal factors may distort many ratios. For example, over-the-counter (OTC) cold and cough sales may be higher during the winter months than any other time of the year and therefore result in more favorable ratios for the quarter spanning the winter months.

Table 17-6. Financial Ratios

Name	Formula
Profitability ratios	
Gross profit margin	(Sales − cost of goods sold)/total sales
Net profit margin	Net income (after tax)/total sales
Return on assets	Net income/average total assets
Return on equity	Net income/average owner's equity
Liquidity ratios	
Current	Current assets/current liabilities
Quick	Quick assets/current liabilities
Turnover ratios	
Inventory turnover	Cost of goods sold/average inventory
Receivables turnover	Credit sales/average account receivable

Firms may also use different, yet still commonly accepted, accounting methods to prepare their balance sheet and income statement. Therefore, it is imperative to understand how the values used in calculating the ratios were obtained. Remember that standards set by FASB are based on acceptable accounting methods and these methods may vary in how they measure revenues collected (cash vs. credit) or expenses paid (cash vs. accounts payable).

Financial ratios are classified according to the information they provide. Table 17-6 provides a list of selected financial ratios used in various pharmacy settings. Different ratios give different pictures of the company's performance and serve different analytical needs. Profitability ratios, liquidity ratios, and turnover ratios are described below. For further discussion of other financial report ratios, please refer to Stickney et al. (2010).

Profitability Ratios

Since an inherent goal of any business is to be profitable, we can view profitability ratios as measures of overall success in the daily operations of a business. More specifically, profitability ratios provide a method to measure the overall financial success of a company. Examining profitability ratios allows managers to assess the company's level of success in generating profits. The most commonly used profitability ratios in pharmacies are the *gross profit margin* and the *net profit margin.*

Gross profit margin = (sales − cost of goods sold) ÷ total sales

By considering the cost of goods sold (COGS), this ratio provides information on the company's ability to generate gross profits. Higher gross profit margin ratios are desirable because they indicate the availability of funds for the company's other expenses. The typical range for this ratio in retail pharmacy practice is 10% to 40%. Two main factors that influence profitability ratios, and in particular the gross profit margin ratio, are drug prices and reimbursement formulas in third party contracts (see Chapter 19). Pharmacy managers have to monitor reimbursement and drug price changes regularly to ensure a viable gross profit margin ratio.

Net profit margin = net income (after taxes) ÷ total sales

Net profit margin indicates the fraction of net profit that is generated for every dollar of sales. As mentioned earlier, as a profitability ratio, it could be used to determine how well the organization manages its operating expenses. It could also be used to compare the performance of two or more pharmacies within a chain or to assess the performance of a pharmacy against industry performance.

Return on assets (ROA) = net income ÷ average total assets

This ratio provides information on the company's ability to generate profits using the company's assets. As stated in the introduction, profits can only be generated from the company's assets. Therefore, effective use of assets results in a high ROA ratio.

Return on equity (ROE) = net income ÷ average owner's equity

Return on equity, also known as *return on investment* (ROI), is a measure of how well the company can make profits from funds provided by owners or investors. High ROE levels are desirable because investors—similar to companies—are interested in maximizing their profits. ROA and ROE sometimes are used to gauge the manager's performance. All else equal, managers who make better financial decisions are better able to produce higher ROA and ROE ratios for their organizations.

Liquidity Ratios

Liquidity ratios provide information on the business's ability to meet its short-term financial obligations. The most popular liquidity ratios are the *current ratio* and the *quick ratio.*

The *current ratio* is the ratio of current assets to current liabilities.

Current ratio = current assets ÷ current liabilities

An organization with a high current ratio is taking fewer risks in meeting its financial obligations. For example, having a lot of cash in the bank and few debts (*liabilities*) to pay results in a high value for current assets, a low value for liabilities, and therefore a high current ratio. While high current ratio values generally are considered desirable, values greater than 5.0 are considered by some to be too high. This might be a sign of a company that is too conservative, leaving too much of its money in the bank rather than investing it in ways that could help the organization grow (e.g., building new pharmacies or expanding existing services). A low current ratio (<2.0) indicates that the organization has low current assets (especially cash) relative to its current liabilities (often bills that are due in 30 to 60 days). This is not a desirable position for any organization because the inability to pay current liabilities may result in bankruptcy.

An alternative to the current ratio is the *quick ratio* (also known as the *acid test*). For this ratio, *quick assets* are defined as assets that are easily converted to cash. Therefore, inventories and prepaid expenses (such as prepaid rent and insurance policies) are not included in calculating assets. Because the quick ratio considers only assets that are easily converted to cash (and therefore can be used to pay bills, etc.), it provides a better picture of a company's liquidity and its ability to meet its financial obligations.

Quick ratio = (current assets − inventories − prepaid expenses) ÷ current liabilities

The standard quick ratio that any organization strives to obtain is at least 1.0. Simply put, having a quick ratio of greater than 1.0 means that the organization has more quick assets than it has current liabilities. On the other hand, having a quick ratio of less than 1.0 means that the cash that organization has on hand would not be sufficient to pay all its current liabilities, particularly its short-term bills and other obligations.

Now that we have the definition of current ratio and quick ratio, let us calculate these ratios for WHP (see Table 17-2, Year 1). The current ratio at the end of Year 1 is \$450,000 ÷ \$200,000 = 2.25, which appears to be acceptable. However, the amount of quick assets on hand at the end of Year 1 is only \$150,000 (current assets − inventories). The resulting quick ratio is \$150,000 ÷ \$200,000 = 0.75. One concludes from the calculation of these two ratios that WHP has a large inventory (\$300,000) and may have difficulty satisfying its short-term debts. A quick ratio of less than 1 is very alarming. This example also illustrates the point that financial ratios should not be considered in isolation because a single ratio rarely will provide a comprehensive picture of the organization's financial health.

Turnover Ratios

Turnover ratios measure the efficiency with which an organization uses its assets. They are also referred to as *efficiency ratios* or *asset utilization ratios.* The two most commonly used turnover ratios are *inventory turnover* and *receivables turnover.*

Inventory turnover ratio = cost of goods sold ÷ average inventory (at cost)

The inventory turnover ratio measures how quickly, on average, an organization's inventories are sold. The data for this ratio come from two different financial statements. COGS is found on the income statement, and the average inventory comes from the balance sheet. Let us assume that a community pharmacy reported COGS of \$1,200,000 for a given year and an average inventory of \$100,000 over the course of that year. This results in an inventory turnover ratio of 12.0. In other words, the pharmacy is able to sell (and therefore replace) its entire inventory, on average, once a month. If you divide 365 by the inventory turnover ratio, you will have a ratio known as the *days inventory on hand.* This ratio indicates the number of days worth of inventory that is on hand. In the example above, 365/12 = 30.42 days. Clearly, lower values for this ratio would mean more effective inventory management.

Low inventory turnover ratios (6.0 or below) indicate that the organization's inventory is too large for its operations and that cash that could be better spent elsewhere is tied up in inventory. High inventory turnover ratios are generally desirable because this means that the organization was able to sell and replace its inventory with high efficiency and therefore generate higher revenues and profits. Although a high inventory turnover ratio generally is desirable, it can also result in the loss of sales and profits if the average inventory is kept too low. Remember that one can achieve a high inventory ratio by keeping a very small inventory. As the denominator value decreases, the ratio will increase, assuming that all else is unchanged. However, the pharmacy will face chronic shortages during its daily operations that may result in patients switching to other pharmacies for better service.

Receivables turnover ratio = credit sales ÷ average accounts receivable

This ratio measures how quickly receivables (money owed to the organization by others) are turned into cash. A high receivable turnover ratio shows that the organization can collect its receivables efficiently while keeping the total amount it is owed by others at any given time relatively low. If you divide 365 by the receivable turnover ratio, you will have a ratio known as the *average collection period.* The average collection period indicates the number of days (on average) that credit sales remain in accounts receivable before they are collected.

The receivable turnover ratio and the average collection period are particularly important in community pharmacy practice. In the 1950s and 1960s, the majority of expenditures on prescription drugs were paid by patients with cash out of their own pockets. Today, third-party payers [e.g., private insurance, Medicaid, and Medicare Prescription Drug Plans (PDPs)] are responsible for paying the vast majority of these expenditures (see Chapter 19). Unlike patients, who pay their co-payments at the pharmacy when they pick up their prescriptions, third-party payers often take up to 90 to 120 days before they reimburse the pharmacy for prescriptions dispensed. This lag period increases the accounts receivable and depletes the cash reserves of the pharmacy. This becomes a significant problem for independent pharmacies that do not have large cash reserves to cover their expenses (current liabilities) during this period.

Although community pharmacies pay close attention to third-party payer contracts to ensure that they understand the reimbursement timetables, in many instances they are not able to influence the third-party practices. For example, being a pharmacy provider for Medicaid patients is a profitable business for many pharmacies across the nation. However, the contracted pharmacies have very little influence on reimbursement schedules set by the Centers for Medicaid and Medicare Services (CMS).

FINANCIAL REPORTS IN COMMUNITY PHARMACY PRACTICE

Financial reports used in independent pharmacy practice are very similar to those used in chain community pharmacies. Managers in chain community pharmacies pay attention to the same financial ratios and key indicators on balance sheets and income statements. It was with this knowledge that Marco and Diana decided to spend some time with WHP's owner to gain more insight into the preparation and review of financial reports in community pharmacy practice.

Almost all prescriptions filled in a community pharmacy are paid for through a third-party payer, and nearly all of them are adjudicated online. Table 17-7 shows a section of WHP's Daily Plan Payment report. As depicted in this report, the manager is able to monitor the daily number of prescriptions filled for each plan, the total amount paid by each third-party payer, the total co-payments made by patients, and total cost of drug products used to dispense these prescriptions. From this information, the gross margin for each payer

Table 17-7. Whole Health Partners Plan Payment Report for Tuesday, January 2, 2011[a]

Plan ID	Plan Name	Rx's	Rf's	Total Plan Pay ($)	Copay ($)	Cost ($)	Gross Margin (%)
AETNA	AETNA	10	32	851.03	335.30	1,010.18	15
ANTHEM	ANTHEM	7	2	1,096.65	15.00	1,014.49	9
BLCS-D	Blue Cross-D	93	119	14,155.35	432.16	15,316.89	(5)
CIGNA	CIGNA	31	10	1,290.78	562.12	1,426.73	23

[a]Only an excerpt of the entire plan is shown.

can be calculated (as shown in the last column). Daily inspection of this report identifies plans with low reimbursement rates. In addition, when a low gross margin is detected, the manager examines the cost of prescription products dispensed to ensure that the pharmacy has received the best prices from the wholesaler. This is especially true for multisource medications (e.g., generics).

The revenues and expenses from the Daily Plan Payment report are compiled each month and entered into the income statement report (typically by the organization's accountant or bookkeeper, not by the pharmacists themselves). WHP begins its fiscal year on November 1. In addition to the yearly income statement and balance sheet, WHP's accountant prepares a monthly income statement and balance sheet to provide managers with a more precise picture of the financial status of the pharmacy. Before we examine these reports, we have to consider an important point about the preparation of the monthly income statement.

The revenues on the monthly income statement have to be revised once reimbursements have been received from third-party payers. The reason for making adjustments is that most payers make adjustments to each claim and charge the pharmacy administrative fees. Therefore, the actual amount paid to the pharmacy for prescriptions dispensed is almost always lower than the amount indicated on the Daily Plan Payment report. If the manager fails to revise the revenues, the income statement will show artificially inflated revenue. This can have a number of adverse consequences for a pharmacy, including inaccurate financial reports and higher income taxes. In other words, if the revenues are recorded from online adjudications, the pharmacy will pay taxes for revenues it never earned. The pharmacy generally receives the reimbursement check with an Explanation of Benefits (EOB) or Pharmacy Reconciliation Report (PRR) form. This form will show the details of the reimbursement (i.e., beneficiaries' names, prescription numbers, amounts paid for each prescription, and all adjustments and administrative fees deducted). WHP's manager points out that for every $1,000 in third-party reimbursement, the pharmacy may lose $30 to $40 in administrative and other fees. This is a 3 to 4 percent reduction in revenue that should be reconciled on the income statement.

Table 17-8 shows the balance sheet for the last 2 months of WHP's last fiscal year (September and October 2011) and the first month of the next fiscal year (November 2011). After careful examination of the information in Table 17-8, notice that the retained earnings of $825,000 in October is reduced to $798,000 in November. What has caused the retained earnings to drop by $27,000? Did the owners redistribute the funds to themselves as dividends? Table 17-9 depicts the income statement for the last 2 months and the entire 2011 fiscal year. In looking over the yearly income statement (fourth column in Table 15–9), note that WHP recorded a loss of $27,000. In November 2011, the previous year's loss was taken out of the retained earnings. Therefore, the new fiscal year began with $27,000 less in shareholders' equity. Consequently, a reduction in retained earnings on the balance sheet does not provide the reader with concrete evidence of the status of the pharmacy's financial health. Once a change in retained earnings is observed on the balance sheet, one has to further examine the income statement to get a "true" sense of the pharmacy's financial status.

Examining the income statement in Table 17-9, we observe that WHP recorded a significant loss for October 2007. In looking closely at the income and expenses for that month, note that the COGS and total expenses for the month of October are significantly higher than for the previous month. What has caused such a dramatic change in just one month? While there can be many potential reasons for such a change, remember that October is the last month of WHP's fiscal year. Pharmacies often make extra drug purchases and pay more of their expenses before ending their fiscal year. Many managers believe that spending more money at the end of a fiscal year allows them to have more cash throughout the rest of the year to use for financing and investing activities. However, keep in mind that all necessary inventory purchases and other expenses have to take place and be recorded so that the net income for the year is not artificially inflated. This is another reason why it is important to evaluate

Table 17-8. Whole Health Partners Balance Sheet

Assets	**September 2011 ($)**	**October 2011 ($)**	**November 2011 ($)**
Current assets			
Petty cash	1,500	1,500	1,500
Cash in bank	105,000	133,000	75,000
Accounts receivable	680,000	658,000	776,000
Allow for doubtful accounts	(16,000)	(16,000)	(16,000)
Inventory—prescription	378,000	441,000	440,000
Inventory—other	17,000	20,000	19,000
Prepaid federal income tax	33,000	44,000	44,000
Prepaid state income tax	16,000	15,000	15,000
Total current assets	1,214,500	1,296,500	1,354,500
Noncurrent assets			
Automobiles	50,000	50,000	50,000
Machinery and equipment	130,000	130,000	130,000
Office equipment	140,000	140,000	140,000
Leasehold improvements	97,000	97,000	97,000
Accumulated depreciation	(308,000)	(310,000)	(313,000)
Total noncurrent assets	109,000	107,000	104,000
Total assets	**1,323,500**	**1,403,500**	**1,458,500**
Liabilities			
Current liabilities			
Accounts payable	223,000	393,000	369,500
Line of credit—Wells Fargo	60,000	55,000	55,000
Payroll taxes payable	0	30,000	0
Sales tax payable	500	500	1,000
Federal income tax pay—current	90,000	0	100,000
State income tax pay—current	25,000	0	35,000
Total current liabilities	398,500	478,500	560,500
Noncurrent liabilities			
Note payable	40,000	40,000	40,000
Loan payable	50,000	50,000	50,000
Total noncurrent liabilities	90,000	90,000	90,000
Total liabilities	**488,500**	**568,500**	**650,500**
Shareholders' equity			
Common stock	10,000	10,000	10,000
Retained earnings	825,000	825,000	798,000
Total shareholders' equity	**835,000**	**835,000**	**808,000**
Total liabilities and shareholders' equity	**1,323,500**	**1,403,500**	**1,458,500**

Table 17-9. Whole Health Partners Income Statement

	September 2011 ($)	October 2011 ($)	Fiscal Year 2011 ($)
Income			
Sales—current prescriptions	702,000	864,000	9,313,000
Sales—taxables	5,000	8,000	80,000
Total income	**707,000**	**872,000**	**9,393,000**
Cost of sales			
Purchases—prescriptions	623,000	920,000	7,600,000
Purchases—other	400	1,000	18,000
Purchases—supplies	0	600	2,000
Total cost of sales	**623,400**	**921,600**	**7,620,000**
Gross profit on sales	**83,600**	**(49,600)**	**1,773,000**
General and administrative expenses			
Advertising	1,400	1,500	25,000
Automobile	2,900	2,900	25,000
Bank charges	0	600	14,000
Billing services	0	4,000	26,000
Benefits	7,000	7,000	82,000
Depreciation	2,000	2,000	26,000
Dues and subscriptions	150	150	500
Interest expense	4,000	3,800	15,000
Insurance—general	400	8,000	50,000
Legal and accounting	1,000	2,500	29,000
Licenses	500	500	6,000
Maintenance and repairs	0	3,500	7,000
Meals and entertainment	1,000	2,400	22,000
Office expense	1,500	6,500	4,500
Office salaries	52,000	52,000	650,000
Officer salaries	19,000	100,000	422,000
Outside services	9,000	12,000	100,000
Postage	400	400	1,500
Pension plan expense	2,400	50,000	54,000
Promotion	400	400	1,500
Rent	8,000	8,000	95,000
Taxes—payroll	3,800	4,900	70,000
Telephone	1,900	2,600	20,000
Travel	0	0	4,000
Utilities	1,100	1,000	10,000
Total general and administrative expenses	**119,850**	**277,150**	**1,800,000**
Net income	**(36,250)**	**(326,750)**	**(27,000)**

more than a single income statement or balance sheet when evaluating the financial performance of any organization.

FINANCIAL REPORTS IN HOSPITAL PHARMACY PRACTICE

Financial reports used to manage the department of pharmacy in hospitals are often quite different from those used in community pharmacy practice. The budget for a hospital pharmacy department is primarily composed of drug costs and labor (pharmacists, technicians, and administrators) and is a part of the global budget of the entire hospital. Drug costs are generally the larger of the two components, although this varies with the size of the hospital, the size of the pharmacy department, and the types of clinical and distributive services the hospital provides. Interested readers should review the book *Financial Management for Health-System Pharmacists* by Andrew Wilson (2009) for more information about financial statements used in hospitals and hospital pharmacies.

The four management principles discussed in Chapter 2 (plan, organize, lead, and control) are relevant in the financial planning of a hospital's pharmacy department. The financial stability of the department will depend on planning and implementation of financial management programs that span these four principles.

The director of pharmacy is responsible for the creation of policies and procedures to manage expenditures. These include, but are not limited to, group purchasing, utilization review protocols, and cost-effective clinical pharmacy services (Pederson et al., 2009). In their efforts to manage expenditures, hospital pharmacy directors are faced with a set of unique challenges unlike those seen in community pharmacy. While all pharmacies have experienced large increases in the costs of drug products since the 1990s (often greater than 10 percent per year), unlike community pharmacies, hospitals generally cannot pass on higher drug costs to consumers in the form of higher prices for their goods and services. Medicare and other payers often use prospective payment systems in hospitals (see Chapters 19 and 20), in which they are provided with fixed payments based on a patient's diagnosis or the number of lives they agree to provide services for over a given period of time. While community pharmacies generally can improve their profitability by selling more goods and providing more services, hospital pharmacies generally cannot "sell" their goods and services because their payers are paying a set amount regardless of how many drugs the hospital dispenses or clinical services it provides. While community pharmacies generally are considered to be *profit centers,* hospital pharmacy departments are considered to be *cost centers* because they do not generate revenue directly and only help to contribute to their hospitals' overall profitability by using drug therapy and clinical pharmacy services to help lower the overall cost of caring for patients. The director of pharmacy manages the performance of this cost center by evaluating complex financial reports that compare actual with budgeted values and the variance between budgeted and actual costs.

The director of pharmacy uses an expense report prepared on a monthly or weekly basis. In this report, all pharmacy department expenses are categorized into at least five major sections. Each expense is also given a unique code so that not only the pharmacy department but also the hospital's central accounting office can access and monitor expenses. The expense report indicates the amount budgeted for each expense, the actual expense incurred, the variance between budgeted and incurred expenses, and the variance percentage. Table 17-10 shows an abbreviated, simplified expense report for the pharmacy department of a large tertiary-care hospital.

The pharmacy expense report consolidates the expenses for the month and compares the actual expenses against the budgeted expenses for the month. The value of this report lies with the comparisons of the total expense for the current year and the variances for the monthly and yearly expenses for the previous year. This allows the manager to identify potential trends or expenses that could be outliers and evaluate how to bring

Table 17-10. Pharmacy Department Expense Report—Actual Versus Budgeted

	August 2011—Monthly				2011—Year to Date (YTD)				Monthly Last Year		YTD Last Year	
Payroll	**Actual ($)**	**Budget ($)**	**Variance ($)**	**Variance (%)**	**Actual ($)**	**Budget ($)**	**Variance ($)**	**Variance (%)**	**Actual ($)**	**Variance (%)**	**Actual ($)**	**Variance (%)**
Ancillary												
Manager/Supervisor	37,916	37,520	396	1.1	301,204	300,160	1,044	0.3	36,541	3.6	298,587	0.9
Technicians/Interns	68,521	70,250	−1,729	−2.5	568,240	562,000	6,240	1.1	67,526	1.5	562,458	1.0
Pharmacists	210,354	210,500	−146	−0.1	1,682,504	1,684,000	−1,496	−0.1	210,586	−0.1	1,602,485	4.8
Administrative	3,825	3,805	20	0.5	29,864	30,440	−576	−1.9	3,912	−2.3	28,862	3.4
Subtotal ancillary	320,616	322,075	−1,459	−0.5	2,581,812	2,576,600	5,212	0.2	318,565	0.6	2,492,392	3.5
Employee benefits												
Benefits—medical/dental	21,058	21,500	−442	−2.1	175,481	172,000	3,481	2.0	22,015	−4.5	176,982	−0.9
Vacation/Sick leave	9,572	8,500	1,072	12.6	67,524	68,000	−476	−0.7	9,632	−0.6	66,057	2.2
Payroll taxes	72,545	73,000	−455	−0.6	594,214	584,000	10,214	1.7	71,523	1.4	584,672	1.6
Subtotal employee benefits	103,175	103,000	175	0.2	837,219	824,000	13,219	1.6	103,170	0.0	827,711	1.1
Subtotal payroll	423,791	425,075	−1,284	−0.3	3,419,031	3,400,600	18,431	0.5	421,735	0.5	3,320,103	2.9

(continued)

Table 17-10. Pharmacy Department Expense Report—Actual Versus Budgeted (*Continued*)

	August 2011—Monthly				2011—Year to Date (YTD)				Monthly Last Year		YTD Last Year	
Nonpayroll	**Actual ($)**	**Budget ($)**	**Variance ($)**	**Variance (%)**	**Actual ($)**	**Budget ($)**	**Variance ($)**	**Variance (%)**	**Actual ($)**	**Variance (%)**	**Actual ($)**	**Variance (%)**
Direct materials												
IV and irrigations solutions	4,528	7,510	−2,982	−39.7	58,796	60,080	−1,284	−2.1	4,689	−3.6	61,865	−5.2
IV supplies	8,650	6,585	2,065	31.4	51,248	52,680	−1,432	−2.7	8,542	1.2	49,879	2.7
Chemotherapy drugs	72,505	75,000	−2,495	−3.3	632,541	600,000	32,541	5.4	61,535	15.1	602,045	4.8
Noninjectable drugs	165,258	158,652	6,606	4.2	1,284,576	1,269,216	15,360	1.2	151,897	8.1	1,225,483	4.6
Injectable drugs	637,265	625,800	11,465	1.8	5,012,478	5,006,400	6,078	0.1	588,963	7.6	4,701,756	6.2
Office supplies	1,850	1,925	−75	−3.9	13,458	15,400	−1,942	−12.6	1,763	4.7	12,647	6.0
Equipment repair	754	800	−46	−5.8	4,215	6,400	−2,185	−34.1	651	13.7	3,897	7.5
Subtotal direct materials	890,810	876,272	14,538	1.7	7,057,312	7,010,176	47,136	0.7	818,040	8.2	6,657,572	5.7
Other nonpayroll												
Business meetings/travel/meals	564	600	−36	−6.0	3,524	4,800	−1,276	−26.6	423	25.0	4,635	−31.5
Reference materials/subscriptions	358	450	−92	−20.4	3,049	3,600	−551	−15.3	348	2.8	3,524	−15.6
Training expenses	495	350	145	41.4	1,786	2,800	−1,014	−36.2	267	46.1	2,227	−24.7
Other miscellaneous expense	865	650	215	33.1	5,432	5,200	232	4.5	792	8.4	5,189	4.5
Subtotal other nonpayroll	2,282	2,050	232	11.3	13,791	16,400	−2,609	−15.9	1,830	19.8	15,575	−12.9
Subtotal nonpayroll	893,092	878,322	14,770	1.7	7,071,103	7,026,576	44,527	0.6	819,870	8.2	6,673,147	5.6
Total expenses	1,316,883	1,303,397	13,486	1.0	10,490,134	10,427,176	62,958	0.6	1,241,605	5.7	9,993,250	4.7

Table 17-11. Full-Time Equivalents (FTEs) and Overtime Productivity

	Actual	Budget	Variance
Paid FTEs per pay period	39	38	1
YTD paid FTEs	38.5	38	0.5
Overtime analysis			
Overtime dollars per pay period	$3,521	$2,500	$1,021
Percent overtime per pay period	6.5%	5.0%	1.5%
YTD payroll overtime dollars	$98,754	$85,246	$13,508
YTD percent overtime of total payroll	5.9%	4.5%	1.4%

YTD, year to date.

the expenses back to budget. For example, uncertainty on the cost and the release date of newly approved drugs and personnel variances such as staff overtime duc to poor managing of the schedule can be effectively analyzed and corrective action taken. Categories with a positive value for variance (and variance %) indicate that department has spent more money than it had budgeted for those categories. Positive values for variance (and variance %) for year-to-date figures also indicate that department is spending more funds this year as compared with the previous year. Conversely, negative variance values are indicative of lower than budgeted expenditures and certainly desirable from the manager's perspective.

An important element of financial cost analysis in the pharmacy department is the development of productivity assessment reports. Most directors of pharmacy prepare a productivity report for each pay period in which the number of full-time equivalents (FTEs) and the quantity of outputs (such as clinical services provided by pharmacists) are analyzed. These reports are useful because they enable managers to use historical data to create budgets and monitor trends over time.

Besides the pharmaceuticals, labor is the other major expense of a pharmacy. The FTE and overtime report helps the manager determine if the correct number of employees are working for a given pay period, as well as the total for the year. It is important to look at the total expense for the year, as this will smooth out pay period variations in staffing that can take place due to vacation coverage and holidays. Evaluating the amount of labor that is caused by overtime will help the manager determine if the department has the correct mix of full-time, part-time, and per diem employees, which can be used appropriately to decrease the amount of overtime for the department. Table 17-11 depicts the FTE and overtime productivity report of the pharmacy department. The table shows actual versus budgeted and percent variance of FTEs. In addition, the report provides information on the cost of overtime pay for the pay period and year to date. For an in-depth discussion of productivity monitoring in hospital pharmacy practice, see Rough et al. (2010a, 2010b). There are a number of productivity ratios that can be used in the inpatient pharmacy to determine the productivity of the department. Table 17-12 depicts the names and definitions of five of the most commonly used productivity ratios in hospital pharmacy practice.

Finally, the director of pharmacy pays special attention to external financial reports. Professional associations such as the American Hospital Association and the American Society for Health-System Pharmacists publish reports that show the national trends in pharmaceutical expenditures and labor productivity in hospitals (American Hospital Association, 2011; Doloresco et al., 2011). Pharmacy managers can gauge the efficiency of their operations by comparing their

Table 17-12. Productivity Ratios

Patient days	The total number of days patients are in the hospital occupying a bed for a given time period
Case mix index (patient acuity factor)	An indicator of the level of severity of the patients which are classified by disease, diagnostic or therapeutic procedures performed, method of payment, duration of hospitalization, and intensity and type of services provided by the facility for a given time period
Full-time equivalents (FTEs) per occupied bed	A measurement of the number of full-time workers who used to care for each bed occupied by a patient
Drug cost per patient day	The cost of the drugs purchased by the pharmacy divided by the number of patient days of the facility
Labor cost per patient day	The cost of the labor (salary and benefits) divided by the number of patient days of the facility.

financial and productivity ratios and with national averages.

CONCLUSION

Familiarity with basic accounting concepts and preparation of financial reports is essential knowledge for every pharmacist. The financial success of any organization depends on proper management of its funds. Those who understand how organizations finance operations, generate revenue, and allocate financial resources will have an easier task understanding many of the factors that affect their success.

QUESTIONS FOR FURTHER DISCUSSION

1. Marco has found two other pharmacists willing to invest in purchasing an existing community pharmacy. This pharmacy has been open for only 2 years and is located in the lobby of an ambulatory-care clinic affiliated with a 200-bed community hospital. This year, the pharmacy is projected to have sales of $2 million.
   a. To prepare for purchasing negotiations, what financial documents should Marco review? Name specific financial indicators that Marco should pay special attention to as he reviews these documents.
   b. Based on the material in this and other chapters in this book, what strategies should Marco employ to increase prescription volume, increase pharmacy revenues, and ensure the pharmacy's long-term success?
2. A few years after Marco and his associates purchase this pharmacy, the director of the affiliated hospital pharmacy retires. Marco announces this news to Diana and encourages her to apply for the position. Diana begins to update her résumé and prepare a letter of intent.
   a. What type of questions should Diana ask during an interview to gain insight into the pharmacy department's financial status? What key financial indicators should hospital administration share with Diana to convince her of the pharmacy department's financial strengths?
   b. Based on the material in this chapter and other chapters in this book, what strategies should Diana employ to ensure the pharmacy department's long-term success?

GLOSSARY

Bond A long-term debt type of security generally issued by corporations or governments to generate cash. The *coupon rate* is the interest rate paid to the bondholder. The *maturity date* is when the face value of the bond will be paid to the bondholder.

Cost center A unit of an organization for which costs are recorded and analyzed. In general, cost centers add to the overall cost of the organization but contribute to the profits of the organization indirectly. Some examples of cost centers are customer-service centers and research and development departments.

Dividend Distribution of a portion of a company's net income to its shareholders.

Current ratio A liquidity ratio that reflects a company's ability to satisfy its short-term financial obligations.

Quick ratio A liquidity ratio that reflects a company's ability to satisfy its short-term obligations with its most liquid assets.

Inventory turnover A ratio that reflects the number of times in a fiscal year that a pharmacy's inventory is sold and replaced.

Receivables turnover A ratio that reflects a pharmacy's ability to collect its debt and extend credit to its customers.

Gross profit margin Also known as *gross margin*, this represents the amount of money left in a firm once the cost of goods sold is subtracted from revenues. It reflects the company's ability to pay for its other expenses.

Net profit margin A profitability ratio that indicates the fraction of net profit generated for every dollar of sales. It is calculated by dividing net income after taxes by total sales.

Return on assets A profitability ratio reflecting a company's ability to generate net income as a percentage of its total assets.

Return on equity A profitability ratio reflecting a company's ability to generate net income as a percentage of total investments by shareholders.

ACKNOWLEDGMENTS

First and foremost, I am indebted to my administrative assistant, Ms. Cynthia Johnson, for her talented work in the preparation of this manuscript. I would like to thank Dale J. Timothy, RPh, MBA, director of Inpatient Pharmacy at Kaiser Permanente Riverside Medical Center in Riverside, CA, for his contributions to the "Financial Reports in Hospital Pharmacy Practice" Section of this chapter. I would also like to thank Dr. Robert Beeman, owner of Beeman Pharmacies in San Bernardino, CA, for his consultations and contributions to the "Financial Reports in Community Pharmacy Practice" Section of this chapter.

REFERENCES

American Hospital Association. Health Care Statistics and Market Research Data. 2011. Available at www.ahadata.com/ahadata_app/index.jsp; accessed on February 24, 2012.

Bodie Z, Kane A, Marcus A. 2010. *Investments*, 6th edn. New York: McGraw-Hill.

Brealy R, Myers S. 2007. *Principles of Corporate Finance*, 6th edn. New York: McGraw-Hill/Irwin.

Doloresco F, Fominaya C, Schumock G, et al. 2011. Projecting future drug expenditures 2011. *Am J Health Syst Pharm* 68:921.

Financial Accounting Standards Board. 2007. Available at www.fasb.org; accessed on November 12, 2007.

Pederson C, Schneider P, Scheckelhoff D. 2009. ASHP national survey of pharmacy practice in hospital settings: Dispensing and administration—2008. *Am J Health Syst Pharm* 66:926.

Rough S, McDaniel M, Rinehart J. 2010a. Effective use of workload and productivity monitoring tools in health-system pharmacy, part 1. *Am J Health Syst Pharm* 67: 300.

Rough S, McDaniel M, Rinehart J. 2010b. Effective use of workload and productivity monitoring tools in health-system pharmacy, part 2. *Am J Health Syst Pharm* 67: 380

Stickney C, Weil R, Schipper K, Francis J. 2010. *Financial Accounting: An Introduction to Concepts, Methods, and Uses*, 13th edn. New York: Harcourt.

United States Department of the Treasury, Internal Revenue Service. 2011. Available at www.irs.gov/businesses/index.html?navmenu=menu1; accessed February 24, 2012.

United States Securities and Exchange Commission. 2011. Available at www.sec.gov; accessed February 24, 2012.

Wilson AL. 2009. *Financial Management for Health Systems Pharmacists.* Bethesda, MD: American Society of Health-Systems Pharmacists.

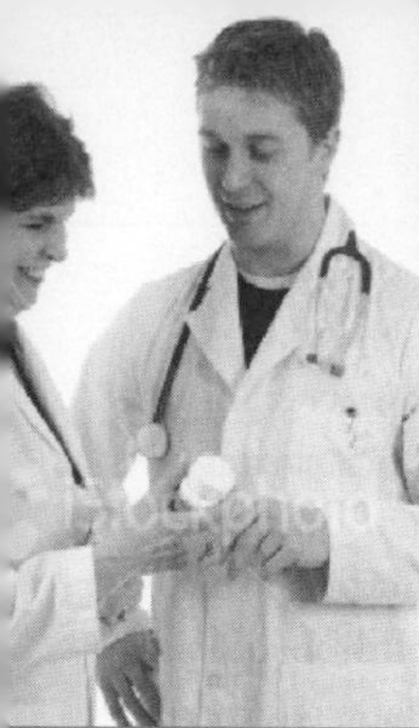

18

BUDGETING

David A. Gettman

About the Author: Dr. Gettman is a professor in the Department of Pharmaceutical, Administrative, and Social Sciences at the D'Youville College School of Pharmacy. He received a B.S. in pharmacy from the University of Montana, an MBA from the College of William and Mary, and a Ph.D. in pharmacy health care administration from the University of Florida. He has practiced pharmacy in numerous settings, including community, hospital, nursing home, hospice, and in the US Navy and Air Force. In addition to pharmacy management, Dr. Gettman has taught pharmacy law, health care ethics, health care delivery, pharmacoepidemiology, pharmacoeconomics, biostatistics, and research design. The author of numerous publications, he has made over 100 presentations to professional health care groups at the state, national, and international levels.

LEARNING OBJECTIVES

After completing this chapter, readers should be able to

1. List and explain five purposes of budgeting systems.
2. Describe the similarities and differences in the operational budgets prepared by pharmaceutical manufacturers, health system pharmacies offering value-added services, community pharmacies selling merchandise, and nonprofit pharmacy organizations.
3. Explain the concept of activity-based budgeting and the benefits it brings to the budgeting process.
4. Describe each of the budget schedules that make up a master budget.
5. Discuss the role of assumptions and predictions in budgeting.
6. Describe a typical pharmacy organization's process of budget administration.
7. Understand the importance of budgeting product life-cycle costs.
8. Discuss the behavioral implications of budgetary slack and participative budgeting.

SCENARIO

Mary Quint, pharmacy student, has just started a 6-week elective advanced pharmacy practice experience (APPE) at Home TPN Care. On this APPE, Mary is working with Anne Smith, Pharm.D., who manages the production and distribution of total parenteral nutrition (TPN).

Home TPN Care is part of a local university's health system that includes a large teaching hospital, several clinics, and numerous ancillary services. Procurement, receiving, insurance verification, claims processing, and cash application operation activities all take place at the Home TPN Care facility, located 5 miles away from its main hospital. Home TPN Care consistently generates a positive net margin that contributes to the health system's margin targets and support of non–revenue-generating activities. Clinical, patient care, quality, and process improvement programs are integrated into the health system's strategic plan.

Home TPN Care is a licensed pharmacy and home infusion provider responsible for providing a wide range of products and services to safely and effectively facilitate care to patients in the convenience and comfort of their homes. Since 2001, Home TPN Care has been providing infusion medications, nutritional therapy, specialty drugs, high-tech infusion nursing, and care management services throughout the region. An interdisciplinary team of pharmacists, nurses, and dietitians, along with technical, administrative, and support staff, provides pharmacy manufacturing (i.e., compounding), equipment management, dispensing, delivery, and care management services to ensure that patient home regimens are safe and effective throughout the course of therapy. The staff has direct access to up-to-date and complete medical and patient drug information that facilitates effective and efficient collaboration with physicians and other caregivers within the organization. To ensure a smooth transition to home care, Home TPN Care has a training and education team. This team consists of nurses and dietitians who work with patients and the referring health care team to ensure that home care needs are identified prior to hospital discharge and infusion nurses who provide care for patients in their homes.

Although Home TPN Care resides within the home care service division in the health system's organizational structure, an administrative relationship exists between Home TPN Care and the health system's department of pharmacy services. Thus, many administrative, pharmacy practice, and educational activities are collaborative and integrated. There is Home TPN Care representation on several pharmacy department committees. In addition, most of the Home TPN Care's health care professionals hold academic appointments within the university, reflecting a commitment to teaching, experiential training, and research.

Mary Quint has been advised that during this APPE she will need to assist Dr. Smith to develop a master budget, or profit plan, for Home TPN Care. It quickly became apparent that she would need to review the materials she studied in her pharmacy management course about budgeting before she could tackle this important challenge.

CHAPTER QUESTIONS

1. How does a budget facilitate communication and coordination in a pharmacy organization?
2. What is a master budget, and what are the parts of a master budget?
3. What is meant by the term *operational budgets*?
4. How does activity-based budgeting differ from more traditional budgeting methods?
5. How does e-budgeting make use of the Internet?
6. What is the purpose of a budget manual?
7. Is padding the budget unethical?
8. What is budgetary slack, and what problem(s) can it cause?

INTRODUCTION

Developing a budget is a critical step in planning any economic activity. This is true for any type of pharmacy operation, for individual pharmacists, and for governmental agencies that regulate both pharmacies and individual pharmacists. As individuals, we all must budget our money to meet day-to-day expenses and plan for major expenditures, such as buying a car.

Similarly, pharmacies of all types and governmental agencies must make financial plans to carry out routine operations, to plan for major expenditures, and to help in making financial decisions.

■ PURPOSES OF BUDGETING SYSTEMS

A *budget* is a detailed plan, expressed in quantitative terms, that specifies how resources will be acquired and used during a specified period of time. The procedures used to develop a budget constitute a *budgeting system.* Budgeting systems have five primary purposes.

Planning

The most obvious purpose of a budget is to quantify a plan of action. The budgeting process forces people who make up an organization to anticipate or react to changes in the environment. For example, the U.S. Food and Drug Administration's (FDA) approval of capecitabine, an oral form of fluorouracil, in 1998, and imatinib mesylate, an oral agent used in the treatment of chronic myeloid leukemia, in 2001, signaled a new period in budget planning for pharmacies and for those who pay for pharmacy benefits. The introduction of expensive new drug therapies can be of particular concern for small, self-insured employers, for whom drugs with a cost of $25,000 to $50,000 or more per year of therapy for one patient could increase the total costs of providing a pharmacy benefit to their employees by 10 percent or more (Curtiss, 2006).

Planning is also very important at the level of the practicing pharmacist. A good example involves the planning for vaccinations at pharmacy-based clinics. In a recent article, the authors describe a mass vaccination clinic budgeting tool that clinic managers may use to estimate clinic costs and to examine how costs vary depending on the availability of volunteers or donated supplies and on the number of patients vaccinated per hour. The tool can also contribute to planning efforts for universal seasonal influenza vaccination (Cho et al., 2011). For novel vaccines (e.g., rotavirus, respiratory syncytial virus, human papilloma virus, and herpes zoster), another author describes a more tailored planning approach based on the individual characteristics and use of each product (Cannon, 2007).

Facilitating Communication and Coordination

For any organization to be effective, each manager must be aware of plans made by other managers. The budgeting process must pull together the plans, financial as well as operational, of each manager in an organization. For example, pharmaceutical companies who market products with "blockbuster" potential are often developed by groups of researchers and project managers around the world. These managers require coordinated financial information at the local, national, and global levels (Cowlrick et al., 2002).

Moving closer to the level of the practicing pharmacist communication and coordination is also very important. For example, the use of radio-frequency identification tags (RFID) to monitor drug movement is a relatively recent phenomenon, but one that is long overdue. With the increases in drug counterfeiting and diversion across the world, pharmaceutical companies are striving to maintain top safety standards to keep their product in safe hands. Progressively, companies are coming to realize the value of containing data in an e-pedigree that can help them improve the reconciliation processes, such as returns and recalls. Other companies will soon benefit from RFID technologies to increase patient safety, enhance collaboration within the supply chain, and improve business performance (Bodine, 2007).

Allocating Resources

All resources are limited, including those used by pharmacists and pharmacies. Budgets provide one means of allocating resources among competing uses. Hospitals, for example, must make difficult decisions about allocating their revenue among services (e.g., pharmacy, laboratory, and nursing), maintenance of property and equipment (e.g., beds, laminar flow hoods, and vehicles), and other community services (e.g., child care services and programs to prevent alcohol and drug abuse). In particular, allocating resources to pharmacy initiatives to improve patient safety often competes with initiatives from nursing and other areas where dollars are also needed to improve patient care (Tierney, 2004).

Controlling Profit and Operations

A budget is a plan, and plans are subject to change. A budget serves as a useful benchmark against which actual results can be compared. For example, a community pharmacy can compare its actual sales of prescriptions for a year against its budgeted sales. Such comparisons can help managers evaluate the pharmacy's effectiveness in selling prescriptions. Pharmacy managers must be prepared and make changes when facing a financial crisis, such as when facing an unanticipated decline in sales or revenues or an increase in expenses. Managers facing these situations must take the initiative to acquire the necessary data, to translate data into relevant information, to seek benchmarks for comparison, and to take corrective action. Once the crisis has passed, attention must be given to updating and maintaining databases, supporting the staff, and improving morale. Scenario planning can help to identify measures that might be taken should another crisis develop (Demers, 2001).

Evaluating Performance and Providing Incentives

Comparing actual results with budgeted results also helps pharmacy managers evaluate the performance of individuals, departments, or entire corporations. Since budgets are used to evaluate performance, they can also be used to provide incentives for people to perform well. Many health care organizations are beginning to implement pay-for-performance (P4P) programs that tie monetary incentives for pharmacy personnel to hospital quality scores (Gregg et al., 2006).

TYPES OF BUDGETS

Different types of budgets serve different purposes. A *master budget,* or *profit plan,* is a comprehensive set of budgets covering all phases of a pharmacy organization's operations for a specified period of time.

Budgeted financial statements, often called *pro forma financial statements,* project how the pharmacy organization's financial statements will appear at a specified time if operations proceed according to plan. Budgeted financial statements include a budgeted income statement, a budgeted balance sheet, and a budgeted statement of cash flows.

A *capital budget* is a plan for the acquisition of capital assets, such as buildings and equipment. A *financial budget* is a plan that shows how the pharmacy business will acquire its financial resources, such as through the issuance of stock or incurrence of debt.

Budgets are developed for specific time periods. *Short-range budgets* cover a year, a quarter, or a month, whereas *long-range budgets* cover periods longer than a year. *Rolling budgets* are continually updated by periodically adding a new incremental time period, such as a quarter, and dropping the period just completed. Rolling budgets are also called *revolving budgets or continuous budgets.*

THE MASTER BUDGET: A PLANNING TOOL

The *master budget,* the principal output of a budgeting system, is a comprehensive profit plan that ties together all phases of a pharmacy's operations. The master budget consists of many separate budgets, or schedules, that are interdependent. Figure 18-1 portrays these interrelationships in a flowchart.

Sales of Services or Goods

The starting point for any master budget is a *sales revenue budget.* For many pharmacy departments, this budget begins with a sales forecast for prescription drug spending. A pharmacy manager would need to keep abreast of how changes in government expenditures (e.g., Medicare prescription drug coverage) might change the distribution of drug spending among payers and affect aggregate spending (Poisal et al., 2007).

Sales Forecasting

All pharmacies have two things in common when it comes to forecasting sales of services or goods. Sales forecasting is a critical step in the budgeting process, and it is very difficult to do accurately.

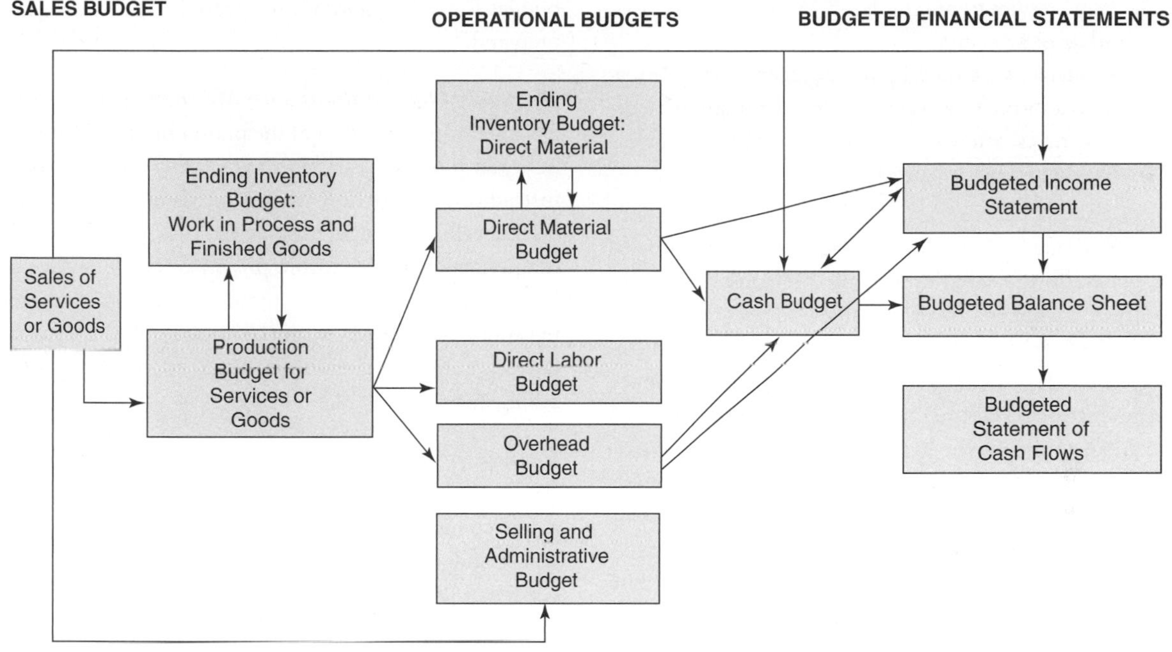

Figure 18-1. Master budget components.

Various procedures are used in sales forecasting, and the final forecast usually combines information from many different sources. Many pharmacy corporations have a market research staff whose job is to coordinate the corporation's sales forecasting efforts. Typically, everyone from key executives to the firm's sales personnel will be asked to contribute sales projections.

Major factors considered when forecasting sales include the following:

1. Past sales levels and trends
    - For the firm developing the forecast (e.g., Walgreen's)
    - For the entire industry (e.g., the chain drug store industry)
2. General economic trends
    - Is the economy growing? How fast?
    - Is a recession or economic slowdown expected?
3. Economic trends in the pharmaceutical industry
    - Changes in the types of goods and services offered by pharmacies
    - Changes in the competitive environment between pharmacies
    - Changes in the demographic characteristics of pharmacy customers
4. Other factors which may affect sales in pharmacies
    - Is an unusually cold winter expected, which would result in increased demand for cold remedies in chain drug stores located in northern climates?
5. Political and legal events
    - Impact of new laws on sales of pharmacy goods and services (e.g., Medicare Part D, Affordable Care Act)
    - Prescription to over-the-counter switches
6. The intended pricing policy of the pharmacy
7. Planned promotional activities
8. Expected actions of competitors

9. New services contemplated by the pharmacy or other pharmacies
   - Medication therapy management (MTM) services may increase the demand for some medications, while decreasing demand for others
10. Market research studies

The starting point in the sales forecasting process is generally the sales level of the previous year. Then budget managers must consider all of the factors described earlier and project the likely impact each will have on sales in the coming year. In many pharmacy organizations, elaborate econometric models are used to incorporate all the available information systematically. Statistical methods, such as regression analysis and probability distributions for sales, may also be used, particularly in large, multiunit organizations. A great deal of effort goes into the sales forecast because it is such a critical step in the budgeting process. Even a slightly inaccurate sales forecast, coming at the very beginning of the budgeting process, will likely disrupt all the other schedules, which comprise the master budget.

Operational Budgets

Based on the sales budget, a pharmacy organization develops a set of operational budgets that specify how its operations will be carried out to meet the demand for its goods or services. The budgets constituting this operational portion of the master budget are illustrated in Fig. 18-1.

Pharmacy Organizations with Manufacturing

A pharmacy organization that conducts manufacturing operations develops a *production budget*, which shows the number of product units to be manufactured. Coupled with the production budget are ending *inventory budgets* for raw material, work in process, and finished goods. For example, home infusion pharmacies plan to have some inventory on hand at all times to meet peak demand while keeping production at a stable level. From the production budget, this pharmacy develops budgets for the direct materials, direct labor, and overhead that will be required in the production process. A budget for selling and administrative expenses is also prepared.

Pharmacy Organizations with Merchandising

The operational portion of the master budget is similar in a pharmacy organization with merchandising, but instead of a production budget for goods, a merchandiser develops a budget for merchandise purchases. For example, a chain drug store pharmacy will not have a budget for direct material because it does not engage in production. However, the chain drug pharmacy will develop budgets for labor (or personnel), overhead, and selling and administrative expenses.

Pharmacy Organizations with Patient Care Services

Based on the sales budget for its patient care services, a service-oriented pharmacy organization develops a set of budgets that show how the demand for those services will be met. Pharmacy departments in hospitals are focusing their efforts on improving the efficiency of product-related functions mainly through automation and redeploying staff to value-added clinical functions. Services added under these transformations include intravenous-to-oral conversion, dosage adjustments for patients with renal impairment, MTM services, and participation in rounds in all areas of the hospital. The introduction of clinical pharmacy services as part of hospital-wide reengineering programs has been associated with positive benefit–cost ratios and a substantial net cost savings (Schumock et al., 1999).

Cash Budget

This budget shows expected cash receipts as a result of selling goods or services and planned cash disbursements to pay the bills incurred by the pharmacy. Pharmacies prepare cash budgets to allow them to anticipate changes in cash flows over a period of time.

Summary of Operational Budgets

Operational budgets differ because they are adapted to the operations of individual pharmacies in various industries. However, operational budgets are also similar in important ways. In each pharmacy, they encompass a detailed plan for using the basic factors of production—material, labor, and overhead—to produce a product and/or provide a service.

Budgeted Financial Statements

The final portion of the master budget, depicted in Fig. 18-1, includes a budgeted income statement, a budgeted balance sheet, and a budgeted statement of cash flows. These budgeted financial statements show the overall financial results of the pharmacy organization's planned operations for the budget period.

Nonprofit Organizations

The master budget for a nonprofit organization includes many of the components shown in Fig. 18-1. However, there are some important differences. Many nonprofit organizations provide services free of charge. Hence, there may be no sales budget as shown in Fig. 18-1. However, such organizations do begin their budgeting process with a budget that shows the level of services to be provided. For example, the budget for a free clinic would show the planned levels of various public services, such as the hours of operation for the outpatient pharmacy. Nonprofit organizations also prepare budgets showing their anticipated funding. A free clinic budgets for revenue from both public (e.g., support from government agencies) and private sources (e.g., donations).

ACTIVITY-BASED BUDGETING

The process of constructing a master budget can be significantly enhanced if the concepts of *activity-based costing* (ABC) are applied. ABC uses a two-stage cost-assignment process. In Stage 1, overhead costs are assigned to cost pools that represent the most significant activities. The activities identified vary across pharmacy organizations, but examples include such activities as purchasing, materials handling, prescription processing, scheduling, inspection, quality control, purchasing, and inventory control.

After assigning costs to the activity cost pools in Stage 1, cost drivers are identified that are appropriate for each cost pool. Then, in Stage 2, the overhead costs are allocated from each activity cost pool to cost objects (e.g., prescriptions, value-added services, and patients) in proportion to the amount of activity consumed. Figure 18-2 portrays the two-stage allocation process used in ABC systems.

Applying ABC concepts to the budgeting process yields *activity-based budgeting* (ABB). Under ABB, the first step is to specify the products or services to be produced and the customers to be served. Then the activities that are necessary to produce these products and services are determined. Finally, the resources

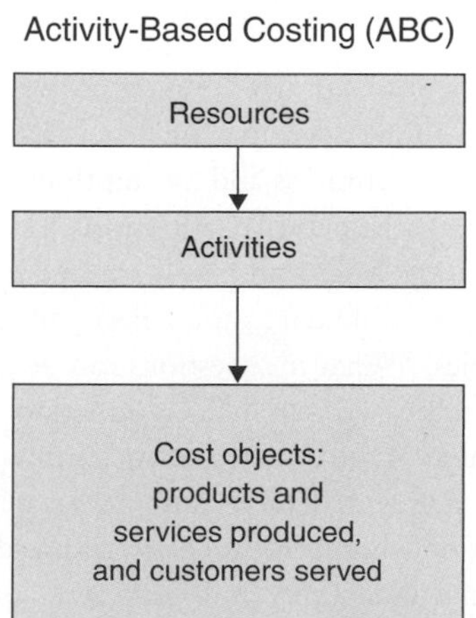

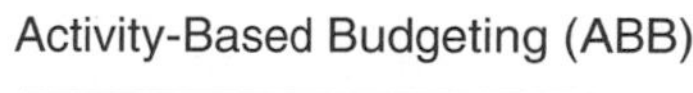

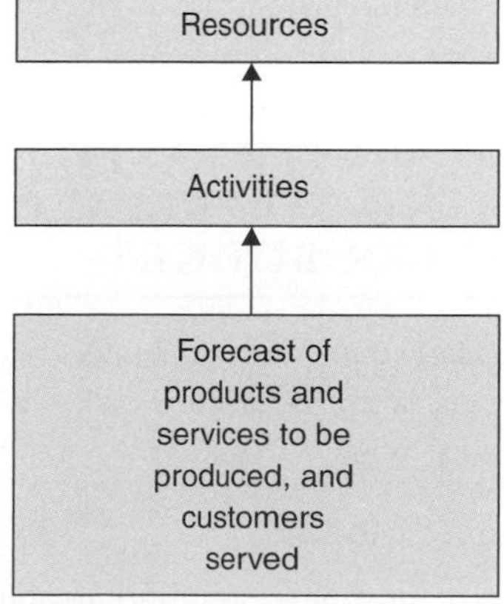

Figure 18-2. Activities-based costing system.

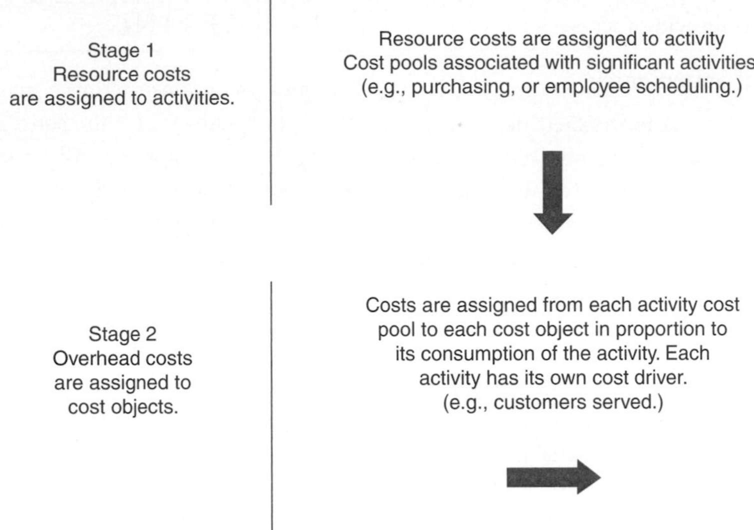

Figure 18-3. Activities-based costing versus activity-based budgeting.

necessary to perform the specified activities are quantified. Conceptually, ABB takes the ABC model and reverses the flow of the analysis, as depicted in Fig. 18-3. As portrayed in the figure, ABC assigns resource costs to activities, and then it assigns activity costs to products and services produced and customers served. ABB, on the other hand, begins by forecasting the demand for products and services as well as the customers to be served. These forecasts are then used to plan the activities for the budget period and budget the resources necessary to carry out the activities.

USING ACTIVITY-BASED BUDGETING TO PREPARE THE MASTER BUDGET

The process of constructing a master budget requires the pharmacy manager to use a variety of schedules that are displayed in Table 18-1.

Financial Planning Models

Pharmacy managers must make assumptions and predictions in preparing budgets because pharmacies, like any other business or organization, operate in a world of uncertainty. One way of coping with that uncertainty is to supplement the budgeting process with a financial planning model. A *financial planning model* is a set of mathematical relationships that expresses the interactions among the various operational, financial, and environmental events that determine the overall results of an organization's activities. A financial planning model is a mathematical expression of all the relationships expressed in the flowchart in Fig. 18-1.

In a fully developed financial planning model, all of the key estimates and assumptions are expressed as general mathematical relationships. Then software programs (e.g., Microsoft Excel) are used to determine the impact of different combinations of these unknown variables. "What if" questions can be answered about such unknown variables as inflation, interest rates, the value of the dollar, demand, competitors' actions, union demands in forthcoming wage negotiations, and a host of other factors. The widespread availability of personal computers and electronic spreadsheet software has made financial planning models a common management tool.

Table 18-1. Schedules Used to Construct a Master Budget

Schedule	Description
Sales budget	Displays the projected sales in units for each quarter and then multiplies the unit sales by the sales price to determine sales revenue
Production budget	Shows the number of units of services or goods that are to be produced during a budget period
Direct material budget	Shows the number of produced units and the cost of material to be purchased and used during a budget period
Direct labor budget	Shows the number of hours and the cost of the direct labor to be used during the budget period
Manufacturing overhead budget	Shows the cost of overhead expected to be incurred in the production process during the budget period
Selling, general, and administrative (SG&A) expense budget	Lists the expenses of administering the firm and selling its units (e.g., prescriptions)
Cash receipts budget	Details the expected cash collections during a budget period
Cash disbursements budget	Details the expected cash payments during a budget period
Cash budget	Details the expected cash receipts and disbursements during a budget period
Budgeted schedule of cost of goods manufactured and sold	Details the direct material, direct labor, and manufacturing overhead costs to be incurred, and shows the cost of the goods to be sold during the budget period
Budgeted income statement	Shows the expected revenue and expenses for the budget period, assuming that planned operations are carried out
Budgeted statement of cash flows	Provides information about the expected sources and uses of cash for operating activities, investing activities, and financing activities during a particular period of time
Budgeted balance sheet	Shows the expected end-of-period balances for the company's assets, liabilities, and owner's equity, assuming that planned operations are carried out

BUDGET ADMINISTRATION

In small organizations, the procedures used to gather information and construct a master budget are usually informal. The pharmacy owner or manager may be the sole person charged with gathering the required information, creating the various budgets, and evaluating their organization's performance against their budget. In contrast, larger organizations use a formal process to collect data and prepare the master budget. Such organizations usually designate a budget director or chief budget officer. This is often the organization's controller (or comptroller in government organizations). The budget director works with departments of employees to specify the process by which budget data will be gathered, collect the information, and prepare the master budget. To communicate budget procedures and deadlines to employees throughout the organization, the budget director often develops and disseminates a budget manual. The budget manual states who is responsible for providing various types of information, when the information is required, and what form the information is to take. For example, the budget manual for a community pharmacy chain may specify that each regional director is to send an estimate of the coming year's sales, by product line, to the budget director by September 1. The budget manual also states who should receive each schedule when the master budget is complete.

A budget committee, consisting of key senior executives, often is appointed to advise the budget director during preparation of the budget. The authority to give final approval to the master budget usually belongs to the board of directors or a board of trustees in nonprofit organizations. Usually the board has a subcommittee whose task is to examine the proposed budget carefully and recommend approval or any changes deemed necessary. By exercising their authority to make changes in the budget and grant final approval, governing boards wield considerable influence on the overall direction their organizations.

e-Budgeting

As pharmacy organizations operate across multiple locations, the Internet is playing an increasingly important role in the budgeting process. e-Budgeting is an Internet-based budgeting tool that can help streamline an organization's budgeting process. The "e" in e-budgeting stands for both electronic and enterprise-wide. Employees throughout an organization and at all levels can submit and retrieve budget information electronically via the Internet. Budgeting software is made available on the Web so that information submitted electronically from any location is in a consistent organization-wide format. Managers in pharmacy organizations using e-budgeting have found that it greatly streamlines the entire budgeting process. In the past, these organizations have compiled their master budgets on hundreds of spreadsheets, which had to be collected and integrated by the corporate controller's office. One result of this cumbersome approach was that a disproportionate amount of time was spent compiling and verifying data from multiple sources. Under e-budgeting, both the submission of budget information and its compilation are accomplished electronically by the Web-based budgeting software. Thus e-budgeting is just one more area where the Internet has transformed how the workplace operates in the era of e-business. Examples of this type of software include OutlookSoft, Cognos, and WebFOCUS.

INTERNATIONAL ASPECTS OF BUDGETING

As the economies and cultures of countries throughout the world become intertwined, more companies are becoming multinational in their operations. Firms with international operations face a variety of additional challenges in preparing their budgets. First, a multinational firm's budget must reflect the translation of foreign currencies into a single currency (i.e., US dollars). Since almost all the world's currencies fluctuate daily in their values relative to each other, this makes budgeting for those translations difficult. Although multinationals have sophisticated financial ways of hedging against such currency fluctuations, the budgeting task is still more challenging. Second, it is difficult to prepare budgets when inflation is high or unpredictable. Over the past 40 years, the United States has experienced rates of price inflation in the range of 2 to 3 percent increases per year, with scattered instances when inflation approached 10 percent. However, in some foreign countries, it is not unusual to experience hyperinflation, with annual inflation rates well over 100 percent. Predicting such high inflation rates is difficult and further complicates a multinational's budgeting process. Finally, the economies of all countries fluctuate in terms of consumer demand, availability of skilled labor, laws affecting commerce, and other factors. Companies with offshore operations face the task of anticipating such changing conditions in the budgeting processes.

BUDGETING PRODUCT LIFE-CYCLE COSTS

A relatively recent focus of the budgeting process is to plan for all the costs that will be incurred throughout a product's life cycle, before a commitment is made to the product. Product life-cycle costs encompass the following five phases in a product's life cycle:

- Product planning and concept design
- Preliminary design
- Detailed design and testing
- Production
- Distribution and customer service

For example, for a pharmaceutical manufacturer to justify a new drug's introduction, the sales revenues it will generate must be sufficient to cover all these costs. Thus, planning these costs is a crucial step in making a decision about the introduction of a new drug. This is particularly true for firms with very short product life cycles. When product life cycles are as short as a year or two, the firm does not have time to adjust its pricing strategy or production methods to ensure that the product turns a profit. Management must be fairly certain before a commitment is made to the product that its life-cycle costs will be covered. Most of a product's life-cycle costs are committed rather early in the product's life. By the time the planning, design, and testing phases are complete, roughly 85 percent of the product's life-cycle costs have been committed, while only about 5 percent actually have been incurred. Given the early commitment that must be made to significant downstream costs in a product's life cycle, it is crucial to budget these costs as early as possible.

BEHAVIORAL IMPACT OF BUDGETS

A budget affects virtually everyone in an organization—those who prepare the budget, those who use the budget to facilitate decision making, and those who are evaluated using the budget. Human reactions to the budgeting process often have considerable influence on an organization's overall effectiveness.

A great deal of study has been devoted to the behavioral effects of budgets. Two key issues that a pharmacy manager should clearly understand are budgetary slack and participative budgeting.

Budgetary Slack: Padding the Budget

The information on which a budget is based comes largely from people throughout an organization. For example, the sales forecast for a community pharmacy chain relies on research and analysis by market research staff, but also incorporates the projections of sales personnel, including pharmacy managers. If a regional sales manager's performance is evaluated on the basis of whether the sales budget for the region is exceeded, what is the incentive for the sales manager in projecting sales? The incentive is to give a conservative estimate, or to *underestimate* the anticipated levels of sales. The sales manager's performance will look better in the eyes of administrators when a conservative estimate is exceeded than when an ambitious estimate is not met.

On the other hand, when an administrator is asked to provide a cost projection for budgetary purposes, there is an incentive to *overestimate* costs. When the actual cost incurred proves to be less than the inflated cost projection, the administrator appears to have managed in a cost-effective way.

These illustrations are examples of padding the budget. *Budget padding* means underestimating revenue and/or overestimating costs. The difference between the revenue or cost projection that a person provides and a realistic estimate of the revenue or cost is called *budgetary slack*. For example, if a pharmacy manager believes the annual utilities cost will be $18,000 but gives a budgetary projection of $20,000, the manager has built $2,000 of slack into the budget.

Why do managers pad budgets with budgetary slack? There are three primary reasons. First, managers often perceive that their performance will look better in their superiors' eyes if they can "beat the budget." Second, budgetary slack is often used to cope with uncertainty. A pharmacy manager may feel confident in his or her cost projections. However, the pharmacy manager also may feel that some unforeseen event during the budgetary period could result in unanticipated costs. For example, an unexpected laminar flow hood breakdown could occur. One way of planning ahead for unforeseen events such as a laminar flow breakdown is to pad the budget. If nothing goes wrong, the pharmacy manager can beat the cost budget. If some negative event does occur, the pharmacy manager can use the budgetary slack to absorb the impact of the event and still meet the cost budget (Dunk, 1995).

The third reason why cost budgets are padded is that budgetary cost projections are often cut by others in the resource-allocation process. Thus, the process of preparing budgets can result in a vicious cycle. Budgetary projections are padded because they will likely be cut, and they are cut because they are likely to have been padded (Leavins et al., 1995).

How does an organization solve the problem of budgetary slack? First, it can avoid relying on the budget as a negative evaluation tool. If a pharmacy manager is beleaguered by a higher level manager every time a budgetary cost projection is exceeded, the likely behavioral response will be to pad the budget. In contrast, if the pharmacy manager is allowed some discretion to exceed the budget when necessary, there will be fewer tendencies toward budgetary padding. Second, pharmacy managers can be given incentives not only to achieve budgetary projections but also to provide *accurate* projections. This can be accomplished by asking pharmacy managers to justify all or some of their projections and by rewarding pharmacy managers who consistently provide accurate estimates as opposed to rewarding managers who perform under their cost projections and punishing managers who exceed their cost projections (Chen and Jones, 2004).

Is Padding the Budget Unethical?

A budget (such as a pharmacy department budget) often is used as the basis for evaluating a pharmacy manager's performance. Actual results are compared with budgeted performance levels, and those who outperform the budget often are rewarded with promotions and/or salary increases. In many cases, bonuses are tied explicitly to performance relative to the budget. For example, the top-management personnel of a department may receive a bonus if departmental profit exceeds budgeted profit by a certain percentage.

Serious ethical issues can arise in situations where a budget is the basis for rewarding managers. For example, suppose a pharmacy department's top-management personnel will split a bonus equal to 10 percent of the amount by which actual departmental profit exceeds the budget. This may create an incentive for the departmental budget officer, or other managers supplying data, to pad the departmental profit budget. Such padding would make the budget easier to achieve, thus increasing the chance of a bonus. Alternatively, there may be an incentive to manipulate the actual departmental results in order to maximize management's bonus. For example, year-end sales could be shifted between years to increase reported revenue in a particular year. Budget personnel could have such incentives for either of two reasons: (1) they might share in the bonus or (2) they might feel pressure from the managers who would share in the bonus.

Put yourself in the position of the pharmacy department manager. Your bonus, and that of your boss, one of the organization's vice presidents, will be determined in part by the department's income in comparison to the budget. When your department has submitted budgets in the past, upper management has usually cut your budgeted expenses, thereby increasing the department's budgeted profit. Moreover, it makes less likely that you and your departmental colleagues will earn a bonus.

Now your boss is pressuring you to pad the expense budget, because "the budgeted expenses will just be cut anyway at the upper management level." Is padding the budget ethical under these circumstances? What do you think?

Participative Budgeting

Most people will perform better and make greater attempts to achieve a goal if they have been consulted in setting the goal. The idea of participative budgeting is to involve employees throughout an organization in the budgetary process. Such participation can give employees the feeling that "this is our budget" rather than the all-too-common feeling that "this is the budget you imposed on us."

While participative budgeting can be very effective, it can also have shortcomings. Too much participation and discussion can lead to vacillation and delay. Also, when those involved in the budgeting process disagree in significant and irreconcilable ways, the process of participation can accentuate those differences.

Finally, the problem of budget padding can be severe unless incentives for accurate projections are provided.

REVISITING THE SCENARIO

Mary Quint, pharmacy student, has been working with Dr. Anne Smith, and now knows that a budget is often used as the basis for evaluating a pharmacy manager's performance. Actual results are compared with budgeted performance levels, and those who outperform the budget often are rewarded with promotions or salary increases. In many cases, bonuses are tied explicitly to performance relative to a budget.

Serious ethical issues can arise in situations where a budget is the basis for rewarding managers. For example, suppose Home TPN Care's top-management personnel will split a bonus equal to 10 percent of the amount by which the actual business unit profit exceeds the budget. This may create an incentive for the pharmacy manager supplying data to pad the profit budget. Such padding would make the budget easier to achieve, thus increasing the chance of a bonus.

Alternatively, there may be an incentive to manipulate the business unit's actual results to maximize management's bonus. For example, year-end sales could be shifted between years to increase reported revenue in a particular year. Budget personnel could have such incentives for either of two reasons: (1) They might share in the bonus or (2) they might feel pressure from the managers who would share in the bonus.

Mary Quint has put herself in the position of Home TPN Care's controller during this APPE and learned a great deal about what it would be like to be a manager like Dr. Anne Smith. Her bonus, and that of her boss, the health system's vice president, will be determined in part by Home TPN Care's income in comparison with the budget. She can see from budgets submitted in the past that the organization's management usually has cut the unit's budgeted expenses, thereby increasing the business unit's budgeted profit. This, of course, makes it more difficult for her business unit to achieve the budgeted profit. Moreover, it makes it less likely that she and her business unit colleagues will earn a bonus. Now her boss is pressuring her to pad the expense budget because "the budgeted expenses will just be cut anyway at the organizational level." Is padding the budget ethical under these circumstances?

CONCLUSION

The budget is a key tool for planning, controlling, and decision making in virtually every organization. Budgeting systems are used to force planning, to facilitate communication and coordination, to allocate resources, to control profit and operations, and to evaluate performance and provide incentives. Various types of budgets are used to accomplish these objectives.

Since budgets affect almost everyone in an organization, they can have significant behavioral implications and can raise difficult ethical issues. One common problem in budgeting is the tendency of people to pad budgets. The resulting budgetary slack makes the budget less useful because the padded budget does not present an accurate picture of expected revenue and expenses.

QUESTIONS FOR FURTHER DISCUSSION

1. Use an example to explain how a budget could be used to allocate resources in a hospital pharmacy.
2. Give an example of how general economic trends would affect sales forecasting in the pharmaceutical industry.
3. Give three examples of how an independent community pharmacy could use a budget for planning purposes.
4. Discuss the importance of predictions and assumptions in the budgeting process.
5. How can the pharmacy department of a large urban hospital help to reduce the problems caused by budgetary slack?
6. Why is participative budgeting often an effective pharmacy management tool?
7. List the steps you would go through in developing a budget to meet your independent community pharmacy expenses.

REFERENCES

Bodine WK. 2007. Working together to strengthen the supply chain. *Pharm Times* 8:90–1.

Cannon HE. 2007. Pharmacy management of vaccines. *J Manag Care Pharm* 13(7):S7–11.

Chen CC, Jones KT. 2004. Budgetary slack and performance in group participative budgeting: The effects of individual and group performance feedback and task interdependence. *Adv Manage Account* 13:183–221.

Cho BH, Hicks KA, Honeycutt AA, et al. 2011. A tool for the economic analysis of mass prophylaxis operations with an application to H1N1 influenza vaccination clinics. *J Public Health Manag Pract* 17:E22–8.

Cowlrick I, Dumon J, Bauleser M. 2002. Managing medical information effectively facilitates the quality and time to delivering the final product. *Drug Info J* 36:825.

Curtiss FR. 2006. Pharmacy benefit spending on oral chemotherapy drugs. *J Manag Care Pharm* 12:570.

Demers RF. 2001. Operational and financial principles of "managing up". *Am J Health Syst Pharm* 58:S7.

Dunk AS. 1995. The joint effects of budgetary slack and task uncertainty on subunit performance. *Account Finance* 35:61–75.

Gregg W, Moscovice I, Remus D. 2006. The implementation of pay-for-performance in rural hospitals: Lessons from the Hospital Quality Incentive Demonstration Project. Available at www.uppermidwestrhrc.org/pdf/pay_for_performance.pdf; accessed on March 5, 2012.

Leavins JR, Omer K, Vilutis A. 1995. A comparative study of alternative indicators of budgetary slack. *Managerial Finance* 21(3):52–67.

Poisal JA, Truffer C, Smith S, et al. 2007. Health spending projections through 2016: Modest changes obscure Part D's impact. *Health Aff* 26:w242.

Schumock GT, Michaud J, Guenette AJ. 1999. Reengineering: An opportunity to advance clinical practice in a community hospital. *Am J Health Syst Pharm* 56: 1945.

Tierney M. 2004. Lessons from patient deaths: An Ontario pharmacist responds to Calgary's patient safety review. *Can Pharm J* 137(8):9.

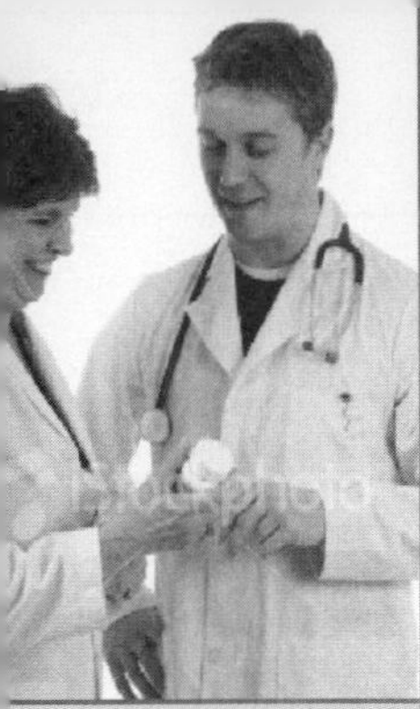

19

THIRD-PARTY PAYER CONSIDERATIONS

Julie M. Urmie

About the Author: Dr. Urmie is an associate professor in the Health Services Research Division at the University of Iowa College of Pharmacy. She received a B.S. in pharmacy from the University of Wisconsin and worked as a community pharmacist prior to returning to the University of Wisconsin for graduate school, where she received an M.S. in pharmacy administration and a Ph.D. in social and administrative sciences in pharmacy. Her teaching interests include insurance and reimbursement in pharmacy, health insurance, the US health care system, health policy, and pharmacy management. Her main areas of research are prescription drug insurance and consumer preferences related to health care use.

LEARNING OBJECTIVES

After completing this chapter, readers should be able to

1. Discuss the history of third-party reimbursement for prescription drugs and its impact on pharmacy management.
2. Understand the basic principles of third-party reimbursement for prescription drugs and define commonly used reimbursement terminology.
3. Evaluate the financial impact of third-party reimbursement on the pharmacy using an average net profit comparison, a differential analysis, and a pro forma analysis.
4. Identify the broad range of factors that a pharmacy manager should consider when evaluating a third-party contract.
5. Discuss issues related to third-party reimbursement for prescription drugs.

SCENARIO

Natalie Hawkins, the pharmacy manager at Good Service Pharmacy in Tipton, IA, opens her mail and sees that Better Health Insurance has sent a new contract. Natalie had heard about the possibility that Better Health might stop using the average wholesale price (AWP) as the basis for their prescription drug reimbursement. She was anxious to see what Better Health was going to use as the basis of their new reimbursement formula.

Better Health is one of the pharmacy's major insurance plans, providing prescription drug coverage for 20% of their patients. Since Better Health significantly decreased their reimbursement rate a few years ago, Natalie worries about the effect of further decreases. As she reads the new contract, she discovers that Better Health is switching from an AWP-based reimbursement formula to a wholesaler acquisition cost (WAC) formula and the new reimbursement rate is WAC plus 2 percent plus a $1.00 dispensing fee. Natalie has no idea how the new reimbursement rate compares with the old reimbursement rate of AWP less 18 percent plus a $1.00 dispensing fee. She worries that the insurer is just trying to decrease the reimbursement.

Natalie wonders whether Good Service Pharmacy should still participate in the Better Health plan. After all, what signal would she be sending to other insurers and pharmaceutical benefit managers (PBMs) if she accepts a very low reimbursement rate? Good Service Pharmacy might become "Poor Service Pharmacy" or even go out of business if all its third-party contracts had such low rates. Then Natalie remembers Mrs. Anderson, a 78-year-old woman with Better Health Insurance, who has been coming to her pharmacy for over 20 years. Natalie has spent many hours over the years talking with Mrs. Anderson about her medications, and she cannot imagine having to tell her that Good Service Pharmacy no longer accepts her insurance. Natalie also worries about the financial impact of losing 20 percent of her patients if she declines the contract. As the pharmacy manager, Natalie knows that it is her responsibility to make a decision about the contract, but as a new manager, she worries about how to make an informed decision that balances the financial needs of the pharmacy with other considerations. Natalie wonders

1. How much will the change in reimbursement affect the net profit on an average Better Health prescription? Will the pharmacy lose money on each Better Health prescription it dispenses? How will moving away from AWP-based reimbursement formulas affect pharmacy profit?
2. Would Good Service Pharmacy be better off financially by accepting or declining the contract? How do you determine whether it is worse to accept a low reimbursement rate or lose about 20 percent of your prescription volume?
3. What other factors need to be considered? Could the contract be renegotiated? Other than prescriptions, what other goods and services do the pharmacy's Better Health customers purchase? Just how many of the pharmacy's Better Health customers would leave if her pharmacy declines the contract, and how much business (both prescriptions and other goods and services) would they take with them.
4. Good Service Pharmacy will likely lose revenue in the future because it will get less money per prescription if it accepts the contract and will lose customers if it rejects the contract. Are there any ways for the pharmacy to make up the lost revenue? Are there any expenses that could be decreased?

OVERVIEW OF THE IMPACT OF THIRD-PARTY REIMBURSEMENT IN PHARMACY

This scenario is a common occurrence in pharmacies of all sizes and types across the country. Pharmacy managers and owners are forced to make difficult decisions about whether to accept or reject third-party plans; pharmacists and patients deal with the consequences of those decisions. A *third party* is defined as an organization that reimburses a pharmacy or patient for all or part of the patient's prescription drug costs. Since most prescriptions dispensed in pharmacies today are paid for by third parties, it is essential that pharmacy managers and pharmacists understand the effect of third parties on pharmacy operations.

Pharmacies have third-party patients and private-pay patients. Private-pay patients, sometimes referred to as *cash patients*, are people who do not have any health insurance coverage or people who have health insurance that does not cover prescription drugs. Some patients with prescription drug insurance may chose to pay cash if the cash price is less than their co-payment; this has become more common due to the prevalence of $4 generic prescriptions or other discount pricing offered by some pharmacies. Other patients may have prescription insurance, but have a deductible or cap in benefits. From the pharmacy's perspective, patients who pay the pharmacy directly for their prescriptions and later are reimbursed by their insurance company often are indistinguishable from private-pay patients. This type of prescription drug insurance, called *indemnity insurance,* used to be common, but it has now been replaced largely by *service benefit plans.* Under a service benefit plan, the patient may pay the pharmacy a predetermined portion of the prescription cost, but the pharmacy is reimbursed directly by the third party for most of the prescription cost.

Third parties may be public or private. Private third parties typically are insurance companies, although other private entities sometimes pay for a patient's prescriptions. For example, some pharmaceutical manufacturers provide free or discounted prescriptions through an indigent care program. Public third parties are government entities that pay for prescriptions through a government program, for example, Medicaid, Medicare Part D, or a state prescription drug assistance program for the elderly. Medicaid is the program to provide health care for the poor. The program is funded jointly by federal and state governments, with each state determining its own prescription drug reimbursement rates. Medicare, the government program that provides health insurance for the elderly and disabled, implemented a voluntary Medicare Part D outpatient prescription drug benefit in 2006. Medicare Part D has had a significant impact on pharmacies because many former private-pay patients now have Part D coverage. Medicare Part D is a mixed public and private third party because the government regulates the benefit, but private third parties deliver the benefit. See Chapter 20 for further description of issues related to public insurance programs.

Many third parties hire pharmacy benefit managers (PBMs) to provide prescription claims processing and other services. Examples of third parties that hire PBMs are insurance companies, employers, Medicare Part D prescription drug plans (PDPs), and state Medicaid programs. PBMs establish pharmacy networks as part of their claims management services, so many pharmacy third-party contracts are with PBMs. In addition to processing claims for prescriptions filled at pharmacies, other services PBMs provide include rebate negotiation with pharmaceutical manufacturers, drug benefit design, formulary development and management, drug utilization management, and disease-state/case management. Some PBMs also offer mail-order pharmacy services.

The past two decades have been a time of tremendous growth in third-party payment for prescriptions. The percentage of prescription drug expenditures reimbursed by a third party increased from 44 percent in 1990 to 79 percent in 2008 (Fig. 19-1). Initially, most of the growth was in private third-party payment, but more recently the trend has been away from private insurance payment and toward public insurance payment; this trend was accelerated by the start of Medicare Part D in 2006. The percent of *prescriptions* paid for by third parties is higher than the percent of *prescription drug expenditures* paid by third parties due to patient cost sharing (e.g., copayments, deductibles). In 2009, 89 percent of prescriptions dispensed at independent pharmacies were paid for by a third party: 30 percent were Medicare Part D prescriptions, 14 percent were Medicaid prescriptions, and 45 percent were other third-party prescriptions (National Community Pharmacists Association (NCPA), 2010: NCPA Digest).

This shift toward more third-party payment for prescription drugs has had a significant impact on pharmacy management. Pharmacies determine what price they want to charge private-pay patients, but as discussed further in the following paragraph, the reimbursement level for third-party prescriptions is determined by a contract between the third party and the pharmacy. Pharmacies usually are not allowed to charge patients more than the contracted reimbursement rate, so, in practice, prescription drug prices are determined by the third-party contract. This decreases the flexibility that pharmacy owners and managers have to price prescription drugs dispensed at their pharmacies.

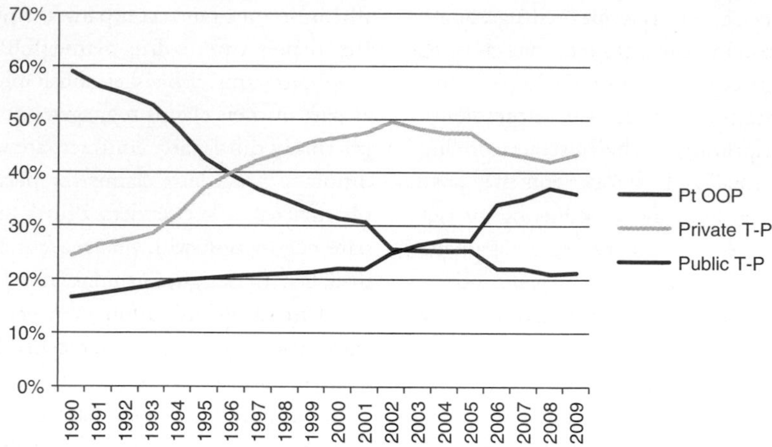

Figure 19-1. Source of payment for prescription expenditures in the United States, 1990–2009. (Data were obtained from the Centers for Medicare and Medicaid Service at http://www.cms.hhs.gov/NationalHealthExpendData/.) *Note*: Pt OOP is direct spending by consumers for prescriptions drugs. It includes prescriptions not covered by a third party and patient cost sharing for third-party prescriptions.

Owners and managers decide what third-party contracts to accept, but once the contract is accepted, the price is determined by the contract between the pharmacy and third party. A significant concern in pharmacy is the level of reimbursement specified in these contracts. The level of reimbursement varies considerably across contracts, so pharmacy managers must make informed decisions about which contracts to accept. An important piece of information to know for each contract is the average *gross margin*, defined as the difference between reimbursed price and the cost of the dispensed product. In 2009, the overall average gross margin on prescription sales in independent pharmacies was 23.8 percent, but the average gross margin for third-party prescriptions was lower: 19.1 percent for Medicaid, 18.6 percent for Medicare Part D, and 20.0 percent for other third parties (2010 NCPA Digest).

Insurers and PBMs usually have pharmacy networks in which pharmacies must accept the third party's reimbursement rate to participate in the network. Most insurers and PBMs require that patients obtain their prescriptions from a network pharmacy, although some will let patients use nonnetwork pharmacies but require them to pay more for their prescriptions. These incentives for patients to use network pharmacies put considerable pressure on pharmacies to participate in third-party networks. There usually are many pharmacies in an area but just a few major third parties, giving each third party considerable bargaining power over the pharmacies because most pharmacies need to be in a network more than a third party needs any particular pharmacy in its network. However, there is some evidence that bargaining power varies across pharmacies (Brooks et al., 1999; Yang et al., 2010). Large chain pharmacies, as well as pharmacies that serve large geographic areas, are likely to have more bargaining power than single independent pharmacies or pharmacies that compete with many others in a small area. The pharmacy access standards that Medicare requires for PDPs participating in Part D may increase bargaining power for pharmacies located in areas with no other pharmacies. For example, if there is only one pharmacy in a rural area of Iowa, and the access standards require at least one network pharmacy in that part of Iowa, then that pharmacy should be able to negotiate better reimbursement terms.

Another concern associated with third-party prescriptions is that they generally cost more to dispense than private-pay prescriptions because of the extra steps involved in dispensing a third-party prescription (Carroll, 1991; Huey et al., 1995; Schafermeyer et al., 1992). For third-party prescriptions, the pharmacy staff must verify patient eligibility, submit and reconcile claims, wait for payment, and comply with third-party rules and requirements, such as formularies. Dealing with third-party issues consumes an estimated 20 percent of pharmacy personnel time (NACDS, 1999). Understanding and knowing how to calculate the cost of dispensing prescriptions are important managerial tools that will be discussed in more detail later in this chapter.

Lower third-party reimbursement combined with higher third-party cost of dispensing means that average net profit is lower for third-party prescriptions than for private-pay prescriptions. This implies that pharmacy owners and managers need to evaluate carefully the financial impact of accepting third-party contracts. Tools for this evaluation are discussed later in this chapter. Pharmacy managers also need to consider many nonfinancial factors when making a third-party contract decisions, and these factors will also be discussed in this chapter.

THIRD-PARTY REIMBURSEMENT FOR PRESCRIPTION DRUGS

The *reimbursement rate*, or price, for a third-party prescription is based on a reimbursement-rate formula that is specified in the contract between the pharmacy and the third-party payer. The reimbursement-rate formula almost universally consists of two parts: the product cost portion and the dispensing fee. The *product cost portion* is intended to pay the pharmacy for the cost of the drug product, and the *dispensing fee* is intended to cover the cost of dispensing the prescription. The total reimbursement rate (product cost + dispensing fee) should be higher than the costs of obtaining and dispensing the drug to provide some profit to the pharmacy. In reality, most third-party contracts currently provide product reimbursements that are higher than the actual pharmacy cost to obtain the drug but provide dispensing fees that are less than most pharmacy's actual cost of dispensing a prescription. This tendency for higher-than-cost product reimbursements may change as third-party payers move away from average wholesaler price (AWP) reimbursement.

Most third-party contracts state that the reimbursement rate for a prescription is the lower of two prices: (1) the price from the reimbursement-rate formula and (2) the usual and customary (U&C) pharmacy price. The U&C price, also referred to as the *cash price*, is the price that the pharmacy would charge a private-pay patient for the prescription.

Understanding the product cost portion of the reimbursement-rate formula requires knowledge of an alphabet soup of acronyms. A list of commonly used reimbursement terms, acronyms, and definitions is provided in Table 19-1. *Actual acquisition cost* (AAC) is the price that the pharmacy pays to purchase the drug product. Third parties would like to base their reimbursement on AAC, but are unable to do so because the AAC is proprietary information that pharmacies do not disclose to third parties. AAC also varies across pharmacies and may change frequently, making it administratively difficult to base reimbursement on AAC. As a result, the product cost portion of the third-party reimbursement rate is an estimate of AAC and is called the *estimated acquisition cost* (EAC).

To establish EAC, most third parties use a standardized drug cost estimate that often is based on *AWP* or *WAC*. Theoretically, AWP is the price that the wholesaler charges to pharmacies, but in reality, AWP is the *list price* rather than the actual price. Just as the sticker price for a car is an overestimate of the price someone actually pays for the car, AWP is an overestimate of the price pharmacies pay for the drug product. A government study found that pharmacies purchase brand-name drug products from the wholesalers at an average rate of AWP less 21.84 percent (OIG, 2001) and generic drugs at an average rate of AWP less 65.93 percent (OIG, 2002). Historically, AWPs have been published for all drug products, so AWP provided a convenient, standardized basis for determining EAC. Third parties did not know the exact amount of discount that pharmacies received, but they recognized that pharmacies received some discount from AWP. As a result, the EAC used by third parties typically has been AWP less some percentage. The percentage off of AWP

Table 19-1. Product Cost Terminology

Actual acquisition cost (AAC)	The price that the pharmacy pays the drug wholesaler or manufacturer to obtain the drug product.
Average acquisition cost (AvAC)	An average of the prices paid by different pharmacies for drug products. Must be determined via pharmacy survey.
Average manufacturer price (AMP)	The average price received by a manufacturer from wholesalers for drugs distributed to the retail class of trade. This price used to be proprietary but the Deficit Reduction Act of 2005 required the Centers for Medicaid and Medicare Services (CMS) make AMPs publicly available.
Average wholesaler price (AWP)	A list price for what drug wholesalers charge pharmacies. This is an overestimate of what the wholesaler actually charges the pharmacy.
Estimated acquisition cost (EAC)	The third party's estimate of what the pharmacy pays the drug wholesaler or manufacturer.
Maximum allowable cost (MAC)	The maximum cost that the third party will pay for a multisource drug. This typically is an average of the generic drug price from several manufacturers.
Wholesaler acquisition cost (WAC)	A list price for what pharmaceutical manufacturers charge drug wholesalers. This is an overestimate of what manufacturers actually charge wholesalers.

steadily declined over time. For example, in the mid-1980s, product reimbursement rates were commonly in the AWP less 5 to 10 percent range, whereas by the mid-1990s, rates often were about AWP less 15 percent (Academy of Managed Care Pharmacy [AMCP], 2007). There are anecdotal reports that some Medicare Part D PDP reimbursement rates in 2006 were around AWP less 20 percent.

Example 1: Reimbursement Formula Using AWP

AWP − 18% + $2.00 dispensing fee

In recent years, third-party payers have begun transitioning away from reimbursement based on AWP. With AWP being a sticker price, there was concern about gaming of the AWP system. In 2009, the two publishers of AWP information (First DataBank and Medi-Span) settled a lawsuit. The plaintiffs in the lawsuit alleged that First DataBank and Medi-Span fraudulently conspired to increase AWP to the detriment of payers and consumers. As a result of the settlement, there was an AWP "rollback" that reduced AWPs for many drug products. First DataBank and Medi-Span also announced that they would stop publishing AWP. With AWP no longer readily available, there is a need for a new reimbursement methodology for prescription drugs.

An alternative way for third parties to establish EAC is by using the WAC. WAC used to be the actual price that drug wholesalers paid pharmaceutical manufactures to purchase drug products, and thus was proprietary information unavailable to third parties. Over the years, WAC has evolved to become an alternative list price. Wholesalers now purchase drug products at some percent off the WAC, and there are some standardized WAC lists available for use by third parties, although the information may not be as accessible as AWPs. The EAC typically will be the WAC plus a small percentage. WAC was used by some third-party payers even prior to the AWP lawsuit settlement, but its use may increase when AWP is no longer published. However, it is a list price and potentially subject to the same problems as AWP, so it may be more of an interim solution as third-party payers try to find a different way to pay pharmacies.

Example 2: Reimbursement Formula Using WAC

WAC + 3% + $2.00 dispensing fee

An alternative replacement for AWP-based reimbursement formulas is average acquisition cost, here called AvAC to distinguish it from AAC. AvAC reflects an average price at which pharmacies purchase drug products. Although AvAC may be a more accurate estimate of a pharmacy's AAC than AWP or WAC, it also is subject to some problems. First, there is no published source of AvAC like there is for WAC or had been for AWP. AvAC typically must be assessed by surveying pharmacies. As a result, it is labor intensive to collect AvAC and difficult to verify the accuracy of AvACs reported by pharmacies. Another issue is that a pharmacy's AAC may be quite different from the AvAC, as different pharmacies negotiate different purchasing terms from their wholesalers. However, this problem is also an issue with WAC- and AWP-based reimbursement. The National Association of State Medicaid Directors (NASMD) (2010) published a white paper on post-AWP pharmacy pricing and reimbursement. They recommended that Medicaid move toward AvAC reimbursement with a single national benchmark being used for AvAC (NASMD White Paper, June 2010). If the federal government measures and publishes AvACs, it is likely that private third-party payers also will move toward this type of reimbursement system.

The EAC for generic drugs sometimes is determined differently from the EAC for brand-name drugs. AWP is a particularly inaccurate estimate of AAC for generic drugs because, as mentioned previously, pharmacies purchase generic drug products at a large discount from AWP. There also often is wide variation in the price for the same generic drug product across different generic manufacturers. One way third-party payers handle this problem is to have a separate reimbursement-rate formula for generic drugs that specifies a larger discount from AWP than for brand-name drugs.

A commonly used alternative method is to specify a *maximum allowable cost* (MAC) for each generic product. The MAC is an average cost to obtain the generic drug product. The federal government calculates and publishes a list of MACs for selected generic drug products. Some third parties use the federal MAC lists, and some establish their own MAC list. The MAC also may be used for all multisource drugs in some third-party plans. *Multisource drugs* are drug products that have at least one generic equivalent available. In this case, the MAC is the reimbursement level for both the brand-name product and the generic equivalent. The result of this type of MAC policy is that the pharmacy needs to collect the difference between the MAC and the brand-name cost from the patient if the patient requests the brand-name product.

The Deficit Reduction Act of 2005 mandated a change to an *average manufacturer price* (AMP)-based reimbursement for their multisource MAC list. AMP is defined as the average price received by a manufacturer from wholesalers for drugs distributed to the retail class of trade. The *retail class of trade* refers to entities that purchase drugs for sale to the general public. Under the final government rules on AMP, this retail class includes chain pharmacies, independent pharmacies, and mail-order pharmacies but excludes other entities such as long-term care facilities and PBMs. The change from AWP- to AMP-based generic reimbursement in the Medicaid program was expected to reduce pharmacy reimbursement for generic prescription drugs dispensed under Medicaid, but implementation of the law was delayed due to legal action by some pharmacy associations. Prior to the change's implementation, the 2010 health care reform law was passed. This law included a change in the formula used to calculate MACs in Medicaid. This change will result in less reduction in pharmacy reimbursement for generic drugs in Medicaid than the formula specified under the Deficit Reduction Act of 2005, but the effects still will need to be monitored. At one time, it was thought that AMP would be a candidate to replace AWP in pharmacy reimbursement formulas, but this now is less likely since the health care reform law limited the public availability of AMP information (NASMD White Paper, June 2010).

As mentioned previously, the dispensing fee is intended to cover the cost of dispensing a prescription. In actuality, determination of the dispensing fee is rather arbitrary, and the amount of the fee usually is lower than the actual cost of dispensing. For example, a 2007 study reported that the average cost of dispensing per prescription was $10.50 (Grant Thornton, 2007) and the 2010 NCPA Digest reported an average cost of dispensing of $11.97 (NCPA Digest, 2010). However, dispensing fees often are in the $0.50 to $6 range, with the higher fees usually occurring in state Medicaid programs. In some cases, a higher dispensing fee will be paid for selected types of drug products (e.g., generic drugs or drugs that are on the third party's formulary). Some third parties also may pay a "bonus" dispensing fee or other incentive if the pharmacy meets specified performance goals (e.g., a targeted generic dispensing rate or formulary compliance rate). For example, assume that a third party pays a $0.50 bonus dispensing fee if the generic dispensing rate at the pharmacy for the quarter is 55 percent. If the pharmacy dispenses 6,000 of that third party's prescriptions for one-quarter and 3,400 of those prescriptions were generic (a generic dispensing rate of 56.7 percent), the third party will reimburse the pharmacy retrospectively an additional $3,000 ($0.50 per prescription × 6,000). If third parties move toward a reimbursement system where the product cost portion of the reimbursement is close to a pharmacy's actual drug cost, then dispensing fees must be adjusted upward to cover the cost of dispensing and provide some profit.

EVALUATING THE FINANCIAL IMPACT OF THIRD-PARTY REIMBURSEMENT

This section describes several ways to examine how third-party reimbursement affects a pharmacy's financial performance. Although other factors are also important and will be discussed later in this chapter, it is essential to understand the impact of different third-party plans on a pharmacy's net profit. One important step in evaluating a third-party contract is to examine the average net profit per prescription. An average net profit comparison may be used to evaluate the effect of a change in reimbursement for a particular third-party plan or to evaluate reimbursement rates across third-party plans and private-pay prescriptions. An important part of this analysis is calculating the average cost of dispensing a prescription.

Recognizing that there are many fixed costs in pharmacies, another evaluation technique that will be discussed is differential analysis. This analysis accounts for the fact that many pharmacy expenses change little as the prescription volume increases or decreases. Finally, pro forma analysis will be discussed. This analysis factors in the different volumes of prescriptions in different third-party plans and includes elements of both the differential analysis and the average net profit comparison.

Calculating the Cost of Dispensing a Prescription

A fundamental pharmacy management tool is calculating the average cost of dispensing a prescription. The cost of dispensing includes the *fair share* of all a pharmacy's costs related to dispensing a prescription *over and above* the cost of the drug product. Knowing the cost of dispensing is necessary to evaluate third-party contracts, and it is also useful in tracking pharmacy expenses. Costs can be separated into two different types of costs: fixed and variable. *Fixed costs* are costs that do not change as prescription volume changes (e.g., computer or other equipment purchases, pharmacy license, and depreciation). A variation is *semifixed costs*, which only change with large changes in prescription volume. An example of a semifixed cost would be pharmacist labor costs. Pharmacists will not be hired or fired for small changes in prescription volume, but if there are large changes in prescription volume, it may be necessary to change the number of pharmacists employed by the pharmacy or reduce pharmacist hours (e.g., full time to part time). *Variable costs* are costs that change directly as prescription volume changes (e.g., prescription vials). When differential analysis is discussed, it will be necessary to identify the average variable costs of dispensing a prescription.

Another way to classify costs is direct versus indirect. *Direct costs* are costs that are completely attributable to the prescription department (e.g., the costs of prescription vials and the prescription department computer). Pharmacist labor is considered a direct expense unless the pharmacist has managerial responsibilities in nonprescription departments. *Indirect costs* are costs that are shared between the prescription department and the rest of the store. Rent, clerical labor costs, utilities, and promotional expenses for the pharmacy are examples of indirect expenses. Methods for allocating indirect expenses to the prescription department are discussed in Table 19-2.

The overall process to calculate a *cost of dispensing* (COD) is to identify the direct and indirect costs associated with the prescription department, allocate the fair share of indirect costs to the dispensing process, and then divide the total prescription department expenses by the number of prescription dispensed during the same time period. It often is convenient to use 1 year as the time frame. To calculate the COD, you will need the most recent income (revenue and expense) statement or a pro forma income statement for the pharmacy and information on the number of prescriptions dispensed during the same time period as the statement. More information on income statements is provided in Chapter 17, and pro forma income statements are discussed later in this chapter. The calculations use the income statement and other relevant information for Good Service Pharmacy that is provided in Table 19-3. This table also contains information about the percentage of expenses allocated to the prescription department. This information will be used to illustrate part of the process of calculating a COD, but it is not typically contained in an income statement and must be calculated separately. Table 19-2 shows the process for calculating the COD for Good Service Pharmacy. It should be noted that although the COD is calculated for the entire prescription department, the COD often varies as the percentage of prescriptions paid for by private or third-party sources changes.

It is useful to know the COD for third-party prescriptions and even the COD for a specific third-party plan, but often the necessary information for these calculations is unavailable or too time-consuming to obtain. In this example, the overall average COD for Good Service Pharmacy of $11.94 per prescription.

Average Net Profit Comparison

The basic formula for calculating an *average net profit comparison* is included in Table 19-4. The average cost of goods sold (COGS) per prescription is subtracted from the average price (for private-pay prescriptions) or average reimbursement rate to give the average gross margin. Gross margin may also be referred to as *gross profit*. The average cost of dispensing is subtracted from the gross margin to yield the average net profit per prescription. The average net profit can be calculated for all prescriptions dispensed at the pharmacy, for selected third-party plans, or for a particular third-party plan before and after a change in reimbursement. The same formula is used on an aggregate basis to conduct a pro forma analysis. Table 19-4 shows an average net profit comparison for the current and new Better Health reimbursement rates from the scenario. In this example, assume that the COD will not change and that the average COD for Better Health prescriptions is the same as for all other prescriptions. Also assume that the average COGS will not change. When conducting an average net profit comparison across different third-party plans, the most accurate approach would be to calculate the average COGS separately for each plan because each plan may have a very different prescription drug mix. In reality, it is often assumed that the average COGS is the same to simplify the analysis. When conducting an average net profit comparison, the need for accurate COGS data must be balanced with practical constraints.

Note: In practice, it may be difficult to determine the average COGS. The information on the COGS that is provided in the computer records often is not an actual reflection of the true COGS. One way to calculate the average COGS is to examine invoices that

Table 19-2. Calculating the Average Cost of Dispensing Per Prescription

Step 1: Identify costs associated with the prescription department

Labor expenses

Labor expenses need to be allocated between the prescription department and the rest of the pharmacy. These expenses typically are allocated based on the percent of time spent in the prescription department. Natalie Hawkins, the pharmacy manager at Good Service Pharmacy, estimates that she spends 75% of her time in the prescription department. Assume that the employee pharmacist and the pharmacy technicians spend 95% of their time in the prescription department, so 95% of their wages are allocated to the cost of dispensing. The other workers spend about 50% of their time in the prescription department. Using these percentages and the wage information contained in the notes under the Income Statement, the total amount of labor costs allocated to the prescription department is $423,165.

Direct expenses

Some expenses are directly related to prescription drug dispensing and should be allocated 100% to the prescription department. For Good Service Pharmacy, the direct expenses that are listed on the Income Statement are prescription vials and the computer. The total of these direct expenses is $17,250. *Note: Other direct expenses that may appear in a pharmacy Income Statement include delivery expenses, professional liability insurance, continuing education expenses, transaction fees, and professional license fees.*

Indirect expenses

The rest of the expenses are indirect expenses that are not obviously linked to a particular department.

Occupancy expenses such as rent, utilities, and other facility costs are often allocated using a square-footage allocation method. Under this method, costs are allocated to the prescription department using the percentage of the store square footage occupied by the prescription department. For Good Service Pharmacy, this percentage is 25.8.

The typical allocation method for other indirect expenses is percent of sales. Since the prescription department generated 75.31% of the total sales, 75.31% of each of the other expenses will be allocated to the prescription department. *Note: The percent of sales allocation method may also be used for occupancy expenses. This method usually results in a higher cost of dispensing than the square-footage allocation method because prescription departments typically generate a large percentage of sales but occupy a small percentage of the store square footage.*

The total of indirect expenses allocated to the prescription department is $237,611 ($18,384 in occupancy expenses and $219,227 in other indirect expenses). All the allocation percentages and amounts are displayed in the far right columns in Table 19-3.

Step 2: Sum all the prescription department costs

Labor expenses	$423,165
Direct expenses	$17,250
Indirect expenses	$237,611
Total expenses	$678,026

Step 3: Divide the prescription expenses by the number of prescriptions dispensed

Average cost of dispensing per prescription: $678,026/56,795 = **$11.94**

Table 19-3. Income Statement for Good Service Pharmacy, 2012

	2012	Sales (%)	Prescription Dept. Allocation for COD	Allocation for COD (%)
Sales				
Prescription sales	3,975,650	75.31		
Other sales	1,303,475	24.69		
Total sales	5,279,125	100.00		
Cost of goods sold	4,006,856	75.90		
Gross margin	1,272,269	24.10		
Expenses				
Labor	586,286	11.11	423,165	
Rent	52,059	0.99	13,431	25.80
Utilities/other facility costs	19,196	0.36	4,953	25.80
Prescription vials/labels	9,750	0.18	9,750	100
Computer	7,500	0.14	7,500	100
Advertising	16,128	0.31	12,146	75.31
All other expenses	274,971	5.21	207,081	75.31
Total expenses	965,890	18.30		
Net profit (before taxes)	306,379	5.80		

COD, cost of dispensing; COGS, cost of goods sold.
Notes:
1. Number of prescriptions dispensed in 2012 = 56,795.
2. Prescription COGS = 76.88% of the total COGS.
3. Labor costs (wages plus benefits): Pharmacy manager = $125,583 (75% in prescription department); employee pharmacist = $115,279 (95% in prescription department); pharmacy technicians = $103,890 (95% in prescription department); and other staff = $241,534 (50% in prescription department).
4. The pharmacy department occupies 25.80% of the store square footage.

the pharmacy receives from the wholesaler. However, the invoice price also may be somewhat inaccurate because the pharmacy may receive an extra price discount or rebate from the wholesaler at the end of the year or during some other time period if the pharmacy reaches target purchase levels.

The net profit comparison of the current and new Better Health reimbursement rates reveals that Good Service Pharmacy is already losing money under the current rate and it would lose even more ($5.78 on an average Better Health prescription) if it accepted the new contract. Although this result would seem to make the decision about accepting the contract clear, this analysis is only one of several relevant financial analyses, and other factors need to be considered. It may also be useful to conduct an average net profit comparison across other third-party plans and private-pay prescriptions at Good Service Pharmacy to see how Better Health compares.

Differential Analysis

Another analysis to consider is a *differential analysis.* The net profit comparison makes it appear as if accepting the new Better Health contract would be a very bad idea because the pharmacy would lose an average of $5.78 per prescription. However, this analysis

Table 19-4. Conducting an Average Net Profit Comparison

Step 1: Calculate the current average reimbursement rate

If the total reimbursement for the Better Health prescriptions and the number of Better Health prescriptions is known, then divide the total reimbursement by the number of prescriptions to obtain the average reimbursement. If either of those pieces of information is unknown, then use the reimbursement-rate formula to obtain an estimate of the average reimbursement. To do this, the following information is needed: (1) the average AWP for prescriptions sold in the pharmacy or (2) the average COGS and the discount from AWP that the pharmacy receives from their drug wholesaler. For this example, assume that Good Service Pharmacy purchases drugs from their wholesaler at AWP − 28% and their average COGS per prescription is $54.24. Given that the new reimbursement formula is based on WAC, you also need to know the average WAC. Use an algebraic maneuver to calculate the average AWP from the average COGS and the purchase formula:

$$\text{AWP} - 28(\text{AWP}) = \$54.24$$
$$0.72\ \text{AWP} = \$54.24$$
$$\text{AWP} = \$75.33$$

Now use this average AWP to determine the average reimbursement under the current reimbursement formula

Current B.H. Formula: AWP − 18% + $1.00

Average reimbursement = $75.33 − 0.18($75.33) + $1.00 = $62.77

Step 2: Calculate the new average reimbursement rate

The new average reimbursement rate is calculated using the average WAC and the reimbursement formula. The average WAC for prescriptions sold in the pharmacy = $58.57. *Note: If you do not know the average WAC but know the WAC purchasing terms from your wholesaler and the average COGS you can use the same methodology as shown above in the AWP example.*

New B.H. Formula: WAC + 2% + $1.00

Average reimbursement = $58.57 + 0.02(58.57) + $1.00 = $60.74

Step 3: Calculate the average net profit

Subtract the average COGS per prescription from the average reimbursement to obtain the average gross margin. Then subtract the average COD that was calculated earlier from the gross margin to obtain the net profit.

Results of an Average Net Profit Comparison

	Formula	Current B.H. Rate ($)	New B.H. Rate ($)
	Price/Reimbursement	62.77	60.74
−	Cost of goods sold (COGS)	54.24	54.24
=	Gross margin	8.53	6.16
−	Cost of dispensing (COD)	11.94	11.94
=	Net profit	−3.37	−5.78

AWP, average wholesale price; WAC, wholesaler acquisition cost.

does not account for the fact that some pharmacy expenses are fixed and will not change if there is a change in prescription volume. Prescription departments almost always have a large percentage of fixed expenses, and this tendency results in economies of scale[1] because the average fixed cost per prescription decreases as the number of prescriptions increases. One example of this is pharmacist labor costs. In general, having a prescription department requires at least one full-time pharmacist, and the average cost of dispensing will be much different if this pharmacist dispenses 20 prescriptions per day or 100 prescriptions per day.

A differential analysis compares the differential (marginal) revenue with the differential (marginal) cost of dispensing a prescription for a selected third-party plan. The differential revenue minus the differential cost is called the *contribution margin.* The differential revenue is the average gross margin, and the differential cost is the variable cost per prescription. The decision rule is to accept all third-party plans if they generate a contribution margin greater than zero. This analysis is particularly useful when deciding whether to accept a contract that would increase the prescription volume, but it also may be used to evaluate continuing with an existing plan if it is framed in terms of losing existing volume. Table 19-5 shows an example of a differential analysis for the new Better Health contract.

The contribution margin under the new Better Health contract is $4.25, suggesting that it should be accepted. The pharmacy would have some excess capacity if it did not accept the new contract, unless it could make up the prescription volume elsewhere. The differential analysis result is contrary to the result of the average net profit analysis, but the pro forma analysis will help to reconcile these opposing results. If this were a new plan, the contribution margin could be multiplied to the number of prescriptions likely to be filled under the new plan and this total added to the old net profit to determine the change in net profit. However, since this is an existing plan, the pro forma analysis is critical, as it captures both the effects of the change in variable expenses and the change in reimbursement.

Pro Forma Analysis

The decision about accepting a third-party contract will be clearly affected by whether 5 or 50 percent of the pharmacy's prescriptions are dispensed under that third-party plan. The *pro forma analysis* incorporates this important factor. A pro forma analysis is a projection of what the income statement for the pharmacy would look like both if the contract is accepted and if it is rejected. In the case of Good Service Pharmacy, if it accepts the new contract, it will maintain prescription volume and therefore have similar costs. However, it will have lower prescription revenue owing to the decreased Better Health reimbursement rate. If it declines the contract, it will have lower prescription volume, resulting in less revenue but also in lower costs. The pro forma analysis provides a comparison of the total net profit under both scenarios.

To conduct a pro forma analysis, it is necessary to construct two income statements using information from the current income statement and knowledge about the pharmacy and the third-party contract being evaluated. Information from the average net profit comparison and the differential analysis will also be needed. An example of a pro forma analysis for Good Service Pharmacy is presented in Table 19-6. The results show that although both scenarios result in less net profit than the current situation, declining the new contract would result in $52,137 less net profit than accepting the contract. However, under the sensitivity analysis, if the manager were willing to reduce the employee pharmacist's hours to part time, declining the contract would be a slightly better scenario.

It is important to note that the pro forma analysis did not incorporate different reimbursement rates for brand-name and generic drugs. If accurate information on percent of generic drugs dispensed under a particular third-party plan is available and it is possible to calculate the different reimbursement rates and COGS for generic and brand-name drugs, it would be useful to incorporate this information into the pro forma analysis. At a minimum, if the third party used MAC

[1] Economies of scale occur when the average cost per unit decreases as the number of units produced increases.

Table 19-5. Conducting a Differential Analysis

Step 1: Calculate the differential revenue (average gross margin)

The marginal revenue is the average gross margin per prescription. Recall from Table 19-4 that the average gross margin under the new Better Health contract is $6.16 per prescription.

Step 2: Calculate the differential cost (average variable cost)

The differential cost is the average variable cost. To calculate this cost, it is necessary to divide the average COD into the fixed and variable components. The most obvious variable costs are prescription vials and labels. If the total prescription vial and label cost is divided by the number of prescriptions, the cost for the vial and label is $0.17 for each prescription. The other direct cost was the computer, but that is a fixed expense. It is assumed that the indirect expenses do not vary directly with prescription volume; for example, the rent and advertising costs will not change just because the prescription volume changes.

Determining whether the labor expenses are fixed or variable is somewhat challenging and may be different for different scenarios; that is, a 5% change in prescription volume will have different effects on labor expenses than a 50% change in prescription volume. For this analysis, the effect of a 20% decrease in prescription volume will be considered because about 20% of the prescriptions are from Better Health Insurance, and it is assumed that the pharmacy would lose all those prescriptions if the contract is declined. The pharmacy currently has two pharmacists, the pharmacy manager and the staff pharmacist, and pharmacy manager believes that the pharmacy needs both of them because of the number of hours the pharmacy is open. As a result, pharmacist labor will be treated as a fixed expense. The pharmacy manager believes that the pharmacy technician hours could be reduced if the prescription volume decreased, so technician labor is treated as a variable expense. Assume that the pharmacy technician labor expenses will be reduced by 20% if the prescription volume is reduced by 20% (a 1:1 ratio), so the average variable technician cost is the total prescription department technician expense divided by the number of prescriptions ($98,696/56,795). *Note: Recall that 95% of the technician time is allocated to the prescription department.* This equals $1.74 per prescription. There are no other variable costs other than the prescription vials and the technician labor, so the total variable cost per prescription is $1.91 ($0.17 + $1.74).

Step 3: Calculate the contribution margin

The contribution margin is the differential revenue (DR) minus the differential cost (DC):

$$DR - DC = \$6.16 - \$1.91 = \$4.25$$

The contribution margin is positive, suggesting that the contract should be accepted.

reimbursement for generic drugs, pharmacy managers should consider the source of the MAC rates and how the MAC rates compare with the pharmacy's AAC for generic drugs. Although MAC rates are set for individual products, third parties tend to have MACs that are generally high or generally low relative to other payers.

OTHER CONSIDERATIONS IN EVALUATING A THIRD-PARTY CONTRACT

Understanding the financial impact of a third-party contract clearly is important when making a decision about whether to accept or decline a third-party

Table 19-6. Conducting a Pro Forma Analysis

Step 1: Constructing the "Accept Better Health Contract" projected income statement

The only information in the income statement that will change if the pharmacy accepts the new Better Health contract is the prescription sales. Recall that the pharmacy dispensed 56,795 prescriptions last year and that 11,359 (20%) of those prescriptions were Better Health. To determine the decrease in prescription sales, multiply the number of Better Health prescriptions by the average decrease in reimbursement per prescription. The average decrease in reimbursement may be obtained from the average net profit comparison in Table 19-4 ($62.77 – $60.74 = $2.03). The total decrease in prescription sales is $23,059 (11,359 × $2.03). Subtracting this amount from the current prescription sales gives the projected prescription sales of $3,952,591. The rest of the income statement can be constructed using the other information in the current income statement.

Note: It was assumed that the total prescription volume, the average COGS, and the average COD did not change. While these assumptions may be inaccurate, it is still possible to obtain an accurate comparison by using comparable assumptions for both scenarios.

Step 2: Constructing the "Decline Better Health Contract" projected income statement

This step is somewhat more complex because several pieces of information will change. The prescription sales, COGS, and operating expenses all will decrease. To calculate the decrease in prescription sales, multiply the current Better Health average reimbursement by the number of Better Health prescriptions ($62.77 × 11,359 = $713,004) and subtract this amount from the current prescription sales to get the new prescription sales of $3,262,646.

To calculate the new COGS, multiply the average COGS by the number of Better Health prescriptions ($54.24 × 11,359 = $616,112) and subtract this amount from the current COGS ($4,006,856 – $616,112 = $3,390,744).

To calculate the new operating expenses, remember that some of the expenses are fixed. Recall from the differential analysis that the prescription vials/labels and technician labor are the variable expenses. The prescription vial/label expense will decrease by the average cost per prescription multiplied by the number of Better Health prescriptions ($0.17 × 11,359 = $1,931). The labor costs will decrease by the average technician cost per prescription (already calculated in the differential analysis) multiplied by the number of Better Health prescriptions ($1.74 × 1,359 = $19,765).

The rest of the income statement can be constructed using the other information in the current income statement.

Step 3: Compare net profit for the two projected income statements

The net profit under the "accept" scenario is $283,320 and the net profit under the "decline" scenario is $231,183 so the pharmacy would make $52,137 more profit if they accept the contract.

Step 4: Sensitivity analysis

Sensitivity analysis is a very important step in doing a pro forma analysis, and it involves changing one or more of the assumptions and seeing how that change affects the results. One assumption was that the pharmacist labor costs are fixed, so an example of a sensitivity analysis would be to change this assumption. The manager estimates that if she reduced the employee pharmacist from full time to half time with limited benefits under the "Decline Better Health Scenario," the labor costs would decrease by approximately $60,000. This would increase the net profit under this scenario to $291,183, which is slightly more than the "Accept Better Health Scenario." The correct conclusion depends on whether the manager is willing to make the decision to reduce the pharmacist's hours.

(Continued)

Table 19-6. Conducting a Pro Forma Analysis *(Continued)*

Note: Other sensitivity analyses are also possible. For example, the amount of other sales and COGS could be decreased under the "Decline Better Health Scenario" to account for lower OTC sales resulting from less store traffic.

Results from the Pro Forma Analysis for Good Service Pharmacy

Sales	**Original ($)**	**Accept Better Health ($)**	**Decline Better Health ($)**
Prescription sales	3,975,650	3,952,591	3,262,646
Other sales	1,303,475	1,303,475	1,303,475
Total sales	5,279,125	5,256,066	4,566,121
Cost of goods sold	4,006,856	4,006,856	3,390,744
Gross margin	1,272,269	1,249,210	1,175,377
Expenses			
Labor	586,286	586,286	566,521
Rent	52,059	52,059	52,059
Utilities	19,196	19,196	19,196
Prescription vials/labels	9,750	9,750	7,819
Computer	7,500	7,500	7,500
Advertising	16,128	16,128	16,128
All other expenses	274,971	274,971	274,971
Total expenses	965,890	965,890	944,194
Net profit (before taxes)	306,379	283,320	231,183

contract, but other factors also have a role in the decision. One factor that needs to be considered is the effect of the decision on pharmacy customers. If the decision is made to reject the contract, customers who have that third party may be forced to go elsewhere to obtain their prescriptions. This may mean angering, distressing, or inconveniencing some pharmacy customers. Many customers may not understand the pharmacy's decision and subsequently direct their anger toward the pharmacy staff. Pharmacists employed by the pharmacy also may be distressed by losing customers with whom they have established relationships.

Pharmacy image is another concern. Some pharmacies want to avoid the reputation of being a pharmacy that "does not accept many insurance plans," and this image may occur if a large third-party contract is declined. Conversely, a pharmacy may want to have an image as a high-quality service pharmacy, and accepting a contract with a low reimbursement rate may jeopardize the pharmacy's ability to provide good service. If the low reimbursement rate means that pharmacists have to dispense more prescriptions, therefore having less time for their patients, then the quality of patient care at the pharmacy may be affected.

Pharmacies also need to consider the impact of the decision on any remaining private-pay customers. If the pharmacy accepts a lower reimbursement-rate contract, it may attempt to make up the lost revenue from other sources. One source of revenue is to raise the private-pay prices, sometimes referred to as *cost shifting.* The problem with this approach is that it may result in the pharmacy being less competitive with other pharmacies, and, perhaps more important, it places the burden of high prescription prices on those who may be least able to afford them. Having a good understanding of the pharmacy's competitors and customer base is necessary to determine the importance of this factor.

Another critical factor to consider is the signal that the pharmacy's decision sends to other third parties. Accepting a low reimbursement rate from one third party may encourage other third parties to lower their rates to comparable levels. As long as pharmacies continue to accept declining rates, the third parties are likely to continue offering progressively lower rates. Conversely, declining a low reimbursement-rate contract may send third-party payers a signal that the pharmacy is not willing to accept poor reimbursement rates.

One last factor to consider is the effect of the decision on other sources of revenue. In the pro forma analysis, it was assumed that other sales would not be affected if they declined to accept the Better Health contract. In reality, if prescription volume decreased by 20 percent, it is likely that other sales would decrease as well. If there is less store traffic, there likely will be fewer over-the-counter (OTC) product sales and fewer sales of other products in the pharmacy. This loss of other sales may be more important for a store where other sales are a large percentage of total sales. OTC or other sales also sometimes are used as a justification to accept a third-party contract with a low reimbursement rate. The argument is that "even though we lose money on each prescription, we will make it up with OTC sales." While prescription customers may purchase some OTC or other products, managers need to be careful with this argument because only the profit on the OTCs will help to compensate for the prescription losses. In one study, researchers found that the average OTC purchase per prescription was $1.24, but pharmacies would have needed an average OTC purchase of $11.27 per third-party prescription to compensate for accepting lower third-party reimbursement (Huey et al., 1995).

Third-Party Contract Terminology

It is important to understand the terminology commonly used in third-party contracts. For a more thorough discussion of this issue, see reference Fridy et al. (2002). Basic elements of a third-party contract include provider rights and responsibilities, transmission of claims process, requirements for pharmacy participation in the third-party network, and third-party rights and responsibilities. Some common provider rights and responsibilities relate to record keeping, collecting patient copayments, complying with third-party formularies, and maintaining professional standards. The reimbursement rate and the timing of reimbursement are described in the section on requirements for pharmacy participation. It also will specify the procedure for changes in the contract. Most changes in the contract occur at the request of the third party. Pharmacies certainly can request changes in a contract, but often are not successful in getting the third party to accept the changes (Fridy et al., 2002). Third-party rights and responsibilities may include the right to inspect/audit pharmacy records and the provision of help-desk support. Pharmacy managers should pay particular attention to the information on audits, since audits often result in the pharmacy needing to pay back money to the third party. Third parties may conduct *desk audits*, where third parties review pharmacy claims data but do not come to the pharmacy, and *field audits*, where a third-party representative visits the pharmacy and inspects pharmacy records and procedures. It is important to understand what information might be inspected in an audit and to make sure that your pharmacy has adequate record-keeping procedures in place.

One thing to consider in a third-party contract is the length of time before the pharmacy will be reimbursed by the third party. If the third party's reimbursement cycle is longer than the pharmacy's payment cycle with its vendors, this may create a cash-flow problem for the pharmacy (see Chapter 17). The length of time before the pharmacy receives payment will also be influenced by the percentage of claims rejected or challenged by the third party. Although electronic "real time" transmission of claims makes it possible to determine at the time of dispensing whether the prescription claim will be accepted, some rejected claims still will be identified during the claim reconciliation process. Having to resubmit rejected claims to the third party or having to try to obtain payment from the patient delays payment for the prescription. One study reported that the median payment time for Medicare PDP claims was 29 days, but almost 41 percent of the December 2006 claims were not paid within 30 days (Shepherd et al., 2007).

A requirement of most third-party contracts with pharmacies is that the pharmacy *accepts assignment.* This clause means that the pharmacy agrees to charge the patient no more than the amount specified by the contract. In other words, a pharmacy that has accepted assignment cannot charge a third-party patient more to make up for a decrease in the third-party reimbursement rate. It is important to be careful that the assignment is confined to payment for prescription dispensing. The pharmacy manager should clarify that accepting assignment does not preclude the pharmacy from charging third-party patients for additional professional services.

Two clauses seen occasionally in pharmacy contracts are the *most favored nation clause* and the *all-products clause.* The most favored nation clause requires pharmacies to extend their lowest price or reimbursement rate to that third party. It is customary for third parties to require that the pharmacy charge the third party its U& C price if it is lower than the third party's reimbursement formula price. However, having to give the third party the lowest reimbursement rate of all the other third-party rates is not customary. The all-products clause requires pharmacies to participate in all the third party's plans if it wants to participate in any one plan. A pharmacy may want to participate in only some of a third party's plans depending on the reimbursement rate and number of customers affected. Some states prohibit all-products clauses. These clauses became especially problematic with the advent of discount cards and more recently with the implementation of Medicare Part D. *Discount cards* are given or sold to people who do not have insurance coverage for prescription drugs. People who have a discount card pay a price that is determined by a reimbursement formula rather than the U& C pharmacy price. As noted earlier, the reimbursement price usually is less than the pharmacy's U& C price, so pharmacies receive less revenue. Some of the discount cards are administered by PBMs and other third parties, and pharmacies may prefer not to accept a third party's discount card even if they accept patients with insurance from that third party. Pharmacies generally do not like discount cards because they lower revenue and further decrease the pharmacy's pricing flexibility.

A final note with regard to third-party contracting is that some pharmacy owners and managers outsource their contracting to an outside organization. Some drug wholesalers offer contract management services to pharmacies, but there are also independent businesses that specialize in third-party network management. These companies may provide valuable and timesaving services, but it is important to assess whether they are making the contracting decisions that best represent the interests of your pharmacy. As discussed in this chapter, there are many factors that go into evaluating a third-party contract, and have a good understanding of how a contract will affect your pharmacy is essential in making strategic decisions about contracts.

Responding to Reductions in Third-Party Reimbursement

As was shown in the pro forma analysis, Good Service Pharmacy's net profit will decrease regardless of whether it accepts or rejects the new Better Health contract. Decreasing third-party reimbursement is a common occurrence, and pharmacies need to develop strategies to maintain their profit levels as reimbursement rates decrease. To accomplish this goal, pharmacy managers need to consider developing alternative sources of revenue or decreasing their expenses.

One source of revenue is to increase prescription volume by attracting new third-party or private-pay customers. As discussed earlier in this chapter, pharmacies tend to have a high percentage of fixed costs, so there usually are economies of scale to be achieved by dispensing more prescriptions. This strategy seems to have been used widely by pharmacies, and although it provides a short-term solution, it may not be a viable long-term strategy because the new private-pay patients may become third-party patients in the future, and the other third-party prescription reimbursement rates also likely will decline over time.

Another strategy for pharmacies to consider is diversifying their sources of revenue. A pharmacy that obtains most of its revenue from prescription drugs is more vulnerable to decreasing reimbursement rates than a pharmacy with other significant sources of revenue. One possible source of revenue is payment for professional and patient care services. Pharmacies may either directly charge patients for these services or bill third-party payers. Medication therapy management (MTM) services under Medicare Part D are one opportunity in this area (see Chapters 20, 25 & 26). It should be noted that obtaining third-party payment for patient care services will likely result in many of the same concerns as obtaining third-party payment for prescriptions (Ganther, 2002). As long as the third-party contract does not prevent pharmacists from charging patients directly for their services, obtaining payment for patient care services is possible for both third-party and private-pay patients. Another source of revenue is sales of items such as OTC products, durable medical equipment, and other health- or non–health-related products. Pharmacies that have the space for additional products may want to consider developing this source of revenue, but it is important to stay informed about ongoing reimbursement changes for these products, particularly in the Medicare program.

Another strategy to preserve net profit when reimbursement rates are decreased is to decrease expenses. The largest prescription department expense is labor, so labor costs are important to evaluate. The most expensive labor cost in most pharmacies is pharmacist labor, so pharmacies need to evaluate carefully how pharmacists are spending their time. Having pharmacists spend their time doing tasks that do not require a pharmacist's expertise is an inefficient use of resources. Pharmacy managers should consider using other pharmacy personnel such as pharmacy technicians and clerks to do some of the tasks associated with the dispensing of prescriptions, for example, counting tablets and reconciling third-party claims. Other pharmacy personnel costs and nonlabor costs of the pharmacy department should also be evaluated.

REVISITING THE SCENARIO

In the scenario described at the beginning of the chapter, the pharmacy manager at Good Service Pharmacy (Natalie Hawkins) was faced with the decision to accept or reject a new contract from Better Health Insurance. The reimbursement rates in the new contract used a new reimbursement formula and Natalie was unsure how the new contract would affect profit margins. She was particularly worried, since the Better Health rates were already low and 20% of the pharmacy's prescriptions were dispensed under Better Health.

1. How much would the change in reimbursement affect the net profit on an average Better Health Prescription? Would they be losing more money on each Better Health prescription they dispense?

   The average net profit comparison showed that the average decrease in net profit from the change in reimbursement would be $2.41. The pharmacy currently is losing money on each Better Health prescription they dispense, but under the new reimbursement rate, the pharmacy would lose even more, an average of $5.78 on each Better Health Prescription.
2. Would Good Service Pharmacy be better off financially by accepting or declining the contract? How do you determine whether it is worse to accept a very low reimbursement rate or lose about 20% of your prescription volume?

   The results from both the differential analysis and the pro forma analysis show that Good Service Pharmacy would be better off financially by accepting the contract. Although the level of net profit in either case would be less than the current level of net profit, the pro forma analysis shows that net profit if the pharmacy accepts the contract would be $52,137 more than the net profit if it declines the contract. In this case, losing 20% of the pharmacy's prescription volume is worse than accepting a low reimbursement rate. The reason for this result is the high percentage of fixed costs in the prescription department. If the pharmacy was willing to make changes to reduce its fixed costs (e.g., reduce pharmacist hours), then the pharmacy might be better off declining the contract.

3. What other factors need to be considered? Could the contract be renegotiated? What effect would signing or declining the contract have on its customers?

   The pharmacy manager knows that if she accepts the contract, the pharmacy risks sending a signal to other third parties that it will accept low reimbursement rates. The pharmacy may also have to raise its cash prices or decrease its level of service to decrease costs, but this may be necessary in either scenario. If she declines the contract, the pharmacy will lose long-term customers and may get a reputation for being a pharmacy that does not accept insurance plans. It may also have to reduce a pharmacist's hours. It is unlikely that the contract could be renegotiated, although Natalie could decline the contract and see how Better Health Insurance responds.

4. Good Service Pharmacy will lose revenue regardless of whether the new Better Health contract is accepted or rejected. Is there any way for Good Service Pharmacy to make up the lost revenue? Or decrease its expenses?

   The pharmacy could raise cash prices to make up for the lost revenue, or it could try to attract new customers to generate new prescription volume. It also could try to generate revenue from pharmacist services or selling more products (e.g., OTC products or durable medical equipment). Its largest expenses are labor costs, so the best way to decrease its cost of dispensing would be to decrease its staffing levels.

   In the end, Natalie decides to continue to accept Better Health Insurance. The financial impact of losing 20% of the pharmacy's business was substantial, and she was not willing to lose Mrs. Anderson and other Better Health customers. However, she is very worried about what other third parties will do in the future and how she can make up the lost revenue. She decides that developing other sources of revenue is a better option for the pharmacy's future than reducing the pharmacy staff, so she decides to try to implement and obtain payment for some pharmacist services. This includes participating in any available Medicare Part D medication therapy management services. She also hopes to expand the pharmacy's sales of durable medical equipment. She also plans to closely monitor profit margins as other third-party plans move away from using AWP-based reimbursement formulas.

CONCLUSION AND FUTURE THIRD-PARTY REIMBURSEMENT ISSUES

What should be apparent is that the decision to accept or reject a third-party contract is often very difficult. Even after the pharmacy manager answered the questions listed in the scenario, she still has to use her judgment about accepting the new Better Health contract with its low reimbursement rate. It is important to understand and use the tools that were described in this chapter, but they do not necessarily yield an easy answer. Regardless of the manager's decision, the pharmacy faces lower net profit unless it finds other sources of revenue or decreases its expenses.

A third-party payer issue that will continue to be important is declining reimbursement rates. Private third-party reimbursement rates are likely to continue to decrease. Medicare Part D PDPs are now major players in the third-party prescription drug market, and there is concern about their low reimbursement rates. There are some opportunities to obtain reimbursement for MTM services from Medicare drug plans, but these reimbursement levels also need to be evaluated by managers. As third-party payers move away from AWP-based reimbursement, it will be critically important to monitor profit levels under the new reimbursement systems, whether they be based on WAC, AMP, or AvAC.

Decreasing Medicaid reimbursement rates are also an issue. Whenever states are faced with budget shortfalls or rapidly rising prescription drug costs in the Medicaid program, there is renewed pressure to decrease pharmacy reimbursement rates. The change to AMP-based reimbursement for generic prescription drugs dispensed through Medicaid is a trend that needs to be monitored carefully. Some state Medicaid programs may increase generic drug dispensing fees or make other changes to compensate pharmacies for the lost revenue from the new AMP-based reimbursement, but they are not required to do so. Other third parties may also use the new federal AMP-based MAC list for their generic drug reimbursement, potentially broadening the impact of this change. Any AvAC list that becomes publicly available has also the potential to be widely used by third-party payers.

Another trend that should be monitored is performance-based pharmacy reimbursement. Performance-based reimbursement is rapidly being integrated in other areas of health care, particularly Medicare, and it is likely that this trend will spread to pharmacy reimbursement. Organizations such as the Pharmacy Quality Alliance (PQA) (www.pqaalliance.org) are in the process of developing quality measures for community pharmacies. It is anticipated that third parties may begin to incorporate these quality measures into their pharmacy reimbursement. This may result in increased revenue for pharmacies that are able to demonstrate that they provide high quality care, and even further reductions in reimbursement for those who do not.

It is crucial that pharmacy managers understand the impact of third-party payers on their pharmacies, as well as understand and use the decision-analysis tools described in this chapter to evaluate carefully third-party contracts. It is also important that pharmacy managers and owners manage expenses carefully and think creatively about developing new sources of revenue. Third-party payment for prescriptions will continue to be an important issue in pharmacy in the future, and pharmacy managers need to be aware continually of changing reimbursement levels and other third-party issues.

REFERENCES

Academy of Managed Care Pharmacy (AMCP) Task Force on Drug Payment Methodologies. 2007. *AMCP Guide to Pharmaceutical Payment Methods*, Version 1.0. Alexandria, VA: AMCP, October 2007.

Brooks JM, Doucette WR, Sorofman BA. 1999. Factors affecting bargaining outcomes between pharmacies and insurers. *Health Serv Res* 34:439.

Caroll NV. 1991. Costs of dispensing private-pay and third-party prescriptions in independent pharmacies. *J Res Pharm Econ* 3:3.

Fridy K, DeHart RM, Monk-Tutor MR. 2002. Negotiating with third-party payers: One community pharmacy's experience. *J Am Pharm Assoc* 42:780.

Ganther JM. 2002. Third-party reimbursement for pharmacist services: Why has it been so difficult to obtain and is it really the answer for pharmacy? *J Am Pharm Assoc* 42:875.

Grant Thornton. 2007. *Cost of dispensing study. Grant Thornton report commissioned by Coalition for Community Pharmacy Action.* Washington, DC: Coalition for Community Pharmacy Action, January 2007.

Huey C, Jackson RA, Pirl MA. 1995. Analysis of the impact of third-party prescription programs on community pharmacy. *J Res Pharm Econ* 7:57.

National Association of Chain Drug Stores (NACDS). 1999. *Pharmacy Activity Cost and Productivity Study.* Alexandria, VA: NACDS, November 1999.

National Association of State Medicaid Directors. 2010. Post AWP Pharmacy Pricing and Reimbursement. Washington, DC: June 2010.

National Community Pharmacists Association. 2010. *NCPA Digest.* Alexandria, VA: October 2010.

Office of the Inspector General (OIG). 2001. Medicaid pharmacy: Actual acquisition cost of brand name prescription drug products. Report A-06-00-00023. Washington, DC: OIG, August 2001.

Office of the Inspector General (OIG). 2002. Medicaid pharmacy: Actual acquisition cost of brand name prescription drug products. Report A-06-01-00053. Washington, DC: OIG, March 2002.

Schafermeyer KW, Schondelmeyer SW, Thomas J, et al. 1992. Analysis of the cost of dispensing third party prescriptions in independent pharmacies. *J Res Pharm Econ* 4:3.

Shepherd MD, Richards KM, Winegar AL. 2007. Prescription drug payment times by Medicare Part D plans: Results of a national study. *J Am Pharm Assoc* 47(6):e20.

Yang X, Brooks JM, Urmie JM, Doucette WR. 2010. Retail pharmacy market structure and insurer-independent pharmacy bargaining in the Medicare Part D era. In Avi Dor (ed.) *Advances in Health Economics Health Services Research*, Vol. 22. Bingley, United Kingdom; Emerald Group Publishing Limited, 2010.

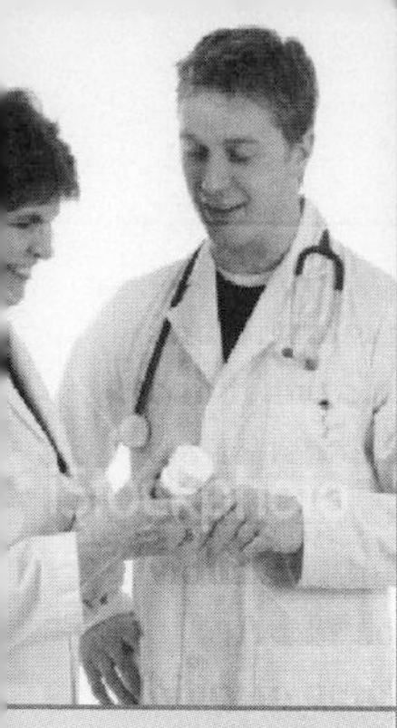

20

IMPACT OF HEALTH POLICY ON HEALTH CARE DELIVERY

Julie M. Urmie

About the Author: Dr. Urmie is an associate professor in the Health Services Research Division at the University of Iowa College of Pharmacy. She received a B.S. in pharmacy from the University of Wisconsin and worked as a community pharmacist prior to returning to the University of Wisconsin for graduate school, where she received an M.S. in pharmacy administration and a Ph.D. in social and administrative sciences in pharmacy. Her teaching interests include insurance and reimbursement in pharmacy, health insurance, the US health care system, health policy, and pharmacy management. Her main areas of research are prescription drug insurance and consumer preferences related to health care use.

LEARNING OBJECTIVES

After completing this chapter, readers should be able to

1. Understand the health policy process in the United States and how pharmacists can get involved.
2. Describe resources to understand and stay current on health policy issues relevant to pharmacists.
3. Describe the Medicare program, including Parts A and B, Medicare Advantage, and Medigap plans.
4. Describe Medicare Part D and discuss its effects on pharmacies.
5. Describe the Medicaid program and understand the dual role of states and the federal government.
6. Explain how health care delivery and financing will be changed by the Affordable Care Act of 2010 (commonly referred to as "health care reform").
7. Discuss federal and state legislation that is of interest to pharmacists.
8. Discuss challenges and opportunities for pharmacists in Medicare, Medicaid, and under health care reform.

SCENARIO

Joshua Anderson is a newly licensed pharmacist who just started working at Badger Pharmacy in North Central Wisconsin. Bob Smart, the pharmacy owner, recently returned from a pharmacy association meeting and is eager to talk to Joshua about what he has learned. Bob says "Joshua, I need to sit down this week and write a letter to our state legislator about H.R. 3546. You should write one too. It is critical to Badger Pharmacy's survival that this legislation passes! Have you seen the latest set of Medicare Prescription Drug Plan (PDP) contracts? Not to mention all this talk about health care reform. I just don't know how it will affect Badger Pharmacy. Oh, and legislation has been introduced again to reduce Medicaid reimbursement in Wisconsin. I sure hope the pharmacy association can lobby successfully to defeat that bill." Joshua thinks to himself "What on earth is he talking about. I hate politics—I'm here to help patients with their medication therapy and learn how to manage a pharmacy, not be a politician. Why should I get involved? Oh, and who's "bill" and why do we need to defeat him?" However, as a new employee Joshua is eager to make a good impression so he wants to learn more. Joshua wonders what is the best way to learn more about the health policy process. He vaguely remembers learning about Medicare and Medicaid in pharmacy school, and he knows he needs to understand the basics in case patients ask him questions, but he does not understand how pharmacists can influence government programs. He does remember that Medicare Part D seemed very complicated. He also remembers his parents talking about a health care reform law being passed, but he does not understand how it relates to being a pharmacist. He certainly never learned how to write a letter to a legislator.

HEALTH POLICY IN THE UNITED STATES

As the role of all levels of government in health care delivery continues to increase, so does the percent of prescriptions paid for by government programs. In 2010, independent pharmacies reported that 44 percent of dispensed prescriptions were covered by government-administered programs such as Medicaid and Medicare (National Community Pharmacy Association, 2010). This is much higher than the 21 percent of dispensed prescriptions covered by government programs in 2000 (NCPA-Pharmacia Digest, 2002). Medicaid, a program that provides health care assistance to those with low incomes and assets, has been an important third-party payer for prescription drugs since it was created in the 1960s. Medicare Part D, implemented in 2006 to provide assistance to the elderly in obtaining prescription medications, has greatly increased the percentage of prescriptions paid for by government programs. Although the prescription drug programs (PDPs) that administer Medicare Part D benefit are private companies, they must comply with rules published by the Centers for Medicare and Medicaid Services (CMS). Under the Affordable Care Act of 2010 (referred to by many as "health care reform"), government involvement in health care will continue to increase with the expansion of Medicaid and government-run health insurance exchanges. This increased government involvement in health care makes it critical for pharmacists to understand the public policy process and how they can be involved.

The first step in being involved in the public policy process is to understand how it works. Constituents such as pharmacists have an opportunity to influence the process in many ways at various stages. The first step in the public policy process involves the legislative branch, consisting of the House of Representatives and the Senate. Constituents can work with their elected federal or state legislators to get a bill introduced. Pharmacy associations routinely do this, but individual pharmacists also may suggest bill topics to their legislators. Once a bill has been introduced into the House of Representatives or Senate (at the federal level or state level), pharmacists can contact their legislators to urge them to vote for or against the piece of legislation. Pharmacists can also support the lobbying efforts of pharmacy associations by contributing to their political action committees (PACs). Once a bill has been passed by both the House of Representatives and Senate, it must be signed by the president (or governor at the state level) to become a law.

After the bill becomes a law, it is turned over to the executive branch for implementation. At this stage, opportunities are still there for constituents to influence the process. Laws are usually assigned to a government agency to be implemented, such as the federal Department of Health and Human Services (HHS) or a state Department of Regulation and Licensing. These agencies publish proposed rules for implementing the law. The rules may not contradict the law, but they can and often do expand the scope of the law. The department charged with implementing many federal laws related to health care is the HHS. The CMS is an important agency within HHS since they publish rules related to Medicare and Medicaid. For all agencies, proposed rules are published in the Federal Register, followed by a period where constituents can submit comments about the proposed rules. After considering the submitted comments, the government agency publishes final rules for implementing the law. Most states follow a similar process when publishing rules for state laws. It is important to understand that the published rules are much easier to change than the law itself. The heads of government agencies are appointed by the chief executive (e.g., president, governor), so when there is a new chief executive, there are also likely to be many new agency heads. A new administration sometimes results in different philosophy for an agency, which may mean new rules and guidance for existing laws. For example, each year CMS provides guidance to Part D plan sponsors who want to participate in Medicare, and that guidance can change from year to year. An example is the CMS 2005 guidance regarding Medicare Part D formularies (CMS, 2005). This guidance was issued after the final rules were published and after many of the Part D plans had already submitted premium bids to CMS. The guidance required Part D plans to cover all or substantially all drugs in six therapeutic classes and was more restrictive than the original CMS rules regarding Part D formularies.

The third branch of government, the judicial branch, also is involved in the policy process. Courts often hear cases involving the interpretation of laws. There are opportunities for constituents to influence the policy process through the legal system. Pharmacy associations and pharmacists have sued to block implementation of various laws. For example, two pharmacy associations successfully sued to block the implementation of AMP based pricing for generic drugs in Medicaid (NCPA Original Complaint). This lawsuit delayed implementation of the law until a change in the law could be made via the legislative process. The Affordable Care Act of 2010 is a recent example where the legality of the individual mandate, the portion of the law that requires most people either purchase health insurance or obtain it from their employers, has been challenged in the courts. All three stages of the public policy process are important. The final section of this chapter further discusses how pharmacists can get involved.

MEDICARE

Medicare is a federal government program that began in 1965. Medicare is an insurance program that covers health care services for people aged 65 and older, disabled individuals, and people with end-stage renal disease. Individuals qualify for Medicare if they are US citizens or permanent legal residents; it is open to all individuals aged 65 and older without regard to income or health status. Some individuals under 65 years of age with permanent disabilities qualify for Medicare after receiving Social Security Disability Income (SSDI) payments for 24 months. Some Medicare beneficiaries are also eligible for Medicaid; these individuals are called *dual eligibles* (see Table 20-1). Originally, Medicare consisted of two parts: Part A that covers hospital costs and Part B that covers outpatient costs (see Tables 20-2 and 20-3). Most outpatient prescription drugs were not covered until Medicare Part D was added in 2006. When Medicare first started, it was a government insurance program where the government acted as an insurer and reimbursed providers directly when they provided care to Medicare beneficiaries. However, in 1997, Medicare Part C was implemented to provide

Table 20-1. Dual Eligibles

Medicare beneficiaries who are also eligible for Medicaid are called *dual eligibles.* They account for 15 % of Medicaid enrollees (Kaiser fact sheet on dual eligibles, May 2011). Medicare is the primary payer for these individuals; Medicaid pays for services that are not covered by Medicare. A key service that is covered by Medicaid and not by Medicare is long-term nursing home costs. Medicaid also pays the Medicare Part B premium and the Medicare cost sharing for services covered under Parts A and D. Dual eligibles receive their drug coverage from Part D plans (see the Medicare Part D section for more information). Medicare beneficiaries become eligible for Medicaid by having low incomes and limited assets. A frequent pathway for Medicaid eligibility among Medicare beneficiaries is for them to "spend down" their resources paying for health care or long-term care. The Affordable Care Act of 2010 established the Federal Coordinated Health Care Office to improve coordination of Medicare and Medicaid services for dual eligibles.

an alternate pathway for Medicare beneficiaries. Under Medicare Part C, later renamed Medicare Advantage (MA), Medicare beneficiaries have a choice to sign up for private insurance coverage via a MA plan. If the beneficiary chooses a MA plan instead of the original Medicare, the government pays a portion of the premium for the MA plan. Beneficiaries get their care from providers affiliated with the MA plan and the MA plan pays providers for this care. Under this pathway, the government is a purchaser of insurance rather than directly being the insurer. A diagram of the two pathways is provided in Fig. 20-1.

Original Medicare

Under the original Medicare pathway, beneficiaries can receive Part A and Part B services from any provider who accepts Medicare. The government sets the reimbursement rates and pays the providers. One problem with the original Medicare pathway is that there are many gaps in coverage and significant cost sharing for the beneficiaries. As a result, beneficiaries risk

Table 20-2. Medicare Part A

Everyone in Medicare is automatically enrolled in Part A and there are no monthly premiums. Part A covers inpatient hospital stays, short-term skilled nursing home facility care following a hospitalization, and hospice care. Beneficiaries pay a deductible and coinsurance for Part A services and there is no limit on beneficiary out-of-pocket expenses. Part A is funded by a payroll tax. The money collected from current workers is put in a trust fund to pay the Part A expenses of people currently enrolled in Medicare.

Table 20-3. Medicare Part B

Medicare Part B, sometimes called Supplemental Medical Insurance (SMI) is voluntary, but almost all Medicare eligible beneficiaries do enroll. People who choose to enroll are charged a monthly Part B premium and there are penalties for late enrollment. Services covered under Part B include physician visits, outpatient services, preventive services, and home health visits. Durable medical equipment (DME) is also covered under Part B. This is of interest to pharmacy managers since some pharmacies are DME suppliers for Medicare. Very few prescription drugs are covered under Part B. There is a Part B deductible and coinsurance for most Part B services. General tax revenue pays for about 75 % of Part B services; beneficiary premiums make up the remainder.

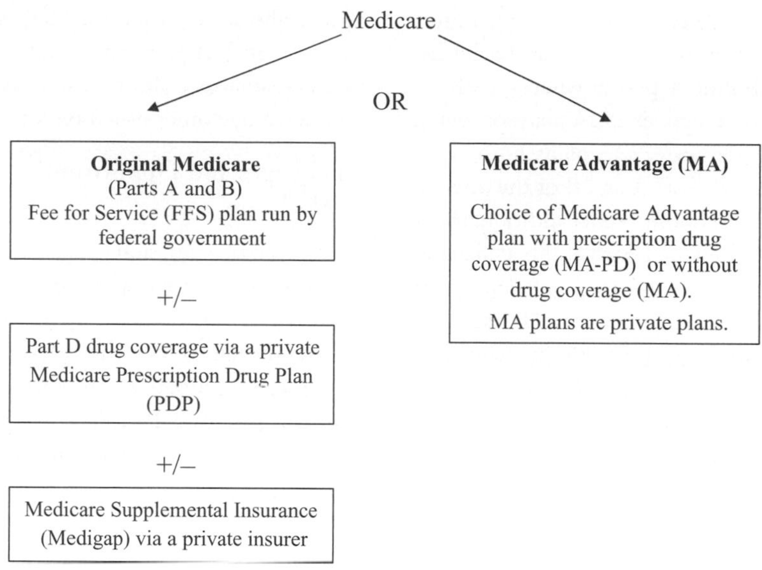

Figure 20-1. Medicare pathways diagram.

significant out-of-pocket costs unless they sign up for a Medicare supplemental plan, sometimes called Medigap plans. These plans are sold by private insurance companies but are heavily regulated by the federal government. Medigap coverage may be purchased by the beneficiary, or it may be provided as retiree coverage by a former employer. If Medicare beneficiaries choose to sign up for Part D, they receive coverage through a privately operated company called a Medicare prescription drug plan (PDP).

From a beneficiary perspective there are both advantages and disadvantages to receiving coverage via the original Medicare pathway. An advantage is that they are free to see any Part A and Part B providers who accept Medicare. This pathway is also more stable than the MA pathway where private plans enter and leave the Medicare market. A disadvantage under this pathway is that beneficiaries may have up to three different insurers paying for their care: the government as the insurer for Part A and B, a private PDP as the insurer for Part D drug coverage, and a private Medigap insurer. Having multiple payers may create confusion for beneficiaries. Another disadvantage is that this pathway is often more expensive for beneficiaries. They face significant cost sharing under Parts A and B, particularly if they do not have a Medigap plan. They must also typically pay premiums for Part B, Part D, and Medigap coverage, although a former employer may provide some Part D and Medigap coverage via a retiree plan. Out-of-pocket costs under the original pathway typically far exceed costs for most MA plans, although this could change if government payments to MA plans are reduced and they increase their premiums or decrease their benefits.

Medicare Advantage

Under the MA pathway, beneficiaries may choose from an array of MA plans; the specific plans available depend on where the beneficiary lives. When the MA pathway first began, plans were typically offered by health maintenance organizations (HMOs), and most of them served only a small geographic area. However, private fee-for-service (FFS) MA plans are also available. Enrollment in these plans has grown rapidly in recent years. The MA FFS plans are typically national plans that are available to beneficiaries throughout the country. Beneficiaries who enroll in an MA plan must typically stay in that plan for at least 1 year. Each year, there is an open enrollment period where beneficiaries are allowed to switch between MA plans or switch back to the original Medicare. MA plans must cover all services covered under Part A and B of the original Medicare, plus they may choose to offer additional benefits, such as vision and dental benefits. If beneficiaries want prescription drug coverage, they can sign up for an MA plan that offers Part D coverage. These plans are called Medicare Advantage Prescription Drug Plans (MA-PDs). Since MA plans have much less cost sharing and typically offer more benefits above and beyond the Part A and B services, beneficiaries who enroll in an MA plan do not need to purchase a Medigap plan. MA plans receive payments from the government that are partially based on a benchmark premium set by the government. MA plans can charge beneficiaries an additional monthly premium. The generosity of coverage and premiums paid by beneficiaries fluctuate depending on the generosity of the government payments to the MA plans.

An advantage of the MA pathway is that beneficiaries receive all their Part A, B, and D (if selected) coverage from the same plan. MA plans typically have less cost sharing and offer additional benefits compared to the original Parts A and B coverage, so MA plans are generally less expensive for beneficiaries than the original Medicare, particularly since they do not need to purchase a separate Medigap plan. MA plans also are more flexible and can adapt to market changes more quickly than original Medicare. As noted above, a disadvantage of the MA pathway is that MA plans enter and leave markets depending on the plan's profitability. In time periods when MA reimbursement has been reduced by Congress, there have been problems with MA plans exiting the Medicare market (Berenson, 2001). In most MA plans, beneficiaries are restricted to providers within their plan's provider network so they have less choice of providers than in original Medicare. From a societal perspective, MA plans are focused on controlling short-term health claims costs for beneficiaries enrolled in their plan. This goal is sometimes at odds with the government's goal of decreasing long-term health care costs for the Medicare population. For example, an MA plan may be reluctant to cover a service that increases short-term costs but may improve long-term outcomes or reduce long-term costs.

Challenges and Opportunities for Pharmacists in Medicare

While pharmacies and pharmacists pay particular attention to the prescription drug coverage in Part D, there also are opportunities and challenges for pharmacists related to the other parts of Medicare. Reimbursement for inpatient pharmacy goods and services through Medicare Part A is a significant challenge. Medicare Part A has a prospective payment system where inpatient reimbursement is predetermined based on a patient's diagnosis, not the actual amount of care used while they are in the hospital. Under this type of a reimbursement system, the hospital pharmacy becomes a cost center rather than a revenue-generating center. Inpatient pharmacies are challenged by increasingly expensive new medications and biologics. In some cases, the cost for the drug product may consume a significant portion of the total Medicare reimbursement. However, there are opportunities for inpatient pharmacists to help hospitals reduce costs and improve outcomes under this type of a payment system. For example, they may help reduce adverse drug events while patients are in the hospital and participate in medication reconciliation between the outpatient and inpatient settings. Helping with transitions between settings will become important especially under the episode based payment pilot program that is being implemented as part of health care reform.

Pharmacists also face challenges when billing Medicare Part B for the outpatient services that they provide, such as diabetes education or management of anticoagulation drug therapy. Currently, pharmacists generally may not bill for their outpatient services under Part B, except as "incident to" physician services. A change that pharmacists would like to see implemented in Medicare is to give provider status under Part B. Legislation that would allow pharmacists to bill for their services under Part B would be a major victory for pharmacies and pharmacists. Pharmacies also have the opportunity to be a Medicare supplier for durable medical equipment (DME) since DME is covered under Part B, but a challenge is the competitive bidding program for DME and the pilot testing of competitive bidding for diabetes supplies.

MEDICARE PART D

Overview

The Medicare Prescription Drug, Improvement and Modernization Act (MMA) of 2003 was signed into law in December of 2003. It added outpatient prescription drug coverage to Medicare beginning in January of 2006. The drug coverage is not included in Medicare Part A or Part B, but is in a separate Medicare Part D. The Part D coverage is voluntary and available to anybody enrolled in Medicare Parts A or B. People who are in the original FFS Medicare program get their Part D coverage from private plans called Medicare Prescription Drug Plans (PDPs). This coverage is sometimes called "stand-alone" coverage because it is not linked to parts A and B. Beneficiaries in the MA program have their Parts A, B, and D coverage through MA-PDs. Beneficiaries who do not have other creditable coverage for prescription drugs must sign up for Part D coverage within 7 months when they are first eligible or they are required to pay late enrollment penalties. Most beneficiaries have the opportunity to change plans once per year during an open enrollment period, but dual eligible and other low-income beneficiaries may change plans at any time. The funding structure for Part D is similar to Part B; general tax revenue covers approximately 75 percent of the costs, and premiums paid by the beneficiaries cover the remainder. Medicare Part D has been successful at increasing the percentage of Medicare beneficiaries with prescription drug coverage. As of September 2011, approximately 90 percent of Medicare beneficiaries had prescription drug coverage, where 60 percent enrolled in Part D plans (Kaiser Fact Sheet November 2011b). Of the beneficiaries in Part D plans, more were in PDPs than MA-PDs (64 percent vs. 36 percent) (Kaiser Fact Sheet November 2011a).

Part D Plans and Premiums

All Part D plans are operated by private companies. Plans that want to participate in the program submit bids to CMS each year and must follow rules established by CMS. They must also participate in regions of the United States that are determined by CMS. Plans do not have to participate in all regions, but they must participate in all areas of any region they choose to operate. Most PDPs offer plans in all regions. The size of the regions varies from one to seven states. There have been large numbers of plans that have participated each year. In the early years, there were 40 to 50 PDPs in most regions, but that number has decreased in recent years as CMS implemented rules aimed at reducing the number of plans. The number of MA-PDs varies more by region, but beneficiaries in most regions may choose from at least five MA-PDs. Beneficiaries can sign up for any plan in their region. Premiums across plans vary widely and some plans have substantially increased premiums since the start of Part D in 2006 (Neuman and Cubanski, 2009). Beneficiaries are able to change plans during the open enrollment period and therefore could switch to a less expensive plan, however, one challenge is that there seems to be evidence of some plan "stickiness" where beneficiaries are reluctant to switch plans (Neuman and Cubanski, 2009). This reluctance may be due to the difficulty of evaluating the large number of plans.

Benefit Designs and Formularies

All PDPs and MA-PDs must offer plans with the defined standard benefit or coverage that is actuarially equivalent to the standard benefit. Under the standard benefit, beneficiaries pay a deductible ($310 for 2011), then pay 25 percent coinsurance until they reach the initial coverage limit ($2,840 in total drug costs for 2011). After they exceed the initial coverage limit, they are in the coverage gap (often referred to as the "doughnut hole") until they reach the catastrophic coverage limit ($6,448 in total drug costs for 2011). Prior to 2011, PDP beneficiaries paid 100 percent of their drug costs while they were in the coverage gap. PDPs or MA-PDs also may offer plans with enhanced coverage.

Historically, CMS has limited the total number of distinct plans that an organization may offer to 3 or less. CMS did not want to limit the number of organizations participating in Part D in order to increase competition between organizations, but they limited the number of plans offered by each organization to somewhat lessen the confusion. Some organizations offered enhanced plans with some coverage of drugs in the gap, but that coverage eroded over time and in 2010 there were no PDPs offering coverage of brand name drugs in the gap. A few MA-PDs still offered some gap coverage of brand name drugs due to the relatively generous funding of MA plans. Under the Affordable Care Act of 2010, gap coverage will be phased in until 2020 when there will be no coverage gap. Starting in 2011, pharmaceutical manufacturers must pay 50 percent of the costs for brand name drugs in the gap. The Part D plan pays 7 percent of generic drug costs in the gap for 2011; over time their share will increase to 25 percent of brand name drug costs in the gap and 75 percent of the generic drug costs in the gap.

Most plans have deviated from the standard benefit structure to offer different but actuarially equivalent coverage. While the standard benefit uses 25 percent coinsurance, most plans have opted to use a tiered co-payment approach. Some of the co-payments are substantial; the average nonpreferred co-payment for 2010 plans was $76 (Hargrave et al., 2009). Some plans have also eliminated the deductible. Each plan is allowed to establish their own formulary, although Part D formularies are heavily regulated by CMS. The CMS formulary rules are designed to prevent the Part D plans from designing their formularies such that they attract healthier beneficiaries or discourage sicker beneficiaries from joining their plan. For example, plan formularies must include all or substantially all drugs in six therapeutic categories: antidepressants, antipsychotics, anticonvulsants, anticancer agents, immunosupressants, and HIV/AIDs. CMS must also review and approve all formularies. As a result of the differences in benefit design and formularies across plans, it is critically important that beneficiaries chose the plan that best meets their needs. One very useful tool is the Medicare plan finder tool available on the www.medicare.gov Web site. This tool allows people to enter the list of prescription drugs they are taking and reports their costs for each plan available in their region.

Low Income Assistance

There is considerable assistance available to low-income beneficiaries enrolled in Part D plans. Dual eligibles have no coverage gap, no deductible and have very small co-payments. They also pay no monthly premiums, assuming they sign up for a "benchmark plan" that has monthly premiums below a level established for each region. Prior to Part D, they received outpatient prescription drug coverage from their state's Medicaid program. Once Part D was implemented in 2006, they began to receive their drug coverage via Part D. Dual eligibles who do not sign up for a plan are randomly assigned to one of the benchmark plans in their region. This can be problematic if they are randomly assigned to a plan that does not include their medications on its formulary. Other low-income beneficiaries who are not dual eligibles may also qualify for reduced premiums, co-payments, and deductibles. The assistance for low-income beneficiaries is quite good, but one challenge has been getting eligible beneficiaries signed up for the extra help. Another challenge is that the number of benchmark ($0 premium) plans available to low-income beneficiaries has declined in recent years (Kaiser Fact Sheet on Low-Income Assistance under the Medicare Drug Benefit, Dec. 2009).

Medication Therapy Management

The MMA of 2003 contained language requiring that Part D plan sponsors provide medication therapy management (MTM) services for targeted beneficiaries. Targeted beneficiaries are those who have multiple chronic conditions, use many prescriptions drug, and have high drug costs. Having MTM services specifically mentioned in the law was a victory for pharmacy associations who had lobbied for inclusion of pharmacist's clinical services. Although the law does not require that MTM be offered by pharmacists, having MTM required for targeted beneficiaries represents an opportunity for a pharmacy profession seeking to expand payment for pharmacist services. The law was quite vague in terms of MTM requirements, leaving it up to CMS to publish more specific rules to govern MTM services in Medicare Part D. Pharmacy organizations hoped that CMS would publish rules with extensive MTM requirements, but initially, CMS concluded there was a lack of evidence on the most effective types of MTM programs and therefore decided to give the Part D plans maximum flexibility to design their own MTM programs.

As a result, from 2006 to 2009 most Part D plans relied on their own employees to provide MTM and they provided minimal levels of MTM (CMS Medicare Part D MTM Programs, 2011). MTM services are an administrative cost for Part D plan sponsors, so they have no incentive to spend money on MTM services unless they lower costs within the plan year. However, beginning with the 2010 plan year, CMS issued new MTM rules that increased MTM requirements for Part D plans. The new rules had the goal of increasing the number of Part D enrollees eligible for and receiving MTM services. The new rules included: (1) changing the definition of targeted beneficiaries by lowering the annual cost threshold, (2) requiring opt out enrollment where all targeted beneficiaries are automatically enrolled unless they inform the plan that they do not want to receive MTM services, and (3) requiring a minimum level of MTM services. This minimum level included an annual comprehensive medication review with an interactive component. It also mandated interventions to resolve medication-related problems. The rules do not address payment levels for MTM that are determined by the Part D plan sponsors. The new rules have expanded opportunities for community pharmacists to provide MTM services.

Challenges and Opportunities for Pharmacists in Medicare Part D

A significant challenge for pharmacists since the start of Medicare Part D has been low reimbursement from Part D plans. Many Medicare beneficiaries who signed up for Part D were either previously uninsured or received their drug coverage from Medicaid. As discussed in Chapter 19, gross margins typically are higher on cash paying prescriptions and Medicaid prescriptions than Medicare Part D prescriptions, so this switch meant less profitability for many pharmacies. One study found that prescription gross margin per dual-eligible claim in 313 Texas independent pharmacies decreased from 26 percent prior to part D (under Medicaid) to 17.0 percent after the start of Part D (Winegar et al., 2009). Furthermore, a government report found that the average Medicare PDP reimbursement to pharmacies yielded a gross margin of $11.40 (OIG, 2008). Given that community pharmacy costs of dispensing often are in the $11 to $12 range (National Community Pharmacy Association, 2010), participation in Part D is not very profitable for many pharmacies. Another concern with Part D, particularly in the early years, was slow reimbursement from the Part D plans. In 2006, pharmacies reported significant delays in receiving payment from Part D plans (Shepherd et al., 2007). This problem has improved with the passage of the Medicare Improvements for Patients and Providers Act (MIPPA) of 2008, which included a requirement that Part D plans reimburse electronically submitted clean claims within 14 days. The passage of this law is an example of pharmacy organizations successfully lobbying for legislation to address a pharmacy concern.

Another challenge for pharmacists has been dealing with the complexity of the program. Dealing with the large number of Part D plans with their very different reimbursement, benefit designs, and formularies consumes a significant amount of pharmacy staff time. Many patients have been confused by the large number of plans and their complexity. As a result, they often seek out pharmacist advice in selecting a plan. This process is made more difficult by CMS rules that prohibit pharmacists from recommending a particular plan to patients. Pharmacists are allowed to provide information about Part D plans, but not recommendations as to which plan a patient should choose. Another challenge is that pharmacy staff are on the front lines in explaining various aspects of patients' prescription drug benefits. The coverage gap in Part D has been particularly confusing for patients. An interesting development was the CVS Pharmacies' purchase of the company that sponsors CCRx Part D plans in December of 2010. The CCRx plans have been leaders in promoting community pharmacist involvement in providing MTM, so it will be important to monitor how the CVS purchase affects the CCRx plans.

There are also some important opportunities associated with Medicare Part D. A key opportunity is the requirement that targeted beneficiaries receive MTM services. The new CMS rules that went into effect in 2010 considerably increased opportunities for community pharmacists to provide and receive payment for MTM services. CMS is beginning to measure outcomes associated with the MTM services, so pharmacists have the opportunity to further demonstrate the effect that their services can have on patient outcomes. Private plans often follow where Medicare leads, so it is possible there will be a spillover effect of the Medicare MTM to other third-party plans. Another benefit of Medicare Part D has been increased prescription volume. We know that insurance coverage increases an individual's use of prescription drugs, so the large number of people that gained insurance coverage via Part D likely yielded increased prescription volume for pharmacies. A final opportunity is that being a public program, pharmacists have the opportunity to lobby for changes in the program. Pharmacy organizations were successful in supporting legislation to improve Part D payment times and they are currently lobbying for other changes in Part D such as further expansions in MTM.

MEDICAID AND CHILDREN'S HEALTH INSURANCE PROGRAM

Medicaid

Medicaid is a health insurance program for low-income individuals which began in 1965. It is jointly funded and run by the federal and state governments. Each state operates its own Medicaid program, so although states must follow federal guidelines, Medicaid programs vary considerably between states in terms of their covered population, covered services and provider reimbursement. One hallmark of Medicaid is *categorical eligibility*, meaning that people must be low income and in certain categories to be eligible to enroll in Medicaid. Historically, only Medicare beneficiaries, pregnant women, children, and parents with dependent children have been allowed to enroll in state Medicaid programs, but this categorical eligibility will change in 2014 as a result of the Affordable Care Act. Another important characteristic of Medicaid is that it is an *entitlement* program, meaning that state must enroll anyone in their Medicaid program that meets the eligibility requirements at the time they become eligible. This creates strain on state budgets during an economic downturn when the number of people eligible for Medicaid increases, but state has less tax revenue available to pay for the program.

Funding for Medicaid is provided via an unlimited federal match (i.e., as the state spends money on health care services for Medicaid enrollees, the federal government pays a percentage of the costs). The percentage paid by the federal government varies from state to state and is higher in states with a larger low-income population. Medicaid programs are required by the federal government to provide a basic set of services, including inpatient and outpatient hospital services, physician services, laboratory services, and long-term care services. Programs receive matching funds from the federal government for covering optional services, such as prescription drugs and dental benefits. State Medicaid programs generally offer a comprehensive set of benefits. While prescription drugs are an optional service, all states currently cover them. A major cost for state Medicaid programs is long-term care. Since Medicare covers very little long-term care, Medicaid pays the majority of long-term care costs for dual eligibles.

Children's Health Insurance Program

The CHIP began in 1997 as a way to increase the percentage of children with health insurance. CHIP covers children who are low income, but who do not have a low enough income to qualify for Medicaid. The following link provides an excellent summary of the complementary role of Medicaid and CHIP in insuring low-income children (http://www.kff.org/uninsured/upload/7698-05.pdf). In 2011, CHIP covered approximately 6 million children (Kaiser fact sheet on the role of Medicaid and CHIP, 2011c). Like Medicaid, CHIP is jointly funded and run by states and the federal government. Also like Medicaid, CHIP must provide a comprehensive benefit package to enrolled children. The federal government provides a higher matching rate for CHIP than it does for Medicaid, but unlike Medicaid, federal funding for the CHIP program is capped. States have an allocation of funds that can be used for their CHIP program each year, once that money is spent, states no longer receive matching funds for the rest of that year. Also unlike Medicaid, CHIP is not an entitlement program, so states do not have to enroll all eligible children. This means that eligible children may be put on a waiting list if the state runs short on funds. State CHIP programs typically have done a better job than state Medicaid programs with investing in outreach and making the enrollment process for CHIP user friendly. The Children's Health Insurance Program Reauthorization Act of 2009 (CHIPRA) reauthorized CHIP and expanded it to cover additional low-income children. It also established bonus payments for states that simplify enrollment procedures and successfully enroll eligible children in Medicaid. This is an attempt to bring some of the more successful outreach efforts from CHIP into Medicaid.

Challenges and Opportunities for Pharmacists—Medicaid and CHIP

A very important aspect of Medicaid for pharmacy managers to understand is pharmacy reimbursement. Each state sets its own pharmacy reimbursement levels, under federal guidelines. Since the reimbursement is determined by the state legislatures, pharmacist involvement in the process is critical. Lobbying by pharmacy associations, pharmacies, and pharmacists can influence the process. A challenge with Medicaid reimbursement is that during times of state budget shortfalls, one of the first places legislators look to make cuts is in the Medicaid program. States are often unable or unwilling to reduce services or impose stricter eligibility requirements, so provider reimbursement is a frequent target for reductions. Pharmacies may choose not to participate in their state's Medicaid program, but if they do not participate they may not dispense any prescriptions for Medicaid patients. Another challenge is that many state Medicaid programs require that pharmacies dispense prescriptions to Medicaid even if the patient cannot afford to make their co-payments. Some state Medicaid programs also have extensive prior authorization requirements that may increase pharmacy workload.

State Medicaid programs also provide some opportunities. Some state Medicaid programs pay for pharmacist services above and beyond prescription dispensing. For example, Iowa Medicaid pays for pharmaceutical case management for high cost Medicaid beneficiaries, and Wisconsin Medicaid pays enhanced dispensing fees for pharmacist services to resolve drug-related problems. Another opportunity is that pharmacists are able to lobby state legislators to make changes in their state's Medicaid program. This is in contrast to private insurance programs, where the only recourse available to pharmacies facing low reimbursement is to stop accepting the low-reimbursement plan. Pharmacists and pharmacy associations in some states have successfully lobbied to block proposed reductions in pharmacy reimbursement, or to add reimbursement for pharmacist services. Pharmacies also are a good place to provide enrollment information for people who are potentially eligible for their state's Medicaid or CHIP program. CHIP programs generally have fairly extensive outreach programs and may be willing to provide pamphlets to the pharmacy.

HEALTH CARE REFORM

After years of discussions and legislative proposals, a major health care reform was passed into law in 2010. The goals of the Patient Protection and Affordable Care Act (ACA) are to expand health insurance coverage, provide additional protections for patients, control costs, and improve health care delivery systems. The law significantly increases the government's role in health care, so it is important to understand the basics of the law as well as challenges and opportunities for pharmacists. For an excellent summary of the basics of the law, see the Kaiser Family Foundation Summary of the New Health Care Reform Law, available at http://www.kff.org/healthreform/upload/8061.pdf.

The law has two basic ways that try to decrease the number of people who lack health insurance: (1) provide incentives for people to purchase insurance and (2) reduce barriers to the purchase of health insurance. As an incentive to purchase insurance, it imposes an individual mandate that requires most people to have qualifying health insurance coverage or pay a penalty. The reason for this mandate is to encourage people who might choose to be uninsured (e.g., the young and healthy) to purchase coverage. Exceptions to the penalty will be granted under some circumstances, including any consumer whose cost for the lowest cost plan option exceeds 8 percent of their income. This mandate is one of the most controversial pieces of the health care reform law and has been challenged via the judicial system. The law uses multiple approaches to reduce barriers to purchasing health insurance, control costs, and improve health care delivery systems. These approaches are briefly summarized below.

State-Based American Health Benefit Exchanges

These state-based exchanges will function as an insurance market to make it easier for individuals and small businesses to shop for and purchase private health insurance coverage. The state run exchanges must follow federal guidelines, but states will also have flexibility in how they operate their exchanges. Credits will be available to individuals and families with income between 133 and 400 percent of the federal poverty level to help them purchase coverage. Plans that are sold on the exchanges must fall into one of five categories: catastrophic coverage, Bronze, Silver, Gold, and Platinum. The catastrophic plan is available only in the individual market to people aged 30 or younger or those who are exempt from the mandate. The other four plans must cover the "essential" health benefits at varying levels of coverage. All plans must limit out-of-pocket expenses for patients, and out-of-pocket limits are lower for people up to 400 percent of the federal poverty level (FPL). A key question is how essential health benefits will be defined. The exchanges begin on January 1, 2014, and at that time all new policies sold outside the exchange must also fall into one of the benefit levels defined earlier. Each state will operate their own exchanges, but if states fail to initiate the exchanges, the federal government will step in to run them.

Changes in Rules for Health Insurers

The ACA significantly changes the rules for how private health insurance companies operate. First, it will require guaranteed issue and renewability for individual and small group health insurance policies sold both within and outside the exchanges. Guaranteed issue means that insurers must agree to insure all applicants, regardless of their health status. Guaranteed renewability means that once a policy is sold, the insurer must continue to sell the policy to the insured individual, regardless of any changes in their health status. Health insurers must also use a modified community rating system for pricing policies. Premiums are only allowed to vary based on age, geographic area, family composition, and tobacco use. They will not be allowed to vary based on health status. All of these changes will be implemented in 2014. A few states had some of these rules in place prior to the ACA of 2010, but for insurers in most states these rules will be a major change. These changes will make it easier for people with chronic medical conditions to purchase health insurance, but will also raise the cost of insurance for healthier individuals. Another change for insurers is that as of 2011, all health insurers are required to spend a minimum amount of premiums on medical services and quality improvements relative to administrative and overhead costs. Large group plans must spend 85 percent and individual and small group plans must spend at least 80 percent. Insurers who do not meet these levels are required to pay rebates to consumers, although many insurers have asked for and received waivers to bypass this requirement.

Medicaid Expansion

The ACA makes some major changes to Medicaid. The most significant change is the elimination of categorical eligibility. Beginning in 2014, all non-Medicare eligible individuals, except undocumented immigrants, with incomes up to 133 percent of the FPL will be eligible for Medicaid. All newly eligible individuals must receive a benchmark benefit package that is equivalent to the essential health benefits package defined under the exchange rules. Initially, the federal government will pay 100 percent of the costs for the newly eligible individuals, but that will phase down to 90 percent of the costs for 2020 and later. However, it is important to note that 90 percent exceeds the current federal match rate so states will pay a lower percentage of the costs for the newly eligible individuals than they will pay for individuals who were eligible under pre-2014 criteria.

Effects on Employers

Employers with 50 or more full-time employees who do not offer health insurance and who have at least one employee who receives a premium credit to purchase insurance on the exchange will have to pay a fee of $2,000 per full-time employee, except that the first 30 employees are excluded. Employers with more than 200 employees must automatically enroll employees into their health insurance plans, although employees will be given an opportunity to opt out of this coverage if they do not want the health insurance offered by their employer. Small employers with 25 or less employees and average annual wages of less than $50,000 will receive a tax credit if they provide insurance for their employees. Pharmacy owners and managers need to be aware of how these changes will affect their pharmacy.

Changes for Medicare

The ACA makes several important changes to the Medicare program. Within Medicare Part D, it started phasing out the coverage gap in 2011 and will fully close the gap by 2020. It will also increase Part D premiums for higher income beneficiaries. Beginning in 2011, it eliminated beneficiary cost sharing for preventive services. Within the MA program, it will restructure payments to MA plans to try and remove some of the historical overpayment of plans in some areas and underpayment of plans in other areas. It will also begin paying bonuses to MA plans that provide high quality care. From a cost control perspective, the ACA is testing some new payment structures in Medicare. Beginning in 2013, it is testing a bundling approach to payment where payment is linked to episodes of care. For example, the payment for hospitalization for a heart attack also will cover care during the postdischarge period. There will also be new Accountable Care Organizations (ACOs) in Medicare, where groups of practitioners can join together to provide care to beneficiaries in the original Medicare program. If they provide high quality coordinated care and save money for Medicare, they will share in the savings, but if the care they provide is costlier for Medicare, they may risk having to pay a penalty. The ACO initiative begins in 2012.

The CLASS Program

The financing of long-term care is a significant challenge in the United States. Most Americans do not have long-term care insurance, and many end up spending down their resources to qualify for Medicaid (which generally covers long-term care). The ACA attempted to partially address this problem with the Community Living Assistance Services and Supports (CLASS) program. The goal of the program is to provide resources to allow people with multiple functional limitations to stay in their homes longer before entering a nursing home. Working adults will make voluntary premium contributions to this program via payroll deductions or direct payments. People will be automatically enrolled in the program unless they choose to opt out. People who are enrolled in the program will be eligible for benefits if they have paid monthly premiums for at least 5 years and have been employed during 3 of those 5 years. Exact benefits have yet to be determined, but the law specifies that people who meet eligibility criteria will receive a cash benefit that can be used to purchase community support services or pay nursing home costs. Since the program is voluntary, it remains to be seen what percentage of people will participate. Other concerns are whether the funds generated from the collected premium will be sufficient to pay costs and whether the benefits will provide sufficient help with long-term care costs. Enrollment is expected to begin sometime after October 2012, and since the premiums are collected through employers, pharmacy managers need to be aware of and monitor implementation of this program.

Challenges and Opportunities for Pharmacists with Health Care Reform

The ACA presents both challenges and opportunities for pharmacists. Overall, it will increase the percentage of people with insurance, which should increase the number of prescriptions dispensed. A critical issue is what benefits are defined as essential benefits. Under the ACA, prescription drugs will be included, but pharmacists must make a case to support inclusion of pharmacist clinical services in the essential benefit package. The expansion of Medicaid will make more people eligible for Medicaid and decrease the number of uninsured, but the net effect of this change on pharmacies depends on the reimbursement levels set by state Medicaid programs. As mentioned in Chapter 19, reimbursement formulas in state Medicaid programs currently are in flux due to the movement away from average wholesale price (AWP)-based reimbursement. The effect on pharmacies also depends on whether more state Medicaid programs expand their payment for MTM or other pharmacist clinical services. The closing of the Medicare Part D coverage gap is an improvement to the benefit and should decrease the time pharmacists spend working with patients who are facing the gap. The incentives for ACOs in Medicare may provide some additional opportunities for pharmacists to get involved with integrated care organizations. There also are some incentives in the ACA to expand the medical home model. This model has a strong focus on primary care, and offers opportunities for pharmacists who may collaborate with other practitioners to manage prescription drug therapy. A final opportunity for pharmacists is that the law contains incentives that promote MTM services. First, MA plans are given a list of programs that they can implement to receive a bonus; one of these programs is to have an MTM program that is more extensive than required under Part D. Second, some grants and contracts to implement MTM programs will be available, although the amount of money is unknown at this time. A requirement of this grant program is that the MTM services be provided by a licensed pharmacist.

■ OTHER FEDERAL AND STATE LEGISLATION OF INTEREST

Although specific bills introduced at the federal or state levels are not discussed here due to their fast-changing nature, it is important to recognize general categories of legislation that are likely to continue to be important in the future. One type of legislation is regulation of pharmacy benefit managers (PBMs). Health insurance companies have historically been heavily regulated by states, with PBMs having minimal regulation. There has been legislation passed in some states to regulate PBMs. It is likely that additional legislation related to PBMs will be introduced at the state or federal level in the future. Another type of legislation is collective bargaining for pharmacies. For the past several years the National Community Pharmacy Association (representing independent pharmacy owners) has been advocating for legislation to allow independent pharmacies to join forces to collectively bargain with third parties. Attempts through 2011 to pass this legislation at the federal level have been unsuccessful, but there will likely be similar attempts in the future. There is also interest at both the federal and state level in limiting the use of mail-order pharmacies. Pharmacy associations are particularly opposed to plans that mandate use of mail-order pharmacies.

Another key area of legislation of interest to pharmacists is mandated benefit laws. Many health care providers and consumer groups have lobbied successfully to pass laws requiring specific health care services be covered. Autism treatment and chiropractic care are examples of services that some states require health insurance plans to cover. Most of this legislation has been at the state level, but some federal mandates also exist (e.g., coverage of reconstruction following a mastectomy). Pharmacists and pharmacy associations have lobbied (successfully in a few cases) to mandate pharmacists as a covered provider or pharmacist clinical services as covered benefits. Sometimes benefits are mandated for a specific population (e.g., Medicaid, state employees, or large group plans) and sometimes they are mandated for all insurance plans. The exception is that state benefit mandates may not be imposed on self-funded plans. These plans are regulated at the federal level. At the federal level, pharmacists have lobbied for legislation to expand payment for MTM services.

Finally, there is a broad range of health policy issues where pharmacists and pharmacy associations may choose to get involved. Examples include reimportation of prescription drugs from other countries, controlled substances policies, electronic medical records, drug shortages, counterfeit drugs, generic substitution, medication disposal, competitive bidding for DME, and pharmacy compounding. Pharmacy organizations that represent specific pharmacy groups may focus on issues that are of interest. For example, the National Community Pharmacy Association (NCPA) has opposed chain pharmacy mergers with PBMs (National Community Pharmacy Association, 2011), while the American Association of Colleges of Pharmacy (AACP), which represents academic pharmacy, has supported legislation related to pharmacist student loan repayment programs. Although pharmacy organizations at times have different areas of focus, in recent years they have tried to present a united front on many issues that are of critical importance across all areas of pharmacy.

CONCLUSIONS

With the increasing role of government in health care, it is critically important that individual pharmacists understand and become involved in the health policy process. There are many ways this can be accomplished. Pharmacy organizations are a key resource for information about health policy issues of interest to the pharmacy profession. Almost all pharmacy associations' Web sites maintain a government affairs or advocacy section where viewers can find information about current health policy issues. Most pharmacy association Web sites allow members to sign up to receive legislative updates via email. Most pharmacy association Web sites also describe ways in which their members can get involved in the health policy process. One type of involvement is to contribute to the political action committee (PAC) of a pharmacy association. PACs use their resources to lobby legislators about legislation of interest. An easy and very important way to get involved is to write letters to your state or federal legislators stating your views on current legislation. Most pharmacy associations have information on how to contact your legislators and some provide sample letters on topics of interest. Pharmacists can learn more about pending and past federal legislation by searching www.thomas.gov, and many states have similar Web sites. National, state, and local pharmacy association meetings are also places to learn about current legislation affecting pharmacists.

Once a law is passed, a government agency will publish proposed rules for implementing the law. These rules are published in the Federal Register and all interested parties have an opportunity to submit written comments on the rules. Pharmacy associations typically submit comments on rules of interest to them, but individual pharmacists may also submit comments. Once the law is implemented, it may still be challenged in the courts. Some pharmacy organizations have also a legal fund that goes to support legal efforts to change legislation via the court system or support pharmacist initiated lawsuits. Finally, although pharmacy associations are an excellent source of information of issues important to pharmacists, sometimes it also is helpful to get a broader view of health policy issues. The Kaiser Family Foundation is a nonprofit organization (www.kff.org) that is an excellent source of health policy information. They have free daily and weekly email health policy updates that are a great way to get current health policy information from a variety of different perspectives. No matter what area of pharmacy practice you are in, staying informed and involved in health policy is essential. The future of the pharmacy profession depends on it.

REVISITING THE SCENARIO

Joshua Anderson, the new pharmacist at Badger pharmacy, was confused when the pharmacy owner shared with him his concerns about current legislation. He felt like he did not understand the health policy process or why it was important to pharmacy. Joshua now understands the growing role of government in health care, which in turn creates a greater need for pharmacist involvement in the policy process. He now knows more about each of the main public insurance programs and understands the basics of the 2010 health care reform law. He knows that pharmacy associations are a great resource to get information on current health policy issues of interest to pharmacists and he plans to write a letter to his congressman in support of H.R. 3546. Who knows, he might even run for congress someday!

REFERENCES

Berenson RA. 2001. Medicare + Choice: Doubling or Disappearing? *Health Aff (Millwood)* web exclusive: W65–W82.

Centers for Medicare and Medicaid Services. 2011. 2011 Medicare Part D Medication Therapy Management (MTM) Programs. Available from www.cms.gov; accessed on April 12, 2012.

Centers for Medicare and Medicaid Services. 2005. Medicare Modernization Act Final Guidelines—Formularies; CMS Strategy for Affordable Access to Comprehensive Drug Coverage; Guidelines for Reviewing Prescription Drug Plan Formularies and Procedures." Available from www.cms.hhs.gov/pdps/FormularyGuidance.pdf; accessed on April 12, 2012.

Hargrave E, Hoaddley J, Summer L, Cubanski J, Neuman T. 2009. *Medicare Part D 2010 Data Spotlight: Benefit Design and Cost-Sharing.* Menlo Park, CA: Kaiser Family Foundation.

Kaiser Family Foundation. 2011a. *The Medicare Prescription Drug Benefit: Fact Sheet.* Menlo Park, CA: Kaiser Family Foundation.

Kaiser Family Foundation. 2011b. *Dual Eligibles: Medicaid's Role for Low-Income Medicare Beneficiaries: Fact Sheet.* Menlo Park, CA: Kaiser Family Foundation.

Kaiser Family Foundation. 2011c. *Health Coverage of Children: the Role of Medicaid and CHIP.* Menlo Park, CA: Kaiser Family Foundation.

Kaiser Family Foundation. 2009. *Low-Income Assistance under the Medicare Drug Benefit: Fact Sheet.* Menlo Park, CA: Kaiser Family Foundation.

National Community Pharmacy Association. 2002. *NCPA-Pharmacia Digest.* Alexandria, VA.

National Community Pharmacy Association. 2010. *NCPA Digest.* Alexandria, VA.

National Community Pharmacy Association. 2011. *Original NCPA and NACDS Complaint Against CMS.* Available at http://www.ncpanet.org/pdf/legal/amp-origcomplaint.pdf; accessed on October 1, 2011.

Neuman P, Cubanski J. 2009. Medicare Part D update-lessons learned and unfinished business. *N Engl J Med* 316(4):406–414.

Office of the Inspector General. 2008. Review of the relationship between Medicare Part D payments to local community pharmacies and the pharmacies' drug acquisition costs. *United States Dep Health Hum Serv* A-06-07-00107.

Shepherd MD, Richards KM, Winegar AL. 2007. Prescription drug payment times by Medicare Part D plans: Results of a national study. *J Am Pharm Assoc* 47(6):e20.

Winegar AL, Shepherd MD, Lawson KA, Richards KM. 2009. Comparison of the claim percent gross margin earned by Texas community independent pharmacies for dual-eligible beneficiary claims before and after Medicare Part D. *J Am Pharm Assoc* 49:617–622.

SECTION V

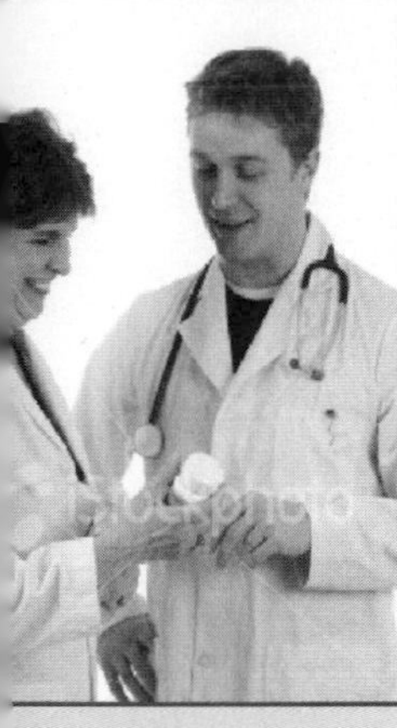

MANAGING TRADITIONAL GOODS AND SERVICES

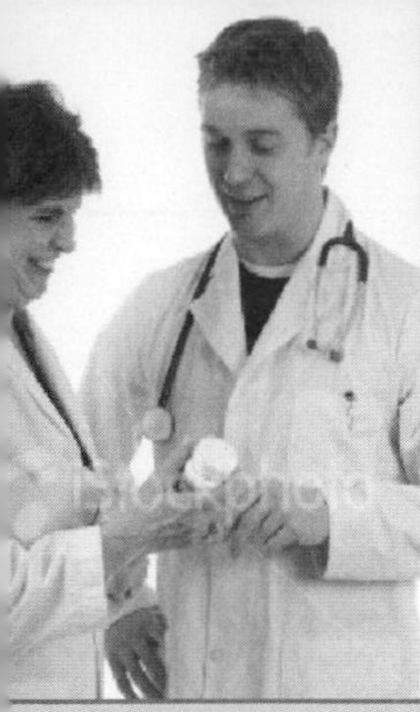

21

MARKETING THEORY

John Bentley

About the Author: Dr. Bentley is an associate professor in the Department of Pharmacy Administration and a research associate professor in the Research Institute of Pharmaceutical Sciences, at the University of Mississippi School of Pharmacy. He received a B.S. in pharmacy and an MBA from Drake University, an M.S. and a Ph.D. in pharmacy administration from The University of Mississippi, an M.S. in biostatistics from The University of Alabama at Birmingham (UAB), and is currently working on his Ph.D. in biostatistics at UAB. In the professional pharmacy curriculum, Dr. Bentley teaches elements of research design, biostatistics, epidemiology, and drug literature evaluation. At the graduate level, he teaches several applied statistics courses. He has conducted research in a variety of areas including quality of life; medication use, misuse, and outcomes; pharmaceutical marketing; patients' evaluation of health care providers; direct-to-consumer advertising; practice management; and ethics and professionalism. His statistics research interests include statistical mediation analysis and longitudinal data analysis. Dr. Bentley was named a fellow of the American Pharmacists Association in 2009.

LEARNING OBJECTIVES

After completing this chapter, readers should be able to

1. Define marketing and describe its societal contributions.
2. Discuss the purpose of marketing within a business.
3. Identify orientations toward the marketplace that organizations might take when conducting marketing activities.
4. Differentiate among the concepts of needs, wants, and demands.
5. Define the concept of exchange and state its importance to marketing.
6. Describe the marketing mix and apply it to the marketing of services.
7. Describe different types of product offerings, and define the distinguishing characteristics of a service.

8. Define expectations, satisfaction, quality, value, and loyalty and describe their role in purchase behavior and the profitability of organizations.
9. Explain the concept of relationship marketing and apply it to pharmacy management.

SCENARIO

Jim Smyth and Sue Davidson co-own and manage West Side Pharmacy. While looking over the books for the last year, both pharmacists begin to recognize that their pharmacy is struggling to meet its financial objectives. Jim and Sue decide to ask the staff pharmacist and the technicians to help brainstorm ideas for improving the pharmacy's financial performance. During the after-hours impromptu staff meeting, the following questions were asked: "Are there any health-related goods that we should add to the line of products we sell?" "What other services can we provide that people in our community need or want?" "What types of services can we develop given our resources?" "Should we provide the services in our pharmacy or at some other location?" "How will our services be different from Corner Pharmacy on the other side of town?" "What should we charge for our services?" "How do we let people know that we are offering these services?" "How will we know if our patients value the goods and services we provide?" "What kinds of relationships do we need to establish with our patients to be successful?" "Should we start a customer loyalty program?"

These are all marketing-related questions, and this chapter and Chapter 22 will focus on providing information to help pharmacy managers begin to address these questions. This chapter will describe and discuss some of the basic building blocks of marketing that are essential for developing and implementing a marketing plan. Chapter 22 will provide the reader some practical tools necessary for marketing pharmacy goods and services.

CHAPTER QUESTIONS

1. What is marketing, and what is its purpose in a business setting and in a pharmacy setting?
2. What are the different philosophies that may be used to guide the marketing efforts of a company?
3. What is the difference between needs, wants, and demands?
4. What is the marketing mix?
5. What characterizes the different types of offerings that a business makes to its customers?
6. How do the concepts of expectations, satisfaction, quality, value, and loyalty relate to each other, and what is their importance to marketing?
7. What is relationship marketing, and how can it be used to enhance pharmacy practice?

INTRODUCTION: WHY MARKETING?

Smith (1996) has observed that marketing has received a "bad rap." Despite its contributions to society (Wilkie and Moore, 1999) and to our high standard of living (Smith, 1996), marketing has many critics. Perhaps, these criticisms stem from the common perception that marketing is the "art of selling products" (Kotler and Keller, 2012). As will be discussed, this is a very myopic view of what marketing is all about. Other criticisms stem from perceptions that many marketers are unethical. While some marketers fail to act according to ethical principles, such a criticism may be levied against every endeavor, including pharmacy. The bottom line is that marketing is an activity that is misunderstood by many. In the opinion of some, marketing is an often-overlooked activity that is critical to the success of any organization (Smith, 2002).

Marketing is not just an activity performed by large, multinational corporations. Indeed, the principles of marketing are just as applicable to small, independently owned pharmacies as they are to large corporations.[1] Marketing is also critical to the profession of pharmacy. Marketing and pharmacy practice have a long history of coexisting with each other. Marketing tools have been used to help pharmacists address many issues in a variety of practice settings, such as what to charge for a prescription drug, whether to add a pharmacokinetic monitoring service or a new clinical specialist at a hospital, which over-the-counter (OTC) products to carry, and whether to use a wholesaler for all products or order directly from manufacturers.

As pharmacy continues to evolve, marketing's role grows in importance. Since the articulation of the concept of pharmaceutical care (Hepler and Strand, 1990), many innovative pharmacy services have been described and implemented, ranging from comprehensive medication therapy management (MTM) services to specific disease management services, such as diabetes care, lipid management, tobacco cessation, and anticoagulation management. However, concurrent with the development and implementation of these services has been a continued growth in the literature documenting inappropriate use of medications, suggesting that a significant need still exists for services that are directed at reducing the negative consequences associated with drug therapy.

So why are these needs not being met? Concerns regarding prescriber, patient, and payer demand often are considered significant barriers to the provision of patient-centered pharmacy services (McDonough et al., 1998a). Understanding customers'[2] needs and using that understanding to create, deliver, and communicate value are key components of marketing. While many practitioners are interested in obtaining the necessary clinical knowledge and skills to deliver MTM services, many would argue that marketing knowledge and skills are equally important. Rovers and colleagues (1998, p. 136) succinctly summarize this point by noting that "pharmacists must build the demand and supply for pharmaceutical care services simultaneously."

As pharmacy continues its evolution from a product-focused to a service-centered practice, marketing, now more than ever, is critical to the success of the profession. The importance of understanding the nuances of marketing to the success of pharmaceutical care is recognized by Hepler and Strand (1990, p. 541), who noted that "a pharmaceutical-care marketing strategy · · · would differ fundamentally from the usual strategy developed for selling drug products." In order for innovative pharmacy services to be successful in helping patients achieve optimal therapeutic outcomes, pharmacy practitioners must be able to understand the important role of marketing. This chapter will define many of the terms and concepts that are critical to understanding how to incorporate marketing effectively and efficiently into management of the pharmacy enterprise.

MARKETING: DEFINITIONS AND CONCEPTS

Since the goal of this chapter is to introduce the reader to the basic building blocks of marketing, it becomes necessary to first define what *marketing* is. According to the American Marketing Association (AMA)

[1]Marketing principles can also be applied at the personal level: for example, marketing your clinical services as a pharmacist to consult with a physician on drug therapy, or even in the development of friendships and romantic relationships!

[2]While some authors appropriately argue that the terms *consumer, customer, patient,* and *client* have fundamentally different meanings, they are, for the most part, used interchangeably in this chapter. A discussion of the meaning and symbolism of these terms is best handled in another setting.

(Lotti and Lehmann, 2007), "marketing is the activity, set of institutions, and processes for creating, communicating, delivering, and exchanging offerings that have value for customers, clients, partners, and society at large." Included in this definition are several concepts that will be explored in subsequent sections of this chapter, namely, the concepts of exchange and value. Other concepts, such as the four P's of the marketing mix (i.e., product,[3] price, place [distribution], and promotion) and the concept of relationships are implicit in this definition. For now, it is important to recognize that this definition explicitly recognizes that marketing is about more than simply selling products.

Each of these preceding points suggests a broadened view of the domain of marketing, a notion that the discipline of marketing struggled with beginning in the 1960s. To many at that time, including the AMA, marketing was recognized as a set of *business* activities that existed to consummate *market* transactions between producers of goods and services and consumers (Hunt, 2002). Others proffered that marketing should be broadened (1) to include nonbusiness organizations and (2) that the societal implications of marketing activities also should be included in the domain of marketing (Hunt, 2002). After considerable debate, in 1985 the AMA adopted the following definition of marketing (Keefe, 2004, p. 17): "Marketing is the process of planning and executing the conception, pricing, promotion, and distribution of ideas, goods, and services to create exchanges that satisfy individual and organizational objectives." The emphasis on *exchange* and the inclusion of *ideas* clearly demonstrate that marketing has been broadened to include nonbusiness organizations. The 2007 AMA definition of marketing (Lotti and Lehmann, 2007) takes this idea a step further by making no reference to marketing as a business function, implying that nonbusiness organizations (and other entities) can implement marketing activities and processes. The literature is replete with examples of how the principles of marketing have been used by charitable organizations, academic institutions, social issues groups, political candidates, and health care institutions. Hunt (2002, p. 11) remarked that "today it is noncontroversial that marketing has an important role to play in nonbusiness organizations."

While some argue that the 1985 AMA definition of marketing did not fully encompass the social role of marketing (Hunt, 2002), other literature (e.g., see Hunt, 1976) and the emergence of the societal marketing concept (see next section) clearly demonstrate that a broadened view of the marketing domain includes the societal implications of marketing activities. Indeed, the 2007 definition explicitly recognizes this social role by focusing on offerings that have value not only for customers, clients, and partners but also for society at large.

The preceding discussion implies that marketing includes business and social aspects. Kotler and Keller (2012) distinguished between social and managerial definitions of marketing. While these definitions shed additional light on the domain of marketing, they also serve to introduce several additional concepts that will be explored later in this chapter, namely, needs and wants. Although exchange is considered the core concept in marketing, these other concepts play a central role. Kotler and Keller's (2012, p. 5) social definition reads: "Marketing is a *societal process* (emphasis added) by which individuals and groups obtain what they need and want through creating, offering, and freely exchanging products and services of value with others." There is little question that marketing fulfills a social role. Several authors have suggested that marketing exists to create a higher standard of living (Kotler and Keller, 2012; Smith, 2002).[4]

[3]As will be discussed later in this chapter, the concept of product in marketing can refer to any item of value offered by an organization, including tangible goods, services, and even concepts or ideas.

[4]While an in-depth discussion of this issue is beyond the scope of this chapter, the reader is referred to an article by Wilkie and Moore (1999) for an intriguing and insightful discussion of marketing's contribution to society.

From a managerial perspective, Kotler and Keller (2012, p. 5) defined marketing as "the art and science of choosing target markets and getting, keeping, and growing customers through creating, delivering, and communicating superior customer value." Marketing plays a demand management function within the organization, focusing partially on methods to stimulate demand but also, more important, on methods for how to control demand to meet the objectives of the organization. To serve a group of customers or a target market adequately, organizations must direct activities so that the right product is sold in the right quantity at the right place at the right price and at the right time. Because pharmacy is in the business of peoples' health, Smith (2002) suggests that some of these factors assume much greater importance than the stimulation of sales.

MARKETING SCIENCE

While there are many conceptions of what a theory is, a noted theorist in marketing suggests that the purpose of theory is to increase *scientific* understanding (Hunt, 2002). This argument, coupled with the title of this chapter, implies that at least some aspects of marketing can be fitted with the label of science. For this reason, it is worthwhile to briefly explore the question as to whether marketing is a science.

Like the broadening of the marketing debate, the debate as to whether marketing is a science has a rich history. Some authors have argued that marketing is a science, whereas others have argued that marketing is an art (e.g., see Hunt, 1976, 1983; Peter and Olson, 1983). One's view of the scope of marketing is critical to answering this question. While an understanding of the nature of science is also critical, it is beyond the scope of this chapter, and the reader is referred to an excellent discussion by Hunt (2002). With respect to the scope of marketing, Hunt (1976) has proposed that all marketing content can be classified into one of eight classes or cells. One criterion that is used to define these cells is whether the marketing content is positive or normative. *Positive* marketing attempts to describe, explain, predict, and understand marketing phenomena; the focus of the analysis is descriptive—what is. *Normative* marketing attempts to prescribe what an organization, individual, or society should do; the focus is prescriptive—what ought to be done.

If one defines the scope of marketing as only normative efforts designed to assist marketing decision makers (e.g., What methods can we use to sell more product? How much should we charge for this product or service?), then marketing is not a science. However, if one considers an expanded scope of marketing to also include the positive dimensions, then marketing can be considered to be a science. As a science, what does marketing purport to do? The concept of exchange once again becomes critical because "marketing science is the behavioral science that seeks to explain exchange relationships" (Hunt, 1983). Marketing as an academic discipline has undergone significant transformation over the years (e.g., see Wilkie and Moore, 2003), and researchers in the field have become increasingly specialized.[5]

Since this chapter is more interested in the application of marketing principles to pharmacy, little more will be mentioned of the science side of marketing. The focus for the remainder of this chapter will be on the technology of marketing, or its applied side. However, it is important to remember that just as the "practice" of medicine and the "practice" of pharmacy are steeply rooted in a scientific knowledge base, so too is the "practice" of marketing. While the sheer quantity of the "product" of marketing science (i.e., the laws, principles, and theories that serve to unify, explain, and predict marketing phenomena) may be less than the quantity of the "product" of the sciences underlying medicine and pharmacy, this should not suggest that marketing is any less of a science. The scientific method is not any less appropriate to marketing than it is to other disciplines (Hunt, 2002).

[5]Readers interested in the science of marketing are referred to the work of McAlister et al. (2010), who have developed a compilation of scholarly articles published in marketing-related journals.

COMPANY ORIENTATIONS TOWARD THE MARKETPLACE

For many years, marketing authors have sought to clarify the role of marketing in an organization. In essence, questions have arisen as to the type of philosophy that should guide the marketing efforts of a company. When deciding on a philosophical orientation, one needs to consider how much weight should be given to the interests of the organization, customers, and society. Kotler (2003) has described six competing concepts that organizations use as guides in the conduct of marketing activities.

The emphasis of the *production concept* is efficiency in the production and distribution of goods and services. The key assumption about consumers is that they are interested primarily in product availability and low prices. A production concept can also guide the efforts of service organizations, where the goal might be to handle as many cases as possible in a given period of time. As Kotler observes, such an orientation may lead to customer comments concerning the impersonal nature of the service delivery. A pharmacy dedicated to dispensing as many prescriptions as possible, often without regard to providing patient education or even to reviewing medication appropriateness, is practicing the production concept.

The *product concept* focuses on making good products, often as defined in the eyes of the producer, and improving them over time. The key assumptions about buyers are that they appreciate well-made products and that they can evaluate product quality. A company guided by the product concept often is focused on designing a great product (or service) and often gets little or no input from those who will benefit from its product. Kotler (2003) acknowledges that managers following this philosophical orientation might commit the "better mousetrap" fallacy. A phrase that epitomizes a product concept orientation is "If you build it, they will come." A pharmacist who develops a smoking-cessation program that has as its sole focus the use of a technologically advanced reminder system for patients who are using nicotine-replacement therapy and believes that patients will enroll in the program and pay for the services with little other effort on his or her part is being guided by the product concept.

The *selling concept* emphasizes actions directed at stimulating consumers' interest through aggressive sales and promotion efforts. Although promotion is an important part of the marketing mix, and its use can be a critical tool in creating, delivering, and communicating value to customers, managers guided by the selling concept assume that consumers must be coaxed into buying products; the focus is on hard selling, and little concern is given to customers' needs, wants, and postpurchase satisfaction. This is a common approach and is cited as a reason why the public often identifies marketing with selling and advertising (Kotler, 2003). A pharmacy that engages in an overly aggressive campaign, including the use of advertising, sales discounts, and high-pressure personal selling, is practicing the selling concept.

The *marketing concept* was proposed as a challenge to the previously discussed concepts.[6] Rather than focus on the needs of the organization or the seller, the marketing concept suggests that the needs of the buyer are paramount. The marketing concept holds that "the key to achieving its organizational goals consists of the company being more effective than competitors in creating, delivering, and communicating superior customer value to its chosen target markets" (Kotler, 2003, p. 19). Smith (2002, p. 9) succinctly summarizes the meaning of the marketing concept from the perspective of the pharmaceutical manufacturer: "The marketing concept states what seems obvious now but was not always practiced: It is easier to change the products and activities of the individual manufacturer to fit the market than it is to convince the entire market to use the products and services as the individual marketer prefers them."

A company guided by the marketing concept takes care to select appropriate *target markets* (i.e., distinct

[6]For an excellent review of the marketing concept and its implementation, referred to as market orientation, see Kohli and Jaworski (1990).

groups of buyers who may benefit from a given product or service mix), is focused on the needs of its customers, attempts to integrate a marketing orientation (a focus on customers' interests) into all segments of the company, and does these activities with an eye toward achieving organizational goals and objectives, notably generating profits through the creation of customer value (Kotler, 2003). The last point regarding profitability through creating customer value is not specific to for-profit firms. This precept is also important for nonprofit organizations, which instead may strive to generate funds through creating, delivering, and communicating value to their stakeholders to continue their useful work.

Increases in market diversity, changes in technology, and the need for enhanced marketing productivity have led some marketing scholars and practitioners to propose a fifth concept that moves beyond the more traditional marketing concept (Sheth et al., 2000). While companies guided by the marketing concept focus on segments of consumers known as *target markets*, the *customer concept* suggests that companies direct separate offers, services, and messages to individual customers (Kotler, 2003). Computers, the Internet (including social media), database software, and factory customization all have enabled such an approach to marketing. The customer concept calls for a focus on individual customer needs, sometimes leading to customization of the product or other elements of the marketing mix. The functions of the company should be integrated around customer value-added activities, and profitable growth is achieved through enhancement of customer loyalty and by focusing on the creation of lifetime value for individual customers (Kotler, 2003; Sheth et al., 2000).

A sixth orientation with respect to marketing thought and organizational philosophy has been proposed because of changes in our surroundings, such as deterioration of the environment, resource shortages, poverty, and neglected social services (Kotler, 2003). The previously discussed orientations give considerable weight to the interests of either the organization itself or its customers, but companies guided by these concepts still often act in ways that may not be in the best interests of society or consumers. Kotler (2003, pp. 26–27) has labeled this sixth orientation the *societal marketing concept*, which "holds that the organization's task is to determine the needs, wants, and interests of target markets and to deliver the desired satisfactions more effectively and efficiently than competitors in a way that preserves or enhances the consumer's and the society's well-being." Thus, social and ethical considerations also must guide marketers' decisions; company profits, satisfaction of consumers' wants and needs, and the public interest; often conflicting end points must be balanced.

Recognizing marketing's central role in the organization and the many forces that have shaped marketing and business practices in the past decade, Kotler and Keller (2012) proposed the *holistic marketing concept*. In essence, this philosophical orientation combines many of the features of the marketing concept, the customer concept, and the societal marketing concept. The term *holistic* communicates both the importance and complexity of marketing activities within an organization.

NEEDS, WANTS, AND DEMANDS

The marketing concept and the definitions of marketing discussed previously suggest that marketers must attempt to understand the needs, wants, and demands of their target markets. Briefly, a *need* is a state of felt deprivation. Needs are basic human requirements. People have physical needs (e.g., food, clothing, and shelter), social needs (e.g., the need for affection and the need to belong), and individual needs (e.g., the need for self-expression). A *want* is a desire for a specific satisfier of a need. Thus, needs become wants, and these wants are shaped by culture and individual personality. A need for food can translate into wanting pizza; a need for affection may result in wanting a hug. A *demand* is a want that is backed by an ability to pay. Many people may want a vacation at a luxurious resort, but only a relative few are able and willing to purchase such a vacation.

One problem faced by health care providers is that people often do not want their goods or services. This situation is called *negative demand* (Kotler and Keller, 2012), and pharmaceutical products often are labeled as *negative goods* (Smith and Kolassa, 2001). Negative demand occurs when a major part of the market dislikes the product and may even pay a price to avoid it. There are numerous examples of negative goods besides pharmaceutical products and services, including automobile repair services, legal services, and dental work. One way to manage negative demand is to try to better understand people's true motivations for purchasing a product. For example, people purchase drill bits not because they want drill bits but because they want holes (Smith, 1996). In the same way, most people use medications not for the sake of using medications but because those medications provide benefits by alleviating, eliminating, or preventing a disease or symptoms. For example, using medications properly can allow a person to return to work or to perform activities that he or she enjoys doing. It is important to talk to patients to find out why they are using a product, what needs or wants they expect to meet by using a product, and what concerns they have about using the product. Thus, good marketing to manage negative demand is consistent with good pharmacy practice.

From the health economics literature, *need* is defined as "the amount of medical care that medical experts believe a person should have to remain or become as healthy as possible, based on current medical knowledge" (Feldstein, 1999, p. 83). Economists are quick to point out that need is only one factor affecting the demand for care; demand for medical care is determined by a set of patient and provider factors, including a patient's need for care (Feldstein, 1999). Thus, demand for care can be *greater than* the need; likewise, demand for care can be *less than* the need. Some might argue that certain lifestyle drugs such as Viagra are good examples of the former; MTM services are a good example of the latter.

Another important issue is the idea that a marketer's responsibility is primarily about meeting or responding to people's stated needs. Some have argued that this is too limited a view of a marketer's role (Kotler and Keller, 2012). Frequently, customers do not know what they want or need in a good or service. Think about the many goods and services available today, such as cellular telephones, 24-hour discount brokerage accounts, and Internet service providers. Did most consumers want (or need) these things *before* they were available? For health care providers, this situation is all too common because most patients do not have the skills and knowledge that health care professionals have. Thus, health care providers often recognize a patient's need for a health-related good or service that the individual patient does not recognize.

For example, assume that Mary Cooper enters a pharmacy wanting to purchase St. John's wort because her friend told her that it would help her feel better. After talking briefly with Mary, the pharmacist realizes that her symptoms are more grave than communicated initially. Given this additional information, the pharmacist refers Mary to a mental health care provider for further evaluation and treatment. In this case, the customer (Mary) stated a solution, not a need. The pharmacist appropriately recognized Mary's need and was able to help her by appropriately influencing her wants and demands.

The job of a marketer (and the job of a health care professional as well) is not only to understand and respond to people's *expressed* needs but also to help customers learn more about what they need and want. In essence, marketers also must understand and respond to people's *latent* needs. Narver et al. (2004) call the former a *responsive* market orientation and the latter a *proactive* market orientation. Marketers do not create needs, but they do help consumers to understand their latent needs and to translate needs into wants. An understanding of this issue is helpful in explaining pharmacy's current experiences with patient-centered services.

There is little question as to the need for patient-centered pharmacy services given the well-documented negative outcomes associated with drug therapy. McDonough et al. (1998a, p. 89) noted that a common misconception among pharmacists is that "patients neither want nor will be willing to pay for pharmaceutical care." While this may be true of *some* patients, this certainly is not true of *all* patients. Part of the problem lies in the fact that many patients are unaware of their needs and possible solutions (i.e., their needs are latent). McDonough (2003, p. 275) argues that "a key reason why patients do not demand pharmaceutical care is that they do not understand the concept." Patients have to see the value of the service. It is up to the profession to help translate latent needs into wants and demands.

THE CORE CONCEPT OF MARKETING

Central to marketing is the concept of *exchange*, referred to as the "core concept of marketing" (Kotler, 2003). It is the unifying concept in marketing not only for marketing practice but also for marketing science. An *exchange* is a process of obtaining a desired product from someone by offering something in return. When two parties in an exchange process reach an agreement, a transaction takes place. A *transaction* is a trade of values between two or more parties. Although the items of value often are money and a tangible good, this does not have to be the case. The items of value can be just about anything as long as they hold value for one of the parties. Thus, services, ideas, experiences, events, places, material, organizations, effort, and information all can be items of value in a transaction (Kotler, 2003).

In a *transfer*, one party gives an item of value to another party while receiving nothing tangible in return. Giving to a charitable contribution is an example of a transfer. At first glance, transfers appear fundamentally different from transactions. However, in most cases, the giving party often expects something in return, such as gratitude, a change in the recipient, a positive feeling, or even a tax deduction. When observed in this light, transfers, like transactions, can be understood through the core concept of exchange. Indeed, marketers have included transfer behavior in their domain of study (e.g., see Mathur, 1996).

THE MARKETING MIX

Along with the concept of exchange, the 1985 AMA definition of marketing explicitly mentions several concepts that have come to be labeled as the *marketing mix*. A marketing mix is a set of tools an organization uses to pursue its objectives with respect to its target market. Although it has received criticism (e.g., Day and Montgomery, 1999) and other frameworks and classifications have been proposed (e.g., Van Waterschoot and Van den Bulte, 1992), McCarthy's (1960) schema has stood the test of time. He proposed that the tools of the marketing mix be classified into four broad groups: product, price, place, and promotion. These concepts have come to be called the *four P's of marketing*. While customer responses may be influenced by many variables outside the direct control of a company, the four P's represent variables within a company's control that can influence customer responses.

Depending on whom one reads, other P's have been added to the marketing mix. Perhaps, most notably, positioning is often included as a fifth P. The following section provides a brief introduction to the variables in the marketing mix. Chapter 22 will provide more details concerning marketing-mix decisions.

Product

Product refers to an organization's offering. It is not limited to tangible goods but, as described earlier, can be any item of value or combination thereof. Thus, to marketers, the term *product* has a very broad meaning. In the delivery of patient care, the product most often provided is a service. The next section will explore some fundamental differences between physical goods and services and will explore briefly some special considerations needed for the marketing of services.

Problems can emerge when organizations narrowly define their product (or business). Theodore Levitt (1960) labeled this *marketing myopia*. Marketing myopia is often a result of the application of the product concept as a philosophical guide to marketing activities. This is common when a firm defines its business by a product rather than in terms of what customer needs are filled by its activities. Common examples include the railroad and movie industries. These industries nearly disappeared because they assumed that they were in the railroad and movie businesses, respectively, rather than the transportation and entertainment businesses. As other businesses emerged (e.g., the airline and automobile industries and the television and theme park industries), those in the railroad and movie businesses faced a fight for the consumer's dollar against competition generated by unanticipated sources. Pharmacists and pharmacies also need to determine why people use their goods and services. To simply say that they are in the business of dispensing medications prescribed by physicians is too myopic.

Another problem related to marketing myopia occurs when a single product becomes an organization's reason for being. The product of an organization is an offering that presents the consumer with a set of benefits that can be used to satisfy needs. Many different products (often seemingly disparate products) may be capable of meeting customer needs. If a company becomes too wrapped up in its product, it may miss the opportunity to fulfill the needs of the market. Pharmacist-delivered MTM services are a type of product that has the potential to fall victim to such a problem. Although MTM services are valuable for patients, for the profession, and for society, this does not imply that such services should be and will be a success. Just because pharmacists have the requisite clinical knowledge and skills to provide these services is not enough. Pharmacists must understand that these services represent an offering with a set of benefits that helps to meet the needs of customers and society. Pharmacists (and the profession) must be able to create, deliver, and communicate the value of what they do. Keep in mind that others (e.g., physicians, nurses, and information from the Internet) can also provide the benefits that pharmacists are purporting with MTM services. What seems like a relatively simplistic point is the key to widespread acceptance of pharmacist-delivered MTM services.

Price

A producer should set a price after considering several variables, including the cost function (i.e., the cost of producing, distributing, and selling the product, including a reasonable return for effort and risk), competitors' prices, and the demand for the product (including the target market's perception of the benefits) (Kotler and Keller, 2012). To a consumer, *price* is what is given up or sacrificed to obtain a product (Zeithaml, 1988). Some researchers have distinguished between an *objective* price (the actual price of a product) and a *perceived* price (what is encoded by the consumer, e.g., "expensive" or "cheap") (Zeithaml, 1988). It is also important to recognize that from the perspective of the consumer, the monetary price charged by a producer is not the only cost associated with buying a product (Lovelock and Wright, 2002; Zeithaml, 1988). Nonmonetary outlays include the costs associated with the time, effort, and discomfort that are related to the processes of searching for, purchasing, and using the product. For example, if a consumer has to travel a long distance to purchase a product, a sacrifice has been made that adds to what the consumer has given up to acquire that product.

While pricing decisions about drug products and other merchandise can be difficult for pharmacists, the pricing of patient care service raises additional considerations. Perhaps, the most significant issue that must be addressed by the profession and its practitioners is the reluctance of pharmacists to request compensation for the services they provide (McDonough and Sobotka, 2003). Some pharmacists feel that they must give their services away initially to develop demand for them in the future. However, consumers generally are reluctant to start paying for something that they have been able to obtain for free in the past. Most consumers are willing to pay lawyers for legal advice and auto mechanics for service primarily because (1) they have expertise that most consumers do not have and (2) they have a tradition of charging for their services exclusive of charging for the goods they also might sell. While pharmacists have expertise in drug therapy not held by most consumers, they have had a difficult time obtaining payment for their professional services. This is likely because pharmacists, unlike lawyers, auto mechanics, and many other service professionals, do not have a history of charging for their services separate from their goods. When consumers obtain a prescription drug from a pharmacy, they are provided one price that has not been broken down into a "good" and a "service" component. This causes consumers to assume that either (1) there are no services that accompany prescription drug products or (2) the services that come with these products are included with the price of the drug.

Place

Place, or *distribution,* refers to any activity designed to create utility by having the product available when and where targeted customers want to buy it. Many companies are considered successful because of their ability to deliver value in the distribution of products and services. Indeed, companies such as FedEx have made significant contributions to the success of many other companies that rely on prompt, efficient, and affordable delivery of goods (Siecker, 2002). In today's world of overnight delivery, telecommunications, and the Internet, speed and convenience are important elements in determining the distribution strategies of many firms (Lovelock and Wright, 2002). For a pharmacy, *place* may refer to providing a private area for counseling and providing other professional services (McDonough et al., 2003) or evaluating whether providing services at the work site for an employer group is feasible.

Promotion

Promotion activities seek to inform, remind, and persuade the target market about an organization and its offerings. Promotion activities also encourage members of the target market to take action at specific times. While advertising may be an important promotional tool, other tools in the promotion mix include sales promotion, public relations (including publicity), direct marketing, and personal selling.

Many pharmacies have used these tools successfully to spread the word about new and existing goods and services. Newspaper, radio, and television advertisements are used commonly by pharmacies. Pharmacies also employ promotional tools such as telephone book listing, coupons, newsletters, brochures, prescriber and patient mailings, health screenings, and presentations to civic groups. Some pharmacies have worked with the media to inform the public about their participation in public health events such as the Great American Smokeout or Talk About Prescriptions Month.

With respect to MTM services, promotion plays an essential role in the translation of needs into wants and demands. Depending on the individual situation, all elements of the promotion mix may have a role in communicating the value of a patient care service, and pharmacists should evaluate each of them for implementation and use. McDonough and Doucette (2003) provide an excellent discussion of the use of personal selling, a practice that can be very effective but often is not considered by pharmacists for a variety of reasons, including pharmacists' discomfort with this role.

Positioning

Positioning is "the act of designing the company's offering and image to occupy a distinctive place in the minds of the target market" (Kotler and Keller, 2012, p. 276). Positioning is about what a marketer can do to the mind of the target consumer; it is not about what marketers do to the product attributes per se. For example, Volvo's core positioning is safety and durability; this is what the company hopes its target market will think of when they think of a Volvo automobile. Because the target market for many pharmacies does not understand what MTM services are, pharmacists have a great opportunity to position these services in the minds of consumers. These pharmacists can position themselves as innovators, medication experts, caring practitioners, and as partners in meeting health-related needs (McDonough et al., 1998b; McDonough et al., 2003).

REEXAMINING THE FIRST P: PRODUCT

To a marketer, the term *product* means more than just a physical good. In pharmacy, physical goods (e.g., drugs and durable medical equipment) usually are combined with a service. Indeed, Shepherd (1995, p. 53) observed that "pharmaceutical products require a service component." However, in pharmacy, it is not uncommon for a service to be provided without a physical good.

Kotler and Keller (2012) described five categories of offerings that are distinguished based on how much the service component is part of the offering:

- *Pure tangible good.* The offering consists primarily of a tangible good, such as toothpaste, toilet paper, or napkins.
- *Tangible good with accompanying services.* The offering consists of a tangible good accompanied by one or more services; as the sophistication for use of the good increases, the more dependent its sale is on services.
- *Hybrid.* The offering consists of equal parts of goods and services, such as the purchase of a meal at a restaurant (consists of food and service).
- *Major service with accompanying minor goods and services.* The offering consists of a major service accompanied by other services and supporting goods, such as the purchase of airplane transportation (primarily a service accompanied by some tangibles such as food and drinks).
- *Pure service.* The offering consists primarily of a service, such as attending an orchestra performance or psychotherapy.

Christensen et al. (1993) differentiated among three types of services associated with patient care provided by pharmacists. Although there are some differences, their classification scheme in many respects resembles Kotler and Keller's (2012) categories, which are applicable to all goods and services, not just those related to pharmacy.

- *Dispensing services.* These are services associated with dispensing a prescription that are obligatory under board of pharmacy regulations. These services include accurately filling a prescription order, clarifying orders, not dispensing an order that contains obvious errors that would be identified by a "reasonable and prudent" pharmacist, and communicating drug-use instructions as required by state statutes and regulations.
- *Dispensing-related value-added pharmaceutical services.* These are services that extend beyond *routine* dispensing activities required by law. These services include activities such as selecting appropriate drug products, monitoring refill behaviors, and consulting with other health providers about a patient's drug regimen (beyond routine clarification questions).
- *Nondispensing-related value-added pharmaceutical services.* These are services that are not associated with the dispensing of a prescription and are not required by law nor inherent in the fee charged for a prescription. These services include screening programs (e.g., osteoporosis, lipids, and blood pressure), weight management programs, in-service training provided to health care providers, and discharge counseling in an inpatient setting.

The preceding discussion may lead one to ask: What is the difference between a physical good and a service? Several authors have attempted to define characteristics that distinguish goods from services. While there is some debate as to which characteristics best represent the fundamental differences, it is important to recognize that any list represents generalizations that may not be applicable to all services (Lovelock and Wright, 2002). The following list contains nine basic differences that can help to distinguish services from physical goods (Lovelock and Wright, 2002)[7]:

- Customers do not obtain ownership of services.
- Service products are intangible performances.
- There is greater involvement of customers in the production process.
- People may form part of the product, including other patrons.
- There is greater variability in operational inputs and outputs, making it more difficult to standardize and control.
- Many services are difficult for customers to evaluate.
- There is typically an absence of inventories.
- The time factor is relatively more important.
- Delivery systems may involve both electronic and physical channels.

---

[7]For an alternative view regarding the meaning and importance of these differences, see Vargo and Lusch (2004a).

Each of these differences may affect the design of a marketing program. For example, a major consideration in service delivery is matching demand levels and capacity. This is so because services are perishable and cannot be inventoried. One mechanism that can be used to better match supply and demand is the use of reservations (e.g., hotel and airline industries) and appointments (e.g., for MTM services). As another example, because of the greater variability inherent in the production of a service, service organizations need to pay special attention to the standardization of the service-performance process or risk damaging the quality of the service provided. One mechanism that can be used is a service blueprint, which is "a visual map of the sequence of activities required for service delivery" that specifies not only the elements of service operations that are visible or apparent to the customer (including the customer's own actions) and those aspects that are hidden from the customer but also the linkages between these elements (Lovelock and Wright, 2002, p. 153). Such a blueprint can help to identify fail points, or points in the process where there are significant risks for problems. In health care, protocols and practice guidelines are commonly used to standardize care to enhance quality.

The differences between services and physical goods contribute to the distinctive nature of service performances. This distinctive nature has led several authors to propose that the traditional four P's of the marketing mix are insufficient as a set of marketing tools for service businesses (Booms and Bitner, 1981; Kotler, 2003; Lovelock and Wright, 2002).[8] Additional elements must be included in the marketing mix, and our view of the tools that form the traditional components must be modified because of the fundamental differences between goods and services. Building on the work of Booms and Bitner (1981), Lovelock and Wright (2002) have proposed the "eight P's" of integrated service management[9]: (1) product elements; (2) place, cyberspace, and time; (3) promotion and education; (4) price and other user outlays; (5) process; (6) productivity and quality; (7) people; and (8) physical evidence. Notice that the first four are closely related to the traditional four P's of the marketing mix, with some modifications because of the distinctive nature of services, the changing environment, and other enlightened recognitions by marketers. The last four variables deserve additional discussion.

Process

The creation and delivery of product elements require that special attention be given to the design, implementation, and evaluation of processes. A *process* is the method and sequence in which a service is created, produced, and delivered. The service blueprint can be useful in understanding and designing processes. For a pharmacy, the focus may be on the entire process of dispensing a prescription starting with presentation of the prescription by a patient (or a telephone order from a nurse or physician) all the way through verifying patient understanding of the medication (Holdford and Kennedy, 1999). Alternatively, a pharmacy may focus on a specific component of the process, such as what steps will be taken if one learns during a patient history that he or she smokes cigarettes.

Poorly designed processes may lead to ineffective service delivery, causing customer frustration and dissatisfaction, as well as employee frustration and dissatisfaction. For example, long waits at checkout lines in a retail environment caused by poorly designed systems that fail to anticipate customer flow are troublesome

[8]Services marketing, coupled with other streams of marketing literature, such as relationship marketing, resource management, and market orientation, has led some (e.g., see Vargo and Lusch, 2004b) to argue that marketing, as an academic discipline and as a business practice, has shifted from a goods-dominant view, largely based on discrete transactions, to a service-dominant view, where relationships play a central role. One could argue that pharmacy has experienced a similar evolution.

[9]Others have proposed similar frameworks for all of marketing, not just services marketing. For example, Kotler and Keller (2012) add four additional P's (processes, performance, people, and programs) to the traditional four P's of marketing to align with the holistic marketing concept.

for customers in line as well as the few employees who are running registers.

Productivity and Quality

Productivity focuses on the efficiency in the transformation of service inputs into outputs, whereas *quality*, in this context, refers to the degree to which a service meets the needs, wants, and expectations of customers. Service firms must attempt to balance these elements. Improving productivity may help to keep costs down, but cuts in service levels may adversely affect perceptions of quality. Similarly, while service quality may be critical for building customer loyalty, investing in quality improvement without understanding the impact on incremental costs and revenues can have negative consequences for profitability. From a managed-care pharmacy perspective, efforts to increase efficiency by limiting the use of certain medications may lead to a significant decrease in quality perceptions not only by patients but also by network providers.

People

People provide most services; thus, the selection, training, and motivation of employees are critical tasks for service firms. Interactions with employees can have a significant impact on perceptions of service quality. Pharmacy managers need to pay special attention to all members of the pharmacy staff, not just pharmacists and technicians. Clerks, maintenance staff, volunteers, students, and anyone else who has contact with customers need sufficient training. In addition, other patrons may form part of the service experience, and firms often need to take these individuals into consideration. For example, the behavior of other patrons at an amusement park may have a dramatic effect on the quality of one's experience and one's level of satisfaction, and the presence of a caregiver may alter the service experience during an MTM session.

Physical Evidence

The appearance of the physical environment where the service is delivered (including buildings, landscape, employees, and furnishings), signs, printed materials, and other visible and tangible cues may provide evidence to customers concerning the service quality of an organization. Pharmacy managers should ask such questions as follows: Do we have adequate parking? Is the appearance of the pharmacy neat, and does it imply a professional image? Is our signage consistent? Is our equipment up to date?

EXPECTATIONS, SATISFACTION, QUALITY, VALUE, AND LOYALTY

Several terms have been used repeatedly in the preceding sections of this chapter. Although exchange is considered the core concept in marketing, these other concepts (i.e., expectations, satisfaction, quality, value, and loyalty) also play a critical role in understanding what marketing is all about.

Expectations

Critical to understanding customer satisfaction and perceived service quality is a clear understanding of expectations. *Expectations* are internal standards used by customers when evaluating a product or service. While they may initially influence a decision whether or not to purchase a product and from whom, they also play a critical role in consumers' judgments of service quality and satisfaction. Conceptual models have suggested that expectations consist of several different elements: desired service level, adequate service level, predicted service level, and a zone of tolerance (Zeithaml et al., 1993; see also Parasuraman et al., 1994a).

The *desired service level* is defined as what customers hope to receive and reflects a combination of what customers believe can and should be delivered. As customers realize that they cannot always get what they desire, they hold another, lower level of expectation that reflects the minimum level of service they are willing to accept, called the *adequate service level.* The *zone of tolerance* represents the difference between adequate and desired levels and recognizes that customers are willing to accept some variation in service delivery. The range they are willing to accept is the zone of tolerance, suggesting that expectations are not a single level but are best characterized by a range of levels bounded by desired and adequate service levels. If a performance falls outside the range and below adequate levels, customers will likely be frustrated and dissatisfied. If performance exceeds desired levels, it will likely surprise and please the customer, leading to customer delight (Lovelock and Wright, 2002). Finally, there is a *predicted service level*, which reflects the level of service customers believe that they are most likely to get. This predicted service level directly affects how the adequate service level is defined for that occasion.

The desired service level can be elevated or lowered based on personal needs and enduring beliefs about what is possible. The adequate service level can be influenced by a number of factors, including the perceptions of service alternatives and situational factors (e.g., emergencies and catastrophes). Explicit and implicit promises made by the service provider, past experiences, and word-of-mouth communications are proposed to influence the desired service level directly and affect the adequate service level indirectly through the predicted service level (Zeithaml et al., 1993).

Marketers can have a significant role in influencing consumer expectations. Setting expectations in the mind of the consumer that are too high can create significant problems, such as possibly setting up the customer for frustration, disappointment, and dissatisfaction. On the other hand, setting expectations too low may lead to difficulties in attracting new customers. Indeed, a significant problem facing the profession of pharmacy is that many patients do not expect to receive MTM services. In planning their marketing communications effort and promotion mix, organizations (including pharmacies) must attempt to set a balance with respect to customer expectations.

Satisfaction and Quality

Some authors use the terms *quality* and *satisfaction* interchangeably. However, there are some notable differences. While there are different conceptualizations of satisfaction (Schommer and Kucukarslan, 1997), in marketing, the most common approach is based on the confirmation/disconfirmation of expectations model.[10] Thus, Kotler and Keller (2012, p. 128) define *satisfaction* as "a person's feelings of pleasure or disappointment resulting from comparing a product's perceived performance (or outcome) to expectations." Thus, if performance is worse than expected (negative disconfirmation), the customer will be dissatisfied. If performance matches expectations (confirmation), satisfaction will result. If performance exceeds expectations (positive disconfirmation), the customer will be highly satisfied and possibly delighted.[11] There are vast differences between satisfied and completely satisfied customers (e.g., see Lovelock and Wright, 2002). For example, completely or highly satisfied customers are much more likely to remain loyal to a business and spread positive word of mouth about the company.

As with satisfaction, there is a rich history concerning the concept of quality. A broad definition of *quality* is superiority or excellence. Researchers note a difference between *objective quality* (i.e., measurable and verifiable superiority on some predetermined ideal standard) and *perceived quality* (Zeithaml, 1988). Perceived quality is a global assessment made by a consumer that is posited to exist at a higher level of abstraction from a consumer's perceptions of a product's specific attributes (Zeithaml, 1988). *Service quality* is defined as "customers' long-term cognitive evaluation of a firm's service delivery" (Lovelock and Wright, 2002, p. 87) and results from a comparison of expectations and perceptions of service performance (Parasuraman et al., 1988). Since service quality represents a global impression rather than an encounter-specific evaluation, consumers are posited to update their perceptions of service quality following their interactions with service providers.

Service quality has been conceptualized to contain multiple dimensions (Parasuraman et al., 1985). One

[10] For an interesting and somewhat alternative view of the concept of satisfaction, see Fournier and Mick (1999).

[11] For a provocative discussion of customer delight, see Oliver et al. (1997) and Rust and Oliver (2000).

measure of service quality, the SERVQUAL scale (Parasuraman et al., 1988), identifies five such dimensions:

- *Tangibles*—the appearance of a firm's physical facilities, equipment, personnel, and communication materials
- *Reliability*—the ability of the firm to perform the promised service dependably and accurately
- *Responsiveness*—the willingness of the firm to help customers and provide prompt service
- *Assurance*—the knowledge and courtesy of employees and their ability to convey trust and confidence
- *Empathy*—the caring, individualized attention the firm provides to its customers

Another useful distinction made by service quality researchers is between technical quality and functional quality. *Technical quality* refers to customer perceptions about what is received from a service (e.g., Was the outcome of the service successful?), and *functional quality* refers to customer perceptions about how a service was performed (e.g., Did the service provider demonstrate concern and inspire confidence?) (Kotler, 2003). Perceptions of both functional and technical quality are important determinants of service quality, suggesting that service providers need to focus on being "high touch" as well as "high tech." In pharmacy, there is some evidence that functional quality has a greater impact on consumer perceptions of service quality than technical quality (Holdford and Schulz, 1999).

Both service quality and customer satisfaction are based on comparisons of expectations and performance. Are these really different constructs? There has been considerable debate in the marketing literature concerning this issue. One way that these two concepts have been distinguished is by examining the type of expectations that are used as the comparison. For service quality assessments, the focus is on desired and adequate service levels. For satisfaction evaluations, the focus has been on predicted service levels (Parasuraman et al., 1988; Spreng et al., 1996; Zeithaml et al., 1993). Another way these concepts have been distinguished is that service quality is a global judgment or assessment, whereas satisfaction is transaction specific (Parasuraman et al., 1988). This suggests that customer satisfaction leads to service quality. However, others have suggested that service quality leads to customer satisfaction. In an effort to work around this debate, Parasuraman et al. (1994b), building on the work of Teas (1993), suggested that both service quality and customer satisfaction can be examined meaningfully at the individual transaction level and be thought of as global (or overall) assessments that are formed following numerous transactions.

Regardless of this theoretical debate, there is considerable evidence that enhancing customer satisfaction and service quality can lead to positive outcomes for the organization and the consumer. As mentioned earlier, highly satisfied customers are more likely to exhibit loyalty, which means a consistent stream of revenues over a period of years for the firm (Lovelock and Wright, 2002). These customers may also be more forgiving when there is a service failure and may make fewer demands and fewer mistakes as they gain experience as consumers of a company's products or services, thus reducing the firm's operating costs (Lovelock and Wright, 2002). Positive word of mouth is also a key effect of high levels of satisfaction and perceived service quality. This outcome is extremely important to providers of professional services such as pharmacists. Satisfied customers also means less negative word of mouth, which can travel faster (and farther) than positive comments. All these behavioral impacts can help to improve the bottom line of the company, namely, profitability (Zeithaml et al., 2001).

Value

Many marketers believe that the fundamental role of marketing is to create value for customers (Lovelock and Wright, 2002). But what is *value,* and how is it different from perceived quality? When customers evaluate a product or a service, they consider the benefits it offers (i.e., what they get) relative to the costs (i.e., what they give up). The benefits of a product or service include fulfilling a functional need, making a process more convenient, and providing an emotional payout such as prestige or a boost to self-esteem. Costs to a consumer include not only monetary costs but also the

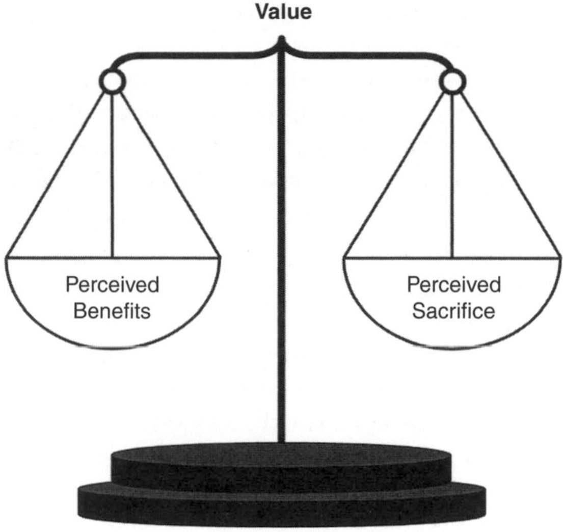

Figure 21-1. A conceptualization of value.

nonmonetary outlays associated with the time, effort, and discomfort related to the processes of searching for, purchasing, and using the product (including costs associated with a product or service failure). *Value* is conceptualized as either the ratio (Kotler, 2003) or the difference (Lovelock and Wright, 2002) between the perceived benefits and the perceived costs (i.e., perceived sacrifice). Figure 21-1 is a useful approach to visualizing how a customer may calculate value.

To increase the value for a customer, marketers can increase the benefits derived from the core product, enhance or provide supplementary services, or reduce the monetary costs or nonmonetary outlays associated with acquiring and using the product (Lovelock and Wright, 2002). Alternatively, a marketer can increase costs to the customer as long as there is a corresponding greater increase in benefits or an offset to some other outlay. Consumers paying a premium price to save time or gain greater comfort are an example of the latter. Marketers still can enhance value for customers by reducing benefits, as long as there is a corresponding greater decrease in costs. It is important to recognize that a consumer's perception of the value of a product may be different before and after consumption, indicating that an individual's perceptions of benefits and costs may be altered by product use and what happens after product use.

Quality and value are not the same thing. The concept of value is more individualistic and personal than quality and thus is theorized to exist at a higher level of abstraction in the mind of the consumer. In addition, quality is usually conceptualized as part of the "get" component, whereas value involves a trade-off of get and give components (Zeithaml, 1988). Because they are related, it is not surprising that efforts directed at increasing quality (or customer satisfaction for that matter) also can lead to increases in perceived value, which may contribute to increased consumer intentions and behaviors and ultimately to improved profitability, as discussed earlier. An important consideration is that perceptions of quality and value exist after as well as prior to service delivery or product use. These preuse perceptions may be based on word-of-mouth messages (e.g., what acquaintances have said) or may be based on the promotional message of the firm. For pharmacists, this suggests that both effective provision of MTM services and appropriate use of the promotion mix are necessary for communicating value to prospective members of the target market. Pharmacists must understand how to use both sides of the value equation if they want to both attract and retain customers.

Loyalty

Loyalty has received a considerable amount of attention from both marketing theorists and practitioners. Most would agree that there are positive consequences associated with a loyal customer base. However, there are some areas of disagreement with respect to customer loyalty.

Part of the debate has been with respect to how loyalty should be conceptualized and subsequently measured. Historically, the concept has been thought of as a behavioral outcome, namely, repurchase or switching intentions and behaviors (Oliver, 1999). Others have argued that loyalty has psychological meaning. For example, firm adoration, identification with the firm, and willingness to assist the service provider and other customers are thought to be part of the loyalty construct (Jones and Taylor, 2007; Oliver, 1999). To better understand the concept, some have suggested viewing loyalty in service provider–consumer relationships in the same manner as pro-relationship behaviors that develop in friendships and even romantic relationships (Jones and Taylor, 2007).

In addition to issues of conceptualization and measurement, marketers also have debated the antecedents of loyalty. The role of satisfaction in the development of loyalty has received the most attention. While there is most likely a relationship between these two variables (satisfaction begets loyalty), the relationship is not perfect; many customers may be satisfied or even highly satisfied yet fail to display repurchase behaviors (Oliver, 1999). Others have demonstrated that it is not just the level of satisfaction that plays a role in determining loyalty but the strength (degree of certainty) with which a customer expresses his or her satisfaction (Chandrashekaran et al., 2007).

Oliver (1999, p. 41) states that ultimate loyalty requires that "the consumable must be subject to adoration." The object or service must be lovable. The negative demand associated with most pharmaceutical products and services suggests that ultimate loyalty may be an elusive goal. This should not suggest that pharmacy cannot learn from the growing body of knowledge regarding loyalty. Because of its known relationship to firm performance, at the very least, pharmacy should be concerned with customer retention and repurchase intentions, even if such conceptualizations fail to recognize the psychological dimensions of loyalty. Related to this issue is a useful recommendation based on the work of Reichheld (2003), who suggests that firms need to be aware of only a single-item measure when thinking about the concept of loyalty: "How likely is it that you would recommend [Company X] to a friend or colleague?" This single-item measure has been shown to be related to the revenue growth rate of firms in several industries.

The recipient of loyalty attitudes and behaviors should also be considered. As mentioned earlier, some have conceptualized service loyalty to be similar to loyalty in interpersonal relationships like friendships. This suggests that the pharmacist, rather than the pharmacy, may be the subject of loyalty attitudes and behaviors (pharmacist-owned loyalty).[12] Such loyalty can be beneficial to the firm if the specific pharmacist continues his or her tenure with the pharmacy. Pharmacy employers need to understand this concept and the importance of good human resources management; management and marketing do not exist in isolation.

Collecting Customer Data

To create, deliver, and communicate superior customer value requires that a company understands its target market's expectations as well as its customers' assessments of satisfaction, quality, and value. Relying on customer complaints (or a lack of them) as evidence that a business is satisfying needs and meeting expectations is notoriously flawed. Studies show that most dissatisfied customers never complain to the company; rather, they buy less or switch to another company (Lovelock and Wright, 2002). Therefore, companies need to take a more active approach in gathering data about improving their products or services. Some examples of how such an effort can be implemented include the following (Lovelock and Wright, 2002):

- *Posttransaction surveys.* The goal of this approach is to collect data concerning customer satisfaction and perceptions about the service experience immediately after (or within a few days of) the encounter. Questions usually are specific to the immediate past transaction or experience, although some more global questions may be included. You probably have been asked to fill out such a questionnaire at a recent visit to a restaurant or during a stay at a hotel. Doucette and McDonough (2002) provide an example of a survey used for a weight control and wellness program at a pharmacy.
- *Overall evaluation surveys.* While posttransaction surveys focus on consumer evaluations of the most immediate encounter, the focus when conducting

[12]For an interesting application to sales representatives, see Palmatier et al. (2007).

an overall evaluation survey is on global impressions of a firm. This can include "customers" overall satisfaction with the firm, as well as "their overall impressions of the firm's service quality, product quality, and price" (Parasuraman et al., 1994b, p. 122). These evaluations should reflect customers' accumulated experiences over time. For this reason, as well as the costs associated with conducting these studies, Lovelock and Wright (2002) recommend that these surveys be administered less frequently than post-transaction surveys. Larson and MacKeigan's work regarding a measure of patient satisfaction with pharmacy services (Larson and MacKeigan, 1994; MacKeigan and Larson, 1989) and with pharmaceutical care (Larson et al., 2002) are examples of this approach. An example outside of pharmacy is the SERVQUAL scale (Parasuraman et al., 1988).

- *Mystery shopping.* This technique involves sending individuals posing as ordinary customers to gather information and provide feedback about service experiences. This technique allows for gathering information on individual employees and can be used to award superior performance or as an indication of the need for additional training. This approach may not be as useful for pharmacies that have few new customers because employees may be able to identify the mystery shopper. Consideration should be given to how employees might react to this deceptive practice. Suggestions include informing employees that this may be happening at some time, informing them on the criteria on which they will be assessed, and evaluating performance over a series of encounters rather than a single visit (Lovelock and Wright, 2002).
- *Noncustomer, new customer, and declining/former customer surveys.* Surveys of these groups may be useful for identifying unmet needs, expectations and image (e.g., noncustomer surveys), reasons for patronage (i.e., new customers), and information about a firm's deficiencies (i.e., declining and former customers).
- *Focus groups.* A more qualitative approach to gathering customer data is the use of focus groups, or groups of customers who are assembled by a researcher for an in-depth discussion on a specific topic. The group is led by a trained moderator who is responsible for keeping the group on task. Focus groups can be useful in learning about customers' needs and expectations, determining how customers evaluate a firm's performance, gathering in-depth information about service problems, or obtaining feedback about a proposed product or service. Pharmacists should be cautioned about projecting results from a focus group to an entire market segment. Bislew and Sorensen (2003) provide an example of how focus groups might be used in a pharmacy setting.
- *Employee data.* Companies should not discount the value of the information that can be obtained from talking and *listening to* employees. Employees have first-hand experience with customers that may lead to improvements in the product or service delivery. Surveys, focus groups, and one-on-one interviews all can be used to collect data from employees.

RELATIONSHIP MARKETING

While the concepts inherent in relationship marketing are not new, it has only been within the past 30 years that the practice and science of marketing have grown aware of the relevance of relational exchanges. The concepts discussed throughout this chapter have significant meaning in a relationship-marketing paradigm. Indeed, an understanding of many of these concepts, such as expectations, satisfaction, perceived quality, value, and loyalty, may be even more critical in a relationship-marketing paradigm because they are key to maintaining long-term collaborations and retaining customers. So what is relationship marketing? There has been considerable debate in the marketing literature concerning an appropriate definition of relationship marketing (e.g., see Parvatiyar and Sheth, 2000). One useful definition has been provided by Lovelock and Wright (2002, p. 102), who define *relationship marketing* as "activities aimed at developing long-term, cost-effective links between an organization and its customers for the mutual benefit of both parties."

Key to understanding relationship marketing is appreciating the distinction between discrete transaction-based exchanges and relational exchanges. Weitz and Jap (1995, p. 305) note that "· · · the growing interest in relationship marketing suggests a shift in the nature of general marketplace transactions from discrete to relational exchanges—from exchanges between parties with no past history and no future to exchanges between parties who have an exchange history and plans for future interactions." Thus, in the practice of transactional marketing, each transaction is viewed as a separate event, or a one-shot deal. The fact that one transaction has occurred does not predict that a future transaction will occur (Gummesson, 2002); the focus of both parties is to make the most of each individual transaction. However, a customer may use the same supplier repeatedly, possibly because of high switching costs, not because he or she is committed to that individual supplier (Gummesson, 2002).

While purely discrete transactions are rare, and while there are numerous benefits to both customers and producers who operate in a relationship-marketing paradigm, neither of these should imply that all forms of transactional marketing are inherently bad or wrong. Indeed, several authors have noted that transactional marketing can be a functional option for some marketers and customers based on the characteristics of the situation and the players involved (Gummesson, 2002; Kotler, 2003; Sheth et al., 2000). These characteristics include the time horizon of the customer, the level of customer involvement, the costs associated with switching to another organization, the level of customer interest in establishing a relationship, and the ability of an organization to implement such an approach efficiently (i.e., the cost and revenue implications must be understood).[13] In their synthesis of the relationship-marketing literature, Palmatier et al. (2006) find that relationship marketing is more effective when relationships are more important to customers, such as in the context of service offerings and business-to-business relationships, and when relationships are established with individuals rather than with the firm as a whole.

Other authors have noted that transactional marketing still can be customer centric, focusing on the needs, wants, and resources of individual consumers and customers rather than on those of mass markets or segments (Sheth et al., 2000). Sheth (2002) has argued that the future of relationship marketing includes the selective and targeted use of relationship marketing coupled with transactional marketing efforts depending on the characteristics of the customer segment.

The basic concepts of relationship marketing have historical roots dating back to the earliest merchants (Berry, 1995; Sheth and Parvatiyar, 1995). However, the concept of relationship marketing as we know it today gained popularity beginning in the early 1980s (Sheth, 2002).

What Does Relationship Marketing Entail?

Gummesson (2002) outlines the fundamental values of relationship marketing:

- *Marketing management should be broadened into marketing-oriented company management.* This value is similar to the marketing concept's call for an integrated marketing orientation throughout an organization. Firms practicing relationship marketing must have an understanding of the importance of marketing throughout the whole organization, *not just for the marketing department.* This is consistent with the 2007 AMA definition of marketing as well as the holistic marketing concept of Kotler and Keller (2012). Effective relationship marketing requires a customer-centric focus (Sheth et al., 2000).
- *Long-term collaborations and win-win.* A key to relationship marketing is a focus on collaboration, viewing suppliers, customers, and others as partners rather than as combatants. This belief implies that relationships will create mutual value, leading to an extension of the duration of the relationship. This also implies that relationship marketing encourages retention marketing over attraction marketing.

[13]For insight into why consumers in general may choose not to engage in relationships with retailers and service providers, see Noble and Phillips (2004) and Ashley et al. (2011).

Table 21-1. Coproduction, Cocreation of Value, and Shared Decision Making

A fundamental value of relationship marketing is the involvement of the customer in the production process. Coproduction has also been labeled as one of the hallmarks of the service-centered view of the discipline of marketing (Vargo and Lusch, 2004b). Coproduction means the involvement of the customer in the creation of value (i.e., cocreation). Examples of consumers as coproducers abound outside of healthcare. Some of these examples are considered somewhat firm centric (e.g., self-service applications such as ATMs and supermarket self-checkouts), while others are truly value cocreation experiences (e.g., certain video games, General Motors' OnStar service, and communication networks that allow for customer-to-customer (C-to-C) interaction) (Prahalad and Ramaswamy, 2004). The Internet, including social media, has fostered the growth of C-to-C communication and other innovations (e.g., online auctions and "price-naming" applications) that allow customers to personalize experiences.

In medicine and pharmacy, the concepts of coproduction and cocreation of value are reflected by a patient relationship rooted in shared decision making (Prahalad and Ramaswamy, 2004). Involvement, information sharing, expression of preferences, and mutually agreeable treatment plans by providers and patients are key traits of a shared decision-making model (Charles et al., 1997). Joint development of treatment plans by patients and providers should lead to improved satisfaction and also enhance adherence to the treatment plan (Guadagnoli and Ward, 1998; Mead and Bower, 2002). The shared decision-making model is also central to several emerging practice models, such as the patient-centered medical home (Epperly, 2011). Pharmacists are educated to seek and use patient input when making treatment recommendations and also to help patients learn to manage treatment plans with respect to unique needs, situations, lifestyles, and behaviors. Relationship marketing and the process of coproduction are not only consistent with these practices but require them!

- *All parties should be active and take responsibility.* The producer is not the only player in a relationship. Indeed, in many business-to-business relationships, the customers initiate innovation and force suppliers to change their products or services. With respect to services, customers are often involved in the production of the service, suggesting a critical interactive role, depending on the situation. See Table 21-1 for further discussion.
- *Relationship and service values instead of bureaucratic-legal values.* This value does not suggest that laws should be broken but instead implies that flexibility rather than rigidity should guide the management of customer relationships. Customers are individuals and should be treated as such.

Service firms and other businesses use a variety of approaches to maintain and enhance customer relationships, such as treating customers fairly, offering service augmentations, and treating each customer as if he or she were a segment of one (Lovelock and Wright, 2002). Significant to maintaining relationships in the delivery of services is the fulfillment of promises made to customers. Bitner (1995) outlined three essential activities to attracting, building, and maintaining service relationships:

- *Make realistic promises in the first place.* Through the eight P's of integrated service management, an organization makes promises to its target market regarding what they can expect. As discussed previously, companies must strike a balance between setting expectations too high (possibly setting up the customer to be disappointed) and setting expectations too low (which may lead to a failure to attract customers). McDonough et al. (2003, p. 217) suggest that "it is better to overperform than to over-promise."

- *Enable employees and systems to deliver on promises.* Process and people, two of the eight P's, are critical to the fulfillment of promises. Promises are easy to make, but without the right people using the right processes and tools, they are difficult to keep. Resources must be available, and people must have the training and motivation to serve customers.
- *Keep promises to customers when delivering services.* Every time a customer interacts with the organization (through its employees or a technological interface), an opportunity exists to keep or break a promise. These encounters, called *moments of truth,* form the basis for how a service relationship is built. Depending on the service and the situation, a single negative encounter (failure to meet a promise) can be enough to sever a relationship or at least cause a weakening of the relationship, even a long-lasting relationship. The provider's response to a service failure (i.e., service recovery effort) may be critical in maintaining satisfaction and repurchase intentions (Bunniran et al., 2011). Pharmacies should have a service-recovery plan for dealing with these situations (see Chapter 13). On the other hand, a series of positive encounters (repeatedly meeting promises and exceeding expectations) can lead to customer trust in the organization and a feeling of commitment to the relationship with the organization (Morgan and Hunt, 1994).

What Are the Consequences of Relationship Marketing?

The definition of relationship marketing stresses that its practice is mutually beneficial for an organization and its customers. Benefits to the organization, such as customer loyalty, referrals, and profitability (Palmatier et al., 2006), are manifested through improvements in marketing productivity and by making marketing more effective and more efficient (Sheth and Parvatiyar, 1995). As an example, loyalty programs are a common relationship-marketing tactic (see Table 21-2). By focusing on individual customers (rather than on mass markets or market segments), and by increasing the involvement of the customer in the marketing effort, relationship marketing should be *more effective* in meeting customer needs and wants. Furthermore, focusing on customer retention, reducing some of the wasteful practices associated with mass marketing, and letting the customer become a more active participant in the production process (i.e., letting customers perform some of the tasks historically performed by marketers—think ATMs) may lead to increases in *marketing efficiency.*

The point with respect to customer retention may need some elaboration. Estimates suggest that at least 65 percent of the average company's business comes from its present satisfied customers (Schoell and Guiltinan, 1990). Other evidence indicates that attracting new customers is significantly more expensive than retaining existing ones (Kotler and Keller, 2012). There is empirical evidence that shows that as customers remain in relationships for longer periods, they are more profitable to the firm (Sheth and Parvatiyar, 1995). These findings lead to the conclusion that focusing on customer retention rather than customer acquisition should be a less expensive (and more profitable) way to conduct business.

Relationship marketing also has significant benefits to the customer (Berry, 1995; Bitner, 1995). Certainly customers benefit economically (e.g., pricing incentives) when engaged in a relational activity and typically receive higher value when a company consistently fulfills promises. Long-term relationships can also reduce both stress and risk for customers as the relationship becomes more predictable and trust in the service provider increases. Such relationships also reduce the need to change, an act that most humans prefer to avoid. Remaining in a relationship simplifies one's life, saving time and effort by lessening the need for information search and decision making. Finally, relationship marketing offers social benefits, such as being made to feel important and having a customer–service provider relationship develop into a friendship or part of a social support system. For years, pharmacists have recognized the importance of this last consumer benefit.

Table 21-2. Loyalty Programs and Relationship Marketing

Loyalty programs have been used in many different industries, including pharmacy, for a number of reasons. These reasons include retaining customers, prompting purchases that would not otherwise be made, encouraging the consolidation of purchases (i.e., sometimes referred to as increasing the "share of wallet," which means buying more products from a single seller that would normally be purchased from multiple, competing sellers), and collecting and using data about consumers' purchases and behaviors (Nunes and Drèze, 2006). Airline frequent flyer programs, hotel preferred guest programs, and supermarket reward programs are prominent examples. Such programs have been shown to increase customer share of wallet and lifetime duration (Meyer-Waarden, 2007) as well as accelerate the customer relationship life cycle with a firm for those customers who are light-to-moderate buyers at the beginning of a loyalty program (Liu, 2007). Attaining success in loyalty programs appears to contribute to increased efforts at subsequent goal attainment (Drèze and Nunes, 2011).
Loyalty programs are increasingly common in the chain drugstore industry (Blank, 2009) and have been suggested as a very useful tool for independent pharmacies (Lockwood, n.d.). In addition to the potential benefits listed earlier, loyalty programs in pharmacy practice also have the advantage of encouraging patients to use a single pharmacy for their prescription medications, which may enhance the delivery of MTM services. However, pharmacy managers need to carefully consider the goals of a loyalty program as well as their specific situations when deciding to initiate such a program. In some industries, larger firms may benefit more from loyalty programs than smaller firms, and in some markets the degree of loyalty program saturation may limit the contribution of such program to the bottom line (Liu and Yang, 2009). Common mistakes made when initiating and managing a loyalty program include focusing on purchase quantity rather than profitability, overpromising and underdelivering, simply paying people to buy your product, giving away too much, and encouraging one-time use rather than the use of a program over time (Nunes and Drèze, 2006). Poorly designed and implemented loyalty programs might even create "disloyal" customers. Pharmacy managers also need to consider that pharmacy and health care are different from other services (Berry and Bendapudi, 2007) and thus loyalty programs may have different meanings for patients and other health care stakeholders.

How Does Relationship Marketing Apply to Pharmacy?

Many of the applications of relationship marketing to pharmacy practice and health care are fairly self-evident. In many pharmacy settings, pharmaceutical goods and patient care services are provided to individuals who require attention and treatment over a long period of time because of their chronic conditions. The establishment of a provider–patient relationship is critical to the successful treatment of patients. Indeed, the nature of the therapeutic relationship between pharmacist and patient has been labeled as *foundational* to the conceptualization of pharmaceutical care (Cipolle et al., 1998). Interestingly, the definition of a therapeutic relationship (Cipolle et al., 1998, p. 344), "a partnership or alliance between the practitioner and the patient formed for the purpose of identifying the patient's drug-related needs," refers to several of the elements discussed throughout this chapter. In addition, the discussion of a therapeutic relationship explicitly recognizes that not only does the practitioner have responsibilities but also the patient—a concept not inconsistent with relationship marketing. While the nature of the patient–provider relationship takes on additional ethical meaning within the context of health care, many of the concepts discussed in this section (and throughout this chapter) have direct applications to the delivery of health care and pharmaceutical services.

A few additional points concerning relationship marketing and pharmacy practice are warranted. First, practitioners need to recognize that most pharmacies (and their computer systems) are full of data that can be used for one-to-one marketing and satisfying the unique needs of individual customers. These data can be used not only as part of the production and the delivery of the service but also to communicate with customers, prescribers, and other stakeholders. Second, it is important to consider individuals and organizations other than patients when implementing a relationship-marketing program within a pharmacy. The same principles can be applied to interactions with physicians and other providers, employer groups, third-party payers, computer vendors, wholesalers, and even others within your own firm. Establishing, developing, and maintaining relationships with these stakeholders have the potential to enhance or facilitate relationships with the ultimate customer, the patient. Third, building relationships does not happen overnight; relationships take time to establish and develop. However, practitioners should be encouraged to consider every service encounter as a relationship-building opportunity (Doucette and McDonough, 2002).

REVISITING THE SCENARIO: A SUMMARY

At the beginning of this chapter, we met Jim Smyth and Sue Davidson, who recognized that something needed to be done to enhance the financial position of their pharmacy. Many questions were raised during their impromptu brainstorming session with their employees, and most were related to marketing. To be effective (and efficient), health care providers and pharmacists (including Drs. Smyth and Davidson) need to wear a marketing hat as well as a clinical hat. They must understand how to integrate a marketing philosophy throughout their organizations. They must realize that focusing on customers' needs and learning how to translate those needs into wants and demands are critical steps. They must master the tools of the marketing mix, including the additional considerations required because of the distinctive nature of services. To stay in business, and to continue to reap the intrinsic benefits from helping patients, requires that pharmacists keep an eye on the bottom line, namely, the profitability of the organization (or at least its financial success measured in other terms when considering nonprofit firms). This means that pharmacists must understand the concepts of expectations, satisfaction, quality, value, and loyalty. Finally, while patient-centered pharmacy services already call for the establishment of a therapeutic relationship with patients, the practice of relationship marketing can help to enhance the level of service provided by pharmacists, potentially leading to improved outcomes for patients, improved financial performance for organizations, and rewarding practices for pharmacists.

QUESTIONS FOR FURTHER DISCUSSION

1. What philosophical approach to marketing is most common in today's pharmacy practice environment? Do you think one is more appropriate than the others?
2. What role does marketing play in ensuring the success of pharmacist-delivered MTM services? How can and should the profession (rather than individual pharmacists and businesses) use marketing principles and practices?
3. How can the expectations of patients be changed regarding the delivery of pharmacist-delivered MTM services?
4. How have your perceptions of marketing changed after reading this chapter?
5. Should the application of marketing principles be different for health professionals (compared with other service providers)?
6. Are loyalty programs appropriate for all types of pharmacies?

REFERENCES

Ashley C, Noble SM, Donthu N, Lemon KN. 2011. Why customers won't relate: Obstacles to relationship marketing engagement. *J Bus Res* 64:749.

Berry LL. 1995. Relationship marketing of services: Growing interest, emerging perspectives. *J Acad Market Sci* 23:236.

Berry LL, Bendapudi N. 2007. Health care: A fertile field for service research. *J Serv Res-US* 10:111.

Bislew HD, Sorensen TD. 2003. Use of focus groups as a tool to enhance a pharmaceutical care practice. *J Am Pharm Assoc* 43:424.

Bitner MJ. 1995. Building service relationships: It's all about promises. *J Acad Market Sci* 23:246.

Blank C. 2009. Pharmacy loyalty programs spur sales. *Drug Top* 153(8):21.

Booms BH, Bitner MJ. 1981. Marketing strategies and organization structures for service firms. In Donnelly JH, George WR (eds.) *Marketing of Services*. Chicago, IL: American Marketing Association, p. 47.

Bunniran S, McCaffrey D, Bentley J, et al. 2011. Patient service experiences in community pharmacy: An examination of health criticality, service failure incidents, and service recovery efforts and their influence on patronage outcomes (abstract). *J Am Pharm Assoc* 51:244.

Chandrashekaran M, Rotte K, Tax SS, Grewal R. 2007. Satisfaction strength and customer loyalty. *J Market Res* 44:153.

Charles C, Gafni A, Whelan T. 1997. Shared decision-making in the medical encounter: What does it mean? (or it takes at least two to tango). *Soc Sci Med* 44: 681.

Christensen DB, Fassett WE, Andrews GA. 1993. A practical billing and payment plan for cognitive services. *Am Pharm* NS33:34.

Cipolle RJ, Strand LM, Morley PC. 1998. *Pharmaceutical Care Practice*. New York: McGraw-Hill.

Day GS, Montgomery DB. 1999. Charting new directions for marketing. *J Market* 63:3.

Doucette WR, McDonough RP. 2002. Beyond the 4 P's: Using relationship marketing to build value and demand for pharmacy services. *J Am Pharm Assoc* 42:183.

Drèze X, Nunes JC. 2011. Recurring goals and learning: The impact of successful reward attainment on purchase behavior. *J Market Res* 48:268.

Epperly T. 2011. The patient-centred medical home in the USA. *J Eval Clin Prac* 17:373.

Feldstein PJ. 1999. *Health Care Economics*, 5th edn. Albany, NY: Delmar Publishers.

Fournier S, Mick DG. 1999. Rediscovering satisfaction. *J Market* 63:5.

Guadagnoli E, Ward P. 1998. Patient participation in decision-making. *Soc Sci Med* 47:329.

Gummesson E. 2002. *Total Relationship Marketing*, 2nd edn. Oxford, England: Butterworth-Heinemann.

Hepler CD, Strand LM. 1990. Opportunities and responsibilities in pharmaceutical care. *Am J Hosp Pharm* 47:533.

Holdford DA, Kennedy DT. 1999. The service blueprint as a tool for designing innovative pharmaceutical services. *J Am Pharm Assoc* 39:545.

Holdford D, Schulz R. 1999. Effect of technical and functional quality on patient perceptions of pharmaceutical service quality. *Pharm Res* 16:1344.

Hunt SD. 1976. The nature and scope of marketing. *J Market* 40:17.

Hunt SD. 1983. General theories and the fundamental explananda of marketing. *J Market* 47:9.

Hunt SD. 2002. *Foundations of Marketing Theory: Toward a General Theory of Marketing*. Armonk, NY: ME Sharpe.

Jones T, Taylor SF. 2007. The conceptual domain of service loyalty: How many dimensions? *J Serv Market* 21:36.

Keefe LS. 2004. What is the meaning of "marketing"? *Marketing News* 38:17.

Kohli AK, Jaworski BJ. 1990. Market orientation: The construct, research propositions, and managerial implications. *J Market* 54:1.

Kotler P. 2003. *Marketing Management*, 11th edn. Upper Saddle River, NJ: Prentice-Hall.

Kotler P, Keller KL. 2012. *Marketing Management*, 14th edn. Upper Saddle River, NJ: Pearson Prentice-Hall.

Larson LN, MacKeigan LD. 1994. Further validation of an instrument to measure patient satisfaction with pharmacy services. *J Pharm Market Manage* 8:125.

Larson LN, Rovers JP, MacKeigan LD. 2002. Patient satisfaction with pharmaceutical care: Update of a validated instrument. *J Am Pharm Assoc* 42:44.

Levitt T. 1960. Marketing myopia. *Harvard Bus Rev* 38:45.

Liu Y. 2007. The long-term impact of loyalty programs on consumer purchase behavior and loyalty. *J Market* 71:19.

Liu Y, Yang R. 2009. Competing loyalty programs: Impact of market saturation, market share, and category expandability. *J Market* 73:93.

Lockwood W. n.d. Differentiating independent pharmacy: Natural health, loyalty programs, and a real web presence. *ComputerTalk for the Pharmacist*. Available at http://www.computertalk.com/content/view/209/187/; accessed on May 25, 2011.

Lotti M, Lehmann D. 2007. New definition of marketing. Available at http://www.marketingpower.com/Community/ARC/Pages/Additional/Definition/default.aspx; accessed on May 25, 2011.

Lovelock C, Wright L. 2002. *Principles of Service Marketing and Management*, 2nd edn. Upper Saddle River, NJ: Prentice-Hall.

MacKeigan LD, Larson LN. 1989. Development and validation of an instrument to measure patient satisfaction with pharmacy services. *Med Care* 27:522.

Mathur A. 1996. Older adults' motivations for gift giving to charitable organizations: An exchange theory perspective. *Psychol Market* 13:107.

McAlister L, Bolton RN, Rizley R (eds.). 2010. *Essential Readings in Marketing with 2006–2010 Update*. Cambridge, MA: Marketing Science Institute.

McCarthy EJ. 1960. *Basic Marketing: A Managerial Approach*. Homewood, IL: Irwin.

McDonough RP. 2003. Obstacles to pharmaceutical care. In Rovers JP, Currie JD, Hagel HP, et al (eds.) *A Practical Guide to Pharmaceutical Care*, 2nd edn. Washington, DC: American Pharmaceutical Association, p. 267.

McDonough RP, Doucette WR. 2003. Using personal selling skills to promote pharmacy services. *J Am Pharm Assoc* 43:363.

McDonough RP, Pithan ES, Doucette WR, Brownlee MJ. 1998b. Marketing pharmaceutical care services. *J Am Pharm Assoc* 38:667.

McDonough RP, Rovers JP, Currie JD, et al. 1998a. Obstacles to the implementation of pharmaceutical care in the community setting. *J Am Pharm Assoc* 38:87.

McDonough RP, Sobotka JL. 2003. Reimbursement. In Rovers JP, Currie JD, Hagel HP, et al (eds.) *A Practical Guide to Pharmaceutical Care*, 2nd edn. Washington, DC: American Pharmaceutical Association, p. 222.

McDonough RP, Sobotka JL, Doucette WR. 2003. Marketing pharmaceutical care. In Rovers JP, Currie JD, Hagel HP, et al (eds.) *A Practical Guide to Pharmaceutical Care*, 2nd edn. Washington, DC: American Pharmaceutical Association, p. 203.

Mead N, Bower P. 2002. Patient-centered consultations and outcomes in primary care: A review of the literature. *Patient Educ Couns* 48:51.

Meyer-Waarden L. 2007. The effects of loyalty programs on customer lifetime duration and share of wallet. *J Retail* 83:223.

Morgan RM, Hunt SD. 1994. The commitment-trust theory of relationship marketing. *J Market* 58:20.

Narver JC, Slater SF, MacLachlan DL. 2004. Responsive and proactive market orientation and new-product success. *J Prod Innov Manage* 21:334.

Noble SM, Phillips J. 2004. Relationship hindrance: Why would consumers not want a relationship with a retailer? *J Retail* 80:289.

Nunes JC, Drèze X. 2006. Your loyalty program is betraying you. *Harvard Bus Rev* 84:124.

Oliver RL. 1999. Whence consumer loyalty? *J Market* 63:33.

Oliver RL, Rust RT, Varki S. 1997. Customer delight: Foundations, findings, and managerial insight. *J Retail* 73:311.

Palmatier RW, Dant RP, Grewal D, Evans KR. 2006. Factors influencing the effectiveness of relationship marketing: A meta-analysis. *J Market* 70:136.

Palmatier RW, Scheer LK, Steenkamp JEM. 2007. Customer loyalty to whom? Managing the benefits and risks of salesperson-owned loyalty. *J Market Res* 44:185.

Parasuraman A, Zeithaml VA, Berry LL. 1985. A conceptual model of service quality and its implications for future research. *J Market* 49:41.

Parasuraman A, Zeithaml VA, Berry LL. 1988. SERVQUAL: A multiple-item scale for measuring consumer perceptions of service quality. *J Retail* 64:12.

Parasuraman A, Zeithaml VA, Berry LL. 1994a. Alternative scales for measuring service quality: A comparative assessment based on psychometric and diagnostic criteria. *J Retail* 70:201.

Parasuraman A, Zeithaml VA, Berry LL. 1994b. Reassessment of expectations as a comparison standard in measuring service quality: Implications for further research. *J Market* 58:111.

Parvatiyar A, Sheth JN. 2000. The domain and conceptual foundations of relationship marketing. In Sheth JN, Parvatiyar A (eds.) *Handbook of Relationship Marketing*. Thousand Oaks, CA: Sage, p. 3.

Peter JP, Olson JC. 1983. Is science marketing? *J Market* 47:111.

Prahalad CK, Ramaswamy. 2004. Co-creation experiences: The next practice in value creation. *J Interact Mark* 18:5.

Reichheld FF. 2003. The one number you need to grow. *Harvard Bus Rev* 81:46.

Rovers JP, Currie JD, Hagel HP, et al. 1998. *A Practical Guide to Pharmaceutical Care*. Washington, DC: American Pharmaceutical Association.

Rust RT, Oliver RL. 2000. Should we delight the customer? *J Acad Market Sci* 28:86.

Schoell WF, Guiltinan JP. 1990. *Marketing: Contemporary Concepts and Practices*, 4th edn. Reading, MA: Allyn and Bacon.

Schommer JC, Kucukarslan SN. 1997. Measuring patient satisfaction with pharmaceutical services. *Am J Health Syst Pharm* 54:2721.

Shepherd MD. 1995. Defining and marketing value added services. *Am Pharm* NS35:46.

Sheth JN. 2002. The future of relationship marketing. *J Serv Market* 16:590.

Sheth JN, Parvatiyar A. 1995. Relationship marketing in consumer markets: Antecedents and consequences. *J Acad Market Sci* 23:255.

Sheth JN, Sisodia RS, Sharma A. 2000. The antecedents and consequences of customer-centric marketing. *J Acad Market Sci* 28:55.

Siecker B. 2002. Principles of place, channel systems, and channel specialists. In Smith MC, Kolassa EM, Perkins G, Siecker B (eds.) *Pharmaceutical Marketing: Principles, Environment, and Practice.* New York: Pharmaceutical Products Press, p. 219.

Smith MC. 1996. Pharmacy marketing. In *Effective Pharmacy Management,* 8th edn. Alexandria, VA: NARD, p. 423.

Smith MC. 2002. General principles. In Smith MC, Kolassa EM, Perkins G, Siecker B (eds.) *Pharmaceutical Marketing: Principles, Environment, and Practice.* New York: Pharmaceutical Products Press, p. 3.

Smith MC, Kolassa EM. 2001. Nobody wants your products: They are negative goods. *Product Management Today* 12:22.

Spreng RA, MacKenzie SB, Olshavsky RW. 1996. A reexamination of the determinants of consumer satisfaction. *J Market* 60:15.

Teas RK. 1993. Expectations, performance evaluation, and consumers: Perceptions of quality. *J Market* 57:18.

Van Waterschoot W, Van den Bulte C. 1992. The 4P classification of the marketing mix revisited. *J Market* 56:83.

Vargo SL, Lusch RF. 2004a. The four service marketing myths: Remnants of a goods-based, manufacturing model. *J Serv Res* 6:324.

Vargo SL, Lusch RF. 2004b. Evolving to a new dominant logic for marketing. *J Market* 68:1.

Weitz BA, Jap SD. 1995. Relationship marketing and distribution channels. *J Acad Market Sci* 23:305.

Wilkie WL, Moore ES. 1999. Marketing's contributions to society. *J Market* 63:198.

Wilkie WL, Moore ES. 2003. Scholarly research in marketing: Exploring the "4 eras" of thought development. *J Public Policy Market* 22:116.

Zeithaml VA. 1988. Consumer perceptions of price, quality, and value: A means-end model and synthesis of evidence. *J Market* 52:2.

Zeithaml VA, Berry LL, Parasuraman A. 1993. The nature and determinants of customer expectations of service. *J Acad Market Sci* 21:1.

Zeithaml VA, Rust RT, Lemon KN. 2001. The customer pyramid: Creating and serving profitable customers. *Calif Manage Rev* 43:118.

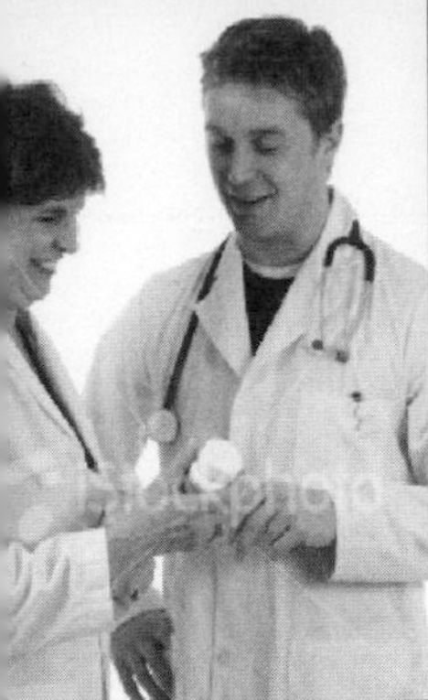

22

MARKETING APPLICATIONS

Benjamin S. Teeter and Salisa C. Westrick

About the Authors: Mr. Teeter is a graduate student in the Department of Pharmacy Care Systems at Auburn University's Harrison School of Pharmacy. He received a B.S. in Public Health from Indiana University and is currently working toward his Ph.D. in Pharmacy Care Systems. His teaching interests include pharmacy management, managing organizational change, and the US health care system. His main research interests include quality improvement in community pharmacy, adoption, implementation, and sustainability of innovations, and how community pharmacies adopt and market patient care services to their clients.

Dr. Westrick is an Associate Professor in the Department of Pharmacy Care Systems at Harrison School of Pharmacy, Auburn University. She received her B.S. in Pharmacy from Chulalongkorn University, Bangkok, Thailand, M.S. in Industrial Technology from Illinois State University, and Ph.D. in Social and Administrative Sciences in Pharmacy from University of Wisconsin-Madison. Her primary research interests are innovation adoption and program evaluation in community pharmacies.

LEARNING OBJECTIVES

After completing this chapter, readers should be able to

1. Describe the role of marketing and its importance in the practice of pharmacy.
2. Describe the essential steps when preparing to market goods or services in a pharmacy.
3. Distinguish between the micro- and macroenvironment of an organization.
4. Conduct a situation analysis for a given organization.
5. Differentiate between mass marketing and market segmentation.
6. Analyze a target market.
7. Apply marketing-mix components to various scenarios.
8. Describe the importance of marketing control.

SCENARIO

Murray Rockefeller earned a Pharm.D. degree 7 years ago. Upon graduation he was presented with the opportunity to become a junior partner of Community Care Pharmacy in Weagle, AL. This pharmacy fills prescriptions, provides compounding services, offers a full line of durable medical equipment, and prepares unit dose blister packages of medications for residents of a local nursing home. For the first 5 years of Dr. Rockefeller's employment, he worked closely with the senior partner and learned about running a pharmacy business. Working side by side with the senior partner ensured the smooth transition of the pharmacy ownership when Dr. Rockefeller became the sole owner of Community Care Pharmacy 2 years ago. Since Dr. Rockefeller assumed ownership of the pharmacy, he has reflected that much of his effort has been focused on maintaining existing services provided by the pharmacy rather than planning for goods and services they might offer in the future.

During the past year, Dr. Rockefeller has realized a significant increase in competition from community pharmacies in the area, as well as lower profit margins from dispensing prescriptions. He knows that he must investigate options to seek additional revenue sources for his pharmacy. These options include offering new goods, as well as developing new services that are needed and wanted by his patients. He also knows that before launching any new good or service he must do extensive planning and evaluate marketing options to ensure success.

CHAPTER QUESTIONS

1. Why is it important that the goods and services a pharmacy provides be consistent with the pharmacy's mission and vision statements?
2. Why is conducting a *S*trengths, *W*eaknesses, *O*pportunities, *T*hreats (SWOT) analysis important, and how can it be used to help shape a pharmacy's marketing efforts?
3. How does setting goals and objectives benefit a pharmacy?
4. What are the characteristics of a good target market?
5. How are the Four Ps applied to a specific marketing effort?
6. Describe pros and cons of each method of advertising.
7. Compare and contrast the four forms of promotion.
8. Describe why monitoring the performance of marketing activities important to a pharmacy's success?

INTRODUCTION

For the past 30 years, health care costs have increased faster than the costs of other goods and services. This has forced the payers of health care (e.g., patients, insurance companies, employers, government agencies) to seek ways to control the costs of health care. These cost control measures have had a direct impact on the practice of pharmacy, as pharmacy benefit managers have been aggressive in reducing their reimbursement rates for prescription drugs (see Chapter 19). Because of reduced reimbursement rates, profit margins generated from dispensing prescriptions, and in turn profit margins for the entire pharmacy's operations, have decreased over time. The reduction in profitability from dispensing, as well as increases in costs of drugs, pharmacist and other employee salaries, and other operating expenses, have forced pharmacies to seek alternative revenue sources. Pharmacies have generated additional revenues in a variety of ways, including selling different lines of goods, and establishing patient care services such as immunizations, health and wellness screenings, and medication therapy management (MTM) services.

Marketing is a necessary and essential function in a highly competitive and resource-constrained environment. To successfully launch any new good or service, a deep understanding of the organization, environment, and market is crucial. This chapter describes how marketing principles (see Chapter 21) can be applied in pharmacy practice, as illustrated through Dr. Rockefeller's scenario. Specifically, this chapter discusses several marketing concepts including situational analysis, market segments, target markets, and the marketing mix, and illustrates how these concepts are applicable in pharmacy practice.

STRATEGIC PLANNING AND EVALUATING BUSINESS OPPORTUNITIES

Strategic planning in pharmacy operations is crucial as it maximizes the organization's future success. Chapter 4 describes the strategic planning process and emphasizes the importance of an organization's vision and mission statement, as they create a sense of purpose and direction for the employees. Also, as previously stated in Chapter 5, a vital step in the development of a business plan is to create a marketing strategy. Therefore, pharmacists should consider what their organization is striving for, as well as the organization's values and overall purpose, and specific steps should be followed in preparing to market a good or service.

The following steps should be taken when preparing to market a good or service in a pharmacy (Hillestad and Berkowitz, 2004; Holdford, 2007). These steps are illustrated in Fig. 22-1. First, the micro- and macroenvironment are analyzed to identify strengths and limitations of the organization's capacity, as well as opportunities and threats in the environment. Second, goals and objectives are formulated using the information compiled in the previous step. The goals and objectives must be consistent with the organization's vision and mission statements. It is possible that the first two steps have already been conducted as part of the strategic plan and business plan development processes. Third, market segments and the target market are identified. At this point, having the organization's goals, objectives, and possible target markets identified, a specific product or service can be developed. Fourth, the organization proceeds to formulate and design the marketing mix for each target market. The last step is to evaluate the extent to which marketing strategies are successful. Information gathered during this final step is crucial as it helps inform the organization and identifies if changes in any components of the marketing process are needed.

REVISITING THE SCENARIO

Dr. Rockefeller now knows that before he can develop new goods and services that his pharmacy should offer to customers, he must consider the vision and the mission of Community Care Pharmacy and ensure that these goods and services are consistent with the organization's overall strategic plan. After reviewing the existing mission and vision statements, he realizes that they do not reflect the direction he would like to take

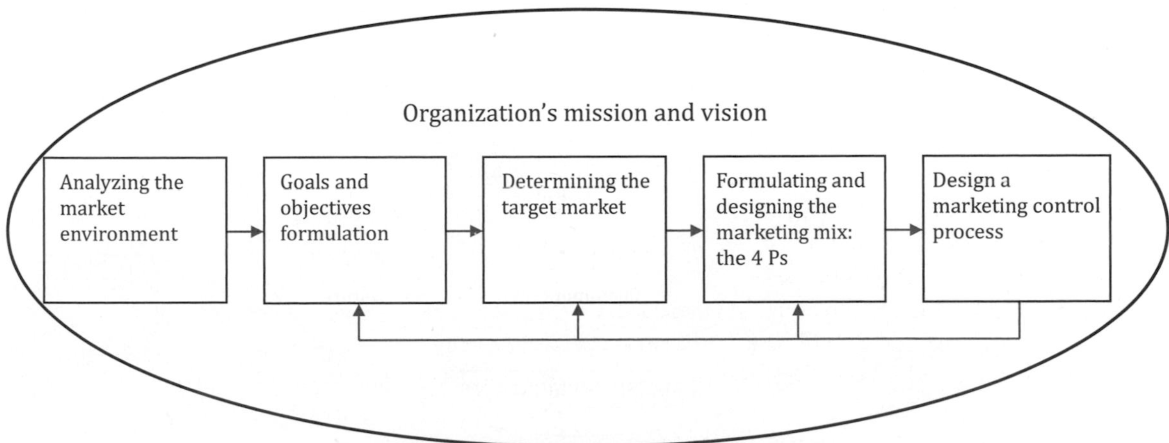

Figure 22-1. Steps in marketing a pharmacy good or service.

the pharmacy under his ownership. He has also come to realize that the pharmacy does not have a strategic plan in place. Dr. Rockefeller schedules a meeting with all of the pharmacy's employees to develop a strategic plan. Soon afterward, Community Care Pharmacy has the strategic plan in place, including updated mission and vision statements.

ANALYZING THE MARKET ENVIRONMENT

Situational Assessment

Before making a decision regarding what goods and services to offer and how to offer them, it is important for managers to analyze their organization's market environment. In essence, organizations interact with two types of environment: the *microenvironment* and the *macroenvironment* (Kotler and Armstrong, 2004) (See Fig. 22-2). Specifically, the microenvironment consists of the organization's internal and external environment. The organizational structure, culture, personnel, and resources are the internal environment whereas the organization's suppliers, customers, and competitors are the external environment. The characteristics of the microenvironment affect the organization's ability to serve its customers. Further, in addition to the microenvironment, organizations should also pay attention to the dynamics of the macroenvironment, as factors embedded within the macroenvironment can influence demand for the organization's goods and services. These factors include demographics, economics, nature, technology, politics, and culture (Kotler and Armstrong, 2004). For example, when considering the demographic environment, an aging population creates demand for chronic care services such as anticoagulation management. Further, at times of economic downturns, there is a need for pharmacists to help patients reduce their overall costs of care. Finally, because technological developments affect how patients interact with health care providers, as well as how patients manage their conditions and illnesses, pharmacists should be aware of both opportunities and threats presented by new technologies.

The situational assessment is an analysis of the organization's environment and of the organization itself (Berkowitz, 1996). This assessment process starts with an analysis of the *S*trengths and *W*eaknesses of the organization, followed by the *O*pportunities and *T*hreats relevant to the organization's future strategy. This process

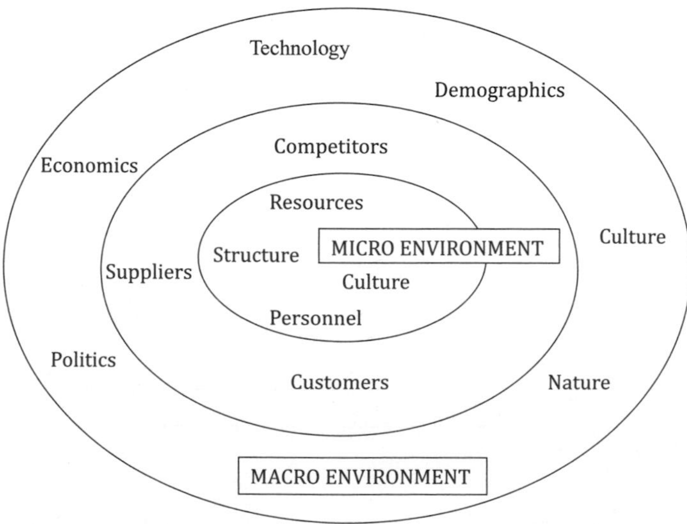

Figure 22-2. The micro and macro environment.

is referred to as the SWOT analysis. Similar to how SWOT analysis can be used in the strategic and business planning processes (see Chapters 4 and 5), SWOT analysis may also be used to develop new goods and services that respond to the opportunities and threats of the organization's environment while recognizing their inherent strengths and weaknesses (Ferrell et al., 2002).

REVISITING THE SCENARIO

Dr. Rockefeller and the employees of Community Care Pharmacy took some time to evaluate the pharmacy's microenvironment and macroenvironment. Community Care Pharmacy is located in the city of Weagle, which is located in Monet County, Alabama. Weagle is the principal city of this county. The county's economy is centered in Weagle as many employers, businesses, schools, and service organizations reside in the city. In fact, the city of Weagle is the largest city in Eastern Alabama. About 15 percent of the population is considered elderly (>65 year old). Weagle is one of the fastest growing metropolitan areas in the South, and has recently been voted as one of the best retirement cities for active adults. The results of their environmental scan of the demographic characteristics of their communities are summarized in Table 22-1.

In reviewing the pharmacy's prescription records, as well as health facts about Alabama [obtained from the Kaiser Family Foundation Web site (www.kff.org)], Dr. Rockefeller discovered that a wide variety of chronic diseases are prevalent among current pharmacy customers, and that state-level health statistics on some health risk factors are concerning (see Table 22-1).

Monet County has a total of 29 community pharmacies. Specifically, there are 10 independently owned pharmacies, 10 chain pharmacies, five grocery store pharmacies, and four mass merchandise pharmacies. Most of these pharmacies (22) are located within the Weagle metropolitan area. Given the growing economy

Table 22-1. Community Care Pharmacy's Community Profile

	Weagle, AL	Monet County, AL	Alabama	United States
Population	54,129	126,092	4,686,900	303,343,300
Median income	$67,745	$57,656	$42,652	$62,363
Education				
High school education	>80%	70%	30%	28.6%
4 years of college	30%	30%	21.5%	27.5%
Health insurance status				
Uninsured	–	14%	14%	19%
Medicaid	–	13%	16%	19%
Medicare	–	18%	15%	15%
Employer-sponsored insurance	–	53%	51%	57%
Prevalence of health conditions				
Diabetes	–	–	12.2%	8.3%
Smokers	–	–	22.1%	18.3%
Overweight adults	–	–	65.9%	60.8%
Overweight adolescents	–	–	36.1%	31.6%
Death per 100,000				
Deaths: stroke	–	40.1	54.5	42.2
Deaths: heart disease	–	201.2	235.5	190.9
Number of community pharmacies	22	29	–	–

in the area, several chain pharmacies have expressed an interest in expanding their businesses in the area.

Strengths and Weaknesses Assessment

To complete an assessment of an organization's strengths and weaknesses, the organization should consider both the current and potential capacity to compete in the market (Holdford, 2007). A *strength* is a resource or capacity of the organization that can be used to achieve its objectives, while a *weakness* is a limitation within the organization that hinders the organization from achieving its objectives. An organization must assess various factors internal to the organization including resources (e.g., financial resources, intellectual resources, location), relationships with patients, reputation among patients, relationships with other healthcare providers, staff, workload, efficiency, management, and culture.

REVISITING THE SCENARIO

Table 22-2 describes the SWOT analysis for Community Care Pharmacy. Dr. Rockefeller and the

Table 22-2. A SWOT Analysis for Community Care Pharmacy

Strengths	• The pharmacy has loyal customers. • The pharmacy has a wide range of services including dispensing, compounding, long-term care, and durable medical equipment. • The pharmacy has a professional image. • All pharmacists have excellent clinical skills and knowledge; all are certified to administer vaccines. • The pharmacy has positive relationships with prescribers in the community.
Weaknesses	• Because the pharmacy has not established advanced pharmacy care services, most staff pharmacists have limited experience in delivering patient care services other than dispensing. • Working relationships with pediatricians in the area have not yet been developed. • Financial resources are somewhat limited and pharmacists' workload has increased.
Opportunities	• A large number of people in the community are enrolled in Medicare. • Elderly population is at risk for influenza, pneumonia, and shingles; but they have limited access to nontraditional vaccination services. • A large number of people in the community are obese and at high risk for developing heart disease, hypertension, and diabetes. • Several companies in the community are self-insured; self-insured employers have expressed their interest in reducing health care cost among their enrollees.
Threats	• There has been an increase in competition among community pharmacies for the dispensing business. • A large chain has recently purchased two independently owned pharmacies and plans to expand their stores to other locations within the community. • One of the self-insured employers in the area has strongly encouraged its enrollees to obtain their chronic medications from an online pharmacy. • Some members of a local physician group have expressed their concern about pharmacy-based disease state management services.

pharmacy staff agreed on several strengths of the pharmacy. One is that the pharmacy has loyal customers. In fact, 60 percent of Community Care Pharmacy's new patients have been referred to the pharmacy by other patients. The pharmacy has been in business for more than 25 years, and every patient receives medication counseling when they pick up their medications. The pharmacy also has a large customer base as it provides a wide range of services including medication dispensing, compounding, serving a local long-term care facility, and providing durable medical equipment. Another strength is that the pharmacy was remodeled 3 years ago; thus it emanates a professional image. Next, all five staff pharmacists at Community Care Pharmacy have excellent clinical skills and knowledge of pharmacotherapy. Three out of the five pharmacists have a Pharm.D. degree and one has completed a community pharmacy residency. All pharmacists are certified to administer vaccines. The excellent skills and knowledge of the pharmacists along with their dedication to patient care have led to positive relationships with physicians and nurse practitioners in the community.

Dr. Rockefeller and his colleagues also recognize the weaknesses of Community Care Pharmacy. Although a wide range of services are provided, much of what pharmacists do is product oriented (e.g., dispensing medications). The pharmacy does not currently offer any patient care services beyond counseling about the medications they dispense, and aside from the pharmacist who completed the residency, the rest of the staff has limited experience in the delivery of patient care services. Furthermore, regarding relationships with prescribers, working relationships with pediatricians in the area have not yet been developed. Lastly, due to low profit margins on prescription dispensing, the pharmacy's financial resources are somewhat limited. Specifically, the pharmacy was forced to lower operating costs by reducing technicians' hours 6 months ago. This has affected pharmacists' workload.

Opportunities and Threats Assessment

An organization must conduct environmental analyses of *opportunities* and *threats.* In scanning the environment, the likelihood and implications of relevant opportunities and threats can be identified. In essence, an opportunity analysis identifies gaps between market demand and what is currently available, as well as changes in the market that enhance the prospects for the organization's goods and services (Holdford, 2007). In contrast, conducting a threat analysis will help the organization identify factors that may prevent the organization from achieving its intended objectives, as well as changes in the market that may reduce the demand for the organization's goods or services. To help the organization identify opportunities and threats, the following questions can be asked (Berkowitz, 1996; Holdford, 2007):

1. What are the changes and trends?
2. How will these changes affect the organization?
3. What opportunities do these changes present?
4. What needs are not being met in the current marketplace?
5. How is the environment changing to the organization's advantage or disadvantage?
6. What potential problems might threaten the success of the organization's plans?

REVISITING THE SCENARIO

Dr. Rockefeller and colleagues analyzed the environment and have identified several opportunities for Community Care Pharmacy (Table 22-2). First, a large number of people are enrolled in a traditional Medicare program with Medicare Part D plans. Since the city of Weagle has been cited as one of the best cities to retire, there has been an influx of relatively healthy, active patients in their 60s and 70s to the area. This group of patients has chronic conditions and needs preventive care services (e.g., immunizations, health screening services). Given Community Care Pharmacy's strengths, they feel that they could easily develop new goods and services that meet the needs and wants of this population. After meeting with the local health department, many people in the area are at risk for influenza, pneumonia, and shingles. However, the ability of local physicians to provide immunizations is limited by their busy schedules, and access to nontraditional immunization providers is limited. The pharmacy staff has also recognized that more than half members of the local population are overweight, many of whom are obese. This group of the population is at high risk for developing heart disease, hypertension, and diabetes and therefore may also be a good group to target new pharmacy goods and services. Based on the discussion with members of the local Chamber of Commerce, many local businesses are self-insured employers and have expressed a strong interest in reducing their healthcare costs. Dr. Rockefeller and his colleagues agreed that these businesses can be targeted as new pharmacy services may help improve their enrollees' health, and therefore reduce health care costs in the long run.

Dr. Rockefeller and his colleagues identified four primary threats to Community Care Pharmacy. A prominent threat is that there has been an increase in competition among community pharmacies in regard to dispensing services. A national mass merchandiser has a 160,000 square feet store two miles from the pharmacy. The mass merchandiser has begun offering many generic prescriptions for $4 for a month's supply, making it difficult for Community Care Pharmacy to compete for price-conscious consumers. The competition for medication dispensing is likely to increase, as a large chain recently purchased two independently owned pharmacies in Weagle and have announced plans to expand their stores in the county. Also, Community Care Pharmacy may lose some patients to mail-order pharmacy in the near future. This is because a large, self-insured employer in the area incentivized their employees to obtain their chronic medications from a mail-order pharmacy by waiving the co-payment on generic medications. Lastly, some local physicians have expressed concerns with pharmacy-based disease state management services, feeling that these services may not be in their patients' best interests.

Now that Dr. Rockefeller and colleagues have completed the SWOT analysis, they realize that additional sources of revenues are needed. They are now ready to identify new goods and services to bring to the market.

Goals and Objectives Formulation

Results of the SWOT analysis should be used to inform the organization in the development of new goods and services. Plans to bring new goods and services to market are commonly described in business plans (see Chapter 5). Business plans should contain a set of goal statements that lead to objectives that an organization wants to accomplish. Goal statements are usually general and abstract (Rossi et al., 2004). They describe a desired state the organization strives to accomplish. Each goal statement may include several objectives. In contrast to goal statements, objectives are specific statements detailing the desired accomplishments of the plan (Rossi, et al., 2004). In other words, objectives are quantitative measures of accomplishment by which the success of marketing strategies can be measured. Objectives might include retention, sales growth, and gains in the organization's share of their market (Berkowitz, 1996). When the organization determines its objectives, it is important that they formulate SMART objectives (Doran, 1981). That is, objectives should be specific, measurable, attainable, relevant, and timely. A specific objective is one that describes exactly what the organization is going to do, with whom, and for whom. A measurable objective is one that can be assessed to determine whether or not the objectives are being met. The objectives that are formulated for the pharmacy should be attainable (reasonable/realistic), considering the pharmacy's availability of resources. Next, the objectives should specify relevant outcomes. Lastly, the objective should be time specific, meaning that each of the objectives has a deadline for its achievement.

REVISITING THE SCENARIO

Dr. Rockefeller and his colleagues utilized the information gained from the SWOT analysis to formulate goals and objectives for Community Care Pharmacy (see Table 22-3 for an example). They agreed that

Table 22-3. Goals and Objectives Formulated by Community Care Pharmacy

Goal 1	To increase pharmacy profitability from providing a new service
Objective 1.1	To attract 100 new patients to the pharmacy by the end of 12 months
Objective 1.2	To increase the pharmacy revenues by 5% within 12 months

given the degree of competition in the dispensing business, Community Care Pharmacy needs to capitalize on its strengths and offer a new service to provide a new revenue source. These objectives will be used to measure the success of the new service.

Determining the Target Market

After an organization's goals and objectives are identified, the next step is to determine the target market. The purpose of identifying the target market is to determine what population the organization is trying to attract (Berkowitz, 1996). Various factors can be used to identify target markets including the organization's capabilities, the competition within the market, the cost of capturing market share, and the potential financial gain from the target group (Berkowitz, 1996).

Targeting the entire market as one target market is referred to as mass marketing. This is when an organization attempts to attract every eligible person to its use of the good or service (Kotler and Clarke, 1986). An organization that utilizes mass-marketing strategies pays little or no attention to differences in consumer preferences (Kotler and Clarke, 1986). However, for most products and services, it is difficult to reach and appeal to all consumers, as they commonly have a variety of needs and may be geographically scattered across a wide area. Because of the limitations presented by the mass-marketing approach, organizations often focus on specific segments of a market, referred to as target markets. In this way, an organization can focus its resources on specific market segments and develop strategies that are tailored to meet the needs of the consumers whom they are aiming to target.

The process to identify the target market includes two steps: market segmentation and target marketing (Kotler and Clarke, 1986). Market segmentation is a process in which a market is divided into distinct and meaningful groups of consumers based on their profiles. For example, the market can be segmented by demographic variables such as income, age, disease categories, sex, health insurance coverage (e.g., cash payers, third-party payers), or buying behaviors. There is no single best way to segment a market, and a market can be segmented in a number of ways. The organization should segment the market in a way that makes the most sense and reveals the most of market opportunities for the types of goods and services they plan to introduce. Once the organization identifies the market segments, they then can evaluate the attractiveness of each segment and choose one or more segments that are desirable (Holdford, 2007). Desirable market segments should be identifiable, accessible, of sufficient size, and responsive to targeted marketing mix strategies (Holdford, 2007).

REVISITING THE SCENARIO

Dr. Rockefeller and colleagues identify target markets for Community Care Pharmacy by reviewing the existing customer databases (e.g., patient profiles, insurance coverage). With the characteristics of desirable market segments in mind, two desired target markets were identified (Medicare enrollees and young, cash-paying customers). Table 22-4 describes characteristics of each group.

After selecting the target markets, an organization must formulate and design elements of the marketing mix that position a good or service in the minds of targeted consumers. Positioning a good or service in this manner is achieved through use of each of the four elements of marketing mix. Since Community Care Pharmacy ultimately aims at attracting two different

Table 22-4. Target Markets Identified by Community Care Pharmacy

Medicare enrollees	This target market consists of elderly people (65 years or older). They have multiple chronic conditions and take multiple medications. Because they are likely to be at risk for preventable infectious diseases, they are candidates to receive influenza, pneumococcal, and zoster vaccines.
Young population who are cash-based payers	This target market is made up of people who are young and relatively healthy. They are employed, well educated, and have income above average. Even though they may have insurance coverage, they are willing to pay out of pocket for certain services. They are interested in prevention services such as immunization services.

target markets, elements of the marketing mix may have to be customized for each market in order to yield the optimal benefits.

THE MARKETING MIX: USING THE 4 Ps

After completion of an organizational SWOT analysis, creation of goals and objectives, and identification of target markets, Community Care Pharmacy is ready to plan the details of the *marketing mix*. The marketing mix is defined as the set of controllable variables that an organization can manipulate and use to reach its goals and objectives (Berkowitz, 1996). These variables are often viewed as the *Four Ps*: product, price, place, and promotion (described in Chapter 21). The forthcoming sections explain how Community Care Pharmacy can apply each of the Four Ps to position themselves in the eyes of their target markets and reach their goals and objectives.

Product

Products are defined as the goods, services, or ideas that are offered by an organization. Goods are tangible and can be touched or examined, while services are intangible and are seen as activities or processes that are offered to help patients solve problems. In pharmacy, over-the-counter pharmaceuticals and prescription medications are examples of goods that are normally sold to consumers. Being that they are tangible, many of their attributes can easily be understood by consumers. On the other hand, marketing services often requires additional effort because their attributes are not as easily examined or understood.

The five key components of services that differentiate them from goods are commonly referred to as the Five Is (Berkowitz, 1996). Since a service is *intangible*, the marketing of a service needs to somehow portray the tangible benefits the patient will receive from the service. *Inconsistency* refers to the fact that services are delivered by individual providers to individual consumers, resulting in inherent variability each time that the service is delivered. *Inseparability* means that a service cannot be separated from its provider. Consumers who feel they are disrespected during the delivery of a service are likely to have a negative impression of the service even if the provider delivered the service correctly. Unlike physical goods, services cannot be *inventoried* and stored until they are ready to be delivered or received. Therefore, attention must be paid to scheduling service delivery at a time and in a manner that is both consistent with an organization's operations, yet meets the consumer's needs and wants. Finally, consumers often evaluate a service based on the *interaction* they have with the person providing the service. Each person a consumer interacts with while receiving a service molds their overall satisfaction with the service. Therefore, each person interacting with consumers has a responsibility to make these interactions as pleasant as possible.

REVISITING THE SCENARIO

Community Care Pharmacy has decided that they are going to address the opportunities the two target markets have provided. With their SWOT analysis, goals, and objectives in mind, Dr. Rockefeller and his colleagues have decided that a vaccination service is aligned with the strengths outlined in the SWOT analysis. For example, all pharmacists are already certified to administer vaccines, and a private area is available in the pharmacy. In addition, a vaccination service seems to be a good fit considering their limited financial resources and workload. The community offers tremendous market opportunities as the elderly population (Target Market #1) in the area has a need for influenza, pneumococcal, and zoster vaccines. Hence, Dr. Rockefeller and his employees decide that Community Care Pharmacy will provide influenza, pneumococcal, and zoster vaccines for this elderly target market. If the service is successful, Dr. Rockefeller believes they will be able to expand the type of vaccines they provide.

Dr. Rockefeller realizes that this service is difficult to classify as purely tangible or intangible. Although the delivery of the service is intangible, the benefit one gains from receiving a vaccination is tangible. Because of this, Dr. Rockefeller concludes that this service is more of a hybrid and believes he can promote the service through advertising. He also realizes the risk of inconsistency in the delivery of a service. For example, while all pharmacists may be certified to administer vaccines, one may have much more experience in providing the service and therefore is much more thorough. He believes his pharmacists are well trained to provide a consistent high-quality service in a polite and respectful manner that is representative of the pharmacy's image and therefore, inconsistency should not be a major issue. His technicians and store employees are also kind and respectful so he is not worried about interactions with patients. Dr. Rockefeller currently has optimal staffing levels but understands that this service may require him to hire another part-time pharmacist. As previously stated, elements of the marketing mix may differ among different market segments. In the case of Community Care Pharmacy, the young population market (Target Market #2) would desire a different product from the elderly market. For example, an influenza vaccination service could be the focus for this target market.

Price

The next step in marketing Community Care pharmacy's new vaccination service is to establish a *price* for the product. In order to ensure the success of any new good or service, organizations must offer them at an appropriate price. There are many factors to consider when setting a price, including the costs of providing the good or service, overall consumer demand for the good or service, competition from other organizations offering similar goods or services, and the use of pricing strategies that appeal to consumers.

Costs of Providing a Good or Service

The first thing to consider when pricing a new good or service is the costs the organization will incur to provide them. In the case of Community Care Pharmacy's new vaccination service, they must purchase vaccines, syringes, needles, a refrigerator, cotton swabs, alcohol wipes, band-aids, and the proper medical waste disposal supplies to comply with state and federal disposal laws. Also included in the cost of providing the vaccination service is the salary and benefits they have to pay their pharmacists, technicians, and other employees involved in providing this service. If Community Care Pharmacy plans to offer this service using an outsourced model (i.e., contracting with another vendor to come to the pharmacy and provide immunizations to their patients), an agreement between their pharmacy and the organization contracted to provide the vaccinations must be made related to how the revenues from this service will be shared. If they plan to provide this vaccination service using their own employees, a decision must be made that relates to how they will compensate their pharmacists. Will they offer their pharmacists additional monetary or nonmonetary rewards? Or will they require their pharmacists to provide vaccinations in addition to their normal dispensing activities without additional compensation? These are important questions that will need to be addressed when pricing the service. Overhead expenses must also be considered when pricing the new vaccination service. The principles used to calculate a pharmacy's cost to dispense a prescription can also the applied to calculate their costs to provide any service, such as the costs to provide an immunization (see Chapter 19).

As seen in Community Care Pharmacy's SWOT analysis, consumer demand for vaccination services appears to be high. The SWOT analysis also shows that there is little competition from other providers in the area when it comes to providing these vaccinations. These two opportunities allow the pharmacy to consider how much profit they aim to gain from providing vaccinations. To merely breakeven from providing the service is not the goal. That being said, pricing the service high may result in failure due to low utilization and an increase in competitors who see the high price as an opportunity to provide the service at a lower cost.

Pricing Strategies

For many goods and services offered in pharmacies, reimbursement rates depend on contractual agreements between third-party payers and the pharmacy. For instance, pharmacies that provide medications and MTM services to Medicare Part D plan enrollees are reimbursed at levels stated in the contract. In this case, pharmacies have limited flexibility in determining prices for services they provide. On the other hand, pharmacists have greater flexibility setting prices for services offered to out-of-pocket payers or services offered through a contractual agreement with self-insured employers.

There are many pricing strategies to consider when determining an optimal price for a new good or service. One pricing strategy that is commonly used is known as *odd pricing*. Odd pricing is the practice of pricing a service just below whole dollar amounts (Berkowitz, 1996). In the case of Community Care Pharmacy, let us assume that their costs of providing an influenza vaccination (including overhead costs and the cost of the vaccine itself) are $20.00. Taking into consideration government regulations regarding the pricing of the service, the usual and customary charge for a similar service by other providers, the pharmacy's cost to provide the service, and the profit desired, Community Care Pharmacy needs the price of influenza vaccination service for cash payers to be at least $20.00. Using the odd pricing strategy, the pharmacy can price this service for out-of-pocket payers at $24.99, just under $25.00. The rationale behind this strategy is that consumers believe products and services priced just under whole dollar amounts ($24.99) are priced at the lowest possible price or that the product or service has been discounted from a higher price.

A second pricing strategy is *bundled pricing*. Bundled pricing is the practice of selling several items or services together for one total price. This is becoming a very common strategy in health care and can be very appealing to consumers (Berkowitz, 1996). If Community Care Pharmacy chooses to do this, the amount of savings to the patient must be seen as a real advantage. For example, because their influenza vaccine is priced at $24.99 and their vitamin supplements are priced at $11.99, bundling them and selling them for $36.98 would not be beneficial. The pharmacy would need to bundle them and sell them at a discount while still covering their costs. A reasonable bundled price for both the good and the service at the pharmacy would be $29.29 (assuming that the cost of the vitamin supplement is under $10). In addition, Community Care Pharmacy can apply a similar strategy by offering a bundled price for influenza and pneumococcal vaccines for those who need both vaccines.

Discounts are another strategy used in the pricing of goods and services in pharmacy. A *functional discount* can be given to a large organization by offering vaccination services to its employees for a lower price than the general public (Berkowitz, 1996; Kotler and Armstrong, 1994). As seen in Community Care Pharmacy's SWOT analysis, there are several large, self-insured organizations in Weagle to whom they could offer such a discount. By offering a functional discount to all employees and retirees of these self-insured employers, Community Care Pharmacy can increase the utilization of their vaccination service. *Seasonal discount* is another pricing strategy commonly used to increase utilization of services. These discounts are given to consumers who purchase goods or services when they are out of season (Berkowitz, 1996; Kotler and Armstrong, 1994). For example, many people wait until the spring and summer months to purchase gym memberships and get in shape. A seasonal discount would offer the same gym membership during the off months for a discounted price. In the case of vaccination service, flu shots are usually offered between September and November and seasonal flu season generally starts in December and lasts through the spring. Even though it is ideal to get vaccinated early, a flu shot in January can still be helpful as there are still 2 or 3 months left in the flu season. To apply this seasonal discount strategy, Community Care Pharmacy may offer influenza vaccine at a discounted price in January or February, if they still have a supply.

Place

The third P in the marketing mix is *place*. This component refers to the distribution of the good or service. In other words, place refers to how and where the product or service is accessed by the consumer. For a chain community pharmacy, the locations and hours that each pharmacy will offer a service are examples of distribution considerations. Some organizations focus on the convenience of accessing their goods and services by providing multiple locations in the area where they compete with the goal of having no customer go out of their way to access what they have to offer. Chain pharmacies such as CVS, Walgreens, and Rite Aid are examples of organizations that employ this strategy. Community pharmacies have also extended their hours of operation to increase access. Many pharmacies are now open 24 hours a day and in most cases, those that are not open for 24 hours have extended their hours of operation and have begun offering their goods and services on weekends.

Intensity of distribution is a key concept that should be understood when thinking about the place component of the marketing mix. Intensity refers to how available the service is to the consumer. The three forms of distribution intensity are intensive, selective, and exclusive (Berkowitz, 1996). Deciding which form of intensity to utilize with a new good or service is vital to its success.

Intensive Distribution

Intensive distribution is a strategy used when the good or service is available from a large number of locations. Everyday products that community pharmacies sell such as toothpaste, eye drops, aspirin, and ibuprofen are examples of products that are intensively distributed. These products can be found in many different locations and therefore consumers will not go out of their way to patronize a specific organization to purchase them. The same is true about automatic blood pressure machines in pharmacies. Since a patient can check their blood pressure for free in many pharmacies around the country, charging a patient to use a "do-it-yourself" automatic blood pressure cuff without pharmacist consultation would result in a service failure.

Exclusive Distribution

Exclusive distribution is the opposite of intensive distribution, and is the strategy used when a good or service is only offered in very few locations. In the Weagle community, most pharmacy goods and services are offered at multiple locations. This is not the case with Community Care Pharmacy's compounding service. Since other pharmacies in the area do not provide compounding services, consumers of this service are required to patronize Community Care Pharmacy to take advantage of this service. This is an example of a service that is exclusive to their pharmacy and therefore, consumers that want to access this service will not find this service at Community Care Pharmacy's competitors' locations.

Selective Distribution

Selective distribution is the strategy used when a product or service is offered in multiple locations, but fewer locations than an intensive distribution approach. It is known as the selective approach because the consumer has the option to shop around and select the location where they purchase the product or service based on the level of support they perceive they will receive. An example of this in the retail setting is designer clothing. Many premier designer clothing brands select high-end retail stores that match the image they want to portray with their brand. This is considered selective distribution because although a consumer may be able to purchase a particular designer brand at a few different stores in their area, they will not find the product everywhere clothing is sold. The consumer has the opportunity to choose which location they purchase the designer clothing based on their evaluation of the options.

REVISITING THE SCENARIO

For a patient to receive vaccination services in the Weagle area they have the option to be vaccinated at Community Care Pharmacy, their primary care physician's office, or the local hospital. The patient has fewer options than an intensively distributed service, but more options than an exclusively distributed service, and therefore will choose the option that best fits their needs and budget. By offering this service in the evenings and weekends (when physicians' offices are closed), and by offering this service on a walk-in basis (most physicians' offices require appointments), Community Care Pharmacy can increase access and utilization of their vaccination service. They also have the opportunity to increase access to this service by occasionally providing vaccinations at a public place such as the local mall, church, or at events like the Monet County Fair in October.

Promotion

The fourth P in the marketing mix and the next step in marketing Community Care Pharmacy's new vaccination service is *promotion* of the service. There are four primary methods used to promote and communicate any good or service to potential consumers. These are advertising, personal selling, publicity, and sales promotion (Berkowitz, 1996). These methods can be used in individually or in combination to promote and communicate goods and services to target markets. In the following section, the four methods will be defined and applied to the marketing of Community Care Pharmacy's new vaccination service to better understand the use of promotion in the pharmacy setting.

Advertising

Advertising can be defined as any directly paid form of nonpersonal presentation of goods, services, and ideas (Kotler and Armstrong, 1994). Traditionally, there have been two primary outlets for advertisements: broadcast media and print media. Broadcast media consists of television and radio advertisements, while print media includes newspaper, magazine, direct mail, and outdoor advertisements. In recent years, Internet marketing has evolved with the emergence of Web 2.0. Web 2.0 refers to the increased number of online applications that are social and participatory. Examples of Web 2.0 applications are Facebook, Wikipedia, YouTube, and Twitter. This new advertising venue has become increasingly popular among health care organizations. It is important to determine where to place advertisements for a new good or service based on the amount of the budget an organization plans to spend and what the organization plans to gain from each venue. Although many pharmacy managers often work with their corporate marketing departments or even an advertising agency to develop advertising materials, it is important to understand the benefits of each form of advertising as well as what makes an advertisement effective.

Broadcast Media

Television advertisements have the ability to incorporate both visual images and sounds with the potential to reach a vast number of consumers. In North America, the majority of advertising dollars are spent on television advertising (The Nielsen Company, 2011). While the costs of television advertising have begun to decrease, it is still considered an expensive form of promotion. The costs of producing television advertisements and purchasing airtime to show them are usually higher than that of other advertising mediums. Advances in technologies, particularly by local cable systems, have made the use of television advertising feasible for many community pharmacies. Community pharmacies now have the ability to select the channel and time of day they would like their advertisements to air. This is the most difficult part of television advertising for many organizations because, to be effective, the organization must know the media habits of their target markets, including what times of day they watch television, and when they do watch, what channels and even programs they view. An advertisement run at 11:00 a.m. will most likely reach a different market than the same advertisement run at 11:00 p.m. The same is true about an advertisement run on a sports network versus an advertisement run on a news network.

Radio advertisements are a popular form of promotion in community pharmacy because radio stations are highly segmented (i.e., the listeners to any particular station often share demographic characteristics) and the production of radio advertisements is relatively inexpensive (Kotler and Armstrong, 1994). Another advantage of radio advertisements is that they can usually be produced in a short amount of time so that the advertisement can be broadcast as soon as possible. For example, if the goal is to reach the most working age consumers, an organization may choose to place a radio advertisement on an early morning or early evening talk show because these are the peak listening times as people drive to and from work. The disadvantages of radio advertising are its lack of a visual component, and given the market segmentation among radio stations, the stations used for advertising must be carefully chosen to assure that the desired target markets are being reached (Berkowitz, 1996).

REVISITING THE SCENARIO

After discussing their options for broadcast media advertising, Dr. Rockefeller and his colleagues believe that a television advertisement is a good investment to promote their new vaccination service. Since one of their target markets is the local elderly population, they have decided to pay to have their advertisement aired during the 5:00 p.m. local news broadcast. Although this is one of the more expensive time slots, they believe that a large portion of the elderly population in the area views this program regularly.

Print Media

Newspaper advertising is used to promote pharmacy goods and services around the world. Newspapers are a good source for health care advertisements because they are seen as highly credible sources of information (The Nielsen Company, 2011). Another advantage of newspaper advertising is the ability to geographically select who will see the advertisement. Even in metropolitan newspapers, the creation of zone editions allows advertisers to target specific geographic locations within a city. The costs associated with newspaper advertisement are also relatively inexpensive compared with broadcast media. A disadvantage of newspaper advertising is its poor production quality and the lack of flexibility and creativity relative to other types of media. Many newspapers require that advertisements fit a particular template and format, limiting a marketer's ability to make their advertisements eye catching and unique.

Magazine advertisements are becoming a popular medium for health care organizations. The number of specialized publications that allow an organization to target specific market segments has increased dramatically. Large chain pharmacies can target health-focused magazines, such as *Men's Health* and *Fitness* for national advertisements. Smaller community pharmacies can target regional magazines as well as national magazines that publish zone and geographic editions. An advantage of magazine advertisements is that they have a longer shelf life than other types of print media. Some consumers choose to keep magazines for weeks, months, or even years, meaning the advertisement may be seen and read multiple times before the magazine is discarded. Another advantage of magazine advertisements is that magazines produce high-quality, colorful ads that attract the reader's attention. As with other forms of advertising, magazine advertisements have their disadvantages. One major disadvantage is the amount of time before the advertisement is seen. Magazines may require that advertisements be received 4–6 weeks before the publication will be on the shelf for consumers to read. This makes magazine advertisements a good option for long-running goods and services, but not so viable for short-term offerings.

Direct mail advertising is the most utilized form of print advertising in North America. It is widely used because of its ability to target very specific markets, such as consumers who live in a specific neighborhood, or patients who are known from pharmacy records to have a particular characteristic or condition. Direct mail advertising allows an organization to target potential consumers by age, income, prior purchasing habits, geographic location, and many other identifiers (Berkowitz, 1996). For direct mail advertising to be effective, the list of recipients must be both well conceived (reaching people known to be part of a pharmacy's target markets) and accurate (a large percentage of direct mail never reaches the intended target due to inaccurate addresses). A disadvantage of direct mail is that many consumers view this type of advertising as junk mail. With multiple organizations using this method, it is hard to make one direct mail advertisement stand out among others. It also has a disadvantage because of the high costs associated with printing these advertisements with bright colors to attract attention, as well as the high costs of postage. Given the costs of both printing and postage, the costs per person reached can be higher than other forms of promotion.

Outdoor advertising, such as billboards and transit ads, is useful as a reminder or introduction to a new product or service. Health care organizations often use this medium to create awareness, but many consumers view this type of advertisement as visual pollution. There are many regulations that affect the availability of billboards in the United States and therefore this form of advertising is most used in metropolitan areas on public transportation.

■ REVISITING THE SCENARIO

Dr. Rockefeller and colleagues at Community Care Pharmacy believe that a print advertisement in the local daily newspaper that is also available online is a good way to reach both target markets (elderly and young population). Further, a print advertisement can reach those who may not be existing customers of their pharmacy. The cost of the advertisement is low and there is a large percentage of the population that receives the daily newspaper and frequents the newspaper's Web site. The local newspaper does not require purchasers of ad space to use a specific template with the design of their advertisements, allowing Community Care Pharmacy to design an advertisement that best fits their needs. Dr. Rockefeller and colleagues have designed a print advertisement (Fig. 22-3) to promote Community Care Pharmacy's new vaccination service with some help from a patient who is an advertising consultant.

There are five main components of an effective print advertisement (Ladd, 2010). The *headline* is the print in the largest font and usually bolded to grab the reader's attention. A headline should be short, direct, and clear so the reader knows exactly what is being advertised. The *copy* further elaborates the headline and explains important information such as price and benefits of the good or service. The *illustration* can be a photo or drawn image that gives the reader a visual portrayal of the good or service. The *sub-headline* can be used to explain specific information that may not be clear in the headline. A common example of a sub-headline is an offer of an item for free with the purchase of another item. Finally, the *signature* is the branding of the organization that produced the advertisement including logos, slogans, and trademarks. This helps the organization to build brand recognition and helps the reader to associate the advertisement with the organization.

WEB 2.0 and Internet Marketing

With the increased use of the Internet and the emergence of Web 2.0, organizations have begun utilizing new methods of advertising. The Internet now allows users to collaborate with colleagues, share information with others, and build new business and social relationships that were much more difficult to create in the past. The use of social media outlets like Facebook, Twitter, and YouTube have increased dramatically. A survey conducted by the Harris Initiative found that almost 9 of 10 (87 percent) of Americans use social media. A similar study conducted by the Pew Research Center found that over a period of 1 year from 2009

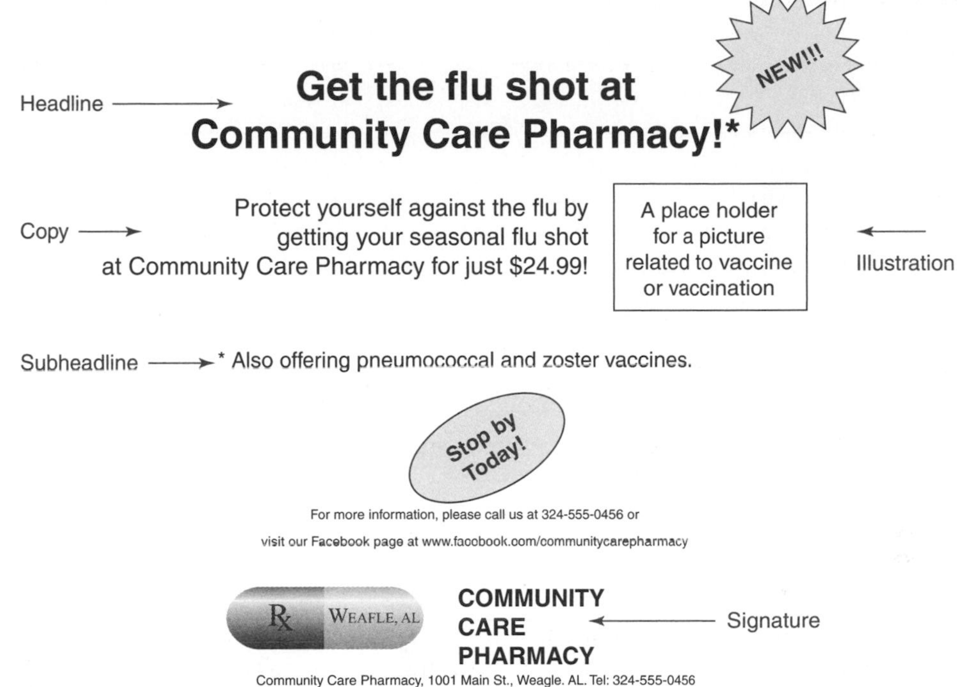

Figure 22-3. Print advertisement for vaccination services offered by Community Care Pharmacy.

to 2010, social media use among Internet users aged 50 and older nearly doubled from 22 percent to 42 percent. Further, 47 percent of Internet users 50–64 and 26 percent of users 65 and older now use social media sites (see Fig. 22-4).

Health care organizations have begun to see this increased Internet social media use as a great opportunity to get their message to their target markets at a relatively low cost (The Nielsen Company, 2011). Social media is not only used widely by large chain pharmacies, but is also a great opportunity for the smaller independent pharmacies to level the playing field. Promotion of Community Care Pharmacy's new vaccination service through social media could be very beneficial as a supplemental advertising strategy. On Facebook, the pharmacy can post "what's on their mind" and let their "Facebook friends" see and share the announcement of their new vaccination service. Twitter can be used with hashtags like "#Pharmacy" or "#flushot" to spread the news when influenza vaccines are being offered. Twitter can also be used to advertise sales taking place at the pharmacy, keeping in mind that Twitter users still tend to fall into their "younger, cash-paying customer" target market. YouTube is a video-sharing site that Community Care Pharmacy could use to create their own commercials explaining the benefits of getting vaccinated. The possibilities are endless when it comes to the use of social media to advertise, and since the majority of these Web sites are free to use, the cost of this form of promotion is relatively inexpensive (primarily the time and effort of staff to create and post the information).

■ REVISITING THE SCENARIO

Community Care Pharmacy decided to use Facebook and Twitter to spread the word about their pharmacy and vaccination services. Customers and patients of Community Care Pharmacy can sign up to be "friends" and "followers". Announcements of new

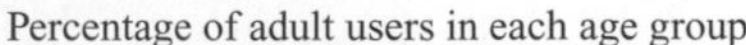

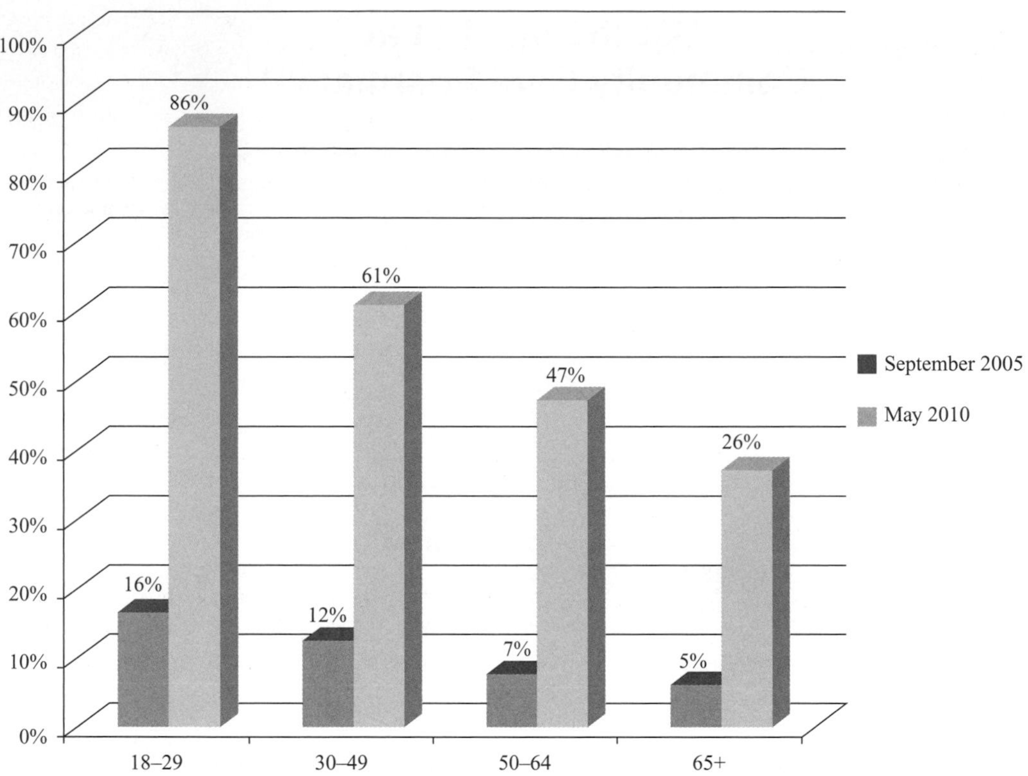

Figure 22-4. Social networking site adoption, 2005–2010. (*Adapted from Pew Research Center's Internet & American Life Project Surveys, September 2005–2010.*)

goods and services offered will be made through these media. Community Care Pharmacy will ensure that their logo appears in both Facebook and Twitter pages to build brand recognition and help readers associate their posts on these sites with their organization.

Personal Selling

Personal selling differs from advertising in that it is a direct, personal form of communication. Advertising is a form of mass communication and therefore it is more difficult to control who receives the message, while personal selling allows the organization to directly target the intended audience (Berkowitz, 1996). Community Care Pharmacy could use personal selling in the form of a salesperson who makes calls to referral physician offices or large self-employed insurers in Weagle to introduce and "sell" the new vaccination service. The advantage of this method is that any questions the receiver of the call may have can be answered immediately, and the service can be fully explained to avoid any confusion. It is also an opportunity to build relationships in the community. A disadvantage to personal selling is the cost, both in time and in money. Employing a salesperson is costly, and if they can only make a few calls per day, the impact the calls have on developing the market may be small.

Personal selling can also be utilized by pharmacists and other pharmacy personnel when they interact with their patients. Any patient who has a prescription filled at Community Care Pharmacy presents an opportunity for the pharmacy staff to describe the benefits of the new vaccination service and answer any questions the patient may have. If the staff identifies a patient as someone who would benefit from the vaccination service, they can offer the service to the patient, schedule an appointment, or provide supplemental information that can be reviewed at the patient's convenience. If the patient elects not to utilize the service, the relationship that the staff and patient have built is still beneficial in that the pharmacy has learned something about why the patient is not interested in receiving the service. This information can be used when developing and marketing future goods and services.

REVISITING THE SCENARIO

After realizing the importance of personal selling, Dr. Rockefeller agrees to visit several physicians' offices (especially those who do not offer vaccination services) to introduce their new vaccination service and request that they refer their patients to Community Care Pharmacy. Further, all pharmacy staff agrees that the vaccination service will be offered to all patients when they pick up their prescriptions.

Publicity

Publicity is a form of communication of goods, services, and ideas that is not paid for directly by the organization (Berkowitz, 1996). Dr. Rockefeller can encourage local newspapers, television, and radio stations to report stories about the importance of vaccinations and places to get vaccinated (such as Community Care Pharmacy). The benefit of publicity is that the audience who reads a newspaper article or watches a report on the local news does not realize that Dr. Rockefeller had to contact these outlets and ask for this coverage. This leads the consumer to believe that the message is coming from a credible source and is unbiased. The limitation of publicity is that there is very little control on who receives the message. There is no way to know when the local news will air the story about the pharmacy or what day the newspaper will print the article. Therefore, it is difficult to know if the target audience is reached. There are costs of using publicity, as someone from the pharmacy typically has to reach out to media outlets to encourage them to produce these stories, requiring resources (especially time) that could be used elsewhere.

Publicity can also work negatively against an organization. A customer who has a bad experience at Community Care Pharmacy can alert the press with negative information about the pharmacy. Web sites like Yelp, Kudzu, and BooRah are used to review organizations and can be sources of good or bad publicity for the pharmacy. It is important for pharmacy managers to monitor these reviews and have a response plan if their pharmacy receives negative publicity.

Sales Promotion

Sales promotions are temporary efforts to encourage consumers to purchase a good or utilize a service. These promotions come in the form of coupons, sweepstakes, rebates, or samples. In health care, the use of promotions such as a free trial of a medication is common, but the use of promotions to influence consumers to utilize a service is not. Community Care Pharmacy may be able use a sales promotion in the form of a rebate by offering patients who utilize their vaccination service some in-store credit to be applied to other purchases in the pharmacy. It is important to maintain the professional image of the pharmacy and to ensure the message that a sales promotion portrays does not negatively impact that image.

MARKETING CONTROL

It is important for an organization to put methods to evaluate the effectiveness of their marketing efforts in place, just as the organization would put methods to evaluate the outcomes of the service in place. Marketing control is defined as the process of measuring and evaluating the outcomes of marketing strategies and, if necessary, taking action to correct the four Ps to

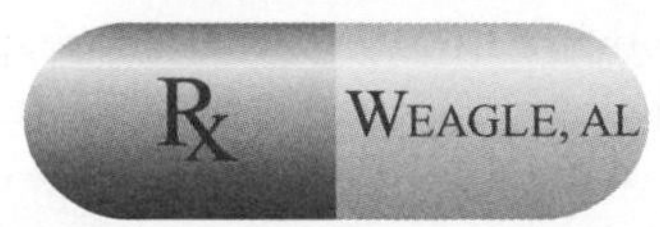

COMMUNITY CARE PHARMACY
1001 Main Street
Weagle, AL
(324) 555-0456

Please take a moment to help us improve your experience with Community Care Pharmacy. We strive to provide the best possible patient care and want to make sure you are informed of our new patient services. When you are finished, please give this questionnaire to one of our staff.

How did you hear about our new vaccination service? (please check all that apply)

- ☐ TV ad
- ☐ Newspaper
- ☐ Facebook
- ☐ Twitter
- ☐ Family Member
- ☐ Friend
- ☐ Other (please list):___________________

How would you rate our newspaper ad?

- ☐ Professional, High quality
- ☐ Average quality
- ☐ Poor quality
- ☐ Never saw it

Why did you choose Community Care Pharmacy to get vaccinated today? (please check all that apply)

- ☐ Flu Season
- ☐ Inexpensive
- ☐ Open late
- ☐ Open on the weekend
- ☐ Just turned 65!
- ☐ Friendly staff

How would you rate our TV ad?

- ☐ Professional, High quality
- ☐ Average quality
- ☐ Poor quality
- ☐ Never saw it

Did you make an appointment today?

- ☐ Yes
- ☐ No, Walk-In
- ☐ No, Other

How would you rate our Facebook and Twitter presence?

- ☐ Frequently updated
- ☐ Adequately updated
- ☐ Poorly updated
- ☐ I don't use Facebook or Twitter

Interaction with our staff has been:

- ☐ Very Pleasant
- ☐ Pleasant
- ☐ Unpleasant
- ☐ Very Unpleasant (please explain):_______

How often do recommend our pharmacy to a friend?

- ☐ All the time
- ☐ Most of the time
- ☐ Some of the time
- ☐ Absolutely not

Additional Comments: ____

Thank You for Helping Us Provide the Best Care Possible!

Figure 22-5. Patient satisfaction questionnaire.

ensure that marketing objectives are met. For a control process to be successful, it is necessary that the regular collection of marketing performance data (e.g., Web site hits, patient questionnaires) be a part of normal pharmacy operations. Specific indicators should be developed and used to track actual performance, such as tracking hits on a pharmacy's Web site and asking new patients where they heard about the pharmacy's services. By tracking actual performance, the pharmacy will be able to compare these measures with expected performance and make corrections to their marketing mix to reach its goals. If need be, corrections can be made to the goals to make them more attainable.

REVISITING THE SCENARIO

To evaluate the effectiveness of their marketing mix, Dr. Rockefeller and his colleagues at Community Care Pharmacy have put in place methods of collecting data on performance indicators to track the performance of their marketing effort. One of the methods they have chosen to employ is a brief questionnaire (see Fig. 22-5) that they request their vaccination service patients to complete. Their plan is to analyze the responses to the questionnaire and evaluate the effectiveness of their marketing mix and determine if/how their marketing efforts should be modified.

CONCLUSIONS

Dr. Rockefeller and his colleagues at Community Care Pharmacy have developed a strategic plan, analyzed their market environment by conducting a SWOT analysis, formulated goals and objectives, determined their target markets, selected their service, prepared their marketing mix, and put controls in place to evaluate the success of their marketing efforts. Although this service is a good start and will put Community Care Pharmacy in a position to reach their additional revenue goals, the competition from other pharmacies in the area will not dwindle. Dr. Rockefeller and Community Care Pharmacy can use everything they have learned through this process to further expand their patient care services and address the market segments they have already identified.

In the ever-changing health care environment, it is vital for pharmacists to expand the scope of their professional services. Pharmacists are in a unique position to provide patient care services in a highly accessible venue and move toward a more influential position in the health care system. Those who chose not to embrace this shift from a dispenser role to a provider role will find it difficult to remain legitimate and keep their businesses viable. Community Care Pharmacy has made an important first step in the continuous effort to stay ahead of the competition and be successful.

QUESTIONS FOR FURTHER DISCUSSION

1. To address the overweight and obese population in Weagle, would it be beneficial for Community Care Pharmacy to offer a weight management service? Why? Why not?
2. On the basis of the SWOT analysis presented, what are other viable opportunities and target markets?
3. What strategies could be used to encourage the working-age (18–65) population to utilize the influenza vaccination service? Would advertising to this population be different from the elderly population? How?
4. Some argue that the use of social media by health care organizations to advertise is unprofessional. Do you agree or disagree? Why?
5. Describe circumstances or examples when sales promotion or discount strategies may negatively impact the professional image of pharmacy.
6. Community Care Pharmacy used a questionnaire to evaluate their marketing effort. What are other ways that can be used to monitor the success of a marketing effort?

REFERENCES

Berkowitz EN. 1996. *Essentials of Health Care Marketing.* Gaithersburg, MD: Aspen Publishers.

Doran GT. 1981. There's a S.M.A.R.T. way to write management's goals and objectives. *Manage Rev* 70(11)35–6.

Ferrell OC, Hartline MD, Lucas G. 2002. *Marketing Strategy,* 2nd edn. Fort Worth: Harcourt College Publishers.

Hillestad SG, Berkowitz EN. 2004. *Health Care Market Strategy: from Planning to Action,* 3rd edn. Sudbury, Mass.: Jones and Bartlett Publishers.

Holdford DA. 2007. *Marketing for Pharmacists,* 2nd edn. Washington, DC: American Pharmacists Association.

Kotler P, Armstrong G. 1994. *Principles of Marketing,* 6th edn. Englewood Cliffs, NJ: Prentice Hall.

Kotler P, Armstrong G. 2004. *Principles of Marketing,* 10th edn. Upper Saddle River, NJ: Prentice Hall.

Kotler P, Clarke RN. 1986. *Marketing for Health Care Organizations.* Englewood Cliffs, NJ: Prentice-Hall.

Ladd AD. 2010. *Developing Effective Marketing Materials: Newspaper and Magazine Print Advertising Design Considerations.* Knoxville, TN: University of Tennessee: Center for profitable agriculture.

Rossi PH, Lipsey MW, Freeman HE. 2004. *Evaluation: A Systematic Approach,* 7th edn. Thousand Oaks, CA: Sage.

The Nielsen Company. 2011. *State of the Media: Trends in Advertising Spend and Effectiveness.* Available from http://www.nielsen.com/us/en/insights/reports-downloads/2011/advertising-spend-effectiveness-q1-2011.html; accessed on March 14, 2012.

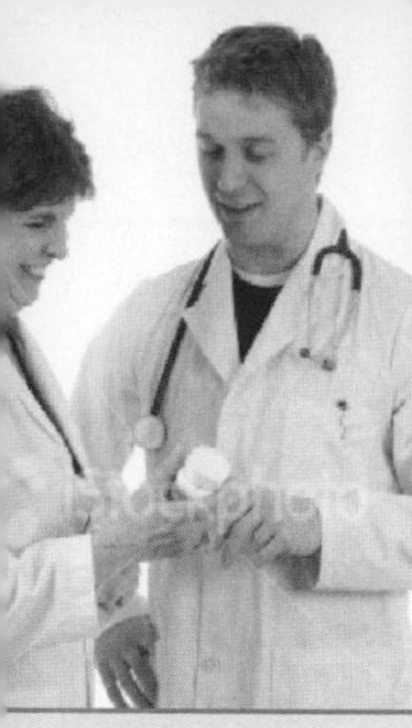

23

PURCHASING AND INVENTORY MANAGEMENT

Donna West

About the Author: Dr. West is Chair and Associate Professor at the University of Mississippi, Oxford, MS. She received a B.S. in pharmacy and a Ph.D. in pharmacy administration from the University of Mississippi. Dr. West teaches pharmacy marketing and medication safety. She also serves as the faculty liaison for the National Community Pharmacists Association student chapter. Her research interests pertain to understanding provider and patient behavior to improve medication use and advance community practice. She is also an American Association of Colleges of Pharmacy (AACP) representative to the Pharmacy Quality Alliance (PQA) and has developed pharmacy education materials related to pharmacy quality.

LEARNING OBJECTIVES

After completing this chapter, readers should be able to

1. Explain the importance, both financially and operationally, of purchasing and inventory management to a pharmacy.
2. List purchasing objectives and inventory management objectives for a pharmacy.
3. Describe procurement and carrying costs for a pharmacy.
4. Calculate inventory turnover rates and use this information to make purchasing and inventory control decisions.
5. Describe three methods of inventory management.
6. Describe the role of technology in improving inventory management in pharmacies.

SCENARIO

It is 5:00 p.m. on a Monday at Community Mental Health Center pharmacy, and for the fifth time today, Marie Parker, Pharm.D., does not have the medication she needs to fill a prescription. She has had to explain to each patient that he will have to come back tomorrow

Table 23-1. Scenario Wholesaler Comparisons

	XYZ Wholesale Drug		Current Wholesaler	
I. Price on Two Drug Products				
Product (No. of Bottles per Month)	**Unit Price**	**Ext. Price**	**Unit Price**	**Ext. Price**
Paxil 20 mg 100s (9)	$210	$1,890	$215	$1,935
Atacand 8 mg 30s (19)	$50	$950	$60	$1,140
Total		$2,840		$3,075
II. Cash discounts	Weekly EFT: 1.25% Weekly prepay EFT: 1.50%		EFT every 7 days: 1.25% EFT every 15 days: 1.00%	
III. Inventory management systems	Perpetual inventory system, Internet accessible; provide inventory management reports		Perpetual inventory system; provide inventory management reports	
IV. Return-goods policy	If the merchandise is salable and returned within 180 days of purchase date, wholesaler will provide a 100% credit. If it is returned after 180 days, only 85% credit will be given. Partial bottles, products that are 3 months after date of expiration, and other selected products are nonreturnable.		Merchandise that is returned within 30 days of invoice date will be credited 100% of original invoice amount (assuming it is in salable condition). If the merchandise is returned after 30 days and is in salable condition, 75% of the original invoice amount will be credited. Partial bottles, controlled/schedule II products, and other selected merchandise cannot be returned.	

to pick up his medication or take his prescription elsewhere. What a day! Meanwhile, the wholesaler delivery person just arrived with today's order—4 hours late! The chief executive officer (CEO) of the mental health center is questioning how much the pharmacy has been spending on medications and pressuring Marie to find a less expensive vendor. Marie decides that she will look into using another vendor. Fortunately, a representative from XYZ Wholesale Drugs dropped off her card last week. XYZ Wholesale Drugs is a large national company with a good reputation. Marie contacts the XYZ representative and describes her current situation. She is constantly running out of products, and with her pharmacy's gross margins shrinking, she needs to obtain drug products at the best price possible. The level of service provided by her current wholesaler seems to be decreasing (e.g., the order is frequently late, and she seldom sees a customer service representative to discuss these issues). Marie asks the XYZ representative some questions and uses this information to compare XYZ Wholesale Drugs with her present wholesaler (Table 23-1). Now that she has all this information, she is not sure what to do.

CHAPTER QUESTIONS

1. Why is balancing supply and demand important to inventory management?
2. What are the advantages of joining a group purchasing organization?

3. How does inventory management affect a pharmacy's profit margins and cash flow?
4. How does the inventory turnover rate indicate how efficient the pharmacist is at managing the inventory investment?
5. How has technology improved the pharmacist's ability to manage inventory?

INTRODUCTION

Inventory usually represents a pharmacy's largest current asset. Inventory also is the least liquid current asset, given that it generally cannot be turned to cash until it is sold to a consumer. The value of inventory to all pharmacies continues to rise owing to the increased variety and expense of pharmaceutical products. Therefore, proper management of inventory has a significant impact on both the financial and the operational aspects of any pharmacy (Huffman, 1996; West, 2003).

Acquisition, procurement, carrying, and stockout or shortage costs are the four general "costs" associated with inventory. Acquisition, procurement, and carrying costs can be calculated accurately and are an important financial consideration in pharmacy management. These three types of inventory costs generally place little direct stress on busy pharmacy staff but can depress the organization's operating margins, if not monitored appropriately. Shortage costs represent failures in customer service and therefore lost sales. These costs may be difficult to quantify but definitely have an impact on any pharmacy.

From a financial perspective, effective inventory management decreases the cost of goods sold (COGS) and operational expenses, resulting in increased gross margins and net profits. For example, saving $100 on the purchase of prescription drugs will increase the gross margin and net profit by $100 (assuming that operational expenses remain constant). Moreover, having less money invested in inventory improves cash flow (West, 2001). A pharmacy that has merchandise that is not selling or an oversupply of product sitting on the shelf has less cash available to pay expenses and/or invest in other business operations. A pharmacy that is able to reduce its inventory by $100 has that much more cash to spend on day-to-day operations, invest in new services, or place in a savings or checking account.

From an operational perspective, effective inventory management is important in meeting consumer demands for both goods and services (Carroll, 1998). Not having a product when needed may cause the pharmacy to lose a sale and potentially a customer. Furthermore, not having a needed product at the right time may cause physical harm to a patient, especially in settings (e.g., hospitals) where lifesaving emergency drugs are needed routinely at a moment's notice.

Inventory management means minimizing the investment in inventory while balancing supply and demand. People use inventory management in their everyday lives. For example, when people shop for groceries, they think about what they would like to eat (i.e., needs and wants) and what items they have on hand (i.e., current inventory). From this, they create a grocery list. This list is revised depending on how much money they have, grocery store specials, storage space, and how quickly the food will spoil. They may compare products and shop at various grocery stores. They eventually make purchases and evaluate how well those purchases satisfy their needs and wants. The process is repeated and reevaluated on a continuous basis. This is similar to how pharmacies purchase their inventory. Pharmacists or their staff create lists of products they need, revise the lists based on current inventory, determine how much money they have to purchase these goods, evaluate any specials from their vendors and their available storage space, and then finally make and evaluate their purchases.

To effectively accomplish the purchasing process, it is important for pharmacy managers to be aware of both purchasing and inventory management objectives (West, 2003). These are distinct yet interrelated functions. Having the right product at the right time at the right price is essential to meeting consumer demand as well as to providing high quality patient care. At the same time, pharmacy managers desire to minimize inventory investment. This chapter will first discuss purchasing functions and then inventory management functions.

Table 23-2. Purchasing Objectives

1. To obtain the right products
2. To obtain products in the right quantity
3. To obtain products at the right time
4. To obtain products at the right price
5. To obtain products from the right vendor

Source: Tootelian and Gaedeke, 1993.

PURCHASING

Some pharmacists perceive that purchasing is just a routine function necessary to keep inventory on the shelf. However, since most pharmacies literally spend millions of dollars every year to acquire medications and other goods, purchasing is actually a substantial investment process. It involves buying the *right products* in the *right quantity* at the *right price* at the *right time* from the *right vendor* (Tootelian and Gaedeke, 1993), as listed in Table 23-2. Many pharmacies, especially in hospitals and other health care facilities, have a designated person or purchasing agent whose responsibility is to order and receive products.

Right Product

Having the right products is an essential purchasing objective. To determine the product mix, the pharmacy manager should consider how much space is available to stock products and how much money is available to invest in products. Having products on the shelf that are not selling because they are not needed in the institution or wanted by pharmacy customers is a waste of resources and leads to obsolescence costs. Opportunity costs are realized because this space and money could be used to supply products that are more likely to be needed and wanted by consumers. Space should be allocated to items generating the greatest sales, and items that are not selling frequently should be given a lower priority.

Deciding what products to stock is also a marketing question. Determining the real and perceived needs of the pharmacy's patients, patrons, and prescribers is an important consideration when deciding what to purchase. The pharmacy manager should evaluate the following factors when deciding what products to order (Huffman, 1996; Tootelian and Gaedeke, 1993; West, 2003):

- *Past usage.* Pharmacy managers should review drug usage reports, as well as new and refilled prescription orders, to determine what to stock.
- *Target market.* The area where the pharmacy is located and the patient populations it serves will affect product selection. A pharmacy located in a children's hospital will need different products than a pharmacy located in a mental health facility. Likewise, a community pharmacy located next to a pediatric clinic likely will need more liquid antibiotics than other pharmacies. Prescribing behaviors of area physicians can provide insight into what drug products are needed.
- *Pharmacy image and goals.* Pharmacy managers should consider the pharmacy's image and business goals. Product selection should complement the pharmacy's image. For example, a pharmacy that is attempting to establish itself as a diabetes care center should maintain a greater inventory of specialty diabetes products. Similarly, pharmacies that promote high levels of service and never being out of needed medications will need to maintain higher inventory levels or obtain more frequent deliveries from vendors.
- *Formularies.* In hospitals and other health care institutions, formularies often drive the decision of what goods to stock (Carroll, 1998). A formulary is essentially a list of preferred drugs for use in that institution that are selected based on a combination of clinical and economic benefits. Pharmaceutical products that are placed on a formulary should be well stocked because these are the products that prescribers will be encouraged to use. Alternatively, products that are not on the formulary may not need to be stocked at all. In general, nonformulary items can be specially ordered, if needed. Pharmacy managers also must consider intravenous tubing, needles, and other supplies that may be needed at their institutions.

Formularies may also influence drug-purchasing decisions in the community pharmacy setting. Products that are more prominent on third-party payer formularies may need to be stocked to a higher degree than products that are not paid for by third-party payers in the area.

- *Industry data.* Pharmacy journals and magazines contain a wealth of information that can be used to provide insight into what drug products should be selected. Pharmacists commonly use "top 200 prescribed drug product lists" to monitor trends in prescription drug use (Drug Information Online, 2011). In addition, these publications commonly alert pharmacy managers to new products or product changes that may affect patron and prescriber needs in the future.
- *Industry representatives.* Both drug company and wholesaler representatives can provide valuable information about available products. These representatives often have industry trend data and are familiar with prescribing habits in the local geographic area. Moreover, industry representatives have information about new and soon-to-be-released products.
- *Consumer information.* Asking patrons, prescribers, and employees is another way to determine what to stock. Monitoring consumer requests for products is also helpful.

Right Quantity at the Right Time*

As stated previously, having too much product ties up a pharmacy's money without providing an adequate return on investment. On the other hand, having too little product may result in lost sales and profits when the product is not available when consumers want to make a purchase. Not having enough product available also inconveniences pharmacy staff and customers, and may result in the loss of customers in the future. Thus, not only having the right product is critical to inventory management, but also having the right quantity at the right time is also essential.

The right quantity means having just enough product on hand to cover consumer demand at any given time. Determining the right quantity for any given product is difficult, if not impossible, given that demand may fluctuate unexpectedly. However, it is still important for pharmacy managers to track consumer demand for their products and monitor trends that may affect their use. While managers may not always have the right quantity on hand, use of this information helps them to anticipate fluctuations in demand (e.g., increasing the supply of antibiotics and certain over-the-counter medications during winter months).

In general, there are three types of stock to consider. *Cycle stock* is the regular inventory that is needed to fulfill orders. *Buffer,* or *safety, stock* is additional inventory that is needed in case of a supply or demand fluctuation. *Anticipatory,* or *speculative, stock* is inventory that is kept on hand because of expected future demand or expected price increase (e.g., flu vaccine in the fall and winter months). Buying anticipatory stock is risky, and therefore, pharmacists usually do not carry much anticipatory stock and place higher markups on such anticipatory stock. These types of stock are important to consider when deciding how much to order and when to order (Silbiger, 1999).

In order to estimate the minimum quantity of goods needed to meet demand, the pharmacy manager or purchasing agent should know the following information for each item stocked:

1. How much is on hand?
2. At what point to reorder?
3. How much to order?

How do pharmacy managers determine *stock depth* (i.e., the point where it is reasonably certain that the item will be available on demand)? Establishing stock depth (product quantity) involves consideration of

1. An item's rate of sale (average demand)
2. The length of time between stock checks (review time)

*Parts of this section are excerpted, with permission, from West DS. 2003. Purchasing and inventory control. In Jackson R (ed), *Effective Pharmacy Management CD-ROM,* 9th edn., Sec. 17. Alexandria, VA: National Community Pharmacists Association Foundation.

3. The period of time between placing and receiving an order (lead time)
4. A safety stock to account for variations in average demand during the buying time (review time plus lead time)

Thus the formula to set the *reorder point* is

$$\text{Reorder point} = [(\text{review time} + \text{lead time}) \times \text{average demand}] + \text{safety stock}$$

This basic formula has been used to develop an *economic order quantity* (EOQ) model (Carroll, 1998; Huffman, 1996; Silbiger, 1999; Tootelian and Gaedeke, 1993). While the EOQ model may be difficult to derive and calculate, it is often incorporated into computer software used by many pharmacies to manage their inventory and make purchasing decisions. The EOQ model describes the level of inventory and reorder quantity at which the combined costs of purchasing and carrying inventory are at a minimum. The formula is as follows:

$$Q = \sqrt{\frac{2(c)(D)}{(I)(UC)}}$$

where

Q = economic order quantity
c = procurement cost per order
D = demand for the product expressed either in dollars or physical units
I = inventory carrying costs
UC = unit cost of the item

Another factor determining how much to order is the budget. Hospital pharmacy directors may estimate this year's budget by increasing last year's budget by a certain percent (e.g., 5 or 10 percent). This budget estimate will provide a guide for how much money can be spent each month to order product. Community pharmacy managers also evaluate the profit-and-loss statement to determine whether too much product is being bought compared with the amount of sales.

Using an *open-to-buy budget* helps to control the total dollar investment in inventory (Carroll, 1998; West, 2003). It limits the manager to a set predetermined dollar amount of purchases during a given time period. The basic steps of this purchasing technique are listed below (Huffman, 1996; West, 2003). This procedure is repeated on a monthly basis.

Step 1. Forecast purchasing budget for each month in the next fiscal year based on sales and COGS data from the preceding year.

Step 2. Each month's forecasted sales are then multiplied by the COGS percent to calculate the monthly unadjusted purchasing budget.

Step 3. At the end of each month, the month's actual sales and purchases are recorded. Next month's purchases are then adjusted based on the past month's actual sales and purchases. If sales were greater than predicted, then next month's purchasing budget may be increased to accommodate for the increased sales. Alternatively, if the sales were lower than expected, then the purchasing budget for the next month would be decreased.

Right Price

Once the right product is selected, it is important to acquire it at the right price. Purchasing pharmacy products (especially prescription drugs) is not unlike purchasing a car in that the "list" or "sticker" price is often different from the final price that pharmacies actually pay. For pharmacy products, the list price and the terms of sale have an impact on the overall acquisition cost. *Terms of sale* pertain to discounts and dating (Huffman, 1996; West, 2003).

Discounts

Discounts describe the reduction(s) in price, whereas *dating* pertains to the period of time allowed for taking the discounts and the date when the invoice becomes payable. Although there are a number of discounts, three main discounts are described below.

QUANTITY DISCOUNTS Quantity discounts have traditionally been offered as an incentive for purchasing large quantities of single products or a special grouping of specific products offered by a manufacturer (West, 2003). For example, a wholesaler may sell one bottle of a drug for $100. A quantity discount may apply so that if the pharmacy orders a dozen bottles at one time, a 2 percent discount is given. Thus the pharmacy that orders 12 bottles will pay a total of $1,176, or $98 per bottle, resulting in a total saving of $24 than if the 12 bottles had each been purchased separately. These discounts, based on a quantity of the same product being purchased on the same order, are described as *noncumulative quantity discounts* (Huffman, 1996; Tootelian and Gaedeke, 1993; West, 2003).

The purchasing agent or pharmacy manager should be aware of these special discounts and adjust ordering to take advantage of them. Assuming that the product purchased is salable in the pharmacy, quantity discounts can decrease the actual acquisition cost of the drug product. However, managers should also balance the savings generated by quantity discounts with the costs of storing and carrying excess inventory, the risks of not being able to sell the extra products, and the opportunity costs that come with spending money on inventory that could have been used in other ways.

Some vendors offer quantity discounts to pharmacies if their total purchases reach a target monetary amount during a specific time period. These discounts involving a variety of products on separate orders over a period of time are termed *cumulative quantity discounts* or *deferred discounts* (Huffman, 1996; Tootelian and Gaedeke, 1993; West, 2003). For example, generic drug manufacturers often offer rebates to pharmacies that are based on the amount of generic product purchased during a given time period (e.g., quarterly or yearly). Similarly, hospital pharmacies, community pharmacies, and others negotiate discounts based on volume purchasing. The pharmacy receives a discount based on the volume purchased in a specified time period. A hospital or institutional pharmacy may be able to negotiate lower prices because a pharmaceutical product is placed on its formulary. The pharmacy can estimate that a certain amount of volume will be purchased or the product will get a percent of the market share. In exchange for this market share or volume purchasing, a discounted price is negotiated.

Cash discounts Cash discounts are small discounts offered for the prompt payment of invoices (Huffman, 1996; Tootelian and Gaedeke, 1993; West, 2003). The discount is stated as a percentage of the amount remaining after all other discounts have been deducted from the bill. A common discount is "2/10, net 30," which translates into a 2 percent discount if the invoice is paid within 10 days of the date of the invoice, otherwise, the net amount is due in 30 days.

Pharmacy managers should be aware of these discounts and take advantage of them, especially because they are not required to purchase excess inventory to do so. Many managers state that they do not take advantage of cash discounts because they do not have enough cash on hand to pay their invoices quickly. One thing that these managers could do is to take out a short-term loan or line of credit to obtain the cash needed to take advantage of the discount. In most cases, the savings provided by the cash discount more than makes up for the interest expense on the borrowed money.

Electronic funds transfer (EFT) is now being used by pharmacies to take advantage of cash discounts and even prepay for purchases. An example of this is displayed in Table 23-1 (West, 2003). Prepayment requires the pharmacy to pay a week or month ahead of actual purchases based on its average weekly or monthly purchases over the last 3 to 6 months. In exchange for prepayments, vendors offer additional cash discounts to pharmacy managers, allowing them to reduce their COGS further. Vendors offer Web-based systems that allow pharmacy managers to view their account information and invoices online in real time. This allows accounts payable to be monitored closely and invoices to be paid quickly online in real time. In addition, these systems reduce procurement costs for the pharmacy by decreasing personnel time and bookkeeping expenses.

Serial discounts Serial discounts occur when multiple discounts are applied at the same time. Serial discounts accumulate as shown in Table 23-3. In this example, the pharmacy manager is able to obtain the product at approximately $12 less than the original list price by taking advantage of both quantity and cash discounts.

Table 23-3. Example of Serial Discount

Invoice Price	**$100**
10% Quantity discount	$100.00 × 0.1 = $10.00 $100.00 − $10.00 = $90.00
2% Cash discount	$90.00 × 0.02 = $1.80 $90.00 − $1.80 = $88.20

Dating

The other purchase term that needs to be considered is the dating of the invoice. *Dating* refers both to the time before the specified amount of discount may be taken and to the time at which payment becomes due (Huffman, 1996; West, 2003). There are three general types of dating: (1) *prepayment,* where the pharmacy pays for the merchandise before it is ordered and delivered, (2) *collect on delivery* (COD), where there is no time before a discount may be taken and payment becomes due, and (3) *delayed* or *future dating,* where the invoice is due sometime in the future (West, 2003). When no specific dating has been placed on the invoice, it is usually assumed that payment is due 10 days from the last day of the month in which the purchase was made. This is often specified by the term EOM (end of month) in the invoice. Two other terms related to the dating of invoices and statements for merchandise include *AOG,* meaning "arrival of goods," and *ROG,* meaning "receipt of goods." For example, "2/10 ROG, net 30" means deduct 2 percent within 10 days after receipt of goods or otherwise pay net within 30 days after receipt of goods.

Right Vendor

Being able to obtain the right product at the right time at the right place depends on the vendor. Pharmacy managers should be careful when selecting a vendor. Although a pharmacy can select a single vendor or multiple vendors, it is advised that pharmacies have a primary vendor and a secondary vendor. Establishing a positive relationship with a vendor can be helpful because it may lead to prompt delivery, special buying opportunities, special pricing information, and prompt resolution of problems. A secondary vendor is advised for times when product is not available from the primary vendor owing to drug product shortages and to obtain special pricing opportunities.

Among the many effective mechanisms used by vendors to market their products to pharmacies are salespersons, service representatives, and account representatives. These individuals try diligently to maintain good communications with their clients. Many wholesaler representatives, for example, visit or telephone major purchasers every 2 to 4 weeks. The salesperson or representative serves as an important source of market information; consequently, many pharmacy managers make it a practice to talk with salespersons and representatives who call on them. In addition, talking with the representative keeps them aware of new programs and services offered by the vendor.

While favorable pricing and purchase terms are important considerations when selecting vendors, additional criteria should also be used (Tootelian and Gaedeke, 1993; West, 2003) (Table 23-4). Selecting a vendor with a good reputation is desirable. Accuracy and fill rates are also important considerations. Pharmacy managers should select vendors that provide quality products and services and have few out-of-stock situations. It is important to select vendors with prompt and reliable delivery. An inconsistent delivery service likely will result in the pharmacy not having the right products at the right times. Moreover, it is suggested that pharmacy managers evaluate their vendors periodically to ensure that they are receiving competitive prices and discounts. Many pharmacies seek bids from wholesalers periodically (e.g., every 3 years) to ensure competitive pricing and quality service.

Types of Vendors[†]

The most common type of vendor for pharmacies is the wholesaler. Wholesalers or distributors are often known as *middlemen.* They search the marketplace

[†]Parts of this section are excerpted, with permission, from West DS. 2003. Purchasing and inventory control. In Jackson R (ed), *Effective Pharmacy Management CD-ROM,* 9th edn., Sec. 17. Alexandria, VA: National Community Pharmacists Association Foundation.

Table 23-4. Criteria to Select Vendors

- Are they reliable and dependable? What is their order accuracy? Do they have a good reputation?
- Will they provide drug pedigree information and certify that the drug is not stolen, diverted, or counterfeit?
- Will they negotiate price and purchase terms with the pharmacy? Will they help to ensure contract compliance when ordering?
- What is their delivery schedule?
- Are they innovative?
- Do they provide financing and credit options?
- Do they have good customer relations? How often will a representative call on the pharmacy? Can I develop a positive business relationship with this supplier?
- Do they offer any value-added services? Will they help with advertising and promotion, provide inventory reports and analyses, or assist with pharmacy layout and design? Do they offer a private-label line of products?
- What technology do they offer to help with purchasing and inventory management?

and buy a wide assortment of products from thousands of different manufacturers and vendors. They then sell the products to pharmacies for use and resale. Most present-day wholesalers can be described with the term *full-service wholesalers* (Huffman, 1996; West, 2003).

The full-service wholesaler's most important function for the pharmacy manager is to serve as a buying agent. This means that the wholesaler anticipates the pharmacy's needs, goes into the market to obtain the necessary goods, and has them available at the appropriate time (West, 2003). This assembling of merchandise is a gigantic task involving thousands of different items that wholesalers store until the goods are wanted by a pharmacy. From a pharmacy manager's standpoint, it is much more efficient to do business with a full-service wholesaler that carries many products from many different vendors than to have to purchase products from each vendor separately. Most wholesalers offer just-in-time (JIT) delivery that allows for next-day or even same-day delivery, thereby reducing the pharmacy's risk and improving the pharmacy's cash flow.

In addition to assembling various product lines, full-service wholesalers render other valuable programs and services that may be offered complementary or for a fee. The account representative may provide information on marketing and merchandising techniques, assist with pharmacy layout and design, and provide customized inventory management reports and information on the availability of new products.

Programs offered by wholesalers include offering private-label products, repackaging services, and backorder programs to improve inventory management for the pharmacy. A backorder program means that the pharmacy can order a product on backorder, and as soon as the wholesaler receives the product, the pharmacy's backorders get top-priority filling status and are shipped before the day's regular orders. Some wholesalers offer programs where products are delivered on consignment, meaning that the pharmacy does not have to pay until the product is sold. This reduces the amount of money the pharmacy has invested in inventory. Some wholesalers also offer pharmacy ownership programs and third-party assistance services. Ownership programs assist people with buying a pharmacy by providing special financing for the initial inventory, store layout design consulting, and other services. Third-party assistance services include third-party contracting, pharmacy benefit management audit assistance, and tools to help with other third-party reimbursement issues. It is important to note that one of the reasons wholesalers offer these services to pharmacies, often at no cost, is that the success of the wholesaler is predicated on the success of the pharmacy. Programs and services that wholesalers can offer to help pharmacies sell more items will ultimately benefit the wholesalers themselves.

Some large pharmacy chains perform many of the wholesaler's service functions within their own organizations. These chains must assume wholesaler functions, such as purchasing, storing, financing, and delivering products to each of their units. While these chains serve as their own primary "vendor," they often still use full-line wholesalers as secondary vendors to obtain selected products or in special circumstances.

Pharmacies in practically every practice setting participate in some type of group purchasing organization (GPO) or central purchasing organization (Carroll, 1998; West, 2003). The purpose of a GPO is to pool the buying power of pharmacies together to obtain better prices and discounts from vendors. With profit margins being squeezed and drug budgets being scrutinized, pharmacies are looking for ways to decrease the cost of goods. A GPO negotiates with wholesalers and manufacturers for better pricing. One caveat to remember is that participating pharmacies must order products according to the terms of their GPO contract to receive special pricing and drug cost savings. If the pharmacists or technicians are not cognizant of the contract when they order, they may select the needed product at random from the list of potential sources. If the selection is not compliant with the contract, the pharmacy will not receive any negotiated prices.

Hospitals and hospital pharmacies are commonly members of GPOs, using the purchasing power of hundreds of hospitals to negotiate the best acquisition costs through competitive bidding. These hospital GPOs typically "bid out" almost every type of good used within the hospital, including equipment, supplies, and drugs. GPOs may also contract wholesaler services to select the wholesaler with the best combination of services, dependability, and costs. The GPO's central office organizes these bids and contracts through formal processes. Highly skilled representatives and professionals within these member hospitals represent the buying groups in the bidding and selection process. For example, GPOs commonly seek the advice of clinical pharmacists regarding comparative drug efficacy and future trends in drug therapy.

A *pharmacy buying group* is defined as a pharmacy organization whose purpose is to seek better drug prices for its members (e.g., community pharmacies, hospital pharmacies, and long-term care facilities) based on their collective buying power. Most, if not all, wholesalers are connected with one or more buying groups. The wholesaler will work with the pharmacy to find the best buying groups to join. Also, the pharmacist may identify a buying group with competitive pricing and then select a wholesaler that has a relationship with that buying group. Most buying groups charge a monthly or annual fee to members.

Another option used by pharmacies is to purchase directly from a pharmaceutical manufacturer. However, many manufacturers have substantial minimum purchase requirements, making it less favorable to buy from the manufacturer. Pharmacies may be receiving discounts based on volume purchased from the wholesaler; thereby giving an incentive to the pharmacy to buy most of its products from one wholesaler. Wholesalers also offer next-day delivery and other value-added services that help pharmacy managers minimize inventory costs. Thus most pharmacies do not purchase products from manufacturers very often.

Pharmacies, particularly those with formularies (e.g., hospital pharmacies) that purchase large volumes of select drug products, may negotiate prices directly with manufacturers. Bids for these products are sought from manufacturers, and then a contracted price is agreed to between the pharmacy and the manufacturer. While the contract involves a pharmacy and a manufacturer, distribution of the product usually involves a wholesaler (Carroll, 1998). The pharmacy will order the product from the wholesaler and receive the price that has been negotiated with the manufacturer. The wholesaler then bills the manufacturer the difference between the list price and the negotiated price (often called a *chargeback*), and in return, the manufacturer credits the wholesaler's account.

PURCHASING PROCESSES

Usually, a designated person (e.g., purchasing agent or pharmacy technician) will submit an order via telephone, fax, or computer and receive order confirmation. It may seem that the purchasing function ends when the order is made and the merchandise arrives at the pharmacy; however, this is not the case. The products need to be counted, checked for damage, and stocked on the shelves (West, 2003). When an order arrives, a pharmacy technician or other designated individual should physically count each item in the shipment and compare it with the invoice. Handheld devices that use bar coding technology are being used to facilitate this process. The designated person can scan the bar codes of all items in the tote to create a list of exactly what is in the tote. This list then can be compared to the invoice. The products should also be checked for any damage or short expiration dates. The vendor should be notified immediately if there is any discrepancy or any damaged products. On receipt, the products need to be moved to a temporary storage area or stocked on the shelves. Proper storage of inventory is vital. Improper storage can result in product that no longer can be sold, resulting in losses of inventory, sales, and profits. When new products are added to the shelves, the technician should rotate the stock, placing the newest stock behind the older stock bottles. This will ensure that the oldest stock is used first, hopefully before it becomes outdated. As discussed later in this chapter, within most community and hospital pharmacy software systems, options are available for the software to count incoming and outgoing products and automatically order product to replenish stock based on models such as the EOQ. However, it is important to remember that these systems only work as good as the inputting of information, including the reduction of inventory through all channels including theft and obsolescence.

■ INVENTORY MANAGEMENT

Inventory refers to the stock of products held to meet future demand. Pharmacies hold inventory to guard against fluctuations in demand, to take advantage of bulk discounts, and to withstand fluctuations in supply (e.g., late deliveries) (West, 2003). There are four costs associated with having inventory: acquisition costs, procurement costs, carrying costs, and stock-out costs (Carroll, 1998; Huffman, 1996; Silbiger, 1999; Tootelian and Gaedeke, 1993; West, 2003).

The *acquisition cost* is the price the pharmacy pays for the product. *Procurement costs* are the costs associated with purchasing the product: checking inventory, placing orders, receiving orders, stocking the product, and paying the invoices. *Carrying costs* refer to the storage, handling, insurance, cost of capital to finance the inventory, and opportunity costs. Another carrying cost is the cost of loss through theft, deterioration, and damage. Procurement and carrying costs must be balanced. For example, increasing the average order size and decreasing the number of orders placed decrease procurement costs but increase carrying costs. The fourth cost is the *stock-out cost,* which is the cost of not having a product on the shelf when a patient needs or wants it. This is frustrating to the pharmacist who has to explain why the product is not available and is an inconvenience to the patient and prescriber (Carroll, 1998).

Inventory management is the practice of planning, organizing, and controlling inventory so that it contributes to the profitability of the business (Huffman, 1996; West, 2003). The goals of inventory management are to minimize the amount invested in inventory and the procurement and carrying costs while balancing supply and demand (Huffman, 1996; Tootelian and Gaedeke, 1993; West, 2003). Inventory management is a key factor to success in a pharmacy because efficient inventory management can keep costs down, improve cash flow, and improve service. Alternatively, inventory mismanagement results in increased operating and opportunity costs.

Evaluating Inventory Management

The most common ratio used to determine how well a pharmacy is managing its inventory is the *inventory turnover rate* (ITOR). It can be calculated for the entire pharmacy, for departments (e.g., prescriptions or over the counter (OTC) products), and even for individual products. The ITOR is expressed as a ratio and is calculated by using the following formula (Tootelian and Gaedeke, 1993; West, 2003, 2010):

$$\text{ITOR} = \text{COGS} \div \text{average inventory value (at cost)}$$

$$\text{ITOR} = \text{COGS} \div [(\text{beginning inventory value} + \text{ending inventory value}) \div 2]$$

Table 23-5. Inventory Turnover Ratio (ITOR) Example

ITOR for Smith Pharmacy for FY 2009 = 8.2

ITOR for Smith Pharmacy for FY 2010 = 9.5

Data for Smith Pharmacy for FY 2011

Sales: $2,000,000	Cost of goods sold: $1,500,000
Gross margin: $500,000	Total expenses: $450,000
Net profit: $50,000	Average inventory: $150,000

ITOR = cost of goods sold/average inventory

ITOR = $1,500,000/$150,000

ITOR = 10

The COGS can be found on the pharmacy's income (profit-and-loss) statement for a given period of time. The average inventory value can be found by obtaining the pharmacy's balance sheets for both the beginning and the end of the period represented on the income statement. The balance sheets should contain the value of the pharmacy's inventory at each point in time. The ITOR indicates the efficiency with which inventory is used. It measures how quickly inventory is purchased, sold, and replaced. Two advantages of increasing the ITOR are that reducing the investment in inventory frees capital for other business activities and increases the return on investment in inventory.

Table 23-5 provides an example of how to calculate ITOR. In this example, the pharmacy's overall annual ITOR is 10. This means that this pharmacy, on average, sells all the inventory that is typically kept in the pharmacy a total of 10 times over the course of a year. This is similar to the national average for independent pharmacies (West, 2010), indicating that the pharmacy manager probably is managing inventory efficiently. Comparing the current year's ratio with last year's ratio also indicates that the manager is improving her efficiency in managing inventory because the ITOR has increased over time. Note that if the COGS remained constant for the year and the average inventory increased, the ITOR would have decreased. This would have indicated that inventory was sitting on the shelf and not selling. The pharmacy manager then would want to determine if she was ordering too much product or the wrong products.

Overall, pharmacy managers need to assess their ITOR. Deciding what is too high or too low is pharmacy dependent. Overall a high ITOR is desirable, as long as the pharmacy is not running out of stock at a level inconsistent with its desired level of service. If out-of-stocks are occurring too frequently, one may interpret the ITOR as being too high. Alternatively, if the pharmacy is carrying too much inventory that is not selling and is not being used, one may interpret the ITOR as too low. Hence cash is being spent to purchase the product, but cash is not flowing in from the sale of the product. The pharmacy manager should consider national or regional benchmarks as well as the pharmacy's trends when interpreting the ITOR. The ITOR is one indicator that should be considered when managing inventory, but it must be interpreted given the context of the pharmacy. For example, an ITOR of 30 may be acceptable if the pharmacy can order and receive items quickly from the vendor and there have not been complaints of shortages. It may also be helpful for the pharmacy manager to look at the ITOR within product lines or departments to facilitate decision making.

As gross margins have continued to shrink in retail pharmacies and drug budgets have gotten tighter in hospital pharmacies, pharmacy managers have been forced to become more efficient in their operations. One way to increase efficiency is to manage inventory properly. Trends have shown that pharmacy managers in various practice settings are making efforts to manage their inventories more efficiently. For example, independent pharmacy owners have increased their overall ITOR from 6.3 in 1995 to 9.8 in 2009 (West, 2010). Moreover, prescription inventory usually turns faster than the overall turnover of merchandise. The ITOR in 2009 for independent pharmacies was 9.8 for all merchandise and 11.7 for prescription inventory (West, 2010). Hospital pharmacies should be striving for an ITOR of at least 14 (Alverson, 2003). JIT deliveries and computerized inventory systems have facilitated this increased efficiency in inventory management, especially prescription inventory.

Another indicator of a pharmacy manager's ability to manage the investment in inventory efficiently is the net-profit-to-average-inventory ratio. This ratio indicates whether the inventory is being used efficiently to make a profit. Pharmacy managers desire to have a ratio greater than 20 percent.

Factors to Consider in Inventory Management

Pharmacy managers must consider multiple factors when evaluating their inventory:

- *Selection of generic products.* Generic drug products usually have a lower acquisition cost, and therefore, by stocking generic products, the amount of money invested in inventory is reduced (Carroll, 1998). For example, a pharmacist may decide not to stock brand name Lasix because generic furosemide is less expensive, thereby reducing the amount of money invested in inventory.
- *Reduction of inventory size.* A pharmacist may decide to have a small front end in his or her store to reduce the amount invested in inventory. He or she may carry only basic product lines (i.e., a smaller numbers of brands and items) as opposed to full product lines (i.e., every brand and every item).
- *Returned-goods policies.* One critical component is the evaluation of returned-goods policies. Many manufacturers and wholesalers have established policies regarding merchandise that may be returned. In exchange for returning unsalable goods, these vendors may provide credit on future purchases, replacement goods, or even cash back to the pharmacy. An example of wholesaler returned-goods policies is provided in Table 23-1. Pharmacy managers should monitor products closely that qualify for the various returned-goods policies, making certain that such returns are made on a regular, periodic basis before time limitations take effect. It is advised to have a staff member responsible for checking the shelves periodically for out-of-date items or items that are not selling. Because the management of return goods is critical, some pharmacies use returned-goods service companies to assist them with managing their returned goods. These companies will evaluate the pharmacy's inventory, return the appropriate products, and often return money from the returned products within 30 to 60 days. These companies charge a fee based on the amount of returns. One major advantage to these companies is that they are aware of each manufacturer's and wholesaler's specific policies and can quickly identify product to be returned.
- *Management of unclaimed prescriptions.* Approximately 1.5 percent of all prescriptions received and/or filled in community pharmacies remain unclaimed (McCaffrey et al., 1998). A pharmacist must be aware of the amount of inventory that has been used to fill these unclaimed prescriptions. It is important for pharmacists to monitor these unclaimed prescriptions and after a specified period (e.g., 14 days) return the stock to the shelf.
- *Monitoring shrinkage.* Inventory shrinkage includes losses owing to shoplifting, employee theft, and robbery. It is estimated that 1.75 percent of annual sales are lost to shrinkage (Kolettis, 2002). The largest source of shrinkage for most retailers is employee theft. It is important to recruit honest personnel and monitor their activities, especially those working in the prescription area of a pharmacy, because theft of controlled substances in pharmacies is increasingly problematic. Equally important; however, is for the pharmacy staff to be observant, say hello to customers, keep displays neat, install security mirrors and cameras, and remove high fixtures to minimize shoplifting. Some pharmacies use technologies such as inventory-control bars, cameras and remote monitoring, and electronic article surveillance to prevent loss of product from theft.
- *Use of formularies.* As stated previously, institutional pharmacies commonly use formularies to facilitate

inventory management (Pearce and Begg, 1992). A formulary allows the pharmacy manager to carry one therapeutic equivalent within a class of drugs instead of each drug product within the class. This allows pharmacy managers to lower their overall investment in inventory.

Methods of Inventory Management

Three methods are used commonly in pharmacy to manage inventory: the visual method, the periodic method, and the perpetual method (Carroll, 1998; Tootelian and Gaedeke, 1993; West, 2003). The *visual method* requires the pharmacist or designated person to look at the number of units in inventory and compare them with a listing of how many should be carried. When the number falls below the desired amount, an order is placed. The *periodic method* requires the pharmacist or designated person to count the stock on hand at predetermined intervals and compare it with minimum desired levels. If the quantity is below the minimum, the product is ordered.

Usually, a designated person is responsible for checking the shelves and placing orders. The pharmacy manager may have a specific checklist, indicating that the person should conduct a stock review weekly or look for expired products monthly, in addition to placing orders and keeping inventory orders to a specific level. This purchasing person will learn the turnover rates for specific products and will develop a skill for purchasing for the pharmacy. This method allows the purchasing person to account for fluctuations in supply and demand. Today, the purchasing person is likely to use a hand-held electronic device into which item numbers and quantities are entered or a hand-held scanning device that scans the barcodes on the product packaging or shelf labels (Carroll, 1998; West, 2003). These devices then can be used to submit an order electronically.

Although the visual and periodic methods are still used today, *perpetual inventory systems* are common in all pharmacy settings. These perpetual systems are computerized inventory management systems. Perpetual inventory management systems are the most efficient method to manage inventory. This method allows the inventory to be monitored at all times. The entire inventory may be entered into the computer, and with the filling of each prescription, the appropriate inventory can be reduced automatically. A perpetual system can tell precisely the amount of inventory on hand for any product at any time. Moreover, the pharmacy manager can quickly assess the value of current inventory.

Computer systems can be used to calculate the EOQ and reorder point so that a product is reordered automatically when the inventory falls below a minimum standard (West, 2003). This type of system reduces procurement costs significantly. Although the computer can be programmed to order products automatically, it is important for pharmacy staff to monitor inventory daily and to make corrections for variances owing to fluctuations in supply and demand.

To maintain a perpetual inventory system, all purchases and sales must be entered into the computer system (Carroll, 1998; West, 2003). A clerk can enter data from purchases, or the computer dispensing system can be interfaced with the computer order system. The interface allows for the inventory to be reduced when a product is dispensed. The sales data can also be entered at the point of sale (POS) by devices that use optical scanning and barcode technology. POS devices are advantageous in that they improve the accuracy of pricing and inventory data. They eliminate the need for price stickers, reduce the frequency of pricing errors, and automatically track inventory.

Regardless of which method is used, most pharmacies also conduct a physical inventory at least annually. This encompasses counting or scanning every item in the pharmacy. Pharmacy staff then can compare the product on-hand quantities in the computer or the value of inventory on the financial statements with what is actually on the shelves. It is important to conduct a physical inventory to verify periodically the accuracy of the pharmacy's financial records. In addition, pharmacy managers should follow state board of pharmacy regulations with respect to inventory counts and control with respect to controlled substances, especially narcotics.

Role of Technology

Based on the preceding description of the purchasing process and perpetual inventory systems, one can recognize the value of technology in inventory management. Thus, computerized inventory management systems are common today in pharmacies in all practice settings. Technology enables pharmacists to manage inventory faster and more accurately.

These computer systems can integrate the management of inventory, information, and costs. The ability to integrate inventory and cost data allows for the generation of a wide array of reports and analyses. Pharmacists use these management reports to identify high- and low-turnover items and determine stock levels for better allocation of shelf space. Examples of inventory management reports include

- *Purchase-trend report*—describes the quantity purchased of OTC products or prescription drug products by month or by quarter.
- *Sales-analysis report*—features a rolling 12-month statement that includes order quantity, shipped quantity, unavailable quantity, returns, credits, and dollars spent.
- *Item-movement report*—lists which items are selling the best.

Many wholesalers will provide the hardware and software for the inventory management system. The most current trend is Web-based systems. These allow pharmacy managers to view in real time the quantity on hand at the wholesaler, the list price, the manufacturer backorder status, and the online catalog. These Web-based systems also enable pharmacy staff to check purchase orders, invoices, and account information in real time. Another advantage is that the pharmacy staff can place orders and view account information from other locations besides the pharmacy. POS systems can integrate with many pharmacy systems. As previously mentioned, POS systems allow product to be deducted from inventory as it is sold or dispensed; thereby, improving inventory management in the pharmacy. POS systems also provide other management efficiencies such as speeding up checkout times with credit card processing and reducing pricing errors.

Pharmacy staff can also order inventory via the Internet, which is termed *e-procurement.* e-Procurement allows the pharmacy to receive immediate item allocation and order confirmation. These sophisticated systems drastically reduce the time and effort spent on procurement. Prices can be updated daily or weekly by using electronic invoice transmission, and returns and credits can be completed electronically. Invoices are then paid by EFT.

It is important to note that Class II (C-II) controlled substances now can be ordered electronically. Pharmacies must first enroll with the US Drug Enforcement Agency (DEA) to acquire a digital certificate. The C-II orders are created using a computerized inventory system, electronically signed using a password-protected digital certificate, and then submitted electronically to the wholesaler.

Clearly, technology is being used to facilitate ordering, receiving, managing, and paying for products. As newer technologies are available, pharmacies will adopt these to improve their inventory management efficiencies. Currently, there is much focus on the use of radiofrequency identification (RFID) microchips to improve product distribution from manufacturer to wholesaler to pharmacy (FDA, 2007). At the factory, a RFID microchip (small computer chip), or "tag," will be attached to a product package. The tag will contain data about where the product was manufactured, when it arrived at the warehouse, and when it was stocked on the shelf. When a product arrives at the store, the RFID reader or sensor can update the store inventory. The sensor can also detect the package leaving the shelf and automatically reorder the product from the manufacturer. RFID tags are different from barcodes in that they have larger memory capacity, allow for data to be added and changed, and do not have to be physically swiped on a scanner to access the stored information. Data can be sent through the air and can penetrate clothing. Hence RFID tags provide a chain of custody for the pharmacy and may help protect against counterfeiting and theft. As manufacturers and wholesalers adopt the use of this technology, pharmacists also will be evaluating the value of the technology for the pharmacy.

CURRENT TOPICS IN INVENTORY MANAGEMENT

Risk Evaluation and Mitigation Strategies and Restricted Distribution

The Food and Drug Administration Amendments Act (FDAAA) of 2007 increased the Food and Drug Administration's (FDA) responsibility with respect to postmarketing surveillance. The FDA can now require risk evaluation and mitigation strategies (REMS) for specific products or product classes. Although REMS strategies vary by drug product, there are elements to ensure safe drug use, including restricting drug distribution. These elements include special training or certification of health care providers who prescribe or dispense the product, special certification of pharmacies or institutions that dispense the product, limited dispensing of the product to certain settings, and patient requirements to have lab tests, enroll in a registry, or agree to monitoring prior to receiving the product. Three examples of restricted distribution include the following:

- OxyContin (controlled-release oral formulation of oxycodone hydrochloride) is used to treat pain and is associated with potentially life-threatening risks. Thus, the FDA and the manufacturer developed a REMS program that requires health care providers who prescribe the product to receive training. Dispensers will have to be trained and authorized as well and will be required to provide a Medication Guide about the product to each patient.
- Onsolis (fentanyl buccal soluble film) has been approved by the FDA with a REMS program. As part of the strategy, the drug product will be only available through a restricted distribution program called the FOCUS program. Pharmacies must be enrolled in the FOCUS program to dispense the medication. The FOCUS pharmacy must confirm that the patient and prescriber are active in the FOCUS program database before dispensing. The pharmacy must also deliver the medication directly to the patient via a secure, traceable courier.
- Vandetanib (an orphan drug for treatment of medullary thyroid cancer) is associated with risk of QT prolongation, torsades de pointes, and sudden death. The REMS program for this product requires prescribers and pharmacies to be certified before they are able to prescribe and/or dispense the product.

Wholesalers have reorganized and positioned themselves to be a specialty supplier for products with REMS. Pharmacies, both institutional and retail, are also reengineering to manage these requirements. Pharmacies are reevaluating their purchasing and inventory management processes for drug products with REMS. It is important for pharmacists to consider the administrative and logistical issues associated with dispensing drug products with REMS requirements. Overall, many pharmacists are concerned with the restricted distribution systems and the possibility of restricting patient access due to the REMS requirements (Bough, 2008; Meyer, 2009). It will be important for pharmacists to stay abreast of the development and implementation of REMS programs for various products.

Specialty Pharmacy

Specialty pharmacies have evolved as there has been a need for the dispensing of drug and biologic products that have high costs or present reimbursement challenges, have special handling or storage requirements, and/or require administration at time of dispensing or other patient support (Suchanek, 2005). Often retail pharmacies cannot bill major medical insurance, or do not have the supplies or personnel to provide an injection or an infusion, or do not have special storage capabilities, or cannot afford the high inventory costs of some drug products (Suchanek, 2005). To fill this need in the marketplace, specialty pharmacies have developed. These pharmacies help control the distribution of specialty pharmaceutical products. Payers often contract with a specialty pharmacy and require beneficiaries to obtain certain products through the specialty pharmacy. To learn more about specialty pharmacies, please see Chapter 34.

It is important to mention that all pharmacies face challenges with respect to purchasing, inventory management, and dispensing as products become more expensive, have REMS requirements, or require other "special" considerations (e.g., storage, administration). For example, hospitals are challenged when a patient is hospitalized and his insurance company requires a drug product to be purchased through a specialty pharmacy or the patient has already purchased the product and needs it to be administered while in the hospital (Kirschenbaum, 2009). If the hospital has to purchase it through the specialty pharmacy, they may not get as good a price as if they had purchased it through their wholesaler. The hospital may allow the patient to bring the specialty product into the hospital; however, there are concerns about product integrity (e.g., how the product has been stored while in possession of patient). Pharmacies need to continue to evaluate their policies and procedures with respect to drug distribution systems.

Integrity of the Drug Supply Chain

This chapter has focused mainly on purchasing and inventory management from the pharmacy's business perspective—having the right products available to sell while reducing the investment in inventory. Yet the distribution of pharmaceuticals from the manufacturer to the pharmacy is being closely scrutinized to ensure product safety. Thus pharmacy staff also must focus on the supply-chain integrity. It is estimated that worldwide drug counterfeiting is a $32 billion business, and 1 to 2 percent of drugs in North America are fraudulent (National Association of Boards of Pharmacy, 2011). It is even possible that drugs dispensed by reputable pharmacies could be counterfeit (National Association of Boards of Pharmacy, 2011).

Pharmacy staff must be aware of the potential for purchasing and dispensing counterfeit products. To ensure that drug products are authentic, pharmacists should choose a reputable vendor with a reliable delivery system. There are large national and regional wholesalers that are considered "authorized distributors" that buy directly from manufacturers. Regulation of drug wholesalers continues to be increased in an effort to ensure supply chain integrity; and therefore, more wholesalers and states are recognizing the importance of the National Association of Boards of Pharmacy wholesaler accreditation program (i.e., the Verified-Accredited Wholesaler Distributors program). Pharmacists should conduct business with accredited wholesalers. There are thousands of secondary wholesalers that purchase products from other wholesalers or repackagers that may or may not be legitimate. If a lesser-known vendor calls with a special deal on a product that appears to be too good to be true, that probably is the case. When a package arrives, the staff person should look for problems such as old or worn packaging, a faded label around the expiration date, missing overt packaging marks, or product or packaging appearance that is different from normal. Pharmacists who suspect that they have purchased counterfeit drugs should contact the FDA Medwatch program, the manufacturer of the drug product, their state board of pharmacy, and their local law enforcement authorities.

To guarantee the integrity of drug distribution in the United States, the FDA is requiring drug distributors to provide documentation of the chain of custody for drug product packages, especially for products at higher risk of being counterfeit (e.g., Lipitor, Celebrex, Nexium, Crestor, Viagra, and other common, expensive brand name drug products). The FDA Counterfeit Drug Task Force recommends the use of electronic track and trace technology to provide an accurate drug pedigree, which is a chain of custody for the product as it moves through the supply chain from manufacturer to pharmacy (FDA, 2007). RFID tags would create an electronic pedigree for each drug bottle. This would make it more difficult for counterfeit products to enter the distribution system. In addition, this pedigree would allow for more efficient and targeted drug recalls. Pharmacies could quickly and accurately withdraw recalled products from their shelves. In March 2010, the FDA issued further guidance to the industry for securing the drug supply chain (FDA, 2010). The FDA is now recommending package-level standardized numerical identifiers (SNIs). The SNI for most prescription drug packages should be a serialized National Drug Code (NDC) where each product package has a unique serial number combined with the NDC code. This serial number will facilitate "track and trace" and authentication systems and can be read by a human or by technology (e.g., barcoding, RFID).

REVISITING THE SCENARIO

Referring back to Marie's predicament, it is easy to see that a number of factors may be influencing her pharmacy's purchasing and inventory control mechanisms. It is apparent that Marie has minimized her investment in inventory to an extent that it may be hurting sales. The pharmacy appears to be having frequent out-of-stock situations, resulting in decreased sales, loss of goodwill, loss of patrons, and possibly harm to patients. Regardless of which wholesaler is selected, Marie should evaluate her purchasing policies and decisions. She should talk with her wholesaler representative and evaluate the inventory management reports to determine which products have a high turnover rate and which products have a low turnover rate. Knowing this should facilitate ordering decisions.

Meanwhile, it appears that Marie is becoming dissatisfied with her current wholesaler. Seeking bids from wholesalers or evaluating other wholesalers periodically is suggested to ensure competitive pricing and quality service. If a new wholesaler is selected, Marie should develop a relationship with the customer representative and examine the services and programs offered by the wholesaler. Marie may also want to select a secondary wholesaler.

Buying goods at the lowest price is another concern. It is difficult to compare prices because price often depends on (1) purchasing volume, (2) rebates and discounts earned, and (3) membership in a GPO. In addition, certain pharmacies, such as disproportionate share (DPS) hospital pharmacies, qualify for other pricing considerations. (*Note:* DPS hospitals qualify for special pricing because they provide a significant amount of care to low-income patients.) Regardless of which wholesaler Marie selects, she should work with her purchasing and accounting personnel to ensure that appropriate discounts are earned. Taking advantage of discounts is one way to reduce costs and improve cash flow for the pharmacy. Marie should also consider participating in a GPO. One of the most significant factors that affect pharmaceutical costs, other than discounts and rebates, is participation in a GPO or a buying group.

These are just a few of the parameters that Marie should consider. There are other purchasing and inventory management activities that Marie could evaluate. For example, she may want to contract with a return-goods company to assist with the return of goods. Another example would be to purchase and dispense more generic drugs because these products reduce the amount of money invested in inventory. Developing a formulary for the community mental health center may be another possibility. Overall, Marie constantly must be aware of the purchasing and inventory management activities. These activities can have a significant impact on both the financial and operational health of the pharmacy.

QUESTIONS FOR FURTHER DISCUSSION

1. What can a pharmacist do to reduce the amount of money invested in inventory in a community pharmacy? In a hospital pharmacy?
2. Describe how you think technology in the future will facilitate purchasing and inventory management in a pharmacy.
3. Discuss the various factors that affect the cost of goods in a pharmacy.
4. What are the current trends in the pharmacy wholesale industry?

ACKNOWLEDGMENT

I would like to acknowledge the National Community Pharmacists Association for releasing copyright on "West DS. 2003. Purchasing and inventory control.

In Jackson R (ed.) *Effective Pharmacy Management, CD-ROM,* 9th edn., Sec. 17. Alexandria, VA: National Community Pharmacists Association Foundation."

REFERENCES

Alverson C. 2003. Beyond purchasing-managing hospital inventory. *Manag Healthcare Exec,* November 1. Available at www.managedhealthcareexecutive.com/mhe/content/printContentPopup.jsp?id=75802&searchString=purchasing; accessed on March 15, 2012.

Bough MA. 2008. Statement of the American Pharmacists Association to the Food and Drug Administration's Joint Meeting of the Anesthetic and Life Support Drug Advisory Committee and the Drug Safety and Risk Management Advisory Committee. American Pharmacists Association, Washington, DC.

Carroll NV. 1998. *Financial Management for Pharmacists,* 2nd edn. Baltimore: Williams & Wilkins.

Drug Information Online. 2010. Pharmaceutical Sales. Available at http://www.drugs.com/top200.html; accessed on August 25, 2011.

Food and Drug Administration (FDA). 2007. FDA Counterfeit Drug Task Force Report: 2006 Update. Available at www.fda.gov/oc/initiatives/counterfeit/report6_06.html; accessed on May 19, 2011.

Food and Drug Administration (FDA). 2010. FDA Standards for Securing the Drug Supply Chain-Standardized Numerical Identification for Prescription Drug Packages. Available at www.fda.gov/RegulatoryInformation/Guidances/ucm125505.htm; accessed on May 21, 2011.

Huffman DC (ed.). 1996. Purchasing and inventory control. In *Effective Pharmacy Management,* 8th edn. Alexandria, VA: National Association of Retail Druggists, p. 355.

Kirschenbaum BE. 2009. Specialty pharmacies and other restricted drug distribution systems: Financial and safety considerations for patients and health-system pharmacists. *Am J Health Syst Pharm* 66(Suppl 7):S13–20.

Kolettis H. 2002. Guarding the Shelves. *Security Magazine.* Available at www.securitymagazine.com/articles/print/76470; accessed on May 21, 2011.

McCaffrey DJ, Smith MC, Banahan BF, et al. 1998. A continued look into the financial implications of initial noncompliance in community pharmacies: An unclaimed prescription audit pilot. *J Res Pharm Econ* 9:33.

Meyer BM. 2009. The Food and Drug Administration Amendments Act of 2007: Drug safety and health-system pharmacy implications. *Am J Health Syst Pharm* 66(supp 7):S3–5.

National Association of Boards of Pharmacy. 2011. Counterfeit Drugs. Available at http://www.nabp.net/programs/consumer-protection/buying-medicine-online/counterfeit-drugs/; accessed on May 22, 2011.

Pearce MJ, Begg EJ. 1992. A review of limited lists and formularies: Are they cost-effective? *Pharmacoeconomics* 1:191.

Silbiger S. 1999. *The Ten-Day MBA,* rev. ed. New York: Quill William Morrow.

Suchanek D. 2005. The rise and role of specialty pharmacy. *Biotechnology Healthcare* 31–5.

Tootelian DH, Gaedeke RM. 1993. *Essentials of Pharmacy Management.* St. Louis: Mosby.

West DS. 2001. *Managing Efficiencies in Pharmacy Cash Flow,* vol. 6. Birmingham, AL: Mylan Institute of Pharmacy, Continuing Education Series.

West DS. 2003. Purchasing and inventory control. In Jackson R (ed.) *Effective Pharmacy Management CDROM,* 9th edn. Sec. 17. Alexandria, VA: National Community Pharmacists Association Foundation.

West DS (ed.). 2010. *2010 NCPA Digest sponsored by Cardinal Health.* Alexandria, VA: National Community Pharmacists Association.

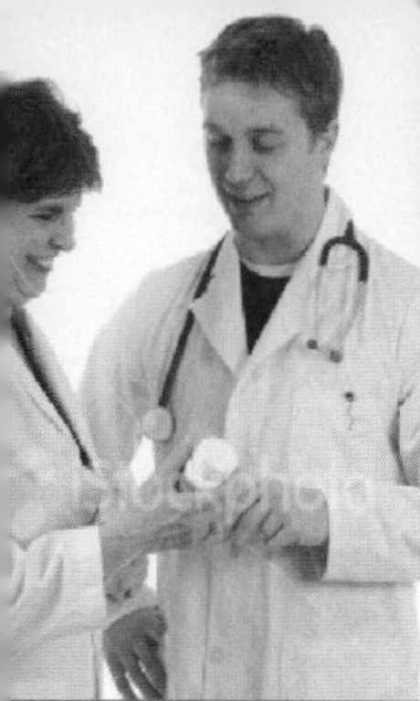

24

MERCHANDISING

Edward Cohen

About the Author: Dr. Cohen received a B.S. in pharmacy from the University of Illinois at Chicago (UIC) and a Pharm.D. from Midwestern University Chicago College of Pharmacy (MWU). After owning an independent pharmacy for many years, he moved into the corporate sector as Director of Pharmacy for Dominick's Finer Foods (a division of Safeway). Today he serves as Senior Manager, Product Development, Corporate Innovations for Walgreens. Dr. Cohen has been recognized nationally for his role in bringing patient care to the forefront of community pharmacy practice. He holds adjunct faculty positions at UIC and MWU, as well as serving on both colleges' advisory committees. Dr. Cohen has served as Chair of the Administration Section of the American Pharmacists Association—Academy of Pharmacy Practice and Management and on the Board of Directors of the Illinois Pharmacists Association.

LEARNING OBJECTIVES

After completing this chapter, readers should be able to

1. Describe the evolution of merchandising in pharmacy from the beginning of the twentieth century to current practices used today.
2. Identify merchandising techniques that enhance the awareness and use of the pharmacy department as a health care destination for patients.
3. Explain how pharmacy layout and merchandising techniques affect consumers' senses.
4. Identify and discuss the implications of ineffective merchandising in a pharmacy.
5. Evaluate the impact of merchandising on the financial success of a pharmacy.

SCENARIO

Mary Quint, a third-year doctor of pharmacy student, was home recently to attend a family gathering. There was much ado about Mary's progress in pharmacy school. Her family was asking numerous questions about school, her classes, her job, and her future. As the conversation continued, Mary found the family involved in a discussion about the different pharmacies in town. The family had a full range of opinions that addressed everything from the location of the store, to the pharmacist, to the store hours.

Mary was impressed with the conversation. She had never thought much about the issues being discussed by her family. It seemed that her pharmacy, Middletown South Pharmacy, is the least liked by her family. Middleton South Pharmacy is perceived to be an "old standard" in the community. It is a traditional drugstore, built on a corner in the center of town. They have limited parking, a smaller front of the store where nonprescription items are sold, a nice prescription department, and an old-fashioned soda fountain is still a busy part of the business. While her family spoke highly of their memories of Middleton South Pharmacy (and particularly of the treats at their soda fountain), they also said that it is "just a regular drugstore" and doesn't offer any of the conveniences and new pharmacist services the other pharmacies are providing.

Her family's favorite pharmacy in town is the new chain pharmacy (Healthway Pharmacy). Healthway Pharmacy is bright and open, making it easy to find items. The staff is friendly and is always doing something to make the store look nice. As people shop, they often find and buy items that they need, as well as items that they had not even planned on purchasing that day. Healthway Pharmacy has many new products, making it enjoyable to shop in the store. The prescription department is large and open with a comfortable waiting area and a private booth to talk with the pharmacist. The pharmacists' offer many patient care services, including health screenings, immunizations, and even classes to teach people about how to make the most of their medicines. The store is easy to access from the major streets in the area and has a large parking area. The store also has a drive-through window by the pharmacy, an in-store medical clinic staffed by a nurse practitioner, and an electronic kiosk to order prescriptions without having to be at the prescription counter. Healthway Pharmacy is open 24 hours a day, 7 days a week. Everyone encouraged Mary to visit Healthway Pharmacy and inquire about getting a job there.

CHAPTER QUESTIONS

1. What are the most prominent merchandising features that drive customers to shop in a particular pharmacy?
2. How does merchandising affect consumer senses?
3. What is the impact of merchandising on the overall operation and profitability of a pharmacy?
4. What are the goals of effective merchandising methods for a pharmacy?
5. Which factors should be considered in the design of the exterior of a pharmacy? In the design and layout of the interior?

INTRODUCTION

The scenario demonstrates the effects of some "invisible" principles of merchandising. The lack of effective merchandising in one pharmacy was enough to send Mary's family to another pharmacy to do business. Many of the physical features of community pharmacies frequently are taken for granted. The exterior design is important to create an identity with customers. The colors and shapes of the outdoor signage add to the pharmacy's identity. Pharmacy managers can plan the ease of entry into the store and everything seen and felt by consumers inside the pharmacy. Merchandising activities used by pharmacy managers can attract customers and make their shopping experience more enjoyable.

Almost every retail store (including community pharmacies) is designed for selling merchandise (Hilditch, 1981). Given the decline in profit margins in the prescription department, the success of a pharmacy's "front end" is crucial to the total financial success of the business.

Drugstores traditionally have been retail establishments where customers can find staple items, basic health care needs, and a pharmacy. Larger chain pharmacies have expanded this definition by promoting and selling large varieties of merchandise that often are well beyond the basic mixture of products found in a traditional drugstore (Francke, 1974). Today, pharmacies are also found in hospitals, clinics, grocery stores, and even large discount stores. The location of the pharmacy within these often very large buildings, as well as the mix, location, and condition of the goods and services the pharmacy offers, is important to the pharmacy's success.

Attracting customers into a pharmacy and inviting them to make purchases while they are there are the main objectives of all merchandising efforts. Pharmacies must consider their design, layout, and merchandise to draw shoppers who will then make purchases. It is important to keep in mind that most of the items sold in a pharmacy can also be purchased in other retail outlets or on the Internet. The proper mix of convenience, price, and service will add to the appeal of the pharmacy.

Pharmacies are working to establish their business as customers' total health care destination. The pharmacy of the future may follow several business models. One model centers on a retail merchandising operation and another centers on health care services. The health care model provides more health related products and less nonhealth related items such as greeting cards and cosmetics. Many pharmacies are expanding their offerings of professional goods and services the pharmacist and staff provide, increasing the offerings of healthier foods, carrying more professional products (e.g., durable medical equipment, blood glucose and other diabetes specialty items, and expanded vitamin and herbal offerings), adding in-store medical clinics for treatment of minor ailments, providing immunizations, and developing services to help better understand their conditions and utilize their medications.

Customers respond to what they see, hear, and feel. Designing a pharmacy to address the everyday needs of our on-the-go society will make the store successful. Merchandising tools are used in every aspect of the pharmacy business, drawing customers to the location, making it easy and comfortable to shop in the stores, and building customer loyalty.

PHARMACY MERCHANDISING TRENDS THROUGH THE 1900s

Early in the last century, people came to drugstores for relief from their ailments. Pharmacists had a handful of drugs, sold mostly in compounded mixtures, and did what they could to ease their patients' discomfort. Drugstores were not merchandised as they are today. Drugstores contained low-cost traditional items that people used every day. Some of the traditional items found in drugstores were cosmetics, magazines, tobacco, stationery, and candy. The prescription business was a small portion of the total sales of the store. Each pharmacy owner built his or her reputation on individual achievements with his or her customers.

With Prohibition during the 1920s, the drugstore fountain replaced the tavern as the new socially acceptable gathering place. Pharmacists and their clerks were busy making milkshakes and other soda fountain creations. During Prohibition, pharmacies became the only legitimate place to purchase alcohol products because they were only available with a doctor's prescription. When Prohibition was lifted in the 1930s, many pharmacies continued to sell liquor, having developed a reputation as legitimate outlets (Higby, 1997).

After World War II (WWII), many new medications came to the market. Pharmacies began filling more prescriptions using prefabricated dosage forms, and thus spent less time compounding medications. Pharmacists began to spend most of their time dispensing prefabricated prescription drug products, making sure the patient received the medication in an efficient manner, with the focus on providing drug products, not drug information. The front end of the store took on a new look and feel as well. Pharmacies began to stock many prefabricated staple items. As a result of filling an increasing number of prescriptions, pharmacists had less time to manage the front ends of their pharmacies. Prescriptions were becoming another commodity in the store, much to the dismay of pharmacists. Pharmacists were looking to transition their practices to have patient safety as their primary concern. By the late 1960s, the profession had taken a firm stand to change and regain the professional stature of the pharmacy (Higby, 1997).

PHARMACY DESIGN, LAYOUT, AND MERCHANDISING

Most consumer purchases in pharmacies are not planned very far in advance. Pharmacy managers use pharmacy design, layout of fixtures, and merchandising of products to affect the purchasing behaviors of their customers. Studies have shown that more than 80 percent of all purchases are made by people who less than a week before their purchases were not planning to buy these particular items (Eisenpreis, 1983). The primary reasons why consumers make unplanned purchases are emergencies (running out of a needed item), latent buying interests brought on by a good price or a new product, and impulse purchases (buying on a whim to try something new or different).

An important contribution to sales success is the store design and layout of merchandise. Getting people into a pharmacy, making it easy to find and purchase both needed and wanted items, and increasing the number of return visits consumers will make to a pharmacy—all can be influenced by design and layout factors. The design and layout of a pharmacy must allow for customer convenience, ease of shopping, and an exciting atmosphere that will promote the selling of both goods and services.

Pharmacy Design

Today's consumers demand convenience, service, and ambience. While pharmacies have not always been known for these attributes, consumers have come to expect a certain atmosphere and comfort level from any retail establishment.

From the 1940s to the 1960s, pharmacy store design and decor did not highlight merchandise or professional activities. Most pharmacies carried a mix of staple items, tobacco, and liquor; had soda fountains; and gave little thought to where the best place might be to locate these items in the store. During the 1970s and 1980s, pharmacy designs transitioned to highlight the products to be sold, resulting in simpler decor and allowing the merchandise to become part of the pharmacy's design.

It is important to select the most appropriate design aspects for a pharmacy without becoming too trendy or rapidly outdated. The target of today's pharmacy designs is the shopper. To determine a pharmacy design, managers first must determine the characteristics and needs of the customers to be served. Customers want pharmacies that are convenient, well organized, and in supply of the goods and services they desire when they need them. Pharmacies that frustrate disappoint, or waste consumer time searching for items will not be patronized.

Women are the key decision makers for the family and make most pharmacy purchase decisions. Today, families have to be efficient with their time and are spending less time planning shopping trips and are making more decisions in the store. Retailers, including drugstores, are making adjustments to their stores to allow people to get in and out quicker.

The size of a pharmacy or pharmacy department commonly is determined by industry averages or by evaluating the sales per square foot of various pharmacy departments. Store managers can obtain industry information on the ideal size for their pharmacies from wholesalers and other vendors, as well as from their professional associations (e.g., National Community Pharmacists Association or National Association of Chain Drug Stores).

Managers can calculate the ideal size of a department (an area within a pharmacy that contains related goods or services) by estimating the total dollar amount of sales from that department and dividing by their expected sales per square foot. While this method is simple to use, it should be applied with care and common sense. Estimates of sales are not always accurate indicators of the need for space for particular types of goods and services. The characteristics of space inside the store (e.g., walls, lighting, and fixtures) and the physical characteristics of the goods and services to be sold in a department both should be considered when allocating space within a pharmacy (Rodowskas, 1996).

Another key point when designing a pharmacy is to make sure that prescription dispensing and counseling sections are in step with the profession. With pharmacists providing an array of counseling, education, and patient care services, additional space for pharmacists to talk privately with patients may be needed. Setting aside and designing an appropriate consultation area and a patient waiting area are important. Many pharmacies also sell items that do not require a prescription, but they often sell better if a pharmacist is available to explain their use to patients (e.g., durable medical equipment, blood glucose monitors, or natural products). These departments often are placed near the prescription department for the convenience of both the patient and the pharmacist.

The Americans with Disabilities Act (ADA) of 1990 has affected almost all businesses, including pharmacies. This federal mandate prohibits discrimination based on any form of disability. To comply with the ADA, pharmacies may be required to adjust counter heights, aisle widths, telephone equipment, doorways, and almost any other physical aspect of their operations. The act allows for reasonableness in designing stores without undue hardship on daily operations. The design goal is to have a store that offers equal access to all products and services for all customers (Laskoski, 1992).

The Heath Insurance Portability and Accountability Act (HIPPA) is a federal mandate designed to protect the confidentiality of patient information. HIPPA considerations in the design and layout of a pharmacy are to ensure that disclosure of protected health information is minimized. Pharmacy managers are to make reasonable efforts to protect the privacy of their patients. Some of the efforts made by pharmacy managers include installation of a partition extending the height of the pharmacy counter, redesigned storage areas for prescriptions that are waiting to be picked up by customers, designated staging areas for patients waiting to be served by pharmacy staff, and private patient consultation areas.

Internal and external environmental factors play a major role in the design and layout of a pharmacy. The age, race, sex, and income levels of consumers are important characteristics that should be addressed. Addressing the needs of a predominant ethnic or age group is beneficial in attracting these potential patrons to a pharmacy. For example, elderly people may be more likely to patronize a pharmacy that has a large section of durable medical equipment.

Designing the exterior of a pharmacy is just as important as design and layout of the interior. When designing the exterior of a pharmacy, one must consider legal requirements, local codes or ordinances that govern materials, the number and sizes of windows, external signage, and the number and placement of doorways.

The exterior design of a pharmacy may need to complement other stores in a shopping center. Many shopping centers place restrictions on the exterior designs of their stores. Pharmacies commonly will try to add defining features (e.g., signage and lighting) that allow their stores to be recognized easily.

The placement of entrances and exits to the shopping center is key to the ease of getting to the pharmacy. The traffic patterns and placement of traffic signals on the roads adjacent to the shopping center affect the convenience of shopping in the pharmacy. Pharmacy managers often negotiate with local officials to have traffic signals at or near the entrance and exit of the center.

The traffic pattern of a shopping center will influence the placement of entrances and exits of the pharmacy. Pharmacy managers wish to maximize the number of patrons that find their store once they are in the shopping center. Pharmacies often desire to be located next to a grocery store or other high-traffic stores to attract cross-shoppers.

Pharmacy Layout

A pharmacy's layout contains numerous cues, messages, and suggestions that communicate to shoppers. A pharmacy manager's goal is to create a mood that welcomes customer traffic, increases time spent in browsing (yet not wasting time searching for needed items), encourages customers to make more purchases than originally planned, and invites them to return to the pharmacy in the future.

The layout or arrangement of in-store fixtures should be designed to move patrons around the pharmacy to obtain the items they need or desire. Ideally, customers should visit as many areas of the pharmacy as possible to increase the probability of impulse purchases.

Pharmacy layout should capitalize on the strengths of the prescription department and pharmacist because they are what make pharmacies unique from other retail outlets. Pharmacy layout should have the prescription department very prominent and visible to patrons in any part of the store (Fig. 24-1). Ideally, consumers should travel past a variety of merchandise on their way to the prescription department. This explains why many prescription departments are located in the rear of a pharmacy. While this layout is popular with pharmacy managers, it is not always popular with consumers. For example, some elderly patrons may find it difficult to walk through the entire store to get to the prescription counter. They may choose to use the drive-through window or frequent a pharmacy that has the prescription counter in the front of the store. The demographics of the population that shops the pharmacy will be very influential to the design of a pharmacy and prescription counter (Walker, 1996).

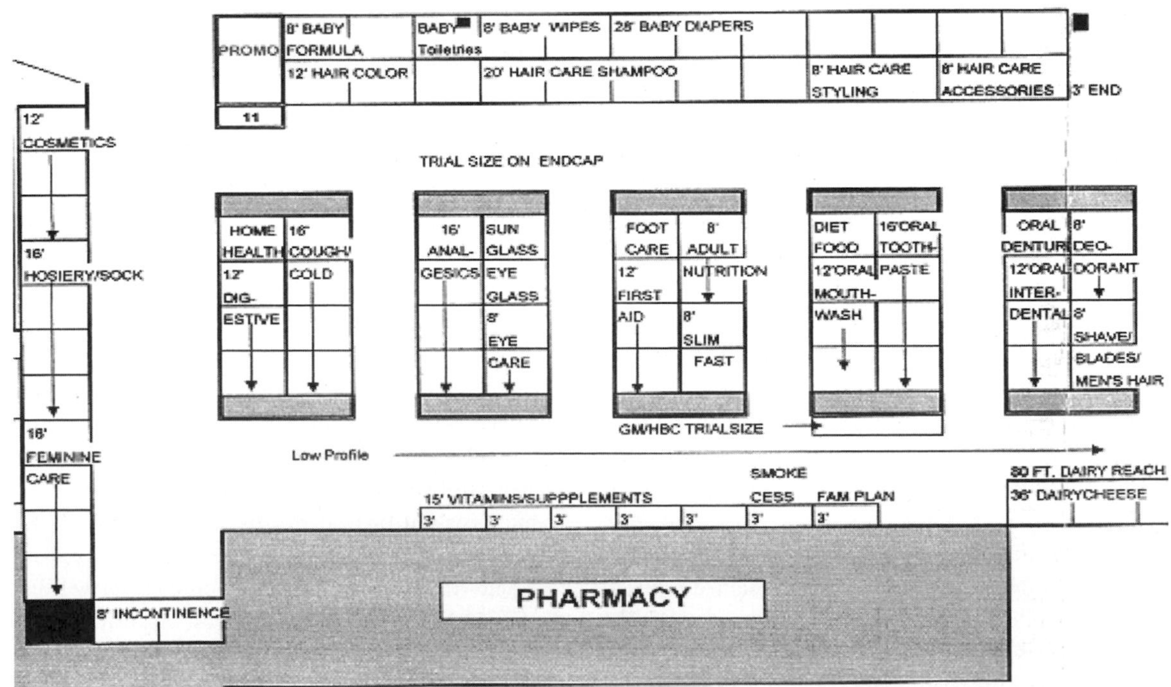

Figure 24-1. Store aisle design.

Gaedeke and Tootelian (1993) discussed two types of store layouts: grid and free flow. In a *grid layout*, all the counters and fixtures are at right angles to one another. Merchandise is displayed in straight, parallel lines, encouraging maximum travel time in the aisles and maximum product exposure. The *free-flow layout* groups merchandise and fixtures into patterns that allow for an unstructured flow of customers. Many of the fixtures are irregularly shaped circles, arches, and triangles. This design is used often in gift and specialty stores, mostly encouraging browsing and impulse buying.

Grid layouts are more common in community pharmacies than free-flow layouts. Aisles are set in straight-line grid arrangements with key departments or service areas located to encourage shoppers to visit the four corners of the store. Departments are arranged to place high-demand items in the rear of the store, promoting traffic past lower-demand and impulse-purchase items. In grid layouts, the prescription department is often located in the back of the store, adjacent to high-demand over-the-counter (OTC) items and other items that may sell better if accompanied by a recommendation from a pharmacist (e.g., durable medical equipment or natural products).

Department placement is done with the intent to entice customers to purchase more than they had intended originally. Some locations in a pharmacy tend to attract more traffic. High-traffic areas are good places to generate additional sales with placement of new product displays or impulse items. In pharmacies, placement of impulse items near or on the prescription counter may increase sales of these items owing to the increased traffic in that area of the store.

In almost any retail business, the risk of theft of merchandise (both by shoppers and by employees) is always present. Pharmacy managers can use store design and layout to minimize losses from theft. High-cost and other items that may be liable to theft generally are placed in open areas where store personnel can observe both the items and shoppers easily. Pharmacies are increasingly using locked cabinets to store items that are liable to theft (e.g., smoking-cessation products and weight-control products). Most states have also enacted laws that require products containing psuedoepherine be kept behind the pharmacy counter despite the fact that it technically has OTC drug status. This has been done to decrease the theft and inappropriate use of psuedoepherine, particularly in the production of methamphetamine. Efforts should be taken not to place high-cost and high-theft items in corners (which are more difficult for personnel to see) or near exits (where it would be easier for shoppers to steal an item leave without being noticed). Many pharmacies use store security personnel, video surveillance equipment, one-way mirrors, and even sensors embedded in products to detect and prevent losses of merchandise.

Pharmacy Merchandising

Merchandising involves the proper placement of goods on pharmacy shelves. The space a pharmacy has for goods to be displayed is limited by the size and design of the store. Pharmacies commonly separate their space into departments or sections that contain major categories of products (e.g., prescription area, cough and cold, headache, and first aid).

Merchandise in a pharmacy tends to flow from one department to the next. This flow is accomplished by placing related departments next to or near each other. *Cross-selling* is the process of selling across departments to facilitate customers purchasing more items than they may have intended originally. Arranging departments in a logical transition from the front to the back of the store will guide shoppers to areas where they may find additional items to purchase. Cosmetics, hair-care products, and health and beauty aids commonly are located near toiletries and feminine hygiene products because consumers who come to a pharmacy to purchase the former products also tend to need the latter (see Fig. 24-1).

Pharmacy aisles are of various lengths and heights. For the convenience of shoppers, aisles tend not be more than 50 feet in length (Raven, 1984). If an aisle is longer, cross aisles should be provided. Cross aisles are a break in a long run of shelving creating an aisle that allows customers to move easily across the store. Cross aisles provide for smooth traffic flow and increase visible space for item placement.

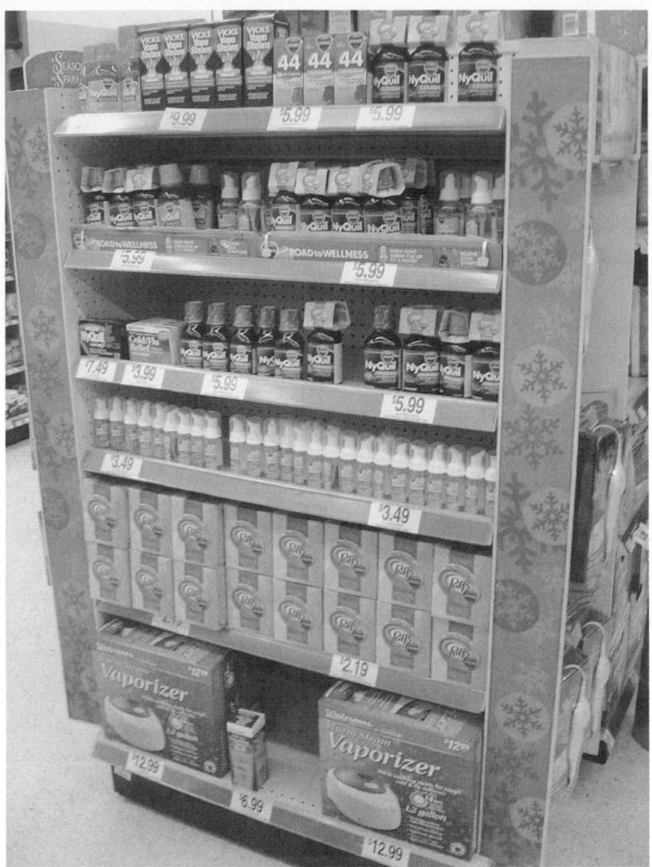

Figure 24-2. End cap.

Many pharmacies use the space at the beginnings and ends of the aisle runs. These spaces often are referred to as *end caps.* End caps often feature displays of promotional and seasonal items, bulk items, impulse items, and new products designed to gain shoppers' attention (Fig. 24-2).

Aisle heights also vary among pharmacies (Raven, 1984). Some smaller pharmacies use a lower aisle height of 54 in. This allows store personnel to see across the entire pharmacy. Larger pharmacies often use fixtures with heights of 60 to 72 in. Higher shelves provide additional space for merchandise and storage. Higher shelves also help consumers to keep eye contact with products in the aisles. Not allowing visibility across aisles is a tool used by retailers to keep the shopper's eye on the items in that section.

When deciding what items and how many of each item to place in a section or a department, pharmacy managers strive for balance between variety and duplication. This balance will vary by and within categories of merchandise. The two considerations to be addressed in achieving such a balance are an understanding of the customers and an analysis of current market trends. Both these considerations address the placement of merchandise to respond to demographics, the type of customer and his or her needs, or market trends, responding to a new or very popular item.

To assist with proper placement of items on shelves, many pharmacy managers use *plan-o-grams.* Plan-o-grams are diagrams that show the placement, space, and management of each item in a particular section of shelves. Plan-o-grams may be produced by manufacturers, wholesalers, corporate pharmacy offices, or the pharmacy staff itself. Plan-o-grams should be based on current sales and market information, as well as on the size and physical characteristics of the items themselves. A properly planned and executed plan-o-gram enables pharmacies to maximize sales and profit opportunities for a given section of space.

Plan-o-grams should arrange products to increase their visibility to consumers. Manufacturers strive to make the fronts and tops of their packaging clearly visible to consumers. A product *facing* is the arrangement of a product one package wide on a shelf. Placement of items on shelves, so that these package facings are visible to consumers, allows for maximum exposure and increases the likelihood of sales. By increasing the facings of a singlc product from two to four, pharmacics have found that sales of that product will increase by 36 percent (Portner, 1996).

When viewing a section in a pharmacy, the most popular items will be placed at eye level for the majority of shoppers (approximately 60 in high). Items placed very high or very low in a section traditionally will be slower-selling items. Customers in North American pharmacies typically scan from left to right when looking at items on a shelf. Items on the shelf should be set vertically, from top to bottom, allowing the customer's eye to scan the shelf across as he or she goes from top to bottom. Pharmacy managers use this concept to cross-merchandise and add items for impulse purchasing. In addition, most customers are right-handed and will grab the item to the right. Consumers commonly find larger-sized products (which generate higher sales and profit margins) kept to the right of smaller-sized products followed by the private label brand.

Pharmacy managers will place some items in more than one department. Fast-moving, high-profit items can be displayed in various departments throughout the pharmacy using a technique known as *cross-merchandising*. For example, displaying facial tissues not only with the paper products but also in the cough and cold section will increase impulse sales of these items.

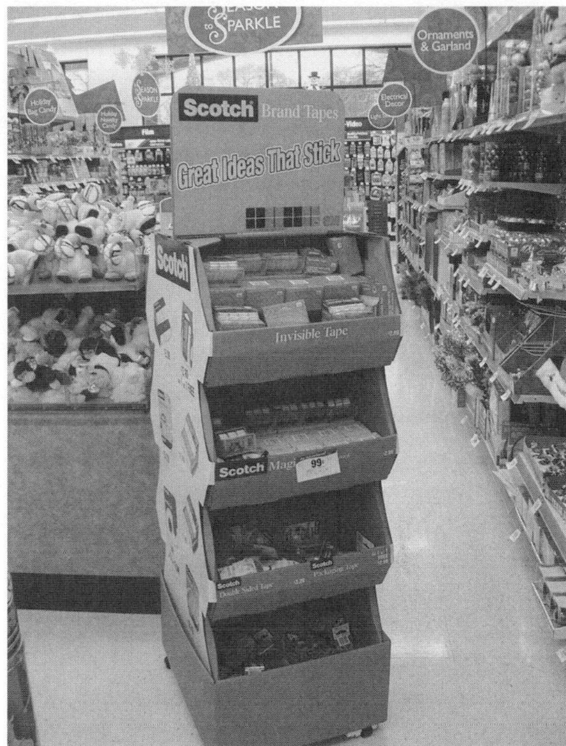

Figure 24-3. Floor stand display.

In addition to placing items in designated sections or departments, pharmacy managers commonly use displays throughout a pharmacy to highlight specific products. Displays often are set in an aisle in front of a shelf to showcase new items or those with special pricing. Floor-stand displays are used to place large quantities of an item on display, making the products easily accessible to consumers. Manufacturers often supply these displays and other promotional materials to pharmacies to highlight their products (Fig. 24-3).

Point-of-purchase materials (signage) also are used to highlight items. Header cards, banners, and price signs are all examples of point-of-purchase materials. These sales aids give product information, demonstrate features, reinforce a sale or special price, and have the ability to generate sales. Other methods used to highlight products are shelf extenders. These are small trays that are attached to a shelf and extend out several inches to highlight an item. Shelf talkers are signs that extend outward from the shelving and "speak" to customers about items or services found in the store.

Merchandising the Prescription Department

The prescription department is the one area that distinguishes a pharmacy from other retail stores that sell similar merchandise. The prescription department should be given a position of prominence in the store. This department usually takes up 300 to 600 square feet of space, having 18 to 24 feet across the front of the department. The prescription department is usually identified with prominent signage or decor to make it easily identifiable to customers to see and use (Fig. 24-4).

Consumers typically view the prescription department as a professional area. When they are able to view the interior of the pharmacy, they should see that this department is clean and well organized. Pharmacy personnel need to exhibit a friendly and professional demeanor because individual attention can distinguish one pharmacy from another.

The front of the prescription department traditionally is used to highlight vitamins and herbal remedies, products that commonly require the advice of a pharmacist for proper use (e.g., glucose monitors), or high-priced specialty items that may be at risk for theft if stocked in a less visible section (e.g., smoking-cessation products). The areas where prescriptions are dropped off or picked up are good places to display new products or impulse-purchase items (e.g., new OTC medications, Chap-Stick, or pill reminders). These areas are also natural spots for small displays of new OTC items that previously were prescription items (e.g., Prilosec™ or Claritin™). The pharmacist's recommendation is one way to increase purchases of these items.

Designing prescription departments with the pharmacist–patient relationship in mind is a

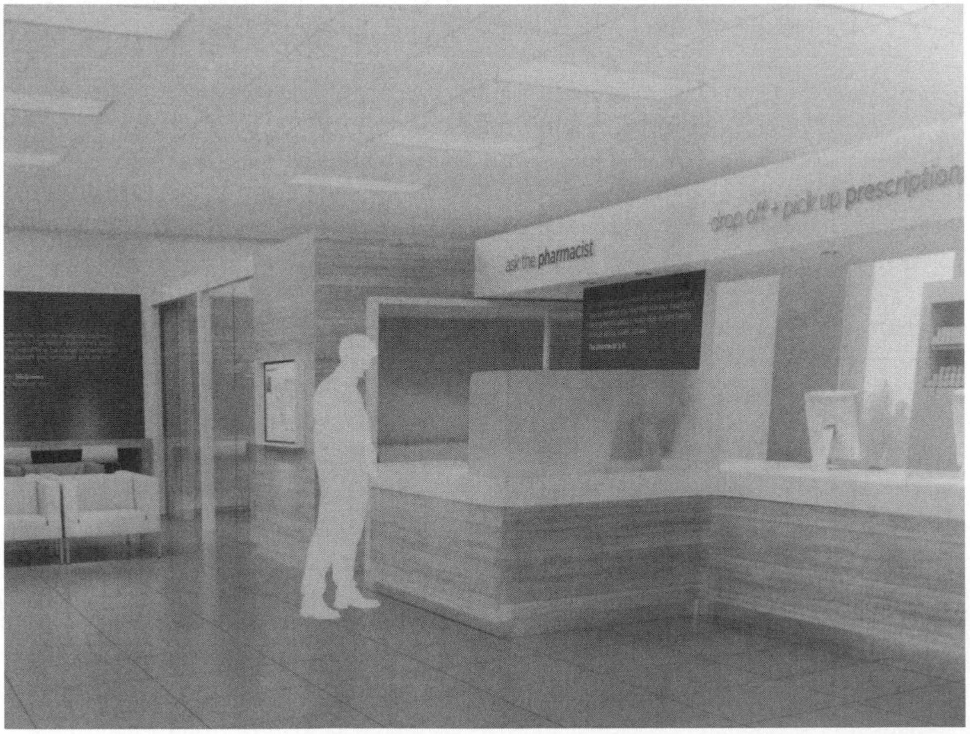

Figure 24-4. Prescription department.

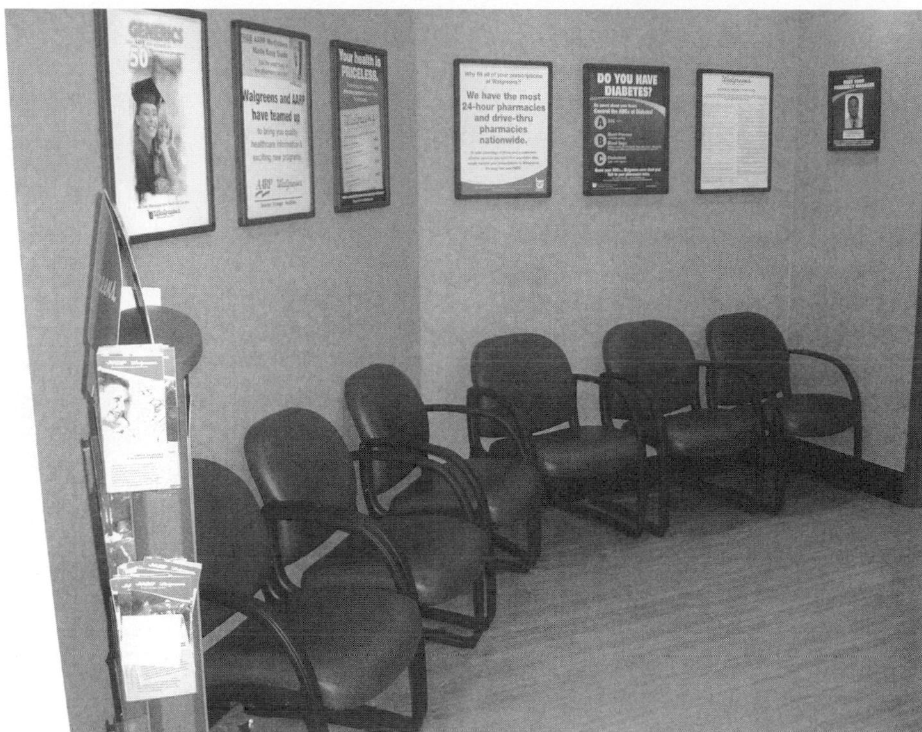

Figure 24-5. Patient waiting area.

merchandising technique intended to have an impact on prescription sales, OTC purchases, and purchases of professional services (e.g., patient education programs, screenings, or immunizations). When pharmacies design prescription departments to be open, patrons feel more comfortable approaching the pharmacy staff with questions. Having the prescription department near other health care items makes the pharmacist's recommendation more likely to result in increased sales of these goods and services.

Some prescription departments are built elevated from the rest of the pharmacy, giving the department an appearance of prominence to the customer. Special lighting may also be used to highlight the pharmacy. The use of brighter lighting in and around the department highlights the pharmacy and draws customers to that area of the store.

Pharmacy design should also include a patient waiting area, a patient consultation area, and in some locations a drive-through window. The patient waiting area provides patients with space away from the sales floor to wait comfortably for their prescriptions. As prescriptions are being filled, customers have an opportunity to view health information or learn more about specific goods or services the pharmacy may offer (Fig. 24-5).

The patient consultation center of the prescription department provides an area for patients and the pharmacist to discuss medications and related patient questions. The consultation center may be as small as an 18-in. window built into the prescription counter or as large as a freestanding patient care center. Patient care centers provide pharmacy staff with a place to offer counseling and medical information and provide screenings for various disease states, therapeutic drug monitoring, and immunizations.

Drive-through windows are seen today in many pharmacies. Patients are able to purchase prescriptions

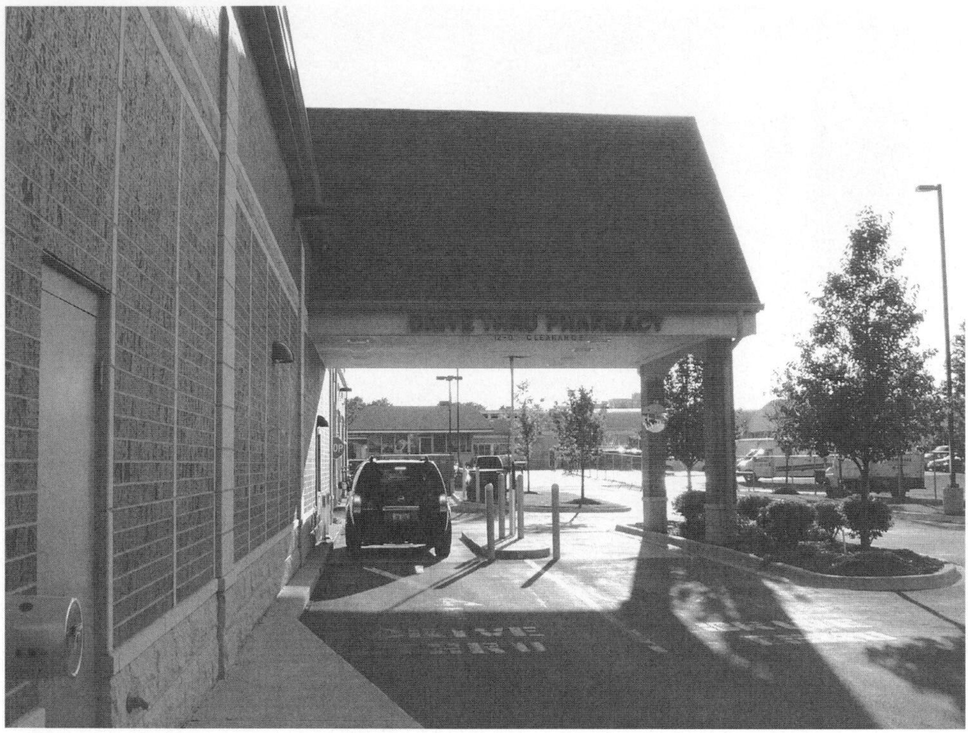

Figure 24-6. Drive-through window.

and limited OTC items without having to leave their cars. Industry measurements have shown that drive-through windows are viewed by customers as an added convenience, increasing stores sales by as much as 7 percent over stores without this convenience (Laskoski, 1992) (Fig. 24-6).

Pharmacies are continually looking for new and better ideas to differentiate themselves from other retail outlets and to offer additional health care services to their customers. Expanding the front end of the store with health related items and services will help differentiate pharmacies from other general merchandisers. Finding a niche area such as compounding, immunizations, or consultative services will develop a different business model based on the needs of their unique customer base. Merchandising these health focused pharmacies places the niche service prominently in the store.

The expansion of health related products and services will attract patients referred to the pharmacy from physicians, hospitals, and health plans. By developing this health care focused model, the pharmacy will develop a greater relationship with the patient and capture more of their health care dollars.

The addition of in-store medical clinics allows customers to receive medical care that is quick, inexpensive, and convenient (Fig. 24-7). Staffed by nurse practitioners and physician assistants that have prescribing authority, patients can choose from a posted list of services provided, receive treatment, and be on their way in less time than at a medical clinic or emergency room. Patients who need OTC or prescription items can pick up these items right in the store.

Retail clinics provide greater access to medical care for common problems. Physicians generally are not happy about this trend and would like to see more

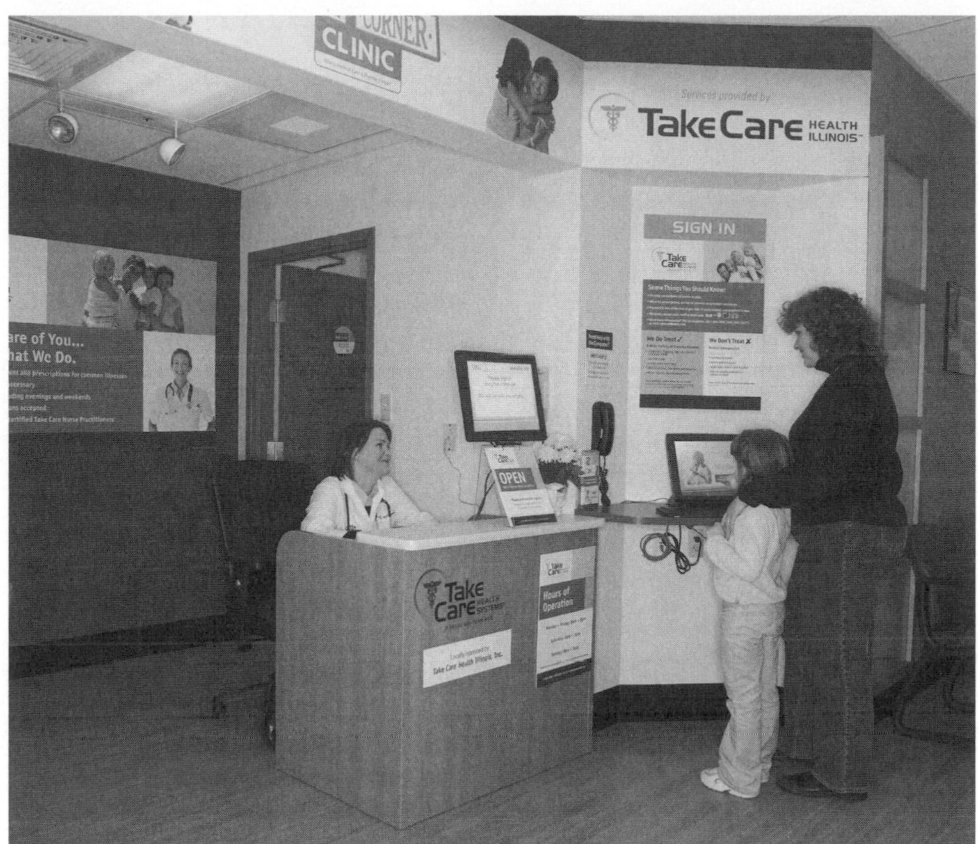

Figure 24-7. In-store medical clinic.

regulations governing in-store medical clinics. Clinics are not intended to replace primary care, and patients who need a higher level of medical attention need to be referred to doctors in a timely manner.

REVISITING THE SCENARIO

Mary Quint, our third-year doctor of pharmacy student, recently visited Healthway Pharmacy. She took some time to understand the factors that made her family so happy to shop there. The pharmacy manager indicated that the store's goal is to create an environment for shoppers that will make the pharmacy easy, fun to shop, and the health care destination of choice for its customers. He explained that the store attempts to satisfy customers' needs by appealing to their senses. What customers see and hear throughout the store is influential to their shopping experience. Customers are assisted by merchandising techniques to find what they need and experience items and services they may not have thought of purchasing. The location is easily accessible to the wide variety of consumers who shop there. All this made Mary think long and hard about continuing to work at Middletown South Pharmacy.

QUESTIONS FOR FURTHER DISCUSSION

1. Given that the female head of household makes the majority of health care decisions for her family, how would you design a pharmacy around the needs of women with families?

2. While customers like the convenience of pharmacies with a drive-through window, what are some potential drawbacks of including them in a pharmacy?
3. How may technology (i.e., smartphones, tablet computers) impact the merchandising practices of community pharmacies?

REFERENCES

Eisenpreis A. 1983. How today's customers shop: What it means to drugstores. *American Druggist* 188:92.

Francke DE. 1974. Accepting things as they are. *Drug Intell Clin Pharm* 8:221.

Gaedeke R, Tootelian D. 1993. *Essentials of Pharmacy Management.* St. Louis: Mosby–Year Book.

Higby GJ. 1997. Pharmacy in the American century: 100 years of change. *Pharm Times* 63:16.

Hilditch J. 1981. Maximizing the value of the sales area. *Pharm J* 227:638.

Laskoski G. 1992. Design: Good, the bad, and the ugly. *American Druggist* 205:38.

Portner T. 1996. *Effective Pharmacy Management: A Comprehensive Presentation of Practical Management Techniques for Pharmacy*, 8th edn. Alexandria, VA: National Community Pharmacists Association.

Raven M. 1984. Drugstore design and layout: Looking at the right angles. *Drug Top* 128:44.

Rodowskas C. 1996. Space allocation and profit maximization. *Pharm Times* 62:70.

Walker G. 1996. Debacle of OTC. *Pharm J* 256:775.

SECTION VI

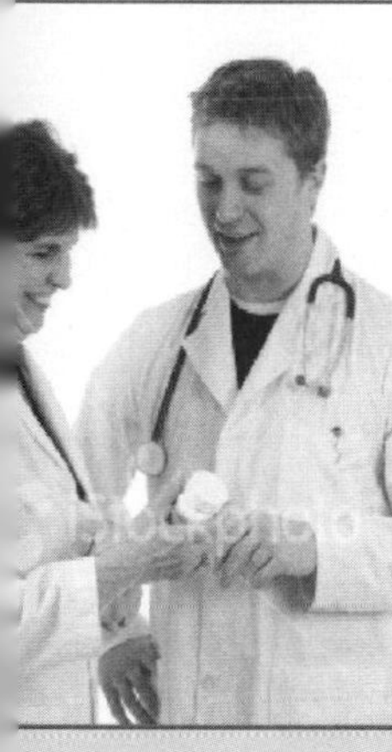

MANAGING VALUE-ADDED SERVICES

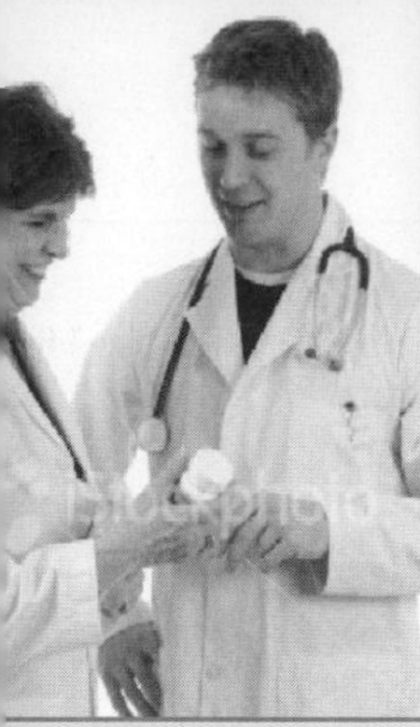

25

VALUE-ADDED SERVICES AS A COMPONENT OF ENHANCING PHARMACISTS' ROLES IN PUBLIC HEALTH

David P. Zgarrick

About the Author: Dr. Zgarrick is Professor and Chair of the Department of Pharmacy Practice in the School of Pharmacy at Northeastern University's Bouvé College of Health Sciences. Dr. Zgarrick received a B.S. degree in pharmacy from the University of Wisconsin and an M.S. and Ph.D. in pharmaceutical administration from The Ohio State University. He has practice experience in both independent and chain community pharmacy settings. Dr. Zgarrick teaches courses in pharmacy management, business planning for professional services, and drug literature evaluation. His research interests are in pharmacist workforce issues, professional service development, and the use of evidence-based medicine by pharmacists.

LEARNING OBJECTIVES

After completing this chapter, readers should be able to

1. Identify factors that should drive the development of value-added pharmacy services.
2. Describe ways that the development of value-added pharmacy services can enhance pharmacists' roles in public health.
3. Describe how the business planning process applies to value-added pharmacy services.
4. Evaluate the market for value-added pharmacy services:
   a. Consumer characteristics and needs
   b. Impact of the internal and external environments
   c. Services already available in the market
   d. Market potential
   e. Consumer willingness and ability to pay for services
5. Evaluate the ability of a pharmacy to provide services that meet consumer needs

SCENARIO

By all accounts, Alan Brouchard, Pharm.D., is a great pharmacist. He graduated at the top of his class in pharmacy school and started a successful career with a pharmacy chain in suburban Chicago. While he enjoyed working with all his patients, he especially liked counseling children and their parents. He had a reputation for being good with kids and informative with their parents, which resulted in many referrals to the pharmacy where he worked.

Last year Dr. Brouchard's wife was offered a job opportunity in Phoenix. While he loved his job in Chicago, his wife's opportunity was too good to pass up, and he knew that there would be positions available in the Phoenix area with his pharmacy chain. He arranged a transfer to another pharmacy in his chain in Sun City (a suburb just northwest of Phoenix). When he arrived, he was anxious to further develop the pediatric services he had started in Chicago. He convinced his pharmacy manager to purchase special equipment to teach children how to monitor their asthma, to remodel the pharmacy to include a private counseling area, and to spend money promoting these services in the local community.

After 3 months, Dr. Brouchard was very disappointed in how his service had been received. On a good week, only one or two persons would come in for his services, and these often were older customers seeking advice for their grandchildren. The pharmacy manager began using the private counseling area to store diabetes supplies (which always seemed to sell as fast as the pharmacy could get them in). Dr. Brouchard did not understand why his services, which were so successful in Chicago, were not nearly as well received in Sun City. He often wondered what he could do to increase the appeal of his services to a larger number of the pharmacy's customers.

CHAPTER QUESTIONS

1. How does an organization's strategic plan affect the kinds of goods and services it offers?
2. How can value-added pharmacy services benefit the needs of populations, in addition to those of individual patients?
3. In what ways is business planning useful in the development of value-added pharmacy services?
4. In addition to patients, who else should be considered consumers of value-added pharmacy services?
5. What information should be gathered before making a decision to offer a value-added pharmacy service? Where and how can this information be gathered?

"BUILD IT AND THEY WILL COME"?

One of the most popular films of the 1980s was *Field of Dreams,* starring Kevin Costner. Costner's character, Roy Kinsella, had moved from a large city to rural Iowa to become a farmer. While working on his farm, he kept hearing a voice that said, "Build it and they will come." At first Roy couldn't figure out what he should be building, or who would come if he did. As the plot progressed, Roy plowed under his cornfield, built a baseball field, and waited for a group of baseball players to come and play. Most of the people in his town thought he was crazy, plowing under valuable corn. Even his wife and family had doubts when they had trouble paying their bills. However, a group of deceased baseball players from the distant past (some Hall of Fame legends, others practically unknown) started coming out of the cornfield every night to play on the field. Roy and his family enjoyed watching these players, but the people in his town still doubted their existence. Eventually, Roy's deceased father showed up to play, and they had a father and son game of "catch" that they both regretted they had not had in the past. By the end of the movie, the players had begun using the field during the day, the people of the town came to see them play, and Roy started charging admission, saving the family farm. Talk about a "Hollywood ending"!

What could *Field of Dreams* possibly have to do with pharmacy in the twenty-first century? On the one hand, if you ask some pharmacists why they offer the goods and services they do, they might just give you an answer similar to if you had asked Roy Kinsella why he built a baseball field in an Iowa cornfield. Maybe it was a voice inside their heads that told them to offer a pediatric asthma consulting service. They may have figured that if they "built" a herbal medicine section in their pharmacy, people would naturally come and purchase these items. Many pharmacists develop goods and services based primarily on their own desires or the needs of their organizations. They may have a personal interest in a particular area or have learned how to provide a specialized service during pharmacy school, residency, or on the job. While offering a good or service based primarily on personal interests or skills may sound like a good thing to do, one very important principle of marketing is being overlooked.

In the real world, Hollywood endings are quite rare. Businesses that develop goods and services based primarily on their own interests, skills, or needs usually end up regretting their time, money, and other resources they had invested. Many of these businesses fail after a short period. This is so because one of the fundamental principles of marketing that is often overlooked by marketers is that the purchase of any good or service or the acceptance of any idea is driven by the *needs of consumers,* not those of the marketer (Kotler, 1997). Contrary to what some people may believe, marketers cannot force consumers to purchase or accept products they do not need. Consumer needs exist regardless of a marketer's products. Successful marketers start by identifying their consumers, evaluating their needs, and developing products (i.e., goods, services, and ideas) designed to meet consumer needs better than their competitors (see Chapters 21 and 22).

All pharmacists and pharmacy organizations are marketers of goods (e.g., prescription and over-the-counter medications, durable medical equipment, candy, greeting cards, and a wide variety of other items) and value-added services [e.g., dispensing prescriptions, delivery, drug utilization evaluation/review, disease-state management, and medication therapy management (MTM)]. A major challenge for any pharmacist or organization is to identify its consumers and evaluate their needs. Pharmacists and pharmacies then must develop products that meet consumer needs, as well as their own personal, professional, and organizational needs. This can be a daunting task, and there is no guarantee of success.

REVISITING THE SCENARIO

At Dr. Brouchard's annual performance review, his pharmacy manager let him know that he would not be allowed to continue to offer pediatric services at the pharmacy. While he was disappointed, he understood why, given the few people who had used the service and the amount of time and money his organization had invested for seemingly little in return. At the same time, he saw that the rest of the pharmacy continued to be successful. Prescription volume was up 10 percent over the past year, and sales of medications for arthritis, diabetes, and heart disease were increasing even faster. Several of the customers he had counseled about their grandchildren had told the pharmacy manager that they were very pleased with Dr. Brouchard's professional manner and advice. He was happy to hear this and thought to himself that if only there were some way, he could continue to offer this level of service to a larger group of patients.

VALUE-ADDED PHARMACY SERVICES AND PUBLIC HEALTH

The profession of pharmacy has long had a profound impact on health. While pharmacists certainly impact the health of individual patients who use drug therapy, they also have the ability to impact the health of the communities they serve. According to the Institute of Medicine (IOM), *public health* is simply "what we, as a society do collectively to assure the condition for people to be healthy (IOM, 2003a)." The primary public health role that many associate with pharmacists is assuring the safe and effective use of medications. For many years this was done primarily through safeguarding the preparation and distribution of drug products. But as pharmacists' roles in health care have evolved over the past generation, so have their opportunities to contribute to society's health and well-being (Capper et al., 2006; Nemire et al., 2010).

Unlike some physicians, nurses and other health professionals who specialize public health practice, the pharmacist's role in public health is not as clearly defined, but is increasingly understood by both health professionals and the public (APHA, 2011). Pharmacists are among the most accessible and available health care professionals. Given the number of pharmacists in the United States (over 280,000, third only to nursing and medicine) and their spread throughout the nation in both urban and rural settings, pharmacists are in an ideal position to both educate patients and advocate for their community's health needs (APhA, 2011c; ASHP 2008). Pharmacists provide health and medication information to both patients and health care professionals. Patients can seek the advice of pharmacists in over 60,000 community pharmacies and in many other practice settings, usually without making an appointment and often at little cost. Pharmacists commonly triage the medical problems of those who seek their advice, particularly in community settings. Pharmacists' ability to refer patients to other health care professionals, or to simply recommend treatment with an over-the-counter product, serve the needs of the public to obtain high quality care while making the most efficient use of health resources.

The IOM establishes three major functions of public health: (1) assessment, (2) policy development, and (3) assurance. Pharmacists have increasingly come forward to play crucial roles in each. In terms of assessment, pharmacists play a unique role in research evaluating the drug use process. Clinical pharmacists and other researchers commonly join forces to determine ideal treatment regimens given clinical, epidemiologic and economic data. Pharmacists and other researchers also work to identify adverse drug events and medications errors (Classen et al., 2005; Lazarou et al., 1998; IOM, 2003b). This and other medication-related research improves health outcomes for individual patients and for society at large. Pharmacists are leaders in their communities, putting them in an ideal position to develop and advocate for policies aimed to improve health. Pharmacists commonly advocate to influence the legislative and regulatory process (see Chapters 20 and 28), especially concerning issues that impact the health of their patients and communities (Matzke, 2011). Pharmacists help assure the health of their communities through activities at a macro level (e.g., administering medication use systems, designing drug benefit plans, educating other health professionals on medication use), as well as at the micro level (e.g., speaking to community groups, developing health education materials, conducting health screening programs) (Hobson et al., 2010). Given the essential roles that medications play in health, pharmacists have come to have a major role in public health preparedness, from serving on local public health boards to emergency preparedness programs designed to assure access to medications and health services after disasters (Woodard et al., 2010; McCrory, 2006).

While pharmacists have long played roles in advancing public health, the formal public health education of pharmacists is a relatively recent development. Curricular guidelines used by schools and colleges of pharmacy now emphasize preparation of pharmacy students to provide both patient-specific and population-based care (AACP, 2004). Accreditation standards for Doctor of Pharmacy programs also state that the graduates must possess a set of minimum skills and attributes to practice, including the ability to provide population-based care (ACPE, 2011). Schools and colleges of pharmacy have responded by integrating public health concepts into the curriculum. Many colleges have developed courses designed specifically to teach public health concepts to pharmacy students (Westrick, 2009; Smith et al., 2008, Sankaranarayanan et al., 2008). A small but growing number of universities have developed joint degree programs, allowing graduates to obtain both the Doctor of Pharmacy (PharmD) and Master of Public Health (MPH) degrees (AACP, 2005).

One particular area of public health where pharmacists have recently taken a major role is immunization delivery. Pharmacists had long educated their patients and the public regarding the risks and benefits of immunizations. Yet millions of Americans who should be receiving immunizations, particularly the influenza and pneumococcal vaccines, were not receiving them, resulting in large amounts of preventable morbidity and mortality (HHS, 2000). Given their accessibility, pharmacists began to promote their role as immunizers. Pharmacy organizations such as the American Pharmacists Association (APhA) developed certification programs to enhance pharmacists' skills as immunizers (APhA, 2011a), and state pharmacy associations advocated for legislative and regulatory changes necessary to give pharmacists the legal authority to immunize. Today pharmacists in all 50 states have the legal authority to immunize under protocols developed with physicians (NABP, 2011). Almost 150,000 pharmacists now provide influenza, pneumococcal, and a variety of other vaccinations to an estimated 20 million patients per year (APhA, 2011b). More importantly, pharmacists stepping forward to provide immunizations have increased the number of Americans receiving immunizations. This has served to improve the health of our society and decrease the complications from preventable diseases (Steyer et al., 2004).

Pharmacists are posed to offer a variety of additional public health services. Pharmacists play a role in increasing the health knowledge of people in their communities (Gazmararian et al., 2010). Given their accessibility, pharmacists can play a valuable role in enhancing the health literacy in underserved and ethnically diverse communities (Vargas et al., 2011; Gerber et al., 2010). Pharmacists can play an active role in disease prevention and health promotion, particularly through their efforts in health education, screening, and wellness programs (Eades et al., 2011). Pharmacists have taken the lead in substance abuse education and prevention and treatment, particularly among health care professionals (Cerulli et al., 2008). And pharmacists have recently stepped forward to take the lead in efforts to protect the environment by offering medication and syringe disposal services (Gray-Winnett et al., 2010).

REVISITING THE SCENARIO

Given the demographic characteristics of Sun City, Dr. Brouchard determined that offering immunization services at the pharmacy could serve the health needs of the community, as well as create a new stream of revenue and source of additional profits. Working with his local public health department, he was able to determine which types of immunizations are most needed by patients in his community (influenza, pneumococcal, herpes zoster (shingles)), and joined a local task force to educate the community about the benefits of being vaccinated. Dr. Brouchard and several staff pharmacists in his chain attended a pharmacy-based immunization delivery certificate program as the first step toward preparing themselves and their pharmacies to offer immunizations.

APPLYING THE BUSINESS PLANNING PROCESS TO PHARMACY SERVICES

One way that many pharmacists identify consumer needs, develop new ideas for new goods and services, and manage the risks involved in any business venture is by using the business planning process (see Chapter 5). Business planning helps decision makers evaluate their markets and environments. It gives managers the freedom to explore new ideas without having to invest their resources in actually developing and offering the product. Using the business planning process does not guarantee that consumers will accept a product, or that the product will meet organizational goals. However, business planning does help managers identify risks and assess the likelihood that a new product will be successful.

Many administrators require their pharmacists to develop written business plans to justify offering a new good or service. This helps administrators decide whether to allocate scarce resources (especially money, time, and personnel) to the development of any new good, service, or idea. One important aspect to keep in mind about business planning is that administrators and pharmacists are under no obligation to implement a plan. If the research done in the planning process indicates that a product will not meet consumer or organizational needs, that it would not be feasible to offer, or that the risks involved are greater than the organization cares to take, a decision can be made simply not to move forward with the plan. While it takes an investment of time to develop a business plan, not implementing a plan that is likely to fail consumes far less time, money, and other resources than developing a new good or service that does in fact fail.

Applying the business planning process to the development of value-added pharmacy services is not that different from how the process is used to evaluate any other good, service, or idea. One of the first steps when starting the business planning process should be to identify the organization's strategic plan and mission statement. Since these documents represent the road map for what the organization wishes to become and how it plans to get there, it is important that the development of any new good or service bears these in mind. One question that almost all administrators will want to have answered is how the implementation of any new value-added service will help their organization achieve the goals set out in the strategic plan.

It is important to recognize that mission statements and strategic plans vary among types of organizations, especially within health care. The mission statement and strategic plan of a not-for-profit children's research hospital likely will be different from that of a for-profit pharmacy chain (Table 25-1). The aspects of a professional service that will need to be emphasized in a business plan will vary as well. The not-for-profit children's research hospital may want to see how a new professional service will result in enhanced clinical outcomes or benefit the greatest number of children at the lowest possible cost. On the other hand, a for-profit pharmacy chain may want to see how the service will expand its market share or enhance its shareholders' value of owning the company.

The next step of the business planning process is to explore the prospects for various types of value-added services. At this point, it is helpful to have several ideas for value-added services that could be implemented. One of the best ways to do this is to observe and speak with pharmacy department customers. This is essential to learn more about their needs and can help business planners learn more about their environments (which will be important later in the process). Other sources for ideas about value-added pharmacy services include colleagues, professional organizations, pharmacy magazines and journals, professional meetings and seminars, the Internet, consultants, books, and full-service wholesalers.

The next step in exploring the prospects for value-added pharmacy services is to learn more about the potential services that have been identified. Many pharmacists start this process by performing a literature review about potential services using electronic databases such as PubMed (National Library of Medicine, 2011) or International Pharmaceutical Abstracts (IPA) (Thomson Scientific, 2011). These databases can identify primary and secondary literature

Table 25-1. Mission and Vision Statements

St. Jude Children's Research Hospital Mission Statement

The mission of St. Jude Children's Research Hospital is to advance cures, and means of prevention, for pediatric catastrophic diseases through research and treatment. Consistent with the vision of our Founder Danny Thomas, no child is denied treatment based on race, religion, or a family's ability to pay (St. Jude, 2007).

Walgreen's Mission Statement

We will treat each other with respect and dignity and do the same for all we serve.

We will offer employees of all backgrounds a place to build careers.

We will provide the most convenient access to health care services and consumer goods in America.

We will earn the trust of our customers and build shareholder value (Walgreen's, 2007).

that provide additional information about services, descriptions of services implemented by others, and research studies that evaluate the outcomes of similar services. Nonmedical Internet search engines such as Google (www.google.com) also may be helpful, but users should be cautioned that finding valuable information can be difficult given the vast amount of information available on the Internet (see Chapter 7).

Professional pharmacy and medical organizations (e.g., the American Pharmacists Association [APhA], the American Society of Health-System Pharmacists [ASHP], the National Community Pharmacists Association [NCPA], and the American Medical Association [AMA]) and health care organizations (e.g., the American Diabetes Association [ADA] or the American Heart Association [AHA]) also provide valuable information about many health conditions and value-added services. This information is important not only in the development of a service but also in justifying the need for a service with consumers and administrators. These organizations also provide treatment guidelines and additional resources that can be used when developing an operations plan for a service (see Chapter 26).

While learning more about potential value-added pharmacy services, it is a good idea for business planners to speak with others about their ideas. Many pharmacists who have already developed value-added services will gladly share what they have learned. Visiting a setting where value-added pharmacy services are already in place not only provides evidence of how these services actually work but also will answer many questions pharmacists may have later in the planning process. Other pharmacists, technicians, and pharmacy employees may have experienced value-added services in their prior practice experiences and may provide insights into how they work. Other health care professionals can provide feedback about additional services that they or their patients may need. Payers [e.g., insurance companies, health maintenance organizations (HMOs), employers, and governments] may be willing to share ideas about value-added pharmacy services that may improve the health of their constituents while saving them money.

Most administrators and organizations do not like to be surprised to learn that their pharmacists are working on proposals for new value-added pharmacy services. It is important to work with administrators and organizations early in the business planning process, not only to keep them informed, but also to learn what they desire from an administrative standpoint. Taking the views of administrative and organizational personnel into account throughout the process increases the likelihood that administrators will support and provide the resources necessary to implement value-added pharmacy services in the future.

REVISITING THE SCENARIO

Dr. Brouchard began to think about what the chain he worked for might want in a professional service. The chain's mission statement said that it was dedicated to providing patients with high-quality customer service while using modern technology. The chain also was open to developing innovative ways to attract new customers and serve its existing customers. The chain's strategic plan stated that it had a rapid expansion plan and that it expected new services to contribute a 15 percent return on investment (ROI) after 3 years. After reading this, Dr. Brouchard knew that his chain was open to developing new services, but that he also would need to show that such services could contribute to profitability in a relatively short time.

With this in mind, Dr. Brouchard thought of some ideas for value-added pharmacy services that he could pursue. He was excited about the possibility of adding immunization services to his pharmacy, but realized that much of their service would occur only from September through December when patients obtained their annual influenza vaccinations. In addition to offering immunizations, he wanted to offer a service that had the potential to consistently serve patients and generate revenue throughout the year. While his pediatric asthma service was not successful, he thought about the possibility of offering the same service to an adult population. He had seen a report on the local news mentioning that the prevalence of asthma had increased greatly in their area over the last several years. Like many other pharmacies serving patients of the "baby boom" generation and older, his pharmacy dispensed many prescriptions for hypertension and hyperlipidemia. And while diabetes was not a specialization he had considered previously, it was difficult to ignore the number of prescriptions the pharmacy filled for diabetes medications, and the amount of diabetes supplies the pharmacy sold. Dr. Brouchard had even read in a pharmacy journal that insurance companies and government agencies were paying pharmacists to provide diabetes education services. He decided to research these ideas and then approach his pharmacy manager to get her thoughts.

Table 25-2. Types of Consumers of Value-Added Pharmacy Services

Patients and caregivers
- Patients with particular disease states
- Patients who have multiple disease states
- Patients who are not well controlled on existing therapy
- Caregivers of children, elderly, and invalid

Physicians and other health care professionals
- Primary care physicians (e.g., family medicine, general medicine, internal medicine, and pediatricians)
- Specialists (e.g., cardiology and endocrinology)
- Physician assistants, nurse practitioners, and nurses
- Dentists, podiatrists, and veterinarians

Payers
- Private insurance companies
- HMOs
- PPOs
- Government programs (i.e., Medicare, Medicaid, and state and local assistance programs)
- Employers

EVALUATING THE MARKET FOR PHARMACY SERVICES

In evaluating potential professional services, it is essential to consider the characteristics of the market where they will be offered. Since any service first must satisfy consumer needs before a pharmacist's personal, professional, or organizational goals can be met, evaluating potential consumers of a service should be the first aspect of the market that is considered.

When pharmacists think of potential consumers of their value-added services, the first (and often only) group they think about is patients. After all, pharmacists interact with patients on a daily basis. While patients are essential to the success of most value-added pharmacy services, pharmacists must remember that groups of consumers other than patients may benefit from pharmacy services as well.

When planning for value-added pharmacy services, pharmacists often classify consumers into one of the three Ps. These three groups are patients, physicians and other health care professionals, and payers (Table 25-2). Pharmacists should consider the characteristics and needs of each of these groups in the business planning process carefully.

While almost all patients that pharmacists interact with have some type of medication-related need (e.g., a drug product, advice about an adverse drug effect, etc.), not all patients may need the same level of service that pharmacists can provide to patients (Hepler and Strand, 1989). It is important for pharmacists to identify subgroups of patients who may benefit more directly from their services. For an asthma service, patients with asthma and other pulmonary conditions likely would have a much higher need for the service than others without these conditions. For a diabetes education service, there are different categories of patients with diabetes on which one may focus (e.g., type I versus type II). In addition to the patients themselves, caregivers (e.g., parents, adult children of the elderly, etc.) should be identified and their needs evaluated. The primary need of patients is health care, the purpose of which is to allow them to live a longer, healthier life. Pharmacists who can convince their patients and caregivers that their services will improve their quality of life will be on their way to developing a successful service.

Pharmacists desiring to implement new professional services must develop relationships with other health care professionals such as physicians, nurses, therapists, and other specialists. For these relationships to be successful, all parties much recognize the others' needs and be prepared to describe how each would benefit from their interactions (Doucette and McDonough, 2002). For example, a pharmacist starting an anticoagulation monitoring service needs patient referrals from cardiologists, internal medicine specialists, vascular surgeons, and other health professionals who prescribe anticoagulation therapy. The pharmacist also will need information about these patients and perhaps even support from the professionals in billing for their services. On the other hand, the health care professionals need information not only about their patients but also about drug therapy. Physicians also are faced with challenges in today's managed-care environment and often need to see many patients per day to maintain their financial viability. Physicians are seeking ways in which they can use other health care professionals to extend their services while maintaining high-quality patient care. Chapter 26 describes ways in which pharmacists can develop and enhance these relationships with other health care professionals.

One group of consumers whose needs often are overlooked by pharmacists is payers. Today, almost all pharmacy goods and services are paid for by someone other than the patient. These third-party payers include insurance companies, managed-care plans, employers, and local, state, and national government agencies. While pharmacists often do not enjoy interacting with third-party payers, most of them have needs that pharmacists are in a unique position to satisfy. Payers generally want to obtain high-quality goods and services at the lowest possible costs. Payers also recognize that they may not always be getting optimal benefits from their expenditures, especially those related to drug therapy. Pharmacists, given their expertise in drug therapy and proximity to their enrollees, are in an ideal position to help payers improve the quality of care while controlling costs, especially through their value-added services. Pharmacists who can demonstrate the value of their services to payers often find that payers are willing to encourage their enrollees to use pharmacy services (Cranor et al., 2003; Kepple, 1998).

Another aspect of the market for any value-added pharmacy services that must be considered is the competition. When identifying competitors, it is important to acknowledge exactly what services the pharmacy will pursue. When identifying competitors for value-added services, pharmacists often limit their search to other pharmacies and pharmacists. While this may be appropriate for traditional pharmacy goods and services (e.g., dispensing drug products), pharmacists considering new value-added services must cast a much broader net. Many value-added services offered by pharmacists are still at the introductory point of their product life cycles. Few, if any, other pharmacies may offer these services in a particular market. Other types of competitors may be very well established. For example, while diabetes education services currently are not offered in many community pharmacies, physicians and certified diabetes educators (CDEs; who can be physicians, nurses, pharmacists, and other health care professionals) have provided this service for a number of years (Zrebiec, 2001).

Recognizing and evaluating competitors is an important part of the business planning process (see Chapter 5). While competitors have an established clientele and represent a potential threat to the success of a new pharmacy service, much can be learned from observing how they provide their services. If a large number of competitors are present in a market, it may be daunting to think about how a new value-added pharmacy service can compete successfully for customers. Competitors represent a challenge, but with proper research and planning, many pharmacists find that these challenges can be overcome. One way is by positioning a value-added pharmacy service in the market such that consumers see it as different from the others. This is often referred to as *niche marketing* (Doucette and McDonough, 2002). A pharmacy that hopes to establish a smoking-cessation service may find that there are a number of established competitors in the market (e.g., physicians, psychologists, support groups, and over-the-counter medications). However, if the pharmacy can provide its service in such a way that consumers recognize that it is more convenient or has higher quality or a lower price than competitors, the pharmacy and its smoking-cessation service still can be successful in the market.

For any value-added pharmacy service to be viable, there must be a sufficiently large number of consumers in the market who may be willing to purchase the service. Investing too many resources into a service that benefits a small number of consumers ultimately will lead to the demise of any business venture. Several sources can be used to determine the size of a market for a professional service. The easiest place for a business planner to start is to review a pharmacy's patient profiles, purchasing and financial records, and other internal data. Knowing how many prescriptions are filled for different classes of medications will help the planner determine which conditions are the most prevalent among the pharmacy's patients. The only downfall of this method is that the information is limited to the pharmacy's current clientele. Many pharmacies would like to provide value-added pharmacy services that attract new patients.

Reviewing the literature to learn the potential size of a market can be helpful, especially epidemiologic studies that describe the incidence and prevalence of a condition. Unfortunately, most of these studies are done on a state, national, or even international level and may not provide information about the prevalence of a condition in a specific geographic location of interest. This disadvantage can be offset in part by combining a literature review with interviews of other health care professionals in the pharmacy's market area. They may be able to provide specific information about the number of patients they and other professionals treat. Another tool that can be used by pharmacists to learn more about the characteristics of a population is geographic information systems (GIS). GIS combines maps with demographic databases (e.g., US Census data) to provide an analysis of the characteristics of a city, a neighborhood, or even a series of blocks around a pharmacy, hospital or other health providers. GIS programs such as SimplyMap have been used by pharmacies and researchers to learn more about the health needs of their surrounding communities (Geographic Research, Inc., 2011).

Perhaps the most direct way to determine the size of a market for a value-added pharmacy service is to perform a market research study. Survey research methods can be used to gather information from potential customers. Not only can this information be used to determine the number of potential consumers in a specific area, but it also can provide additional information about consumers that can be useful in developing a value-added pharmacy service (e.g., if/where they currently obtain this service, their level of satisfaction with the service, and their willingness to obtain the service from a pharmacist). Some of the drawbacks of market research include the specialized knowledge and skills needed to carry out a study properly, the amount of time involved, the relatively high cost of performing this type of research, and the potential biases that are inherent in any type of survey research. Several studies have been published that used market research to determine the size and characteristics of potential consumers of value-added pharmacy services (Larson, 2000; MacKinnon and Mahrous, 2002; Zgarrick and Cohen, 2000).

Even if there are a large number of consumers who might be interested in obtaining a value-added service from a pharmacist, the ultimate question that must be answered is whether these consumers are willing and able to make this purchase. Some consumers (especially patients) may be very interested in obtaining a health service from a pharmacist and actually may say on a survey that they would be willing to pay for this service. However, saying that one is willing to pay does not always result in an actual payment for the service. The consumer may not have the means to pay the price being charged by the pharmacist or may be able to obtain the service from another provider (e.g., a physician) for only a small insurance co-payment.

Other groups of consumers also may be interested in obtaining a value-added pharmacy service and often have the financial resources to do so (e.g., other health care professionals, insurance companies, employers, and government agencies). However, pharmacists often find that these groups may not be willing to pay for these services until the pharmacist can demonstrate the value of the services (Poirier et al., 1999). This has created a "chicken and egg" problem for many pharmacists. Pharmacists state that they cannot show the value of the service unless they are given the opportunity to provide it. At the same time, pharmacists state that they cannot afford to provide the service unless they are paid to do so. Several demonstration projects have been performed to show the value of professional services to various groups of consumers (Bluml et al., 2000; Singhal et al., 1999). Medicare now provides opportunities for pharmacists to receive payment for MTM services through the Part D program (see Chapters 20 and 26).

Several methods can be used to learn more about consumers' willingness and ability to pay for value-added pharmacy services. Getting to know consumers and observing their habits (e.g., what services they will pay for, how much they will pay, and what they expect to receive in return) can be done relatively quickly and easily in most practice settings. Market research and the pharmacy literature also can be used, but it is important to remember that what a consumer says he or she will pay for a value-added pharmacy service on a survey may not represent what he or she actually will pay when presented with the service in the pharmacy. The only way to truly determine what a consumer will pay for a value-added pharmacy service is to offer the service, charge a price, and observe whether the consumer actually makes the purchase. Unfortunately, this can occur only after the decision has been made to offer the service.

REVISITING THE SCENARIO

Dr. Brouchard's research into asthma and diabetes services provided him with a great deal of information. The initial data he gathered from Internet searches and the primary and secondary literature showed him that each service had a great deal of potential. He visited other pharmacies in the Phoenix area that offer these services and came away impressed with the level of service that was being provided and the pharmacists' willingness to share their ideas.

He started looking into the market for each of these services. After checking the pharmacy's dispensing records, he found that there were a large number of patients using asthma medications and even more on lipid-lowering and cardiac medications, but the largest proportion of patients was using oral hypoglycemic drugs. The local physicians he spoke with said that they were having a difficult time keeping up with all the new cases of diabetes they were seeing. Several of them stated that they employed nurses who were CDEs to educate their patients about their disease (especially since Medicare was now paying them to do so) but that it took more than 6 months from the time they made the initial diagnosis until they could get a patient into an education program. Dr. Brouchard imagined that at least some of these patients might be willing to pay out of their own pockets to get this service sooner than to wait more than 6 months to get this education from a nurse. Besides, how well could the nurse explain all the medications that are being used to control this disease?

CAN A PHARMACY MEET THE NEEDS OF CONSUMERS?

Assuming that there is a consumer need and a market for a particular value-added pharmacy service, business planners must ask themselves a very serious question before moving forward. The question is whether they actually can meet the needs of consumers. The answer to this question is not always as easy as it might appear and requires a great deal of introspection on the part of the pharmacist and the organization.

One way that business planners can begin to answer this question is to perform a SWOT (i.e., *s*trengths, *w*eaknesses, *o*pportunities, and *t*hreats) analysis, as described in Chapters 4 and 5. SWOT analysis has applications in both strategic and business planning. In strategic planning, managers perform this analysis on a broad level, looking at the entire organization. In business planning, strengths, weaknesses, opportunities, and threats are evaluated only at the level of the service being considered. Strengths and weaknesses are considered to be internal to an organization and are the easiest to *initially* evaluate. They are also within the control of the organization, such that aspects that initially may be considered a weakness can be addressed and perhaps even become strengths of the organization in the future. Opportunities and threats generally exist external to an organization. Given that they are part of the external environment, they often are more difficult to control. At the same time, they can exert just as much influence over the success or failure of a value-added pharmacy service as internal strengths and weaknesses.

The first internal factor that an organization planning to offer a value-added pharmacy service should evaluate is the resources necessary to provide the service. This starts with the abilities and interests of the staff to provide the service. Many value-added pharmacy services require knowledge and skills beyond those used in traditional dispensing functions. Staff members may need to attend educational or training programs to gain the appropriate knowledge and skills. Some value-added services require that pharmacists become certified to demonstrate their knowledge and skills in an area before the service may be offered. States that allow pharmacists to administer immunizations often require that they become certified before providing this service (APhA, 2011a). Medicare and many insurance companies require that pharmacists become CDEs before they will compensate them to provide diabetes education services. Becoming a CDE involves completing a series of exercises, gaining experience in providing diabetes education to patients, and passing an examination. This process generally takes about 2 years to complete (NCBDE, 2011).

It may go without saying that pharmacists should be interested in providing value-added services if they are to be successful. It is important to match the skills and interests of a pharmacy's personnel with the services the pharmacy intends to provide. If a pharmacist is not interested in providing a service, can he or she be provided with an incentive that may motivate him or her to do so? If not, can another pharmacist be hired who has the interest and skills needed to be successful?

Pharmacies need a number of physical resources to provide most value-added services. This usually begins with the layout of the pharmacy. Many value-added pharmacy services require at least some degree of privacy. Unfortunately, pharmacies that were designed to maximize the efficiency of the dispensing process often do not have a private office or classroom space necessary to provide patient care services. Other physical resources that may be needed to provide a professional service include computer hardware and software, testing devices, medical supplies, and office supplies.

Pharmacies must be willing to commit financial resources to the development of a new value-added service. Working capital is needed to support the purchase of equipment, supplies, and marketing before the service can be offered. Since most services do not bring in enough income initially to cover their costs, money also will be needed to pay employees and continue to purchase needed resources. Business planners must consider how much working capital they will need to start a service and how long they are willing to support the service before it is expected to cover its costs and contribute to organizational profitability.

Another internal resource that cannot be overlooked is support from administrators within the organization. Administrators who "buy in" to the concept of providing value-added services are much more likely to support their development and provide the resources needed to get them off the ground. Pharmacists hoping to gain this support generally work to convince administrators how implementation of value-added services will help the organization reach its overall goals.

Many external factors, such as patient demographic trends, can be viewed as both a threat and an opportunity for the development of a value-added service. The aging of the population and the increased reliance on drug therapy as a medical treatment have greatly increased the number of prescriptions filled in pharmacies (NACDS, 2011). This can be seen as a threat, in that pharmacy staff may not have as much time to provide other nondispensing services. On the other hand, these trends also present opportunities for pharmacists to implement new services that meet the increased patient needs for health information and drug therapy monitoring.

Other external factors that may influence the success or failure of a value-added service include laws and regulations affecting practice (both of pharmacists and of other health care professionals), reimbursement and compensation policies of third-party payers, competition from other pharmacies and health care providers, technology, and the ever-changing needs of health care consumers themselves. While these factors may be difficult for business planners to influence, they are manageable. Pharmacists willing to take a proactive stance regarding these issues (especially though involvement in professional organizations and other groups) are often able to have their voices heard and help to shape the policies that affect their futures.

REVISITING THE SCENARIO

After assessing the market for a diabetes education service, Dr. Brouchard took a closer look at his environment. Within his pharmacy and organization, the outlook appeared to be fairly positive. While he was not a diabetes expert, he spoke with another pharmacist in his chain who had become a CDE. The chain had supported his training and even helped to pay part of the certification fee. Dr. Brouchard always had been willing to learn more, so he decided that he would start the certification process on his own.

The pharmacy already had a private counseling area, and he figured that he could use some of the resources he had obtained for the pediatric asthma service for a diabetes service. When he told his pharmacy manager about his idea, she seemed excited, especially given the potential for the service to attract new customers to the pharmacy. She did stress that her budget to support this service was limited and that he would have to provide more financial projections that she could share with her district manager before she could commit to support the service.

There were threats that could have an impact on the service, but none that he felt could not be overcome. There always seemed to be more prescriptions to be filled, and reimbursements for dispensing were decreasing as a result of the Medicare Part D programs that so many of their patients participated in. However, he knew that his chain was developing new technologies that would speed the dispensing process and that his state had just changed its pharmacy practice act to allow pharmacy technicians to perform more functions. He figured that these changes should help to free up some time that would be needed to develop, market, implement, and ultimately provide a diabetes education service to patients.

Dr. Brouchard investigated first steps he could take in developing a diabetes education service. Through his contacts with the local public health department, he was able to identify senior centers and community groups that were interested in learning more about health-related matters. Dr. Brouchard created a couple of 20-minute health education presentations aimed at the general public, one of them focusing on preventing diabetes, another on living a healthy lifestyle with diabetes. He began to visit local senior and community centers to give these presentations. These presentations included a diabetes screening and risk assessment so that participants could gauge their need for additional health services. Finally, Dr. Brouchard began the process of becoming a CDE. This would allow him not only to bill for services he would provide for his patients, but to also visit local physicians, nurses, and other health care professionals to keep them up-to-date on the latest advances in diabetes therapies.

CONCLUSION

Pharmacies, like any other business or organization, cannot build new value-added services with the hope that consumers will adopt them. Pharmacy managers can use business planning as a tool to evaluate consumer needs, the market, and their own resources before deciding whether to offer value-added services and which services would be most likely to succeed. While using business planning does not guarantee that a new value-added pharmacy service will be successful, the process helps pharmacy managers manage the risks involved in this increasingly important area of their organizations.

■ QUESTIONS FOR FURTHER DISCUSSION

1. What are the dangers of the "build it and they will come" approach to developing professional services?
2. Compare and contrast the types of value-added pharmacy services that most likely would be accepted at St. Jude's Children's Research Hospital and Walgreen's (see Table 25-1).
3. What obligations does a pharmacy have to provide goods and services that benefit their community, in addition to those that benefit individual patients?
4. How would have developing a business plan before he implemented the pediatric asthma service in Arizona helped Dr. Brouchard?
5. Given what you now know, what other professional services also may be viable for Dr. Brouchard to offer at his new pharmacy?

REFERENCES

Accreditation Council for Pharmacy Education (ACPE). 2011. *Accreditation Standards and Guidelines for the Professional Program in Pharmacy Leading to the Doctor of Pharmacy Degree.* Chicago, IL: ACPE.

American Association of Colleges of Pharmacy (AACP). 2004. Center for the Advancement of Pharmaceutical Education (CAPE). *Educational Outcomes.* Alexandria VA: AACP.

American Association of Colleges of Pharmacy (AACP). 2005. Council of Deans and Council of Faculties Joint Task Force. *White Paper on the Role of Schools and Colleges of Pharmacy in Developing and Administering Combined/Dual Degree Programs.* Alexandria VA: AACP.

American Pharmacists Association (APhA). 2011a. Pharmacy-Based Immunization Delivery Certificate Program. Available at the APhA Web site, www.pharmacist.com; accessed on October 13, 2011.

American Pharmacists Association (APhA). 2011b. Pharmacist Immunization Center. Available at the APhA Web site, www.pharmacist.com; accessed on October 14, 2011.

American Pharmacists Association (APhA). 2011c. Public Health. Available at the APhA Web site, www.pharmacist.com; accessed on August 5, 2011.

American Public Health Association (APHA). 2011. Policy Statement: The role of the pharmacist in public health. Available at the APHA Web site, www.apha.org; accessed on August 5, 2011.

American Society of Health-System Pharmacists (ASHP). 2008. ASHP statement on the role of health-system pharmacists in public health. *Am J Health Syst Pharm* 65:462.

Bluml BM, McKenney JM, Cziraky MJ. 2000. Pharmaceutical care services and results in Project ImPACT: Hyperlipidemia. *J Am Pharm Assoc* 40:157.

Classen DC, Pestotnik RS, Lioyd JF, Burke JP. 2005. Adverse drug events in hospitalized patients. Excess length of stay, extra costs, and attributable mortality. *JAMA* 294:2858.

Capper SA, Sands CD. 2006. The vital relationship between public health and pharmacy. *Int J Pharm Educ* 2:2.

Cerulli J, Grassi M, Blustein L, et al. 2008. A student-driven initiative for substance abuse prevention. *American Association of Colleges of Pharmacy Annual Meeting.* 72:NIL.

Cranor CW, Bunting BA, Christensen DB. 2003. The Asheville Project: Long-term clinical and economic outcomes of a community pharmacy diabetes care program. *J Am Pharm Assoc* 43:173.

Doucette WR, McDonough RP. 2002. Beyond the 4 P's: Using relationship marketing to build value and demand for pharmacy services. *J Am Pharm Assoc* 42:183.

Eades CE, Ferguson JS, O'Carroll RE. 2011. Public health in community pharmacy: A systematic review of pharmacist and consumer views. *BMC Public Health* 11:582.

Gazmararian J, Jacobson KL, Pan Y, Schmotzer B, Kripalani S. 2010. Effect of a pharmacy-based health literacy intervention and patient characteristics on medication refill adherence in an urban health system. *Ann Pharmacother* 44:80.

Geographic Research, Inc. 2011. SimplyMap Web-based application. Available at http://www.geographicresearch.com/simplymap/; accessed on October 14, 2011.

Gerber BS, Cano AI, Caceres ML, et al. 2010. A pharmacist and health promoter eam to improve medication adherence among Latinos with diabetes. *Ann Pharmacother* 44:70.

Gray-Winnett MD, Davis CS, Yokley SG, Franks AS. 2010. From dispensing to disposal: The role of student pharmacists in medication disposal and the implementation of a take-back program. *J Am Pharm Assoc* 50: 613.

Hepler CD, Strand LM. 1989. Opportunities and responsibilities in pharmaceutical care. *Am J Pharm Educ* 53:7S.

Hobson EH, Haines SL, Van Amburgh JA. 2010. Meeting the challenge of public health information delivery in the digital age. *J Am Pharm Assoc* 50:214.

Institute of Medicine (IOM) of the National Academies, Committee on Assuring the Health of the Public in the 21st Century. 2003a. *The Future of the Public's Health in the 21st Century*. Washington, DC: National Academies Press.

Institute of Medicine (IOM) of the National Academies, Committee on Quality Health Care in America. 2003b. *Crossing the Quality Chasm: A New Health System for the 21st Century*. Washington, DC: National Academies Press.

Kepple SR. 1998. Pharmacists in Asheville, North Carolina, pick up city paychecks for diabetes services. *Am J Health Syst Pharm* 55:10.

Kotler P. 1997. *Marketing Management: Analysis, Planning, Implementation, and Control*, 9th edn. Upper Saddle River, NJ: Prentice-Hall.

Larson RA. 2000. Patient willingness to pay for pharmaceutical care. *J Am Pharm Assoc* 40:618.

Lazarou J, Pomeranz BH, Corey PN. 1998. Incidence of adverse drug reactions in hospitalized patients: A meta analysis of prospective studies. *JAMA* 279(15):1200–5.

MacKinnon GE, Mahrous H. 2002. Assessing consumers' interest in health care services offered in community pharmacies. *J Am Pharm Assoc* 42:512.

Matzke GR. 2011. Health-care policy 2011: Implications for pharmacists. *Ann Pharmacother* 45:412.

McCrory PH. 2006. Disaster planning lessons learned from Hurricane Katrina. *ASHP Midyear Clinical Meeting* 41:PI-140.

National Association of Boards of Pharmacy (NABP). 2011. *Survey of Pharmacy Law*. Mount Prospect, IL: National Association of Boards of Pharmacy.

National Association of Chain Drug Stores (NACDS). 2011. *The Chain Pharmacy Industry Profile: 2010*. Alexandria, VA: National Association of Chain Drug Stores.

National Certification Board for Diabetes Educators (NCBDE). 2011. NCBDE Web site. Available at www.ncbde.org; accessed on October 14, 2011.

National Library of Medicine. 2011. Pub Med Web site. Available at www.ncbi.nlm.nih.gov/sites/entrez; accessed on October 14, 2011.

Nemire RE, Ward CT, Whalen K, et al. 2010. Public health matters: The role of the pharmacist and the academy. *Curr Pharm Teach Learn* 2:2.

Poirier S, Buffington DE, Memoli GA. 1999. Billing third party payers for pharmaceutical care services. *J Am Pharm Assoc* 39:50.

Sankaranarayanan J, Ridgway JE, Olsen KM, Fletcher CV, Baldwin JN. 2008. Content mapping of public health in the Pharm.D. program for programmatic development. Paper Presented at the Annual Meeting of the American Association of Colleges of Pharmacy. http://www.allacademic.com/meta/p269953_index.html.

Singhal PK, Raisch DW, Gupchup GV. 1999. The impact of pharmaceutical services in community and ambulatory care settings: Evidence and recommendations for future research. *Ann Pharmacother* 33:1336.

Smith KM, Talbert J, Steinke DT. 2008. Design of a public health/pharmaceutical policy course for pharmacy students. *American Association of Colleges of Pharmacy Annual Meeting*. 72:NIL.

Steyer TE, Ragucci KR, Pearson WS, et al. 2004. The role of pharmacists in the delivery of influenza vaccinations. *Vaccine* 22:1001.

St. Jude Children's Research Hospital. 2007. Mission Statement, St. Jude's Web site. Available at www.stjude.org; accessed on October 2007.

Thomson Scientific. 2011. International Pharmaceutical Abstracts Web site. Available at www.thomson.com/content/scientific/brand_overviews/ipa; accessed on October 14, 2011.

US Department of Health and Human Services (HHS). 2000. *Healthy People 2010: Understanding and Improving Health*. 2nd edn. Washington DC: US Government Printing Office.

Vargas J, Dang C, Subramaniam V. 2011. Public health approaches in ethnically diverse populations. *Drug Top* 155:4.

Walgreen's. 2007. Mission Statement, Walgreen's Web site. Available at www.walgreens.com; accessed on October 2007.

Westrick SC. 2009. College/school of pharmacy affiliation and community pharmacies' involvement in public health activities. *American Association of Colleges of Pharmacy Annual Meeting.* 73:NIL.

Woodard LJ, Bray BS, Williams D, Terriff CM. 2010. Call to action: Integrating student pharmacists, faculty, and pharmacy practitioners into emergency preparedness and response. *J Am Pharm Assoc* 50:158.

Zgarrick DP, Cohen E. 2000. Consumer demand for disease management services in a chain of grocery store community pharmacies. *J Am Pharm Assoc* 40:158.

Zrebiec J. 2001. A national job analysis of certified diabetes educators by the National Certification Board for Diabetes Educators. *Diabetes Educ* 27:694.

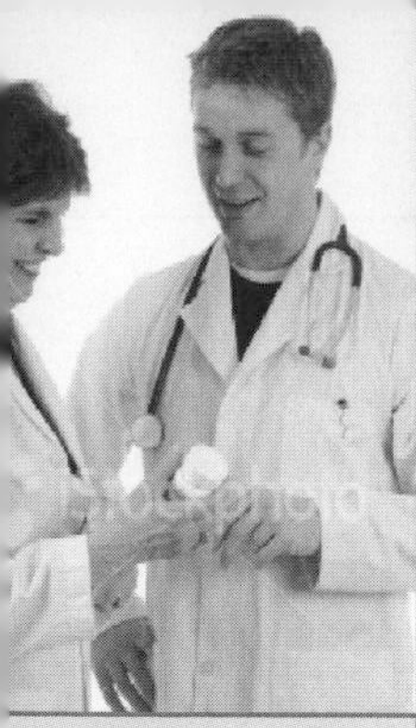

26

IMPLEMENTING VALUE-ADDED PHARMACY SERVICES

Randal McDonough

About the Author: Dr. McDonough is co-owner and Director of Clinical Services at Towncrest and Medical Plaza Pharmacies in Iowa City. He is also an Adjunct Professor (Clinical) at the University of Iowa College of Pharmacy. Dr. McDonough received a B.S. in pharmacy, an M.S. in pharmacy administration, and a Pharm.D. from the University of Iowa College of Pharmacy. At his community practice in Iowa City he has developed and implemented several pharmacy services, including pharmaceutical case management (PCM), medication therapy management (MTM), immunization services, and health screenings. He is board certified in geriatrics and pharmacotherapy. He is invited frequently to speak about practice development and implementation and has published numerous articles and book chapters on these topics.

LEARNING OBJECTIVES

After completing this chapter, readers should be able to

1. Describe the types of value-added services that pharmacists have implemented in their practices.
2. Discuss the components of a value-added service to consider before implementation.
3. Recognize the key components of a policies and procedures manual.
4. Discuss management of the marketing mix during service implementation.
5. Describe the role that collaborative practice agreements have in developing value-added pharmacy services.
6. Describe strategies for pricing and obtaining compensation for value-added pharmacy services.

SCENARIO

Carol Smith, the pharmacist-owner of Care-Rite Pharmacy, is interested in expanding her clinical services. Her pharmacy is located in a city with a population of approximately 100,000 people. Although she has not implemented any specific value-added services in the past, patients and other health care providers recognize her practice as customer friendly and service oriented. She has two full-time pharmacists and two part-time pharmacists who have been working at the pharmacy for a number of years (range 5 to 15 years). Recently, they have completed a strategic plan, a strengths, weaknesses, opportunities, and threats (SWOT) analysis, and a survey of their patients. The results of the patient survey identified their key target market as women 50 years of age and older. Initially, they had wanted to implement a diabetes educational program, but their market research determined that a local hospital sponsored an American Diabetes Association (ADA)-recognized program. The hospital is a strong presence in their community, and the hospital's diabetes educators were not interested in collaborating with local pharmacies. Also, they looked into developing a community-based anticoagulation service, but after some checking into the reimbursement for this type of service, they realized that this service would not be feasible financially. Their market research did show that there was a need in their community for a MTM program. They already had a large percentage of high-risk patients who were taking four or more chronic oral medications and had several chronic medical conditions. Many of these patients expressed a need for assistance with medication management issues. They also serve a large percentage of patients eligible for Medicaid and/or Medicare and they saw an opportunity to provide MTM services for those patients who may be eligible according to their drug plan. Also, they noted that there was not a similar program elsewhere in the community.

CHAPTER QUESTIONS

1. What are the different types of value-added services that pharmacists have implemented in their practices? Describe the medication management process for each.
2. What are the components of a value-added service that pharmacists should consider and plan before implementation?
3. Why is a policies and procedures manual important to successful service implementation?
4. How should pharmacists manage the marketing mix during the implementation of value-added services?
5. How can a collaborative practice agreement help pharmacists implement value-added services?
6. How much do pharmacists typically charge for their value-added services? What strategies have been successful in obtaining reimbursement from patients? From third-party payers?

INTRODUCTION

As discussed in previous chapters, implementing value-added pharmacy services requires a comprehensive strategic plan that includes a mission statement, SWOT analysis, goals and objectives that the practice hopes to achieve, and strategies to achieve the objectives. This plan provides direction for the practice and guides the allocation of resources and efforts. As the scenario demonstrates, the planning process helped Carol, the pharmacist owner, identify a service that fits with the pharmacy's strategic plan, yet has a niche in the marketplace. Pharmacists can implement many types of services in their practices, but it is essential that they do some market research to determine the opportunities and threats in the marketplace to ensure the success of the new service. Also, it is important to assess the pharmacists' motivations and abilities to provide a service. Ultimately, the success of any service depends both on market opportunities and the pharmacists' ability to provide the service.

TYPES OF VALUE-ADDED PHARMACY SERVICES

Value-added pharmacy services can be thought to exist along a continuum (see Fig. 26-1). On one end of the

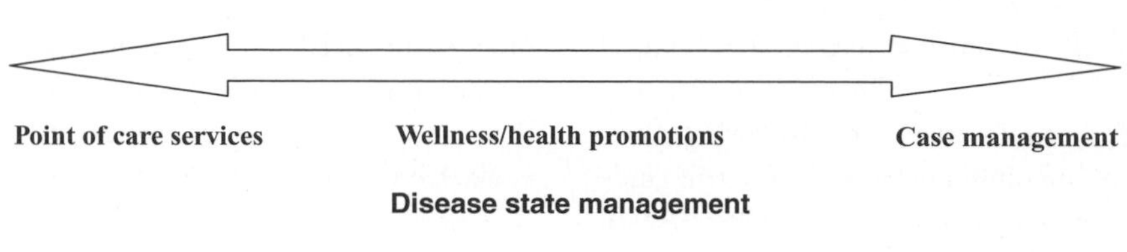

Figure 26-1. Value-added pharmacy services continuum.

continuum, pharmacists are more narrowly focused on drug therapy issues that occur during the dispensing functions (i.e., point of care). On the other end of the continuum, pharmacists provide ongoing drug therapy management services for select individuals who have multiple comorbidities requiring complex therapies (i.e., case management). Other types of services fall between these two ends of the continuum. For example, disease-state management programs, clinical services such as anticoagulation or lipid clinics, and health screening services fall somewhere in the middle of the value-added service continuum. Some services such as MTM can be focused or comprehensive and therefore can fall anywhere within the continuum. Focused MTM services can occur during the dispensing when a drug therapy problem is identified and the pharmacist performs a targeted intervention. Comprehensive MTM service is at the other end of the continuum and the pharmacist provides a comprehensive medication review (CMR), identifies problems with the patient's drug therapy, develops a medication action plan (MAP) and a personalized medication record (PMR) in which they share with the patients, and finally the pharmacist sends her patient workup to the physician or other health care provider.

Regardless of the service being provided, the clinical activities and process of medication management provided by pharmacists implementing value-added services are similar along the continuum. These clinical activities or patient workups have been described elsewhere (McDonough, 1996; Strand et al., 1988, 1992). The medication management process includes collection of pertinent patient data regarding the patient's medical and medication histories, evaluation or assessment of this information, identification of a problem occurring with the patient's medication, development of a plan of action to resolve the problem, and implementation of the plan, including follow-up as needed. Implementing a plan to manage drug therapy typically involves communication with the patient (i.e., patient education), as well as with practitioners (e.g., physicians). Appropriate documentation of patient care activities is an integral component of value-added services.

A number of studies have examined the impact that pharmacists can have delivering drug therapy management services at the point of care during the dispensing process (Christensen et al., 1999; Dobie and Rascati, 1994; Knapp et al., 1998; Rupp, 1988, 1992; Smith et al., 1999). The information that needs to be collected at the point of care may not be as comprehensive as for other services along the continuum. For example, during the dispensing process, it may be determined that the patient has an allergy to a specific medication. By focusing efforts on resolving this problem, data is collected pertaining to this allergy, an alternative is identified, the physician is called, the pharmacist's recommendation is made, the medication is changed, and the pharmacist documents a quick patient note (in the patient dispensing record) to complete the process. While the clinical process in this scenario is narrowly focused, this is an essential and clinically relevant service commonly performed by pharmacists.

Pharmacist' monitoring/screening services and wellness/health-promotion programs are the next level of value-added services along the continuum. These types of services, although relatively narrowly focused, require more patient data collection and may be delivered over an extended period. Documentation may be more comprehensive, with a patient chart being created in addition to the dispensing record. The clinical process remains the same as the point-of-care service but occurs separate from the dispensing function. Examples of ongoing monitoring services include pharmacist-managed anticoagulation services (Ansall et al., 1997; Davis and Sczupak, 1979; Knowlton et al., 1999; McCurdy, 1993; Norton and Gibson, 1996; Reinders and Steinke, 1979) and lipid management services (Furmaga, 1993; Simpson et al., 2001; Tsukuki et al., 1999). Health-promotion/screening programs also have been developed in community pharmacies in areas of smoking cessation (Kennedy et al., 2002), osteoporosis screening (Elliott et al., 2002), and lipid screenings with cardiovascular assessment (Madejski and Madejski, 1996; Tice and Phillips, 2002).

The next types of clinical services along the continuum are those which pertain to disease-state management. These services occur separately from the dispensing function over an extended period but have an added feature of ongoing patient education and an extensive review of drug therapy as it relates to attainment of the patient's therapeutic goals. A comprehensive patient chart is created, patient sessions may last from 15 to 60 minutes, and pharmacists may review the entire medication profile, although their efforts are focused more on the disease state they are following. Pharmacist-managed hypertension (Hawkins et al., 1979; McKenney et al., 1973, 1978; Reinders et al., 1975), diabetes (Baran et al., 1999; Berringer et al., 1999; Coast-Senior et al., 1998; Jaber et al., 1996; Schilling, 1977; Swain and Macklin, 2001; Tiggelaar, 1987), and asthma (Grainger-Rousseau et al., 1997; Herbog et al., 2001; Kneoll et al., 1998; Pauley et al., 1995; Rupp et al., 1992) disease-state management programs have been cited frequently in the literature.

The most comprehensive of drug therapy management services is that of case management. In this situation, pharmacists are responsible for complete patient workups. A thorough patient history needs to be taken, a comprehensive review of all medications is done, and the patient is followed for an extended period. These services also occur separate from dispensing and can be the most challenging for pharmacists. Patients' medical problems can be complex, and multiple physicians often are involved. Several studies have investigated the impact of pharmacists' reviews in high-risk patients in the community setting. (Cowper et al., 1998; Hanlon et al., 1996; Petty et al., 2002).

COMPONENTS OF A VALUE-ADDED PHARMACY SERVICE

Once it is determined which service is to be implemented, it is important to put some thought into what the service will look like and how it will be delivered at the practice. As discussed previously, regardless of the type of service (i.e., diabetes, lipids, asthma, etc.), the medication management processes used by pharmacists remain relatively the same. Some component of the service will require the pharmacist to collect patient clinical information, including laboratory data. The pharmacist also needs to assess the patient information that has been collected and make a clinical decision regarding the appropriateness of the therapy. Patient education is a component of each type of service, but may be emphasized more so with certain services (e.g., wellness programs and services focused on disease-state management). Lastly, some consideration should be given to the clinical outcomes that the pharmacists want to achieve when implementing the service.

Data Collection

Patient data collection is a critical component of any value-added service. The information collected provides pharmacists with important baseline and monitoring parameters for patients. The amount and type of information needed from the patient or other health care providers may differ depending on the service, but nonetheless, this information is the foundation on which the other components of the service are built. Forms can be developed to help pharmacists collect this information (see Figs. 26-2 through 26-4). In addition, some consideration should be given to how this information will be stored (e.g., paper charts or electronic patient database). The information that

Patient History Form

Name: ____________________ Phone: (H) ____________ (W) ____________________

Address: __________________ City: ___________ State: ___________________

Date of Birth: ________ Height: ______ Weight: ______ Gender: ________

Marital Status: ____ Pregnancy Status: ____

Medical Alerts (examples; hearing aids, prosthesis, heart valves, eyeglasses, artificial hips): ____

____

Allergies/reactions:

____________________________ ____________________________

____________________________ ____________________________

Smoking History:

_____ Never Smoked

_____ Packs Per Day for ______Years

_____ Stopped_____ Years Ago

Caffeine Hostory:

_____ Never Consumed

_____ Drinks Per Day

_____ Stopped __________ Years Ago

Alcohol History:

_____ Never Consumed

_____ Drinks Per Day

_____ Stopped ____ Years Ago

Dietary History:

_____ Number of Meals Per Day

_____ Food Restrctions (explain)

Other: ______________________________

____

Since health information may change periodically, I will notify the Pharmacist, to the best of my ability, of any new medications (prescription and non-prescription), any changes in directions of medicines, any new allergies, drug reactions or health condition changes. I authorize any releases of information and insurance benefit payments to the above pharmacy on my behalf.

______________________________________ ____________________

Signature Date

This information is requested by your Pharmacist as required by state regulations so that he/she can provide appropriate pharmacy services to you. This information will be kept confidential.

I do not wish to complete this form and WILL NOT HOLD THE PHARMACY RESPONSIBLE FOR ADVERSE SIDE EFFECTS I MAY INCUR.

______________________________________ ____________________

Signature Date

Figure 26-2. Patient history form.

Care-Rite Pharmacy

Patient Medical History Form

Medical History: Have you or any of your blood relatives had (mark all that apply)

Disease State	Self	Relative
High Blood Pressure		
Asthma		
Cancer		
Depression		
Lung Disease		
Diabetes		
Heart Disease		
Stroke		
Kidney disease		
Mental Illness		
Substance Abuse		
Other		

Medical Problems: Have you experienced or do you have any of the following?

Disease	Yes	No	Disease	Yes	No
Frequent urinay infections			Sores on legs or feet		
Difficulty with urination			Known blood clot problems		
Frequent urination at night			Leg pain or swelling		
Known liver problems			Unusual bleeding or bruising		
Trouble with certain foods			Anemia		
Nausea/Vomiting			Thyroid Problems		
Constipation/Diarrhea			Known hormone problems		
Bloody or black stools			Arthritis or joint problems		
Abdominal pain or cramps			Muscle cramps or weakness		
Frequent heartburn/cramps			Memory problems		
Stomach ulcers			Dizziness		
Shortness of breath			Hearing or visual problems		
Coughing up phlegm or blood			Frequent headaches		
Chest pain or tightness			Rash or hives		
Fainting spells or passing out			Change in appetite/taste		
Thumping or racing heart			Walking or balance problems		

Figure 26-3. Care-Rite Pharmacy patient medical history form.

Care-Rite Pharmacy
Medication History and Medical History

Collected by: ______________________________ **Date:** ________________

Patient Name: ____________ Sex ______ Birth Date ______ Ht _____ Wt _____ LBW _____ Race ______

Prescribed Medications (Rx and OTC)					
Name/Strength	**Dose/Sig**	**Duration**	**Indication**	**Dr**	**Comments**

Past Medications Not Currently Taking (Rx and OTC)					
Name/Strength	**Dose**	**Duration**	**Indication**	**Dr**	**Reason for Stopping**

Figure 26-4. Care-Rite Pharmacy medication history and medical history.

should be collected from the patient includes demographic information, medical history, family history, and medication history. Since some of the information may need to be collected from other providers and health care institutions, an authorization to release medical information should be signed by the patient and kept as part of the chart (see Fig. 26-5). Lastly, pharmacists should ensure that their site is in compliance with the Health Insurance Portability and Accountability Act (HIPAA—See Chapter 28) and reinforce to their patients that the information they provide is confidential and secure at the pharmacy.

Pharmacy-Based Laboratory Monitoring/Screening Services

Although pharmacists can receive objective patient data from local laboratories or from physicians, it may be decided that it is more convenient for the patient and pharmacist if a laboratory monitoring/screening service is performed at the point of care. Several types of monitors and equipment can be purchased by pharmacists and integrated into their practices. For example, pharmacists who implement wellness programs may purchase a body-fat analyzer, a weight scale, or a monitor that measures lipid and blood glucose levels. Alternatively, pharmacists who develop a diabetes program may obtain a device that measures the glycosylated hemoglobin ($A1_c$) of patients. Also, some pharmacists may decide to develop a women's health program and purchase a bone densitometer that measures bone mineral density to determine fracture risk owing to osteoporosis.

Pharmacies implementing monitoring/screening services must become familiar with the Clinical Laboratory Improvement Amendments of 1988 (CLIA). CLIA was enacted to ensure that all medical laboratories meet quality standards. These amendments are administered by the Centers for Medicare and Medicaid Services (CMS), which is responsible for laboratory registration, certificate generation, surveys, and surveyor guidelines for development and training. Tests typically performed by pharmacists in pharmacies (e.g., glucose, lipid panels, hemoglobin $A1_c$, and international normalization ratio [INR] tests) are considered *CLIA-waived* tests. CLIA-waived tests are considered by the Centers for Disease Control and Prevention (CDC) and the Food and Drug Administration (FDA) to be simple to administer and have little risk of error. Currently, 40 tests have been approved for certificate of waiver (COW) (Centers for Medicare and Medicaid Services, 2003).

If a pharmacy is interested in performing waived tests as part of its services, it must complete a COW. Instructions for how to obtain a COW can be found at www.cms.hhs.gov/CLIA. The COW should be sent to the local CMS office. CMS will assign the pharmacy with a CLIA number and send the pharmacy a CLIA fee-remittance coupon. Pharmacies must pay a nominal fee for the COW ($150 in 2011), and the COW must be renewed every 2 years. After receiving the CLIA number, the pharmacy may start providing the service. Pharmacists providing waived tests agree to follow good laboratory practices that include following the manufacturer's instructions on instrument operation and maintenance, performing quality-control procedures, appropriately documenting test data, and storing the monitoring equipment and its reagents properly (Rosenthal, 2000).

In addition to CLIA, pharmacists should be knowledgeable about the Occupational Safety and Health Act (OSHA) that regulates workplace safety. In particular, pharmacists who perform laboratory tests that require finger sticks are at risk from exposure to blood-borne pathogens. Pharmacies that perform these tests should have a blood-borne pathogen exposure control plan (BPEPC) that describes who should be trained about the hazards of blood-borne exposure, precautions that need to be taken to prevent exposure, and what to do when an exposure incident occurs (Rosenthal, 2000). More information regarding OSHA and an example BPEPC can be found at the OSHA Web site (www.osha.gov).

Medication Management Protocols

The next component of a value-added pharmacy service is the medication management that pharmacists will provide once they have collected the patient's

AUTHORIZATION TO RELEASE MEDICAL INFORMATION

Date: ______________________ Date of Birth: ______________________

SSN: ______________________

Patient Name:

____

Address:

____

I, the undersigned, do hereby grant permission for the above named pharmacy to obtain from or release to:

____

(Name of person or institution the information will be coming from)

____

(Address of person or institution the information will be coming from)

The following information from the patient's clinical record:

____

____

____

I understand that this information will be used for the purpose of:

- ❐ Providing information to allow pharmaceutical care to be provided to the patient
- ❐ Providing information to the physician regarding the care provided by the Pharmacist
- ❐ Supporting the payment of an insurance claim
- ❐ Other:

____

This authorization will be valid for the period of twelve months unless otherwise specified below.

I understand that I may revoke this consent at any time by sending a written notice to the above named pharmacy. I understand that any release which has been made prior to my revocation which was made in reliance upon this authorization shall not constitute a breach of my rights to confidentiality. I understand that I may review the disclosed information by contacting the above named pharmacy.

______________________ ______________________

Signature of Patient or Patient's Authorized Representative/Date — Relationship of Authorized Representative

____

Pharmacy Representative/Date

Specific authorization for release of information protected by state or federal law - I specifically authorize by writing my initials beside the category and signing below the release of data and information relating to:

- ❐ Substance abuse
- ❐ Mental Health
- ❐ AIDS/HIV

____

Signature and date of Patient or Patient's Authorized Representative

❐ Release mailed or information sent ______________________

Signature/Date

Prohibition on Redisclosure

This form does not authorize redisclosure of medical information beyond the limits of this consent. Where information has been disclosed from records protected by federal law for alcohol/drug abuse, by state law for mental health records or HIV/AIDS related records, federal requirements (42 CFR Part 2) and state requirements (Iowa Code chs..228/141) prohibit further disclosure without the specific written consent of the patient, or as otherwise permitted by such law and/or regulation. A general authorization for the release of medical or other information is not sufficient for these purpose. Civil and/or criminal penalties may attach for unauthorized discloure of alcohol/drug abuse, mental health or HIV/AIDS information.

Figure 26-5. Authorization to release medical information.

clinical information and laboratory data. During this component of the service, pharmacists will assess patients, determine if they are reaching their goals of therapy, identify and resolve any drug therapy problems, and develop a care plan that helps to guide the pharmacists' follow-up and monitoring of the patients. For some services, protocols may be developed to help guide the pharmacists' therapeutic decisions (e.g., anticoagulation clinic protocols). For others, general decision pathways may be used to guide the pharmacists depending on the clinical situation that may occur during the patient assessment (e.g., lipid management programs). The protocols may be specific (e.g., adjustment of warfarin given a specific target INR) or more general without specific drug therapy recommendations regarding patients' therapy. For example, in comprehensive MTM services, a protocol may be developed to describe what clinical activities the pharmacists will perform at each patient visit, the documents that will be created from the services provided, and the communication/documentation that the pharmacist provides to the physician or prescriber to resolve identified drug therapy problems. The protocols and clinical decision pathways should be evidence based and supported by national guidelines and/or the primary literature. Protocols and clinical decision pathways for many disease states and conditions are gathered by the Agency for Healthcare Research and Quality (AHRQ) and can be obtained from their Web site at www.guidelines.gov.

Patient Education

Patient education is a component of each type of value-added pharmacy service. The comprehensiveness of the education differs though, depending on the service being implemented. For example, pharmacists implementing lipid screenings may see patients for a limited time (during the screening) and provide them with baseline education to help them understand their cardiovascular risk factors, fasting lipid panel results, and lifestyle-modification strategies. On the other hand, pharmacists providing diabetes educational services may provide more comprehensive education by determining the patients' educational needs, providing ongoing educational services to help them achieve their self-management goals, and assessing if the patients are achieving their therapeutic end points. In this situation, there usually will be multiple educational sessions with patients, including comprehensive documentation. In both examples, patient education is a well-defined and integrated component of the service.

Pharmacists can create or identify existing patient educational resources (e.g., patient brochures, educational fliers, and flip charts) to reinforce important educational messages. These resources should be screened for accuracy and completeness. Also, reading difficulty should be assessed to make sure that difficult technical terms are replaced with more patient-friendly language (e.g., instead of blood glucose, use the term *blood sugar*). Another consideration is that some patients may not be able to read at all, especially if English is not their primary language. Therefore, it is not appropriate to simply hand out educational materials without first assessing the patient's understanding and reading ability. Once the educational resources are selected, it should be determined how they will be used as part of the service. Also, adequate copies should be ordered or created, and these should be inventoried periodically to make sure that there are sufficient supplies to meet patients' demands.

OUTCOME MEASUREMENTS

Outcome measurements are covered in more detail in Chapter 9, but pharmacists should determine what outcomes they will be assessing to evaluate the effectiveness of their service. These measures help pharmacists decide if certain aspects of the service need reviewing and altering if outcomes are not being achieved. Clinical outcomes are the most readily apparent and easiest outcomes to assess. These outcomes include objective parameters such as blood pressure, lipid panels, blood glucose, hemoglobin $A1_c$, and weight. Clinical outcomes usually are part of the patient chart and so are easily accessed. Humanistic outcomes (e.g., health-related quality of life and patient satisfaction) can be collected from surveys that become part of the service delivery. If such surveys do become a component of the service, then it should be determined how frequently patients fill out the surveys and how the data will be stored and used. Economic outcomes may require other types of data that pharmacists do not always collect, such as hospitalizations, emergency room visits, or physician visits. If economic outcomes are of interest, then a data-collection tool can be created that routinely requests these types of data. Patient knowledge also may be of interest to pharmacists who are providing comprehensive educational services. For this type of outcome, before and after knowledge-assessment quizzes/tests can be used.

■ REVISITING THE SCENARIO: CARE-RITE PHARMACY AND SERVICE DEVELOPMENT

Data Collection

After performing a SWOT analysis and some baseline market research, Carol and the other pharmacists at Care-Rite Pharmacy have decided to develop a MTM service. One of Carol's pharmacists volunteered to put together a prototype patient chart that will be used by the pharmacists to document their activities. The patient chart contains several forms, including a patient history form that requests some basic demographic information (see Fig. 26-2), medical and medication histories forms (see Figs. 26-3 and 26-4), and an authorization to release medical information that is signed and dated by the patient (see Fig. 26-5). Also, a communication form was created to fax clinical information and pharmacists' recommendations to the physician (see Fig. 26-6). Several copies of each individual form will be kept in separate folders in a file cabinet located in a secure area of the pharmacy. One of the pharmacists will be responsible for making sure that enough copies are always on hand. Completed charts will be kept in a filing cabinet that is arranged in alphabetical order by patient last name.

Pharmacy-Based Laboratory/ Monitoring Service

The pharmacists at Care-Rite Pharmacy decided to purchase a Cholestech LDX portable analyzer to measure the lipid profiles of their patients. They realized that many of their patients who they were targeting for the MTM service had cardiovascular disease. By purchasing the Cholestech LDX analyzer, they are able to assess lipid profiles and glucose levels for those patients who are willing to pay for this additional service. The system was chosen for its ease of use, quick results, and wide range of tests that it offers (i.e., lipid profile, glucose, and alanine aminotransferase (ALT)). The Cholestech LDX lipid profile is considered a CLIA-waived test. Also, the pharmacists sent in their completed application for a COW, paid the biennial fee, and received their CLIA number. All the pharmacists were trained in use of the Cholestech and how to perform quality-control procedures. The pharmacists were taught how to do finger sticks, appropriate procedures on how to minimize exposure to blood-borne pathogens, and proper disposal of used supplies. Each pharmacist was required to perform a test on another pharmacist to demonstrate his or her competency in using this analyzer. Lastly, a cardiovascular risk assessment form was created. The results from the test are added to the form and reviewed with the patient during the 5-minute test (see Table 26-1).

Medication Management Protocols

Owing to the complexities of the patients that the Care-Rite pharmacists were targeting for their MTM service, they determined that there was not one single type of protocol that they could use to assess and manage a patient. For patients who did have cardiovascular disease requiring lifestyle modifications and/or lipid-lowering therapy, however, a general protocol using data from the ATP III guidelines was developed (see Table 26-2). The protocol provided a clinical decision pathway to determine treatment strategies depending on the patients' low-density lipoprotein (LDL) concentration and risk factors. To help in their assessment of patients, the pharmacists used the cardiovascular risk assessment

Care Rite Pharmacy

Physician Communication Form

Physician: ______________________ Fax: ______________ Telephone: ______________

☐ Initial ☐ Follow-up ☐ New Problem ☐ Preventative ☐ Other

Patient Name: ______________________

Birth date: ______________________ Gender: ______________

Pharmacist: ______________________ Date: ______________

Subjective Findings:

Objective Findings:

Assessment:

Plan:

Recommended Pharmacist Follow-up Assessment: ☐ 4 weeks ☐ 8 weeks ☐ 6 months ☐ Other

Pharmacist Signature: ______________________

Physician: ______________________ Date: ______________

☐ I agree with the above recommendations:

☐ Proposed modified plan:

Pharmacist Follow-up ☐ As recommended ☐ Other: ______________________

Physician Signature: ______________________

Figure 26-6. Physician communication form

Table 26-1. Cardiovascular Risk Factors

Positive risk factors

+1 Female ≥55 years old, or premature menopause without estrogen replacement therapy

+1 Family history or premature CHD:
MI or sudden death of father or first-degree male relative (i.e., father, brother, son) <55 years old
MI or sudden death of mother or first degree female relative (i.e., mother, sister, daughter) <65 years old

+1 Current cigarette smoking

+1 Hypertension (>140/90 mm Hg on multiple measurements on several occasions), or currently taking antihypertensive medications

+1 Low HDL cholesterol (<40 mg/dL), confirmed by multiple measurements

Negative risk factors

−1 High HDL cholesterol (>60 mg/dL), confirmed by multiple measurements

Total risk factors = ____________________(positive risk factors + negative risk factor)

Risk Factors	**LDL Goal**
Without CHD, and 0–1 risk factors	<160 mg/dL
Without CHD, and 2 or more risk factors	<30 mg/dL
With CHD or CHD risk equivalents	<100 mg/dL

CHD and CHD risk equivalents

- CHD = myocardial infarction (MI), significant myocardial ischemia (angina), history of coronary artery bypass graft (CABG), history of coronary angioplasty, angiographic evidence of lesions, carotid endarterectomy, abdominal aortic aneurysm, peripheral vascular disease (claudication), thrombotic/embolic stroke, transient ischemic attack (TIA)
- Diabetes mellitus
- Multiple risk factors that confer a 10-year CHD risk of >20%

form. The protocol, although providing direction for pharmacists, did not give specific recommendations regarding which medications to choose if the patients need LDL-lowering medications in addition to therapeutic lifestyle changes (TLCs). By using this protocol, the pharmacists still had some discretion regarding medication options based on patient-specific factors.

Patient Education

The pharmacists of Care-Rite Pharmacy also developed patient educational tools to be used during the patient assessment and patient education components of the MTM service. Because many of the targeted patients have similar medical conditions, education materials were developed for specific disease states, including hypertension, ischemic heart disease, diabetes, asthma, chronic obstructive pulmonary disease (COPD), and so on. Also, educational materials were developed for certain therapeutic classes of medications. The Care-Rite pharmacists also determined that many patients needed individualized education materials, so they implemented a drug information/educational service as part of the MTM service. With this service, patients can ask questions regarding their medical conditions and/or drug therapies. The pharmacists will research and provide an individualized written response for each patient.

Outcome Measures

The main patient outcome measures of interest to the pharmacists at Care-Rite Pharmacy are clinical

Table 26-2. Medication Management Protocol Example

1. Perform fasting lipoprotein analysis and risk factor assessment.
   a. If the patient has 0 to 1 risk factor (10-year risk usually <10%)
      (1) If LDL <130 mg/dL
         (a) Provide education on healthy life habits and risk factor reduction strategies.
         (b) Repeat fasting lipoprotein analysis and risk factor assessment in 5 years.
      (2) If their LDL = 130–139 mg/dL
         (a) Provide education on healthy life habits and risk factor reduction strategies.
         (b) Repeat fasting lipoprotein analysis and risk factor assessment in 1 year.
      (3) If LDL ≥160 mg/dL
         (a) Initiate therapeutic lifestyle changes (TLCs) for 3 months.
            (1) Reduce intake of saturated fats and cholesterol
            (2) Weight reduction
            (3) Increased physical activity
         (b) After 3 months, reassess LDL.
            (1) If LDL <160 mg/dL, continue TLCs.
            (2) If LDL = 160–189 mg/dL, continue TLCs and consider LDL-lowering medications in certain high-risk patients.
            (3) If LDL ≥190 mg/dL, continue TLCs and consider adding LDL-lowering medications.
   b. If the patient has multiple (2+) risk factors and the 10-year risk is 10–20%
      (1) If LDL <130 mg/dL
         (a) Provide education on healthy life habits and risk factor reduction strategies.
         (b) Repeat fasting lipoprotein analysis and risk factor assessment in 1 year.
      (2) If LDL ≥130 mg/dL
         (a) Initiate TLCs for 3 months.
            (1) Reduce intake of saturated fats and cholesterol.
            (2) Weight reduction
            (3) Increased physical activity
         (b) After 3 months, reassess LDL.
            (1) If LDL <130 mg/dL, continue TLCs.
            (2) If LDL ≥130 mg/dL, continue TLCs abd consider LDL-lowering medications.
   c. If the patient has multiple (2+) risk factors and the 10-year risk <10%
      (1) If LDL <130 mg/dL
         (a) Provide education on healthy life habits and risk factor reduction strategies.
         (b) Repeat fasting lipoprotein analysis and risk factor assessment in 1 year.
      (2) If LDL ≥130 mg/dL
         (a) Initiate TLCs for 3 months.
            (1) Reduce intake of saturated fats and cholesterol.
            (2) Weight reduction
            (3) Increased physical activity

(Continued)

Table 26-2. Medication Management Protocol Example *(Continued)*

(b) After 3 months, reassess LDL.
(1) If LDL ≤160 mg/dL, continue TLCs.
(2) If LDL ≥160 mg/dL, continue TLCs and consider LDL-lowering medications
d. If the patient has CHD or CHD risk equivalents
(1) If LDL ≥130 mg/dL
(a) TLCs
(b) LDL-lowering medications
(1) If LDL <100 mg/dL, continue these therapeutic interventions.
(2) If LDL = 100–129 mg/dL, consider other therapeutic options.
(c) If LDL = 100–129 mg/dL
(1) TLCs
(2) Therapeutic options
(d) If LDL <100 mg/dL
(1) TLCs
(2) Control other risk factors

outcomes, patient knowledge, and patient satisfaction. Also, the pharmacists were interested in monitoring physician response to their clinical recommendations. The information collected would be kept in the patient chart. An electronic database was created to store and collate outcome data. One of the pharmacists is responsible for periodically entering data. The information garnered from these efforts would be used to identify areas needing improvement, to market the program to other providers, and to ensure payment from third-party payers.

POLICIES AND PROCEDURES

To help provide an organized approach to service delivery, a policies and procedures manual should be created to guide pharmacy staff during program implementation. The policies and procedures manual is a comprehensive road map to the service, providing information regarding the purpose of the service, patient eligibility, how patients will be evaluated, what happens during each clinic visit, and the documentation that will be kept. Also, a copy of all forms, patient educational tools, patient assessments, and protocols are included in the manual. The policies and procedures manual is a dynamic document that must be updated and changed as new information becomes known or as the program is modified.

The policies and procedures document should be kept at the pharmacy, used as a training tool for pharmacists and other personnel, and referred to as needed during the patient care process. It should be easy to access information in the manual. A table of contents should be included, sections tabbed, and an appendix created containing the forms that will be part of the program. Also, published medical guidelines and key articles from the primary literature should be included in the manual.

REVISITING THE SCENARIO: POLICIES AND PROCEDURES FOR THE CARE-RITE MEDICATION THERAPY MANAGEMENT SERVICES

The Care-Rite pharmacists created a comprehensive policies and procedures document for their MTM service. They determined that the purpose of their program is to

- Manage the drug therapy of high-risk patients. The criteria chosen to define the target population for the program were patients who used four or more chronic oral medications and had at least one chronic medical condition.
- Assess patients for drug therapy problems.
- Resolve drug therapy problems by working collaboratively with patients, physicians, and other prescribers.
- Provide comprehensive and ongoing education to patients and/or family members about common drug therapy problems, therapeutic goals, and the importance of becoming informed consumers of their own health care.

Next, they developed their policies for the program. The policies contained information regarding the evaluation of patients. The initial evaluation will occur after the patient is enrolled into the MTM service either by a health plan, other health care provider or self-referral. A patient chart will be created containing the patient's demographic information and medical and medication histories. The patients will sign an authorization to release medical information form and a lipid clinic contract that outlines the patient's responsibilities in the program. To be eligible for the program, patients must meet the eligibility criteria. Patients must be able to attend clinic appointments, must agree to come in for scheduled follow-up visits at the pharmacy, and should have the capacity to understand their health condition and the implications for therapy. Also, patients must be willing to be active participants in their health maintenance.

It was decided that there will be an initial visit and one to three follow-up visits within a 12-month period. All sessions will include a comprehensive review of medications, vital signs and laboratory values (as needed), patient education (as needed), and physician communication.

The initial session will last approximately 30 to 45 minutes, and the follow-up visits will last approximately 15 to 20 minutes. The follow-up visits will occur at 3 to 6 month intervals depending on the clinical situation. Pharmacists will assess the following information at each visit:

- Patient vital signs
- Dietary considerations
- Patient laboratory values
- Family history
- Medication history
- General activity
- Social history, including alcohol use and smoking
- Health problems
- Compliance with therapy
- Signs and symptoms of intolerance to a drug

Medication and/or dosage changes will be made, if necessary, based on the pharmacists' assessment, and patients will be counseled on these changes. The physician communication form will be used to communicate clinical recommendations regarding drug therapy. Also, patient education will be reinforced and documented. Patients will be instructed on when to return to the clinic, and referrals to physicians will occur as needed. The referrals are based on patient complications of therapy or condition and patient resistance to therapy.

The documentation will occur via a patient chart. Subjective patient information and objective laboratory data will be stored in the chart. Assessments of patients during the clinic visit will be documented in pharmacy progress notes contained in the chart. Acceptance of pharmacy recommendations by physicians will constitute an order change, and this will be documented in the patient record as well. Lastly, patient outcomes (i.e., clinical, knowledge, and satisfaction) will be documented in the patient record.

The other components of the policies and procedures manual include the medication management protocol and detailed instructions on use of the Cholestech LDX analyzer. The appendix of the policies and procedure manual contains copies of the forms and patient educational tools used in the program.

PHARMACIST TRAINING

As with any successful implementation of a pharmacy service, education and training of pharmacy staff prior to the implementation of the service are essential for success. Pharmacists should achieve proficiency in providing the service before the start date of the service. The time needed to train pharmacy staff depends on the complexity of the service and the experience of the staff. Not only do the pharmacists need to be knowledgeable about the service, but they also may need to practice some of the skills required for some services (e.g., giving a flu shot or completing a lipid panel). Therefore, there should be sufficient practice and a demonstration of competence before they work with actual patients. To help illustrate how the education and training can occur, the preparation of pharmacists at Care-Rite Pharmacy for their MTM service will be discussed.

REVISITING THE SCENARIO: PHARMACIST TRAINING FOR THE CARE-RITE MEDICATION THERAPY MANAGEMENT SERVICES

Care-Rite Pharmacy developed a comprehensive pharmacist educational/training program for its MTM service. This educational program had multiple components and activities that the pharmacists needed to demonstrate knowledge of or proficiency in before they were ready for service implementation. Initially, it was determined that a general knowledge of patient care, types and categories of drug therapy problems, and how to perform a patient assessment should be the foundation for the rest of the education. To help improve pharmacists' knowledge of this topic, the pharmacists were responsible for reading several articles on patient care delivery from the primary literature, a general overview of patient medication assessment from a therapeutics textbook, and articles on how to communicate to physicians and other prescribers. The readings were standardized so that the pharmacists were all learning from the same materials. They were given 4 weeks to read all the material and also given 10 standardized patient cases to work up to demonstrate their knowledge. At the end of the 4 weeks, a 3-hour review of the material and cases was scheduled so that the pharmacists could discuss their cases and ask any questions regarding the material.

Carol had hired a local clinical pharmacist who had expertise in ambulatory care as a consultant to assist with the pharmacists' education and skills development. The clinical consultant facilitated the case discussions. The cases that were developed for this program required pharmacists to assess and modify patients' dietary habits and activity levels. Also, they needed to identify and develop plans for resolving drug therapy problems. They practiced writing recommendations to physicians on the physician communication form.

The next component of the pharmacists' education was demonstrating their abilities to perform a finger stick and a lipid panel. The pharmacists first watched a video provided by Cholestech that demonstrated these two activities. Also, a component of the training included information regarding CLIA, the importance of good technique when performing a test, OSHA requirements, and discussions about the reduction of exposure to blood-borne pathogens. The pharmacists were given adequate time to practice using the Cholestech LDX analyzer. Once the practice was over, pharmacists were assessed on their competency to perform the test. A checklist with required activities that needed to be completed during a lipid panel was used as the grading criterion. Once the pharmacists were capable of providing the test, their proficiency with the Cholestech LDX analyzer was documented and stored in their personnel files.

MANAGING THE MARKETING MIX

Once the service is ready for implementation, recruiting patients into the program becomes the next activity. This requires a basic knowledge of marketing principles that were covered in Chapters 21 and 22. Successful implementation of value-added pharmacy services requires that pharmacists manage each of the variables of the marketing mix. An illustration of how Care-Rite Pharmacy managed its marketing mix is provided below.

REVISITING THE SCENARIO: MARKETING THE CARE-RITE MEDICATION THERAPY MANAGEMENT SERVICES

The product that Care-Rite Pharmacy is marketing is its MTM service. As discussed throughout this chapter, much attention has been given to developing each component of the service and planning for its implementation so that it is perceived as a quality service by patients and other providers. Also, pharmacists updated their knowledge regarding patient care and medication assessments and developed proficiency for testing patients' lipid panels. They hope to be perceived as knowledgeable and competent when providing the service. Lastly, protocols, policies and procedures, and standardized forms were all created to ensure consistency in service delivery among the providers.

The next marketing-mix variables that need careful consideration are the place and physical facility. Care-Rite Pharmacy will be providing the MTM service on site at the pharmacy. Therefore, pharmacy staff need to consider the characteristics of their space to provide the service. In preparation for this service, Carol did some remodeling of her pharmacy. She created two semiprivate patient areas using office partitions. One area was designated as the area where lipid testing would be performed. The Cholestech LDX analyzer and its supplies were stored in this area. Also, CLIA and OSHA guidelines were kept there as well. The second patient care area was created in case there were multiple appointments at the same time. Both areas had a small table, three chairs, and a computer terminal as standard equipment.

Price is the third marketing-mix variable. Carol and the pharmacy staff spent considerable time discussing the price of their service. They estimated the length of the time for each session, estimated the costs to provide the service, researched the price of office visits for other providers, and determined the profit level they needed to help them develop a pricing structure for their service. While no local pharmacies provided a MTM service, Carol decided to price the service to be competitive with similar services offered by physicians. The pricing structure for the service is as follows:

- Initial visit: $75
- Follow-up visits: $40 each
- Fasting lipid panel: $50

The pharmacists will monitor patient responses to these prices and their profitability before making any adjustments.

The next marketing-mix component is promotion. Care-Rite has selected several promotional strategies to market their services. Also, Carol has created a marketing budget for the practice. The pharmacists will use press releases in local newspaper to announce the new service. Next, they decided to run an advertisement in the local newspaper twice per month promoting this service. They chose Sundays and Mondays as the days they would place the ads in the newspaper. Sunday was chosen because of the large readership of the newspaper, and Monday was chosen because the newspaper had a special health section on that day. Also, they purchased airtime on their local cable TV and radio to promote the service. They selected channels that attracted viewers and listeners whose demographics matched their target markets (e.g., women over age 50). They placed an ad for the program in a local magazine that was directed toward women, and they created a new ad for their pharmacy in the local telephone directory.

One of the pharmacists began to call on physicians so that he could promote the services face to face. The pharmacist met with some of the local pharmaceutical company representatives to find out which physicians should be identified as key targets for the promotional efforts. Also, the pharmacy created a physician newsletter entitled, "Progress Notes," that would be sent every other month to key physicians. The format of the newsletter includes sections on new drug updates, clinical pearls, and message updates about Care-Rite Pharmacy. The first newsletter was dedicated to the MTM service.

In-store signage and patient brochures were created to help market the program to current pharmacy patients. Pharmacists were instructed to market the program to patients they encountered who were receiving four or more chronic oral medications. A mailing list was created from the pharmacy's computer system from patients taking four or more chronic oral medications. A brochure describing the program was sent to each of those patients. Lastly, bag stuffers and monthly patient billing statements included information about the new program.

Process management, the next marketing-mix variable, refers to how Care-Rite Pharmacy incorporated the new MTM service into its existing practice. Workflow decisions were made regarding patient flow during the service. It was decided that the service would be by appointment only to minimize disruption of the other aspects of the practice. Schedules for pharmacists were created so that one pharmacist was responsible for clinic services while another covered the dispensing area.

The last marketing-mix variable that needs addressing is personnel. Care-Rite's pharmacists and staff were trained and assessed to ensure that they had adequate knowledge and skills regarding all aspects of pharmacotherapy management. Also, pharmacists need to take responsibility for the success or failure for the program. This means that they should continue to identify patient candidates for the lipid management program, use various promotional strategies to increase the community's awareness of the program, and ensure that they have the knowledge and skills to provide quality care to patients. Carol changed the format of her annual evaluations of pharmacists to include reviewing their impact on the MTM service. As a reward for their efforts, she has agreed to cover the costs of their continuing education each year and attendance at one national pharmacy meeting of their choice.

ONGOING MONITORING OF VALUE-ADDED PHARMACY SERVICES

Once the service is implemented, several strategies should be in place to provide ongoing monitoring to ensure program quality and success. Scheduled staff meetings should be considered regularly, especially early during the implementation phase. These meetings should be used to discuss the number of patients who have enrolled, patient and physician acceptance of the service, feedback that has been received, and areas that need improvement. Staff can provide their own feedback on how they perceive the program's effectiveness and how it can be improved. These meetings can be used as educational offerings for the pharmacists to keep their therapeutic knowledge up to date. It is important to keep a time limit on these meetings to minimize disruption of the practice.

Another strategy to ensure program quality is to monitor the outcomes of the service of interest to the practice itself. One of the goals for service implementation is to create new business and generate additional revenues and profits for the pharmacy. The goals should be realistic and challenging to ensure economic viability for the practice. Pharmacists need to be held accountable for their efforts to help the practice reach its goals. Service outcomes that may be of interest to pharmacy staff are number of patients enrolled, revenue generated from the service, number of physician referrals, and profitability of the service (revenues minus expenses). If the service is not profitable, then it needs to be either eliminated or altered (price increases or improved service delivery efficiencies).

An additional continuous quality improvement strategy is to request feedback from patients who have completed the program and physicians who have referred patients to the pharmacy. The feedback could be as simple as a one-page questionnaire asking open-ended questions to provide more qualitative comments about the service. The information that is gathered from these surveys and/or questionnaires can be used to improve patient and physician perception of the service. Furthermore, the request for feedback gives the impression that the practice is proactive toward meeting the needs of patients and other providers.

REVISITING THE SCENARIO: CARE-RITE PHARMACY'S CONTINUOUS QUALITY IMPROVEMENT STRATEGIES

Carol decided to schedule pharmacy staff meetings twice monthly on the second Tuesday and fourth Thursday of each month. Those days were selected to ensure that all staff members had the opportunity to attend at least one meeting monthly. The meetings were scheduled at 11:00 a.m. because this usually is the least busy time for the pharmacy. The time limit for the meetings was 1 hour. The format of the meetings were as follows:

- Review of service outcomes (i.e., patient enrollment, revenue generation, and physician referrals): 5 minutes
- Pharmacists' discussion of program improvements: 15 to 20 minutes
- Review of feedback from patients and/or physicians: 5 to 10 minutes
- Miscellaneous issues: 5 to 10 minutes
- Therapeutic updates for pharmacists: 20 to 25 minutes

Carol is tracking the service outcomes over time and documenting pharmacists' activities to ensure successful program implementation. She informed the staff about the change in their annual evaluations to include reviews of their impact on the program. Also, she developed a patient satisfaction survey that patients are given after completing the program. A one-page physician questionnaire has been developed and is sent to physicians who have had patients enrolled in the service.

COLLABORATIVE PRACTICE AGREEMENTS

Collaborative practice agreements (CPAs) (also referred to as Collaborative Drug Therapy Management—CDTM) are a strategy that pharmacists can use to integrate their value-added services with prescribers such as physicians (Ferro et al., 1998). CPAs are used to formalize relationships between providers. They spell out the responsibilities of each provider and the acceptance of mutually agreed-on drug therapy management protocols. Although CPAs are an important aspect of service implementation, they require that pharmacists develop working relationships with prescribers. The development of collaborative working relationships (CWRs) between providers is a four-stage process, with the final stage usually representing the time when prescribers are most comfortable signing off on a CPA (McDonough and Doucette, 2001).

Although physicians and pharmacists may be aware of one another in a certain community, they may not be collaborating, and they may communicate only during discrete episodes of care (Stage 0: professional awareness). Pharmacists who are interested in developing services that require the sharing of patient information and regular communication with physicians and other providers will need to increase their interaction with these other providers. For example, the owner of Care-Rite Pharmacy could meet with physicians in her community and discuss her desire to start an MTM service. During these meetings, she could provide the physicians with preliminary protocols and communication forms and request their feedback. By increasing her communication and face-to-face interactions, she moves into the next stage of the CWR (Stage 1: professional recognition).

In the professional recognition stage, physicians not only are aware that a pharmacy exists, but they also recognize that the pharmacy can offer services that go beyond dispensing medications. Since not all pharmacies are providing MTM services, Carol has set herself and her practice apart from other pharmacies in her community. Although attainment of Stage 1 is important early in the working relationship, there is still not much information being shared between providers. Therefore, pharmacists need to develop closer and stronger professional relationships with other providers. In Carol's situation, she requested and received feedback from one physician group regarding her protocol. The physicians in this practice, although initially skeptical of this new service, believed that some of their patients might benefit from the pharmacy's education regarding risk factors, medications, and lifestyle modifications. Therefore, it was agreed that they would refer one or two patients to Care-Rite's Pharmacy's MTM service (Stage 2: exploration and trial).

The exploration and trial stage is one in which physicians are ready to try the service. It is important that pharmacy staff are ready and able to perform at a high level because the physicians will be monitoring their patients' progress closely. Following along with the chapter's scenario, Carol's staff was fully prepared to provide high-quality services for the two patients that were referred to the program. They worked up the patients, performed the medication management services, provided the patient education, and communicated back to the physicians after each patient appointment. After the patients completed several appointments with the pharmacists, Carol met with the physicians to seek their input regarding the program. The feedback was positive, and the physicians' recommendations to improve the program and communication flow were integrated into the program. The physicians agreed to refer more patients to the MTM service (Stage 3: professional relationship expansion).

If physicians and other provides are satisfied with the quality and efficiency of a pharmacy service, they may be willing to increase their referrals. It is during this stage that communication between providers becomes more bilateral, and physicians and pharmacists are exchanging information more equally. Also, physicians begin to develop expectations about the pharmacists and the service. It is important during this stage that pharmacists maintain or increase the quality of the service so that physicians see a benefit to referring patients. If pharmacists perform consistently and at a high level, they may earn the right to develop a CPA with the physicians (Stage 4: full collaborative working relationships (CWR)).

In the final stage, the CWR, pharmacists have proven their clinical abilities, performed reliably and consistently, and gained the trust of physicians. Because of this trust, physicians are now willing to sign a CPA. This is the case with Care-Rite Pharmacy. Carol and her pharmacists consistently helped the physicians' patients reach their goals of therapy. The patients became more compliant with lifestyle changes, and they spoke positively of their experience working with the pharmacists. At Carol's next meeting with the physicians, she discussed developing a CPA, and the physicians agreed to sign it and refer patients regularly to her practice.

The requirements for participation in a CPA are often spelled out in a state's Pharmacy Practice Act, resulting in variations in requirements to participate and the types of activities on which prescribers and pharmacists may collaborate. The components of a CPA typically include the information contained in the policies and procedures manual, drug therapy management protocols, and pharmacist/physician responsibilities. Pharmacists should seek input from physicians regarding patient eligibility criteria and drug therapy management protocols. Once this information is agreed to, then physicians and pharmacists should sign an agreement form. A copy of the CPA should be kept at the pharmacy and at the physician practice. An example of a CPA for Care-Rite Pharmacy is shown in Fig. 26-7.

RECEIVING COMPENSATION FOR VALUE-ADDED SERVICES

Developing and implementing value-added pharmacy services can be challenging and time consuming. An equally challenging task is determining an adequate compensation schedule to ensure that the service is economically viable and sustainable. Factors which must be considered when determining a compensation schedule are the pharmacy's costs to provide the service, what competitors may charge for similar services (both other pharmacies and other health care professionals, and what third-party payers may be willing to pay pharmacies for the service.

The first component to pricing value-added services is to determine all the costs associated with providing the service. This can be especially challenging because all costs—fixed and variable need to be considered. These costs include staff time, rent, overhead costs, equipment and technology, paperwork, and the

Management by Care-Rite Pharmacists

1. Care-Rite pharmacists will complete lab orders and coordinate the draw (finger stick) to fit the patient's schedule.
2. The patient's fasting lipid panel, cardiovascular risk factors, and dietary and exercise habits will be assessed.
3. Care-Rite Pharmacists will follow the protocol mutually agreed to by the physician to manage the patient's lipid therapy.
4. Care-Rite Pharmacists will communicate their assessment and recommendations to the physician via fax.
5. The physician will communicate via fax with their response to the pharmacists' recommendations within 24 hours.
6. If the physician agrees to the recommendations, their signature should constitute a new order and the pharmacists will carry out thier orders.
7. Pharmacists will schedule patients for follow-up visits at the designated times discussed in the policy and procedures manual.
8. Ultimately, the physician is responsible for the care of the patient and at anytime can discontinue the patient's involvement in the program.

______________________________ ______________
Physician Signature Date

______________________________ ______________
Pharmacist Signature Date

Figure 26-7. Collaborative practice agreement for the Pharmacy Check-up Program.

costs associated with the process of care (e.g., chart generation, faxing, photocopying, etc). It is important to closely review all aspects of the service to ensure that all costs have been included. The principles used to calculate the cost of dispensing a prescription (see Chapter 19) can also be applied to estimate the costs of providing a value-added pharmacy service.

Once the costs are determined, then prices that will be charged for the services should be set. There are different pricing methodologies that have been used. Fee-for-service pricing is the traditional method of billing for health care. This is when a specific rate is charged for a service based on time or a specific intervention. This method has been criticized because of its inherent incentive to providers to provide more care, even when it may not be warranted. Fee-for-service is focused on payment for actions of the provider, and not on fulfilling patient needs for optimal health and quality of life outcomes. Another pricing method is the Resource-based relative-value scale (RBRVS) in which payment is directly related to the level of service provided to the patient. This method uses ICD-9 codes that identify the diagnosis of the patient, and CPT codes that describe specific types of patient visits. Although CPT codes unique to pharmacists have not been traditionally recognized by Medicare and other payers, this has changed with the advent of medication therapy management services (MTMS) as a component covered by Medicare Part D. Pharmacy-specific CPT codes that are used by some payers for MTMS include

99605—An initial encounter service performed face to face with a patient in a time increment of up to 15 minutes.

99606—For use for a subsequent or follow-up encounter with the same patient in a time increment of up to 15 minutes.

99607—An add-on code that may be used to bill for additional increments of 15 minutes of time to either of the above codes.

Other CPT codes that have been used by pharmacists include 99211, which is a code used by pharmacists providing patient care incident to a physician. Pharmacists may bill for lab tests performed in the pharmacy by using CPT codes 82465 for total cholesterol, 80061 for fasting lipid panel, 85610 for INR testing, 76977T for bone mineral density screening, 83036 for A1c, and G001 for a finger stick. Also, pharmacists who are qualified to provide diabetes education may use G108 for individual patient training or G109 for group training. Pharmacists billing utilizing these codes normally use the CMS 1500 claim form. This form is used to bill medical services to an insurance program and is universally recognized and accepted for physician billing.

Lastly, another pricing methodology is a capitation. This is where a service is provided for a fixed fee, usually per patient per month. This payment methodology may be appealing to the payer because their costs are predetermined at a monthly rate. But the provider is at risk because they need to keep their costs below the total monthly capitated amount if the services are to be profitable and sustainable.

Each pricing methodology can be used within a pharmacy practice depending on the service and needs and wants of the customer/payer. Regardless of methodology chosen, there are some basic considerations to setting a reasonable fee for a value-added pharmacy service. As discussed above, it is important to determine the cost of doing business, but it is also important to determine a reasonable profit. One general rule that has been used by some pharmacists is that the individual providing the service should generate two to three times their salary in revenue. Assuming that a pharmacist earns $60/hour, this may mean charging $2.00 to $3.00 per minute for a value-added pharmacy service. But the reality of the marketplace is that pharmacists will not be paid an unlimited amount based on their time spent with the patient, but rather most payers either have a fixed amount or a ceiling on the amount that they will pay. Since this is the most common scenario that most pharmacists will face, it is essential that they become efficient with the service so that their costs (in particular their time) do not become excessive as to make the service unprofitable.

There are strategies that can be used to make value-added pharmacy services more profitable. First and foremost, the pharmacist has to be efficient. Therefore, patient interviews should be methodical and time efficient. Pharmacists should be current with their knowledge, be able to identify drug therapy problems from the information they collected from the patient, develop an action plan to resolve the problems, and communicate/document all this to the prescriber and patient. It is essential that pharmacists have a good working knowledge of therapeutics if they are to be successful.

Pharmacists also need to look to their technicians to help them become more cost effective. Pharmacy technicians can be used to help triage patients, help to collect patient histories, update current medication lists, scheduling patients, and billing patients and payers. Pharmacy technicians can assist pharmacists with health screenings/lab testing. By utilizing technicians in these functions, pharmacists are freed up to spend their time working directly with patients to identify and resolve drug therapy problems.

It is also important to realize that some services are more time intensive than others, making it more difficult to be profitable. For example, immunizations take a relatively short period of time to perform, the paperwork can be filled out by the patient, and pharmacists are usually reimbursed for an administration fee in addition to the vaccine fee. This makes immunizations particularly easy to implement and profitable. But services such as MTM are time intensive and require a lot of time with the initial meeting with a patient. But if the pharmacist does a comprehensive work-up and has a thorough medical and medication history to draw from, follow-ups can be profitable. Unfortunately the way the marketplace is paying for MTM services, it may only be once a year that pharmacist can be reimbursed for a CMR, which makes it more challenging to be profitable. On the other hand, if the patient can be seen 2 to 4 times in a year, and the pharmacist reimbursed for follow-up visits, then there is a possibility of long-term service viability.

To summarize this section on compensation for value-added services, pharmacists need to know all their costs, know how much they can be paid, and understand each payers billing process. Once these factors are known, then pharmacists can determine the amount of time they can spend with a patient to ensure profitability. Costs need to be minimized as much as possible and efficiencies maximized.

CONCLUSION

Pharmacists are implementing several types of value-added services in their practices. It is important that they follow a systematic process during development and implementation of these services so that the services are of high quality. Regardless of the service being implemented, the process remains the same. First, pharmacists need to determine the essential components of the service (e.g., data collection, medication management, patient education, etc.). Next, they should develop a policies and procedures manual that provides the purpose of the service, patient selection, and a description of each patient visit. Also, it is important that pharmacists are trained to provide quality and efficient care. For a pharmacy to be successful, pharmacists need to manage the marketing mix and develop CWRs with other providers.

Pharmacists can ensure their success with program implementation if they follow these steps. By preplanning and preparing before service initiation, pharmacists can minimize the challenges with any new startup program. As part of their preparation, the development of documentation tools, protocols, and physician communication forms is essential. Lastly, as they develop a trusting relationship with other providers and begin to receive regular referrals, a CPA may need to be created. With this document, pharmacists and physicians will know each other's roles, and an efficient exchange of information begins to occur.

QUESTIONS FOR FURTHER DISCUSSION

1. This chapter emphasized that the process of implementing value-added pharmacy services remains the same regardless of the service. What may be some differences in the forms used, protocols, and CPAs if the service were a diabetes educational program instead of a medication management service?
2. Discuss how the marketing mix may be similar/different from the scenario used in this chapter and a pharmacist implementing a heart failure clinic.
3. Think about a value-added service that you have an interest in implementing. What are the components of the service?

REFERENCES

Ansell JE, Buttaro JL, Thomas OV, Knowlton CH. 1997. The anticoagulation guidelines task force: Consensus guidelines for coordinated outpatient oral anticoagulation therapy management. *Ann Pharmacother* 31:604.

Baran RW, Crumlish K, Patterson H, et al. 1999. Improving outcomes of community-dwelling older patients with diabetes through pharmacist counseling. *Am J Health Syst Pharm* 56:1535.

Berringer R, Shibely MC, Cary CC, et al. 1999. Outcomes of a community pharmacy-based diabetes monitoring program. *J Am Pharm Assoc* 39:791.

Centers for Medicare and Medicaid Services. 2003. What is waived testing? Available at www.fda.gov/cdrh/clia; accessed on June 14, 2003.

Christensen DB, Holmes G, Fassatt WE, et al. 1999. Influence of a financial incentive on cognitive services: CARE project design/implementation. *J Am Pharm Assoc* 39:629.

Coast-Senior EA, Kroner BA, Kelley CL, Trilli LE. 1998. Management of patients with type 2 diabetes by pharmacists in primary care clinics. *Ann Pharmacother* 32:636.

Cowper PA, Weinberger M, Hanlon JT, et al. 1998. The cost-effectiveness of a clinical pharmacist intervention among elderly outpatients. *Pharmacotherapy* 18:327.

Davis FB, Sczupak CA. 1979. Outpatient oral anticoagulation: Guidelines for long-term management. *Postgrad Med* 66:100.

Dobie RL, Rascati KL. 1994. Documenting the value of pharmacist interventions. *Am Pharm* 34:50.

Elliott ME, Meek PD, Kanous NL, et al. 2002. Osteoporosis screening by community pharmacists: Use of national osteoporosis foundation resources. *J Am Pharm Assoc* 42:101.

Ferro LA, Marcrom RE, Garrelts L, et al. 1998. Collaborative practice agreements between pharmacists and physicians. *J Am Pharm Assoc* 38:655.

Furmaga EM. 1993. Pharmacist management of a hyperlipidemia clinic. *Am J Hosp Pharm* 50:91.

Grainger-Rousseau TJ, Miralles MA, Hepler CD, et al. 1997. Therapeutic outcomes monitoring: Application of pharmaceutical care guidelines to community pharmacy. *J Am Pharm Assoc* NS37:647.

Hanlon JT, Weinberger M, Samsa GP, et al. 1996. A randomized, controlled trial of a clinical pharmacist intervention to improve inappropriate prescribing in elderly outpatients with polypharmacy. *Am J Med* 100: 428.

Hawkins DW, Fiedler FP, Douglas HL, Eschbach RC. 1979. Evaluation of a clinical pharmacist in caring for hypertensive and diabetic patients. *Am J Hosp Pharm* 36:321.

Herborg H, Sondergaard B, Froekjaer B, et al. 2001. Improving drug therapy for patients with asthma: 2. Use of antiasthma medications. *J Am Pharm Assoc* 41:551.

Jaber LA, Halapy H, Fernet M, et al. 1996. Evaluation of a pharmaceutical care model on diabetes management. *Ann Pharmacother* 30:238.

Kennedy DT, Giles JT, Chang ZG, et al. 2002. Results of a smoking cessation clinic in community pharmacy practice. *J Am Pharm Assoc* 42:51.

Knapp KK, Katzman H, Hambright JS, Albrant DH. 1998. Community pharmacist interventions in a capitated pharmacy benefit contract. *Am J Health Syst Pharm* 55:1141.

Knoell DL, Pierson JF, Marsh CB, et al. 1998. Measurement of outcomes in adults receiving pharmaceutical care in a comprehensive asthma outpatient clinic. *Pharmacotherapy* 18:1365.

Knowlton CH, Thomas OV, Willamson A, et al. 1999. Establishing community-based anticoagulation education and monitoring programs. *J Am Pharm Assoc* 39:368.

Madejski RM, Madejski TJ. 1996. Cholesterol screening in a community pharmacy. *J Am Pharm Assoc* NS36: 243.

McCurdy M. 1993. Oral anticoagulation monitoring in a community pharmacy. *Am Pharm* 10:61.

McDonough RP. 1996. Interventions to improve patient pharmaceutical care outcomes. *J Am Pharm Assoc* NS36:453.

McDonough RP, Doucette WR. 2001. A conceptual framework for collaborative working relationships between pharmacists and physicians. *J Am Pharm Assoc* 41: 682.

McKenney JM, Brown ED, Necsary R, Reavis HL. 1978. Effect of pharmacist drug monitoring and patient education on hypertensive patients. *Contemp Pharm Pract* 1:50.

McKenney JM, Sliining JM, Henderson HR, et al. 1973. The effect of clinical pharmacy services on patients with essential hypertension. *Circulation* 48:1104.

Norton JL, Gibson DL. 1996. Establishing an outpatient anticoagulation clinic in a community hospital. *Am J Health Syst Pharm* 53:1151.

Pauley TR, Magee MJ, Cury JD. 1995. Pharmacists-managed physician-directed asthma management program reduces emergency department visits. *Ann Pharmacother* 29:5.

Petty DR, Zermansky AG, Raynor DK, et al. 2002. Clinical medication review by a pharmacists of elderly patients on repeat medications in general practice: Pharmacist interventions and review outcomes. *Int J Pharm Pract* 10:39.

Reinders TP, Rush DR, Baumgartner RP, Graham AW. 1975. Pharmacist's role in management of hypertensive patients in an ambulatory care clinic. *Am J Hosp Pharm* 32:590.

Reinders TP, Steinke WE. 1979. Pharmacist management of anticoagulant therapy in ambulant patients. *Am J Hosp Pharm* 36:645.

Rosenthal W. 2000. Establishing a pharmacy-based laboratory service. *J Am Pharm Assoc* 40:146.

Rupp MT. 1988. Evaluation of prescribing errors and pharmacist interventions in community practice: An estimate of "value added." *Am Pharm* NS28:766.

Rupp MT. 1992. Value of community pharmacists' interventions to correct prescribing errors. *Ann Pharmacother* 26:1580.

Rupp MT, DeYoung M, Schondelmeyer SW. 1992. Prescribing problems and pharmacist interventions in community practice. *Med Care* 30:926.

Rupp MT, McCallian DJ, Sheth KK. 1997. Developing and marketing a community pharmacy–based asthma management program. *J Am Pharm Assoc* NS37:694.

Schilling KW. 1977. Pharmacy program for monitoring diabetic patients. *Am J Hosp Pharm* 34:1242.

Simpson SH, Johnson JA, Tsuyuki RT. 2001. Economic impact of community pharmacist intervention in cholesterol risk management: An evaluation of the study of cardiovascular risk intervention by pharmacists. *Pharmacotherapy* 21:627.

Smith DH, Fassatt WE, Christensen DB. 1999. Washington State CARE project: Downstream cost changes associated with the provision of cognitive services by pharmacists. *J Am Pharm Assoc* 39:650.

Strand LM, Cipolle RJ, Morley PC. 1988. Documenting the clinical pharmacist's activities: Back to basics. *Drug Intell Clin Pharm* 2:63.

Strand LM, Cipolle RJ, Morley PC. 1992. Pharmaceutical care: An introduction. *In Current Concepts.* Kalamazoo, MI: Upjohn Company, p. 1.

Swain JH, Macklin R. 2001. Individualized diabetes care in a rural community pharmacy. *J Am Pharm Assoc* 41:458.

Tice B, Phillips CR. 2002. Implementation and evaluation of a lipid screening program in a large chain pharmacy. *J Am Pharm Assoc* 42:413.

Tiggelaar JM. 1987. Protocols for the treatment of essential hypertension and type II diabetes mellitus by pharmacists in ambulatory care clinics. *Drug Intell Clin Pharm* 21:521.

Tsukuki RT, Johnson JA, Teo KK, et al. 1999. Study of cardiovascular risk intervention by pharmacists (SCRIP): A randomized trial design of the effect of community pharmacist intervention program on serum cholesterol risk. *Ann Pharmacother* 33:910.

SECTION VII

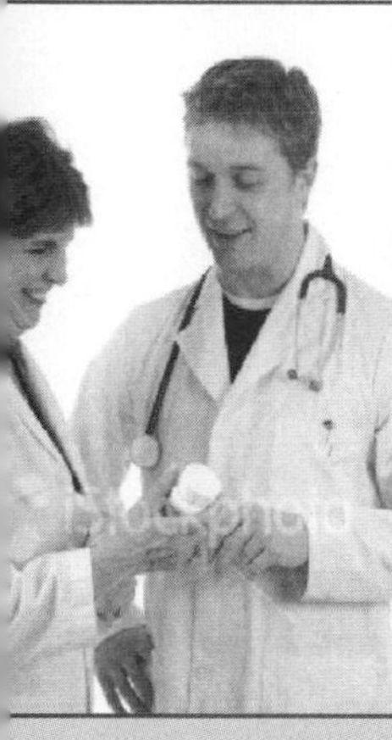

MANAGING RISKS IN PHARMACY PRACTICE

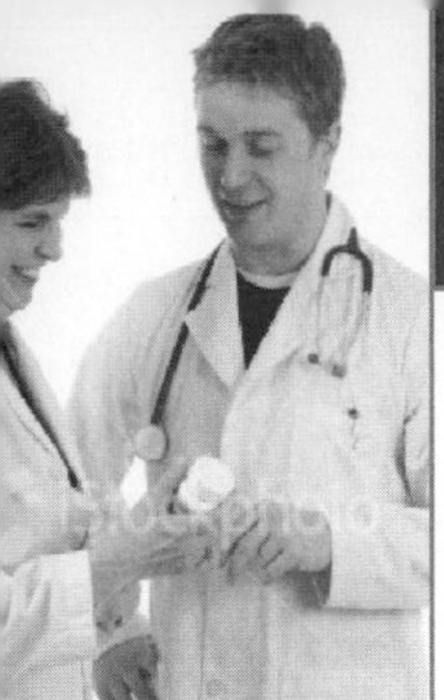

27

RISK MANAGEMENT IN CONTEMPORARY PHARMACY PRACTICE

Kevin Farmer and Donald Harrison

About the Authors: Dr. Farmer is Professor of Pharmacy Administration at the University of Oklahoma Health Sciences Center College of Pharmacy. He received a B.S. in pharmacy and Ph.D. in pharmaceutical sciences from the University of Missouri–Kansas City. Dr. Farmer has experience in community and hospital pharmacy practice settings and marketing research in the pharmaceutical industry. He teaches courses in US health care systems and policy, financial management, and pharmaceutical marketing. Dr. Farmer's research is focused on issues related to medication adherence and health and economic consequences of health and medication health care policies.

Dr. Harrison is Associate Professor of Pharmacy Administration at the University of Oklahoma Health Sciences Center College of Pharmacy. He received a B.S. in pharmacy from the University of Missouri—Kansas City. He received an M.S. in pharmacy and a Ph.D. in pharmaceutical sciences from the University of Arizona. Dr. Harrison has experience in many areas of pharmacy operations—community, institutional, and research. Dr. Harrison teaches courses in research design, biostatistics, and pharmacoeconomics. Dr. Harrison's research interests are in the economic analyses of pharmaceutical services, outcomes research, and strategic planning by pharmacy institutions and businesses.

LEARNING OBJECTIVES

After completing this chapter, readers should be able to

1. Describe the role of risk management in pharmacy practice.
2. Identify critical components that constitute pure risk.
3. Describe the criteria for determining an insurable risk.
4. Discuss how risk management techniques can be used to manage emerging risks that may pose a threat to community pharmacy practice.
5. Describe how increased reliance on information technology and automation may exacerbate certain risks.

6. Describe the factors that affect performance risk of an information technology system used in pharmacies.
7. Characterize the risk of loss associated with the use of information technology in pharmacy operations.

SCENARIO

Bill Halsey, Pharm.D., has spent the past 2 years since graduating from pharmacy school working as a staff pharmacist for a well-respected community pharmacy to refine his skills as a clinically oriented community pharmacist. Bill's dream is to someday return to his hometown and purchase the pharmacy that had inspired him to pursue this career. That day seemed to arise even sooner than Bill expected when he learned that Mr. Simmons, the long-time owner of Corner Drug in his hometown, had suffered a minor heart attack. Mr. Simmons would like to sell Corner Drug and move to a retirement village. Bill quickly scheduled a trip back home to visit with Mr. Simmons and inspect the pharmacy to see what it might be worth. He also evaluated the current state of the pharmacy for providing specialized services in diabetes and geriatrics. Bill was somewhat surprised to see that the pharmacy was essentially in the same condition that it was when he worked there during high school. Mr. Simmons had always enjoyed chatting with his customers, so the pharmacy counter was very small with wide openings on both sides so that he and his employees could easily move in and out of the pharmacy department to interact with customers. The desk where the clerk took care of the insurance claims paperwork and charge accounts was in the corner of the customer waiting area. The computer appeared to be somewhat ancient, and Mr. Simmons joked that the high school students he hired as clerks often had to help him when the computer would start "acting up." Bill was understandably concerned. The delivery car could best be described as a "beater." He had been serving as the Health Insurance Portability and Accountability Act (HIPAA) compliance officer for his current pharmacy and was wondering what, if any, security and privacy measures were in place at Corner Drug. Bill also remembered Mr. Simmons lecturing him on his philosophy of the unnecessary reliance on insurance and wondered how well the pharmacy was protected from harm or loss or liability. Mr. Simmons always told him, "Your customers will never sue you if they love and respect you, so treat them well." Bill was beginning to question himself as to what may lie in store for him if he bought Corner Drug, as he now contemplated several emerging unresolved issues that could threaten the ability of the pharmacy to exist and prosper.

CHAPTER QUESTIONS

1. What is the primary difference between a speculative risk and a pure risk for an individual?
2. What are the common risk threats that pharmacies share with any type of retail business?
3. Is it possible for a community pharmacy to avoid all risks? If not, how should risk be handled?
4. How might HIPAA privacy rules affect a pharmacy's liability insurance coverage and costs?
5. What are four areas of risk that arise when pharmacies increase their reliance on information technology and automation?
6. What are the increased risks brought about by the interaction of information technology with the safety and health hazards this technology poses to employees in the workplace?
7. Which six factors characterize the operational risk associated with information technology and automation in pharmacies?

INTRODUCTION

An element of risk exists in every human activity. One can become injured in an automobile accident on the way to work, become ill from food poisoning eating at a favorite restaurant, or lose thousands in retirement savings when the value of a company's stock declines significantly owing to an unexpected product recall. Pharmacists who own or operate pharmacies always must deal with the risk of business declines or even failure. There are always threats from the economy and the competition, as well as the potential for damage caused by a tornado, fire, flood, or hurricane. Indeed, a degree of risk is inherent in performing a most common task in almost any pharmacy—that of dispensing a patient's prescription. The changing health care environment requires pharmacists to critically examine risks in all aspects of their practice, especially as they look to take on more patient-oriented roles.

Historically, the primary risk exposure for pharmacists was related to traditional business risks (i.e., fire, theft, etc.), coupled with negligence related to prescription-filling errors. Modern pharmacy practice must also consider new risks related to the use of technology and electronic data transmission, patient counseling and drug utilization review requirements, and protected private health information. As the practice of pharmacy continues to evolve, so do the risks associated with the changing environment and scope of pharmacy practice. Pharmacists must be aware of the inherent and evolving risks of delivering health care goods and services and develop risk management strategies to deal with the risks. This chapter will review the concept of risk management and then focus on the new and developing risks associated with modern pharmacy practice in a technology-based environment.

DEFINITION OF RISKS

Risks are associated with negative outcomes. A *risk* is anything that threatens the ability of a person or organization to accomplish its mission. To fully understand risk in one's life or business venture, one must realize that there are several factors related to defining a risk as a threat. A risk may best be described as some *degree of probability* that *exposure* to a *hazard* will lead to a *negative outcome or consequence* such as loss, damage, injury, or death (Ropeik and Gray, 2002). Exposures to some risks are a part of daily life. You could have an auto accident on any given day. For a risk to be a threat, there must be some statistical chance (probability) that a negative event will occur. One may or may not be exposed to a risk that may diminish or eliminate the risk as a real threat. You cannot drown if you are not near water. You cannot suffer an adverse reaction from a drug you have never consumed. To be a risk, it also must constitute a hazard (hence the sports phrase "No harm, no foul"). The severity or consequences also must be negative to be a risk. A drug may have a small probability of anaphylactic shock, but anaphylactic shock may result in death. A new computer virus could destroy all the patient files and records stored in the pharmacy computer system.

From an insurance perspective, there are two basic types of risks: speculative risks and pure risks. A *speculative risk* involves a chance of gain or benefit as well as loss. Speculative risks are not insurable. Gambling is the prototypical speculative risk. When the $1 scratch-off lottery ticket you just bought didn't win the instant $1,000, you knew you had a very good chance of losing your dollar. The individual decides on the amount of risk he or she is willing to assume, including how much money to gamble and at what odds. Choosing to purchase shares of a mutual fund or common stock as an investment also involves speculative risk. Based on an investor's choices and a great number of other factors, his or her investment portfolio can experience substantial gains or suffer significant losses. Operating a pharmacy also involves speculative risk, in that there is no guarantee of success or failure. The number of independent community pharmacies in the United States declined from 31,879 in 1990, to 20,641 in 1998 [U.S. Department of Health and Human Services (DHHS), 2000]. In general, small-business ownership is inherently a risky venture. Data from the U.S. Bureau of Labor Statistics has found that only 45 percent of newly established businesses survive at least 4 years (Knaup, 2005).

Pure risk involves a risk in which there is only the opportunity of sustaining a loss; there is no opportunity for gain. Pure risks are considered accidental, unanticipated, or unavoidable. Illness, death, fire, flood, and most accidents involve pure risk. Insurance is a product designed to assist people in managing their exposure to these unanticipated or accidental risks. Individuals and businesses can purchase insurance for risks involving health, death, and damage to home and business property. Damage to a place of business from fire or a tornado could cause catastrophic loss with little chance of gain for the owner and is therefore an insurable pure risk. The identification and management of pure risks are essential for a business to manage potential threats to its mission.

CRITERIA FOR INSURABLE RISKS

For a pure risk to be insurable, it must meet certain requirements (Schafermeyer, 2007):

- The loss must be measurable in dollar figures, easy to measure, and result in a substantial loss.
- The loss must have a defined time and place.
- The loss must be accidental for the insured. There should be no prospect of gain or profit for the individual.
- The probability of the event occurring in a population can be accurately calculated. There must be a sufficiently large number of homogeneous individuals with similar risks to make losses predictable.
- The insured must have an insurable interest. Compensation cannot be awarded to those not actually suffering the loss.
- The insurance premium must be available for a reasonable cost. One would not want to pay an insurance premium greater than the value of the item insured.

DEVELOPING A RISK MANAGEMENT STRATEGY

What strategies should pharmacists pursue to identify and minimize their risk exposure? A risk management process should be developed to analyze and identify strategies to manage risk threats. A risk management strategy should be designed to protect the vital assets of a pharmacy through coping with uncertainty. This process involves not only identifying risks but also assessing their threat potential and making decisions on managing those risks. Recall the definition of risk in this process—that some type of probability exists that exposure to some type of hazard will lead to a negative outcome or consequence.

THE RISK MANAGEMENT PROCESS

There are five steps that organizations should follow when developing a risk management process:

1. *Establish the context.* What are the goals of the risk management process? What are potential vulnerabilities of the business? Do employees or patients risk injuries? How might the reputation of the pharmacy suffer if a patient was injured owing to a prescription error, or if a patient's health condition was inadvertently made public by an employee? Could costly claims be avoided by not providing certain goods or services?
2. *Identify and analyze risks.* Pharmacy managers should start by analyzing each dimension of their operation. Some examples of risks faced by pharmacies include the activities inherent in their business (i.e., filling prescriptions, counseling patients, and providing professional services). Other risks faced by pharmacies include making deliveries; maintaining the building, sidewalks, and parking lot; preparing sterile products; maintaining a computer system, and protecting patient health information. Problems in any of these could result in substantial losses for the pharmacy.

3. *Evaluate and prioritize the risks.* Pharmacy managers must prioritize their risks because every risk cannot be addressed at one time. Some risks are fairly common yet are not associated with a high degree of loss (e.g., prescription insurance claim rejections and shoplifting). Other risks are much less common yet are associated with substantial losses (e.g., catastrophic damage from a fire, flood, or storm, or harm to a patient associated with a dispensing error). Pharmacies should prioritize managing risks that have the greatest potential to result in substantial losses for their business.
4. *Select an appropriate risk management strategy and implement the technique.* Pharmacy managers must determine which risks could (and should) be avoided. Policies and procedures should be developed for appropriate risk prevention measures. Additional insurance policies or add-on riders should be secured as necessary. *Riders* are supplemental policies that provide additional coverage for something not covered in the original policy at some additional charge. There may be a ceiling or maximum amount the original policy will cover to replace personal property or equipment that may not provide adequate cost replacement for an asset(s). Thought should go into the level of deductibles to appropriately balance risk-sharing issues and risk-transfer issues (see "Techniques to Manage Risks" below). These strategies and the evaluation of which risks to avoid versus those that should be managed should be discussed with consultants or advisors (e.g., attorney, accountant, etc.) of the business operation.
5. *Monitor decisions and update the risk management program.* Pharmacy managers should monitor and update their risk management strategies to meet new challenges, threats, and opportunities. For example, when a pharmacy decides to offer immunizations to their patients, it not only creates new patient care and business opportunities, but it also exposes itself to additional risks (e.g., patients could experience an anaphylactic reaction to the immunization, patients could receive an inappropriate or incorrect immunization, and pharmacy employees could be exposed to pathogens). Once these new risks are identified, managers must create new strategies for their management.

TECHNIQUES TO MANAGE RISKS

Although risk is inherent to some degree in all our activities, there are different types of risks that require different techniques to manage. Each risk should be evaluated individually as to which technique(s) would be the most appropriate for that given risk.

1. *Risk avoidance.* Although avoiding risks may sound like a logical approach, it is often impractical for many risks in a business environment. For example, most pharmacies cannot (and would not want to) avoid dispensing prescriptions despite the inherent risks involved in the process. However, there may be situations where not offering a specific good or service with an unreasonable risk may be the most prudent action. Many pharmacies choose simply not to perform sterile compounding services rather than incur the expense and risks associated with the preparation of these products.
2. *Risk prevention/modification.* Pharmacy managers may not be able to eliminate a risk, but they can take steps to minimize the likelihood of its occurrence. All pharmacies take steps to avoid medication-dispensing errors. This commonly involves the development of policies and procedures to prevent errors and improve patient safety (see Chapters 8 and 29).
3. *Risk absorption/retention.* Pharmacies often choose to retain or absorb some risks. Pharmacies commonly accept losses owing to shrinkage (i.e., shoplifting, employee theft, and unsalable products), usually by losing profits or passing on higher prices to consumers. A deductible on an insurance policy is absorption of risk. Some may choose to pay higher deductibles when losses occur in exchange for lower insurance premiums.
4. *Risk sharing or transfer.* Another technique to manage risk is to share or transfer the risk to another

party. Insurance companies commonly share or transfer the risks inherent in paying for health care for their beneficiaries by entering capitated agreements with providers, paying them a set amount per member per month, regardless of how much or how little their beneficiaries need health services. Another method to share or transfer risk is to purchase reinsurance (insurance for insurance companies). Health care providers can also purchase insurance to share or transfer the risks involved in providing care to patients whose costs may exceed the income provided in the capitated contract.

On an individual level, one can avoid some unnecessary risks (i.e., someone may never go swimming to avoid the risk of drowning), but from a business perspective, this strategy is impractical. One may choose to absorb certain risks if the cost of insurance is very high and the potential loss is small. Foregoing automobile collision insurance on a vehicle of minimal value would be an example (while retaining legally required liability insurance). Risk prevention is an important component of effective risk management strategies and is generally used in tandem with risk transfer. On the most basic level, risk prevention includes the use of smoke alarms, security systems, and theft detection. In addition, for a business such as a pharmacy, employee training programs, education, and established policies and procedures are essential to deal with such risks as prevention of medication errors. With the possible exception of risk avoidance, most instances of conducting risk management will use some combination of each of the techniques of risk prevention, risk absorption, and risk sharing.

BASIC INSURANCE CONCEPTS

A pharmacy, like any other business entity, needs to protect itself, its employees, and its customers from physical and financial harm. No matter how careful a pharmacy is about preventing risks, it is practically impossible to eliminate accidents, such as when a customer or employee slips on the pharmacy's floor. At the same time, insuring for these risks does not eliminate the need for pharmacies to take effective risk prevention measures. Indeed, insurers commonly require that pharmacies have risk prevention measures in place to keep insurance policies in good standing for these risks or to reduce premiums. For instance, insurance for fire damage generally requires a sprinkler system or smoke detectors or alarms.

Common Insurance Terms

Insurance companies often use language that may be confusing to individuals not in the insurance industry. Pharmacy managers should have an understanding of the following terms commonly used in insurance policies (Insurance Information Institute, 2007):

- *Coverage.* The scope (extent) of protection provided under an insurance contract.
- *Coinsurance.* A provision that requires the insured party to share (absorb) some of the costs of covered services or losses on a fixed percentage basis. For example, this may require the insured to pay 20 percent of the replacement costs.
- *Deductible.* The amount (a fixed amount specified in dollars) of an insured loss to be paid (or absorbed) by the policyholder. Deductibles may range from several hundred to several thousand dollars. For automobile collision insurance, $500 deductibles are common.
- *Disability insurance.* A type of health insurance that provides monthly income to the policyholder if he or she becomes unable to work because of an illness or accident.
- *Insured.* The party covered by the insurance contract or persons entitled to benefits under the terms of the policy (e.g., family members may be covered under the employee's employer-sponsored health insurance plan).
- *Liability.* Individual responsibility for causing injury to another person or damage to another's property through negligence.
- *Negligence.* The failure to use reasonable care. The failure to do something a reasonably prudent person would do in similar circumstances.

- *Peril.* Insurance terminology for risk, possible cause of injury, or event causing damage or loss.
- *Policy.* A written contract for insurance between an insurance company and the insured party.
- *Rider.* Term used to describe a document that amends or changes the original policy.
- *Umbrella liability.* A form of insurance protection in excess of the amount covered by other liability insurance policies. It also protects the insured in situations not covered by the usual liability policies.
- *Worker's compensation.* A policy that pays benefits to an employee (or his or her family) for job-related injury or death.

Types of Insurance for a Pharmacy

Depending on the needs of the individual pharmacy, several different types of insurance policies may be required to provide adequate risk protection for the business. The geographic location, type of practice, and services offered will influence the types of insurance needed. The risk management process is a continuous process, and periodic evaluations are necessary to address new or emerging risk threats to the pharmacy. Emerging threats discussed later in this chapter exemplify how recent changes in health care practices (privacy issues) and technology create new and different risk threats to the pharmacy.

Property Insurance

This is one of the most common types of insurance for protecting the property and physical assets of any business entity. These policies generally cover losses owing to fire or lightning and theft and the costs of removing property to protect it from further harm. Property that should be insured includes buildings (leased or owned), equipment, supplies, fixtures, inventory, money, accounts receivable records, computers and other data storage devices, vehicles, and intangible assets (e.g., goodwill and the value of a trade secret). Additional coverage can be purchased for specific "extended perils" such as windstorms, hail, floods, explosions, riots, or other specific events. A pharmacy manager should know exactly what is covered in his or her basic property insurance policy to determine if additional coverage is warranted owing to geographic location or local circumstances.

Liability Insurance (also known as Casualty Insurance)

Liability insurance protects a business entity against claims when it is sued for damages or injuries caused by the negligence of the business or its employees. Liability insurance generally covers bodily injury, property damage, personal injury (including libel and interference with privacy), and advertising injury. Advertising injury may occur when advertising activities cause loss to another person through slander, defamation, libel, violation of privacy, or misuse of a copyright or trademark (Rupp's Insurance & Risk Management Glossary, 2002). The legal expenses involved in a negligence suit (i.e., investigation, settlement, or trial) also should be covered by the policy. In today's litigious society, liability insurance is essential for any business entity, including pharmacies. Even fraudulent lawsuits brought by plaintiffs with little hope of success will result in expenses necessary for the pharmacy to defend itself. When a pharmacy is found to be negligent (such as in a dispensing error), a single judgment could result in a claim into the millions of dollars, resulting in financial ruin for an uninsured pharmacy. Liability insurance does not protect against nonperformance of a contract, wrongful termination of employees, sexual harassment, or race or gender lawsuits.

Business Owner's Policy

Insurance companies commonly bundle property and liability coverage together in the same policy for small-business owners. This policy allows for broader coverage, generally with less expensive premiums, than if property and liability insurance were purchased separately. Small businesses must meet certain criteria to qualify for these policies, such as having fewer than 100 employees and revenues not exceeding set amounts. These policies generally do not include professional liability coverage, worker's compensation, or employee health insurance. These must be purchased separately.

Individual Professional Liability Insurance
Pharmacists frequently purchase individual professional liability insurance policies in addition to what their business or employer may provide. This policy protects the individual against claims emanating from actual or alleged errors or omissions, including negligence, in the course of professional duties or activities. Individual policies are purchased because the business policy limits may not be high enough, and they will not cover the pharmacist outside that workplace. These policies commonly provide coverage of up to $1 million to $2 million per incident.

Key Person Insurance
This is insurance designed to protect a business entity from financial loss if key individuals (very likely the owner or partners) were to die or experience a disability. For instance, if the pharmacist-owner were to die suddenly or become disabled, this policy would pay to find and train a replacement or replace profits the company may have earned if the person had not died.

Umbrella or Excess Liability
It is possible that a lawsuit filed against a pharmacy could exceed the limits of the primary liability protection. For instance, a pharmacy's base liability policy may provide a maximum of $300,000 of coverage, but the pharmacy experiences a lawsuit in which the settlement or judgment reaches $1 million. The umbrella policy would cover the difference between the base liability limits and the judgment amount. An umbrella policy is activated only when the limits of the underlying base policy have been exceeded and exhausted. Umbrella liability policies can add substantial coverage for a relatively small additional cost.

Worker's Compensation
This statutory insurance covers medical expenses, disability income, and death benefits to dependents of an employee whose accident, illness, or death is job related. Businesses are required to provide a safe working environment for their employees. Failure to provide a safe environment makes an employer liable for harm to their employees and may result in damage claim lawsuits from their employees. Worker's compensation can be a costly expense for some types of business in which the risk of injury to the worker is high, such as construction. Examples of injuries related to a pharmacy would be those owing to falls, overexertion, or repetitive motion, such as using a computer keyboard. Coverage rates depend highly on individual state laws and the type of work employees are engaged in.

There are a number of insurance companies that specialize in providing insurance coverage to pharmacies. It is a good idea for pharmacy managers to meet with representatives from these companies to discuss their specific insurance needs and compare policy offerings. Pharmacies may also purchase additional coverage for the specialty services they may offer. Examples include policies for home medical equipment, consultant pharmacist services, and professional liability insurance for pharmacists. As previously mentioned, it is generally a good idea for pharmacists to purchase individual professional liability insurance for more comprehensive protection.

EMERGING RISKS ASSOCIATED WITH MODERN PHARMACY PRACTICE

The health care industry, including pharmacy, is one of today's most dynamic environments. Health care is a technology-rich environment, with pharmacy often leading the way in technological innovations and advancement. For example, pharmacies now commonly use robotics to assist in the prescription-filling process. They have long used computers in the transmission of third-party prescription claims and to share information between pharmacies. Today, prescriptions are increasingly transmitted electronically from the physician to the pharmacy, a process known as *electronic prescribing* (or *e-prescribing*). Although advances in technology may offer many benefits in terms of patient safety and cost reductions, pharmacies need to incorporate these new technologies into their risk management processes. Employees need to be trained to become aware of new patient privacy regulations and requirements. Pharmacists may need to check and verify not only prescription dispensing activities by technicians but also computer input and data review. Ignoring or not understanding the impact of new professional requirements or technologies can place the pharmacy at risk. The Omnibus Budget Reconciliation Act of 1990 (OBRA 90) and the Health Insurance Portability and Accountability Act (HIPAA) are examples of significant changes in pharmacy practice, which present risk factors the pharmacy must consider in risk management.

Omnibus Budget Reconciliation Act of 1990 (OBRA 90)

The OBRA is enacted by Congress on an annual basis. It is used primarily to enact the budget for all the nation's governmental agencies and activities and generally has little to do specifically with pharmacy. However, the OBRA passed by Congress in 1990 (OBRA 90) had implications for pharmaceutical costs and state Medicaid pharmacy programs. In general, OBRA 90 specified what was expected of pharmacists in providing drug therapy to Medicaid patients. By 1993, pharmacists providing medications to state Medicaid recipients were required to provide prospective drug use review (Pro-DUR) and patient counseling and to maintain proper patient records. Most states quickly amended their state pharmacy practice acts to require that all patients receive this level of pharmacy services. Although patients had the option to refuse counseling, pharmacists now had the legal responsibility to provide information to their patients. While most pharmacists welcomed the legal acknowledgment of the professional responsibilities of modern pharmacy practice, OBRA 90 and the resulting changes in state pharmacy practice acts required that pharmacies reassess their risk exposure. Historically, pharmacists and pharmacy liability exposure had been limited to errors (negligence) when a prescription was filled incorrectly. A policy known as the *learned intermediary doctrine* traditionally held that pharmacist had no duty to warn patients against potential adverse reactions or other problems associated with a properly filled prescription. The duty to warn resided with the prescribing physician. However, with the advent of OBRA 90 and new professional standards of practice in pharmacy, courts have begun to abandon this doctrine (Dinardo, 2006; Holleran, 1995). While three-fourths of all claims against pharmacists are still related to dispensing the wrong drug or wrong strength, drug review claims against pharmacists (i.e., checking for interactions, allergies, and other problems), which virtually did not exist before 1991, now account for 9 percent of all claims (O'Donnell, 2005).

The Health Insurance Portability and Accountability Act (HIPAA) of 1996

The HIPAA, which set standards for the privacy of individually identifiable health information, was signed into law in 1996 and went into effect in 2003. The Department of Health and Human Services (DHHS) was required by Congress to promulgate the privacy standards and to set security standards for patient health information [U.S. Department of Health and Human Services (DHHS), 2003]. The standards for security and privacy are interconnected so that meeting the security standards would satisfy privacy concerns (Spies and Van Dusen, 2003). An individual's health information is referred to as *protected health information* (PHI) and is subject to the HIPAA privacy and security rules.

Pharmacies are affected by these rules in two ways. Pharmacies, by definition, deal with PHI (e.g., a prescription itself is PHI). If the pharmacy uses a computer, the information is then electronic and is known as *ePHI* (Barlas, 2004). HIPAA protects all "individually identifiable health information" held or transmitted by a covered entity or its business associate in any form or media, whether electronic, paper, or oral (DHHS, 2003). This covered information includes demographic data, including the individual's physical or mental health (past, present, or future); the health care provided to the individual; and payment information and common identifiers (e.g., name, address, birth date, and Social Security Number) that can be used to identify the individual. Pharmacies must have numerous policies and procedures in place to be in compliance with the HIPPA mandates. These include conducting risk assessments, appointing security and privacy officers to ensure compliance, and implementing policies and procedures to detect and prevent security violations.

There are a host of issues involving HIPAA that can place a pharmacy at risk. These include procedures for handling PHI in the event of fire, theft, system malfunctions, and disaster situations (Spies and Van Dusen, 2003). Even such seemingly benign events such as sticky-note reminders regarding customer requests in the pharmacy area or a technician verbally inquiring at the counter if the Zoloft® for Mr. Jones prescription that came in the morning wholesaler shipment are likely HIPAA violations. Risk exposure involving PHI goes beyond violations of federal law. Personal injury claims (nonbodily injury) are one of the fastest-growing areas of professional liability claims against pharmacists (O'Donnell, 2005). These claims involve libel, slander, or the unauthorized release of confidential records. The release of a patient's PHI constitutes the unauthorized release of confidential records.

Information Technology-Related Risks

The health care sector in general and community pharmacies specifically have become increasingly dependent on information technology. Almost all aspects of goods, services, and activities provided or conducted by community pharmacies have become interlinked with information technology. Many community pharmacies have invested heavily in information technology systems not only to dispense prescriptions and maintain patient records but also to digitize their financial and accounting systems, enterprise resource planning, human resources, and almost every other element of the business. Information technology has benefited community pharmacy in many ways. However, pharmacy's increased dependence on information technology has brought about a relatively new and increasingly important risk known as *information technology-related risk* (ITRR), often referred to as *digital risk.* Hardly a day passes without the report of some business losing confidential client information or having its computer network compromised by unauthorized intruders.

In addition to the usual ITRR that any business must confront, community pharmacies possess patient health, prescription, and financial data that can be an attractive target to unauthorized individuals wishing to gain access to those data. Therefore, risks owing to the implementation of and dependence on information technology potentially can offset the benefits derived if the implementation and management of information technology are not given sufficient attention. The ITRR incurred by community pharmacies can be grouped into several areas:

Strategic Risk

Strategic risk is the first and foremost risk confronted by pharmacies implementing information technology. To make any information technology project successful in the long run, pharmacies must assess the compatibility of the technology with their mission and goals (see Chapter 4). Businesses must make choices between investing in information technology and other types of resources to achieve their overall goals and objectives. Although the purpose of most information technology is to achieve efficiencies and competitive advantages, there are always risks that the organization would have been better off by pursuing other options. The costs of these risks are known as *opportunity costs.* Such risks can even result in failure to meet a pharmacy's goals and objectives and potentially can put the pharmacy at risk for significant financial loss.

Successful implementation of information technology projects can be difficult to achieve. According to the Standish Group's CHAOS Report (2003), an analysis of 13,522 information technology projects found that 15 percent "failed" and another 51 percent were considered "challenged." Further, a survey found that 30 percent of all application projects lasting more than a year "failed to meet business requirements" Lynch (2007). In a survey of 82 Fortune 500 companies, 44 percent of respondents experienced "total abandonment" of an information technology project and another 16 percent experienced "substantial abandonment" (Ewusi-Mensah, 2003). Within community pharmacy, failures of this sort can be numerous and wide ranging. For example, a new (or even existing) information technology system may fail to interface with pharmacy benefit manager (PBM) systems, resulting in an inability to process almost all third-party prescriptions. A pharmacy information technology system's failure to interface with a wholesaler's system may result in an inability to order and receive drugs and other goods in a timely manner. These are only two of many examples of system failures that a pharmacy can experience and that can seriously hinder its financial performance.

Organizational behavior problems can arise when integrating information technology into pharmacy practice. These often occur when stakeholders (i.e., employees and patients who interact with these systems) are not provided appropriate training before or after information technology implementation. The intended outcomes of information technology integration into pharmacy operations can occur only if there is good communication, commitment, cooperation, and coordination among all the stakeholders. Pharmacy managers incur risks associated with the acquisition and implementation of information technology resources when there is denial of the potential adverse events that can occur in the future. Pharmacy managers must "think outside the box" and consider each and every bad situation that can arise from the implementation and increased dependence on information technology.

Performance Risk

Performance risk is the degree of uncertainty inherent in the procurement and application of information technology solutions that may keep the system from meeting its technical specifications or from being suitable for its intended use and the consequences (Browning, 1999). The most important aspects of performance—those contributing most to performance risk—will vary with the needs and desires of the pharmacy (Barker et al., 1998).

Performance risk arises from product complexity. Product complexity involves the number of components, functions, and interfaces in the pharmacy information system. There are several factors that contribute to product complexity:

SYSTEM REQUIREMENTS Specifications required by a pharmacy in its information technology are directly related to the degree of product complexity and performance risk. These challenges result from the various individual tasks pharmacies require of their information technology and the desire to integrate these tasks into a single piece of technology. Pharmacy information systems must handle a multitude of complex and interrelated elements, such as prescription entry, claim processing, prescription pricing, inventory, and financial management (see Chapter 7). These interrelationships make it difficult to balance optimal performance in all these areas and achieve the ultimate design goal of the system (i.e., enhanced operational efficiency and patient safety). For example, the information system must work to adjudicate third-party prescription claims and at same time check therapeutic substitution or drug–drug interaction for a particular patient. Another area of concern to pharmacies is data storage. Pharmacy information systems have become a huge repository of PHI for patients. The need to prevent unauthorized third-party access to sensitive patient data increases the chances of data becoming corrupted or lost due to improper maintenance, inadequate replication (backup), and complex encryption and decryption processes. Therefore, there is a tradeoff between data privacy and longevity data storage.

MODULARITY The ability of important components to function independent of the main application is preferable for information technology systems operated by pharmacies. The system should be decomposable into subsystems that make the product less complex. This provides room for individual component upgrades instead of redesigning the whole system when specifications change in certain areas, such as claim processing.

Operational Risk

Operational risk generally is defined as risk of loss resulting from inadequate or failed internal processes, people and systems, or external events (APRA, 2007; Walker, 2001; Wikipedia, 2007). Information technology operational risks in today's digitized pharmacy are characterized by six event factors:

1. *Internal fraud* is an act committed by at least one internal party (typically an employee) that leads to data theft and/or loss. Information technology creates a tempting environment for employees to create fraud not only because the payoff from such activities can be high but also because the risk of detection is minimal.

   An *intranet* can help a pharmacy operate more efficiently by allowing information to be shared and communicated quickly and reliably. However, having a large number of users increases the intranet's vulnerability to internal threats. Intranet applications and their content may be exposed to a far greater audience than just those authorized users of the intranet. Recent research reports that more than 30 percent of all organizations report at least one security incident beginning within the organization, and an additional 24 percent reported a security incident but could not determine the origin (Allan, 2006). A pharmacy intranet can become more vulnerable as the user base becomes larger and more complex. Pharmacy intranet users commonly include employees, wholesalers, vendors, business partners, and other associated parties such as pharmacy students. Coincidentally, pathways from outside the intranet to the network can become less effective as the gateways needed to protect the organizational assets (mostly data) grow in scope and size. Finally, the degree of protection offered by firewalls can diminish as more and more exceptions to otherwise tight controls to the pharmacy's intranet are granted.
2. *External fraud* is an act committed by a third party that leads to data theft, data loss, and function disruption. People with technology skills can access (hack) the computer systems of pharmacies to steal or manipulate patient information for financial or nonfinancial reasons. For example, cell phone service provider T-Mobile experienced ongoing security problems that led to the publication of celebrity Paris Hilton's personal information and the telephone numbers of many Hollywood stars (Brian, 2005). Even more recently, 100 million users had their private information exposed when unknown intruders gained access to the Sony Corporation's PlayStaytion Network (Osawa, 2011). The cost in security alone, attributed to the attack, was estimated to hurt the company's profit by 14 billion yen (approximately US $182.3 million). One can only imagine the problems that could arise if patient data contained in a pharmacy's database were to be exposed, stolen, or manipulated.

   In general, threats from external users can be classified into one of two groups: information attack and business-functions attack. *Information attack* can lead to Web site defacement, financial data theft, denial of service, and network performance degradation. *Business-function attack* may cause disruption of online refill requests, physician e-prescribing, and inventory management and interference with automated schedule actions. One of the most vulnerable areas of information technology for pharmacies are Web servers for Internet applications (e.g., pharmacy Web sites where patients can go to place refill orders or make other purchases). Web servers that have not been configured specifically to the pharmacy's needs (i.e., default configuration, insufficient input validation, poor encryption, improper cleaning of temporary files, and poor management of user sessions) are susceptible to serious attacks that may compromise these applications.

   Another important tool of pharmacy automation is the barcode, which can be used to increase patient safety, facilitate inventory management, deliver checked prescriptions to patients, and refill automated stock cabinets (see Chapter 23). However, barcodes can be bypassed and are increasingly easy to exploit. To duplicate a barcode, one needs only the font of the barcode, a scanner, and the right software program. Exploitation of the barcode system can place a pharmacy at great risk in maintaining the security of its supply system as the risk of counterfeit drugs becomes increasingly common. To help control this risk threat, radiofrequency identification (RFID) chips are now being developed to help maintain the security of the drug supply system (see Chapter 23).

3. *Computer homicide* is the use of information technology systems to perform a malicious act that results in the death of a patient (Brenner, 2001a, 2001b). A user could access the information technology system and alter a patient's health care or prescription data. Whenever a pharmacy's computer system is compromised, this kind of event could be very probable, and its impact on the pharmacy's business can be profound. While there are no documented incidences of this happening within the pharmacy setting, it is easy to see how it could be carried out. For instance, what if a patient is severely allergic to a drug such as penicillin? It could be possible that a malicious person could gain access via the pharmacy's information technology system to the patient record and alter the patient record such that the allergy is no longer documented? Further, if a prescription were written for penicillin or any penicillin-like product, the contraindication would not likely be caught by the computer software. Although this is a very simplistic example, it is easy to see that without proper pharmacy information technology system safeguards, there is a great potential for significant patient harm or homicide because of the sensitive nature of patient data contained in the pharmacy's databases.
4. *Digital veil* is the term applied when the use of computer and automated machinery to execute business-related tasks creates a unique state of mind among the employees, resulting in complacency and blind trust in automation. This results in a mental disengagement with the work process, as if existing under a veil of digitization.

   In the summer of 1995, the Panamanian cruise ship *Royal Majesty* ran aground off the coast of Nantucket Island. The ship drifted off course because its satellite-based navigational system silently failed, and the crew did not monitor other sources of information that would have warned them they were in danger. Luckily, no one was hurt, but the mistake cost Majesty Cruise Lines $7 million in damages and lost revenue (Azar, 1998). Similar circumstances can occur in today's highly automated pharmacy. Employees can be become complacent, and the resulting mistakes in both patient and pharmacy safety and security can be catastrophic.
5. *The human-automation tradeoff* becomes more prominent as pharmacies become more dependent on automation. Years of experience and situational factors cannot be incorporated into software, which makes it less capable than humans to deal with emergency situations. Machines do not have the problem-solving capabilities that humans do for responding to new types of situations or threats.
6. *System failures* can occur in a multitude of ways once a pharmacy business is automated. System failures can have disastrous consequences. The use of sophisticated and intertwined Web services such as Internet refill request and processing, insurance processing, and inventory management create an overlay data-level network that ties multiple business functions together. If one function crashes, its failure potentially creates a cascading effect, causing other Web services to fail as well. In addition, an attack against a single node supporting a purchase transaction in a supply chain could corrupt databases at several pharmacies, interfere with logistics and third-party shipping organizations, and create errors in financial reports and inventory management. The damage may not be localized to the node that was attacked initially. The damage could extend across a business network, spanning companies.

The examples of system failures just cited are general and can happen in any automated business. However, some system failures are unique to pharmacies because of time and regulation constraints. Automated dispensing devices have become increasingly common to enhance pharmacy efficiency and improve patient safety. Although the implementation of automated dispensing reduces personnel time for medication administration and improves billing efficiency, reductions in medication errors have not been uniformly realized (Murray, 2001). Further, a case study by Perry et al. (2005) provided vivid insight into the operational risk associated with automated dispensing unit failure. Automation failures can test the adaptive capability of practitioners. In this specific case, an automated dispensing unit in an emergency department failed to dispense medications in an emergency situation. The authors assert that the more reliable the technological system is, the less skilled workers become in responding to eventual system breakdowns. Finally, the desire to avert human error by practitioners can lead to fragile automation and unanticipated forms of failure that can be impossible to plan for.

Psychosocial Risk

Psychosocial risk involves the moral and legal issues related to the interaction of information technology and the safety and health hazards that technology poses to employees in the workplace (Burton, 2006). Pharmacies with an increased risk of these conditions also risk higher worker's compensation costs, absenteeism, short- and long-term disability, and decreased productivity. Highly automated businesses, such as pharmacies, may seem like a safe work environment but actually may have hazardous work conditions. Repetitive-motion injuries, known as *cumulative trauma disorders,* are common among employees who deal with automation on a regular basis. The most common cumulative trauma disorder is carpal tunnel syndrome, a painful injury that can debilitate the hands, wrists, and arms. Carpal tunnel syndrome stems primarily from the repetitive motions of typing and computer work (Sheehan, 1990). Other illnesses associated with pharmacy automation and computer usage include neck, shoulder, and lower back pain; headaches; irritability; difficulty sleeping; deteriorated vision; and eye strain (Daniels, 1995; English, 2001; Sodani, 2003).

Electronic Medical Records and E-Prescribing

Electronic health records (EHR) and e-prescribing are becoming increasingly common, and bear special discussion. In a recent study by Grossman et al. (2011), the percentage of office-based physicians utilizing an e-prescribing system more than doubled between 2008 and 2009, from 12.1 percent to 26 percent. In this same study, physicians stressed the importance of having accurate electronic medical records in conjunction with the e-prescribing ability. In California, the adoption of e-prescribing has been varied, from 85 percent in institutions employing more than 51 physicians to only 18 percent in solo practices (Simon, 2011). There is no doubt that a large part of the increased acceptance of e-prescribing and EHR can be attributed to the federal incentive programs, specifically the Medicare Improvements for Patients and Providers Act (MIPPA) and the Medicare or Medicaid Electronic Health Records Incentive Programs (EHR Incentive Programs) (Grossman et al., 2011). The purpose of increased use of EHR and e-prescribing is to attain increased patient safety and increased efficiency (cost savings). However, with the increased reliance on IT, there is an increased concern for the security of PHI and the need for risk-management concern. In fact, in a recent report by the U.S. Department of Health and Human Services Office of Inspector General (DHHS OIG) (2011), there were some serious concerns regarding IT security controls for health information technology (HIT). The report noted that while there were application controls, IT controls were deficient. The specific IT controls cited included encrypting data stored on mobile devices, requiring two-factor authentication when remotely accessing HIT, and patching operating systems of computer systems that process and store EHR (DHHS OIG, 2011).

With the increased concerns regarding HIT, pharmacies must be concerned regarding the exposed risks of this increasingly adopted form of technological communication. In reality, it would serve the pharmacy well to have an information security consultant assess the pharmacies information technology systems for potential risks.

RISK PARADIGM

Risk can be defined either as a negative outcome (e.g., lung cancer is a risk among smokers) or the cause for any negative outcome (e.g., smoking is a health risk). When there are several causes for a single outcome or several outcomes from a single cause, the qualitative assessment of risk becomes complicated. The

Table 27-1. Pharmacy Risk Paradigm

Cause/Effect	Financial Risk	Reputation Risk	Privacy Risk	Human Capital Risk
Strategic risk	Budget constraint; Low or no return			Skill shortage; key personnel loss
Performance risk	Low or no return; patient injury	Loss of customers/ trading partners		
Operational risk	Data theft/loss; patient injury	Loss of customers/ trading partners	Data theft	
Psychosocial risk	Productivity loss; increased health benefits			

quantitative approach in defining risk does not divide the events into causes and outcomes explicitly; rather, a probability is assigned to each possible relationship whose development is undesirable. The impact of the previously discussed four categories of risk associated with integration of information technology in pharmacies can be viewed as probability events (which are also risks) because they happen at a discrete time and have impact on financial and nonfinancial aspects of pharmacies, as described in Table 27-1.

The *qualitative* explanation for risk provides a better understanding of risk in terms of both cause and outcome. However, the identification of causes and predictions of outcomes is better rather than identifying the outcomes and predicting the causes to minimize the risk because the failure rate of information systems projects is high and is an ever-changing field bringing new and advanced solutions almost every year.

REVISITING THE SCENARIO

Bill Halsey clearly saw a huge task in front of him if he was to purchase Corner Drug. He started making a list of all the issues and risks he would have to address. Not only would he need to update most of the fixtures in the store, but he also foresaw problems with the current layout of the pharmacy department from a security standpoint. He would have to purchase a new computer system and install other information technology and then consider the security issues related to this new technology. Two local physicians were interested in having Bill monitor drug therapy for all their geriatric patients. Bill knew that he also would have to develop a training program for the store's employees to meet HIPAA requirements and for counseling and monitoring documentation. One of his first tasks would be to develop a risk management program to assess current and future risk threats and to ascertain which techniques would have to be employed to address the risks. Bill breathed a sigh of relief that his current employer had included him in meetings with his insurance agent and that he had become well versed in insurance terminology and planning. He would have a big job in front of him and a lot of additional learning to do, but Bill thought he was prepared to know where to start and what needed to be done.

CONCLUSION

Just as with human beings in our daily lives, business entities such as pharmacies face risks that may threaten their financial health or ability to exist. Risk management is the process of identifying risks and developing strategies to manage or eliminate negative outcomes for the business. Risk management programs are an important component of business management. Risk management techniques include not only the use of insurance to transfer risk but also implementing strategies to minimize the likelihood of hazards occurring. Pharmacists need to be aware of these potential threats and seek assistance from their professional business consultants and experienced colleagues to develop and maintain appropriate risk management programs. Advice from experienced professionals may be crucial because most pharmacists have little training or experience in these areas.

The use of advanced information technology in community pharmacies continues to rise. Managers must be continually vigilant in safeguarding not only the pharmacy's own assets but also patient data from individuals both within and outside the pharmacy. As pharmacies grow more reliant on information technology and attacks on pharmacy systems grow more frequent and sophisticated, the successful pharmacy manager must manage the various risks brought about by this technology.

QUESTIONS FOR FURTHER DISCUSSION

1. Why is a risk management program an important component of a progressive patient-oriented pharmacy practice?
2. Many pharmacists have argued and fought for expanded roles in patient-oriented medication therapy management (MTM). These newer roles obviously increase the risk exposure of the pharmacists and the pharmacy. Therefore, should they be avoided?
3. A local physician has approached you about the possibility of establishing a paperless e-prescribing system with your pharmacy. What are the risks involved, and how can you minimize those risks?
4. You have decided to establish a Web site that can be used by your patients to order both over-the-counter medications and prescription refills. Would you also like to incorporate inventory management? What are the specific patient security risks? What are the pharmacy data security risks? Are other strategic, operational, performance, and psychosocial risks involved?

REFERENCES

Allan D. 2006. *Web Risk Exposure: Don't Forget Your Intranet. A White Paper from Watchfire.* Waltham, MA: Watchfire.

APRA. 2007. Prudential Practice Guide: LPG 230—Operation risk. Available at http://www.apra.gov.au/GI/PrudentialFramework/Pages/general-insurance-ppgs.aspx; accessed March 19, 2012.

Azar B. 1998. Danger of automation: It makes us complacent. *APA Monitor Online* 29(7).

Barker K, Felkey B, Flynn E, Carper J. 1998. White paper on automation in pharmacy. Available at http://www.ascpfoundation.org/programs/prog_automation.cfm; accessed March 19, 2012.

Barlas S. 2004. Securing electronic HIPAA data becomes hip. *P&T* 29:343.

Brenner S. 2001a. State cybercrime legislation in the United States of America: A survey. *Richmond J Law Technol* Available at http://www.richmond.edu/jolt/v7i3/article2.html; accessed March 19, 2012.

Brenner S. 2001b. Cybercrime investigation and prosecution: The role of penal and procedural law. Available at http://unpan1.un.org/intradoc/groups/public/documents/APCITY/UNPAN003073.pdf; accessed March 19, 2012.

Brian K. 2005. Paris Hilton Hack Started with Old Fashioned Con. *Washington Post,* May 5, 2005; www.washingtonpost.com/wp-dyn/content/article/2005/05/19/AR2005051900711.html.

Browning T. 1999. Sources of Performance Risk in Complex System Development. Available at http://sbufaculty.tcu.edu/tbrowning/Publications/; accessed March 19, 2012.

Burton J. 2006. Psychosocial risk management: What every business manager should know! Available at www.iapa.ca/pdf/2006_hwp_psychosocial_risk.pdf; accessed March 19, 2012.

Daniels C. 1995. Computer ergonomics: Living with computers. Available at www.klis.com/computers + health/; accessed March 19, 2012.

Dinardo JE. 2006. Your liability in filling Rxs correctly. *Drug Topics.* Available at http://drugtopics.modernmedicine.com/drugtopics/article/articleDetail.jsp?id=335300; accessed March 19, 2012.

English T. 2001. One pharmacist's battle with work-related injuries. *Pharmacy Today.* Available at www.medscape.com/viewarticle/406811; accessed March 19, 2012.

Ewusi-Mensah K. 2003. *Software Development Failures: Anatomy of Abandoned Projects.* Cambridge, MA: MIT Press.

Grossman JM, Boukus ER, Cross DA, Cohen GR. 2011. *Physician Practices, E-Prescribing and Accessing Information to Improve Prescribing Decisions.* Washington, DC: Center for Studying Health System Change.

Holleran MJ. 1995. Avoiding civil liability under OBRA 1990: Documentation is the key. *J Pharm Pract* 8:48.

Insurance Information Institute. 2007. Glossary of Insurance Terms. Available at http://www2.iii.org/glossary/; accessed on March 19, 2012.

Knaup AE. 2005. Survival and longevity in the business employment dynamics data. *Monthly Labor Rev.*

Lynch C. 2007. IT Value Methodologies: Do They Work? CIO WebBusiness Magazine, Apr. 10, 2007. Accessed at http://www.cio.com/article/103059/IT_Valu_Methodologie_Do_They_Work_/1; accessed on April 20, 2008.

Murray M. 2001. Automated Medication Dispensing Devices. Available at www.ahcpr.gov/clinic/ptsafety/pdf/chap11.pdf; accessed on March 19, 2012.

O'Donnell JT. 2005. Pharmacist practice and liability. *J Nurs Law* 10:201.

Osawa J. 2011. Sony expects Big Net Loss. Available at http://online.wsj.com/article/SB10001424052702304520804576340750302051690.html?mod=djemTAR_t; accessed March 19, 2012.

Perry SJ, Wears RL, Cook RI. 2005. The role of automation in complex system failures. *J Patient Saf* 1:56.

Ropeik D, Gray G. 2002. *Risk: A Practical Guide for Deciding What's Really Dangerous in the World Around You.* Boston: Houghton Mifflin.

Rupp's Insurance & Risk Management Glossary. 2002. Chatsworth, CA: NILS Publishing.

Schafermeyer KW. 2007. Private health insurance. In McCarthy RL, Schafermeyer KW (eds.) *Health Care Delivery: A Primer for Pharmacists,* 4th edn. Boston: Jones and Bartlett.

Sheehan M. 1990. Avoiding Carpal Tunnel Syndrome: A Guide for Computer Keyboard Users. Available at http://www.midmichiro.com/carpaltunnel.htm; accessed March 19, 2012.

Simon J. 2011. The State of Health Information Technology in California. Oakland, CA: California Healthcare Foundation.

Sodani O. 2003. Computer-Related Injuries Guide. Available at http://www.help2go.com/Tutorials/Computer_Basics/Computer_Related_Injuries_Guide.html; accessed March 19, 2012.

Spies AR, Van Dusen V. 2003. HIPAA: Understanding the security requirements. *U.S. Pharmacist* 28:42.

Standish Group. 2003. CHAOS. Available at www.standishgroup.com/chaos/introduction.pdf; accessed March 19, 2012.

U.S. Department of Health and Human Services (DHHS). 2000. *The Pharmacist Workforce: A Study of the Supply and Demand for Pharmacists.* Rockville, MD: Health Resources and Services Administration.

U.S. Department of Health & Human Services (DHHS). 2003. OCR Privacy Brief: Summary of the HIPAA Privacy Rule. Available at www.hhs.gov/ocr/privacy/hipaa/understanding/summary/privacysummary.pdf; accessed March 19, 2012.

U.S. Department of Health and Human Services (DHHS) OIG. 2011. Audit of Information Technology Security Included in Health Information Technology Standards (A-18-09-30160). Washington, DC. Available at http://oig.hhs.gov/oas/reports/other/180930160.pdf; accessed March 19, 2012.

Walker S. 2001. Operational Risk Management: Controlling Opportunities and Threats. Available at www.connleywalker.com.au/ORM.pdf; accessed March 19, 2012.

Wikipedia. 2007. Operational risk. Available at http://en.wikipedia.org/wiki/Operational_risk; accessed March 19, 2012.

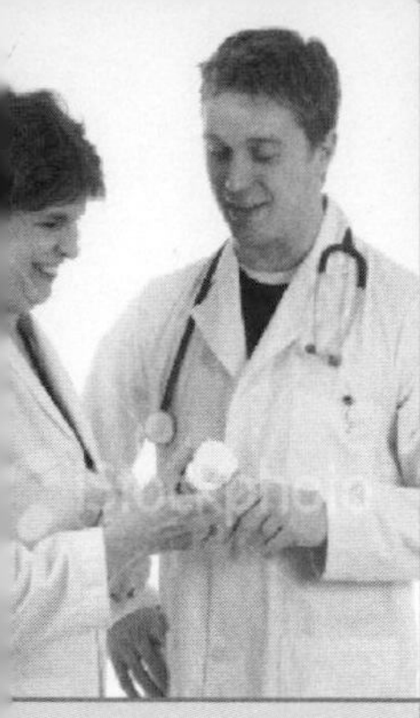

28

COMPLIANCE WITH REGULATIONS AND REGULATORY BODIES

Bartholomew E. Clark

About the Author: Dr. Clark is an Associate Professor in the Pharmacy Sciences Department at Creighton University School of Pharmacy and Health Professions. He earned a B.S. and an M.S. in pharmacy from the College of Pharmacy, University of Illinois at Chicago, and a Ph.D. in social and administrative sciences in pharmacy at the University of Wisconsin–Madison School of Pharmacy. Dr. Clark has practiced in a variety of community and institutional pharmacy settings and has served as professional affairs manager for the National Association of Boards of Pharmacy (NABP). His teaching and research interests include pharmacy practice management, pharmacy law, patient safety, pharmacists' work environments, and the pharmacy benefits management (PBM) industry.

LEARNING OBJECTIVES

After completing this chapter, readers should be able to

1. Describe the reasons for the evolution of pharmacy and drug regulation that have created the current legal environment for pharmacy practice organizations.
2. Summarize and explain the basic provisions of the major pharmacy and drug laws discussed in this chapter.
3. Describe the manager's role in monitoring a pharmacy's compliance with applicable laws and professional standards.
4. Explain the role of the manager in developing and maintaining appropriate policies for the protection of patient privacy.
5. Analyze practice-based situations where laws and/or professional standards may have been violated. In these analyses, consider the implications (statutory, regulatory, and civil) of a manager's actions in resolving any problems presented by these situations and propose appropriate courses of action for the manager.

SCENARIO

Few examples of how much trust is put in the hands of a pharmacist and the extent to which that trust can be betrayed come close to the story of Robert Courtney, a former pharmacist from Kansas City. During the 9 years leading up to his arrest in August 2001, Courtney secretively diluted the chemotherapy drugs of over 4,200 cancer patients to increase the profits of his home infusion pharmacy business. Courtney broke the law while betraying the trust of his patients and damaging the reputation of his profession.

Patients place their trust in pharmacists to do and know things that they themselves do not understand. State and federal laws provide additional layers of protection to shield the public from dangerous and/or contaminated drugs and from dangerous and/or dishonest professionals. As with any system, though, it can be breached. Consider how Courtney accomplished his deception.

Courtney began by diluting chemotherapy drugs for patients who were near death. He started out by diluting the drugs only a bit, thinking no one would notice. Later, he became more bold and diluted medications to the point that only a trace of the prescribed dose remained. He started out cheating "just a little" and then slid down a slippery slope until he was convicted of his crimes and sentenced to 30 years in prison. As stated in a newspaper feature about his case:

"The path to hell leads one step at a time," says Mike Ketchmark, the brash but persistent attorney who successfully litigated a $2.2 billion civil judgment against Courtney. "I think he started from the gray market and realized you could make a whole bunch of money. Then he'd get orders in from people who were on their deathbed, and he'd slice a little bit. Then he realizes he can just continue to cut it, and no one's going to notice. It's a felony once you engage in the gray market; you're then breaking down the barrier of a person's inhibition. You don't go from being John-Boy to Charles Manson overnight" (Draper, 2003).

Although the Courtney case is an extreme example of just how far someone can go in betraying their professional duties and in breaking the law, it is important to understand that Courtney's transgressions started out small and were almost undetectable. Then his moral compass drifted further, and greed became his guide. His patients no longer mattered to him. Their trust in him was betrayed. Laws were broken. Courtney's crimes provide a hideous but poignant example of just how vulnerable patients are and exactly why there are pharmacy and drug laws in the United States to protect them.

CHAPTER QUESTIONS

1. Do you think that statutes and regulations are necessary to protect the public from dangerous drugs and/or incompetent pharmacists? Why or why not?
2. What areas of pharmacy regulation do you find excessive and overly restrictive?
3. What areas of pharmacy practice and pharmacy operations can you identify that you think need to be regulated more closely?
4. How have standards and legal requirements for pharmacists evolved to the point where we see them today?
5. What is the significance of the current state of pharmacy and drug regulation for pharmacy managers?

INTRODUCTION

The purpose of this chapter is not to present a study guide for pharmacy law, an area to which entire texts have been devoted (e.g., Abood, 2010). Instead, its purpose is to provide an orientation to the professional and operational implications of food and drug law, pharmacy law, and professional regulation for pharmacy managers. This orientation should encourage pharmacy managers to think seriously about how the legal and regulatory environment that is external to a pharmacy practice organization can exert substantial influences on both the organization and its members. This encouragement includes a strong recommendation to know, understand, and follow applicable laws and professional standards in the operation of a pharmacy.

This chapter begins with a discussion of standards for pharmacists' professional performance and their importance to a manager. The chapter continues with a brief overview of some key historical mileposts in the development of laws and regulations governing both the quality of drug products (at the federal level) and the conduct of pharmacy professionals (at the state level). The chapter concludes with an examination of how the existence of standards can affect what an organization should and/or needs to do. These concepts are then illustrated by case-study examples that apply the principles presented.

STANDARDS FOR PHARMACISTS' PROFESSIONAL PERFORMANCE AND THEIR IMPORTANCE TO A MANAGER

Webster's Dictionary defines a *standard* as "something established by authority, custom, or general consent as a model or example" and states that *standard* "applies to any definite rule, principle, or measure established by authority (standards of behavior)" (Webster's Online Dictionary, 2012). From a contemporary managerial perspective, standards of conduct for a pharmacist and for the operation of a pharmacy are derived both from laws and from professional standards or values. Standards for professional conduct and the operation of a pharmacy, whether stated formally in statutes and regulations or present in professional codes of ethics, are important for managers to understand and apply. Violations of these standards can affect the licensure status of a pharmacy practice site and/or its pharmacists, may result in litigation if a patient is harmed subsequent to a violation, and in the most serious cases can result in criminal prosecution. Both criminal prosecution and civil liability resulted in the case of Robert Courtney, the pharmacist discussed in the scenario. Courtney was sentenced to 30 years in prison, fined $25,000, and ordered to pay $10.4 million in restitution to the patients and families affected. These penalties were in addition to the civil judgment of $2.2 billion (Stafford, 2002).

What Are Standards and Where Do They Come From?

Before there were laws in the United States for regulating the behavior of professionals, there were standards and codes of ethics established by professional guilds and associations. These codes of ethics stated in a formal way the type and level of professional performance that a guild or association expected from its members. These expectations were derived from the kinds of expert services that society needed from members of that profession. The professional standards in codes of ethics helped to align the highest standards of a profession with society's expectations. Knowing that professionals worthy of their title and status should adhere to their profession's standards, society came to expect no less. Yet, there was and continues to be an inherent tension between the desire of professions to self-regulate and the often justified cynicism of members of the pubic who fear that self-regulation can lead to lax oversight and endanger the public. The result is that we see not only professional standards and codes of ethics that emanate from professional associations (e.g., the American Pharmacists Association (APhA) Code of Ethics and Oath of a Pharmacist) but also federal and state statutes and regulations designed to protect the public from dangerous products and practitioners.

Bledstein (1976) discussed the evolution of the relationship between professionals and those whom they serve and noted that in mid-Victorian America there seemed to be a prevailing sense of insecurity among some members of the population. People who were seeking to expand their cultural horizons looked to professionals even for such things as recommendations concerning what should be considered appropriate reading material.

> A riot of words and a crisis of confidence alarmed a society which began placing its faith in professional persons. In mid-Victorian America, the citizen became a client whose obligation was to trust the professional. Legitimate authority now resided in special spaces, like the courtroom, the classroom and the hospital; and it resided in special words shared only by experts. . . . [T]he

> professions as we know them today were the original achievement of mid-Victorians who sought the highest form in which the middle class could pursue its primary goals of earning a good living, [and] elevating both the moral and intellectual tone of society.... . Americans after 1870, but beginning after 1840, committed themselves to a culture of professionalism which over the years has established the thoughts, habits and responses most modern Americans have taken for granted (Bledstein, 1976, pp. 78–81).

The trust in the professional just mentioned came at a time in the history of American culture long before the existence of the commercial aspects of professional–client relationships sometimes seen today. This dichotomy was discussed by May:

> Contract and covenant, materially considered, seem like first cousins; they both include an exchange and an agreement between parties. But, in spirit, contract and covenant are quite different. Contracts are external; covenants are internal to the parties involved. Contracts are signed to be expediently discharged. Covenants have a gratuitous, growing edge to them that springs from ontological change and are directed to the upbuilding of relationships.
>
> There is a donative element in the upbuilding of covenant—whether it is the covenant of marriage, friendship, or professional relationship. Tit for tat characterizes a commercial transaction, but it does not exhaustively define the vitality of that relationship in which one must serve and draw upon the deeper reserves of another (May, 1988, p. 93).

Why Laws Governing Drugs and Professional Conduct Became Necessary

Despite such lofty expressions of the duties owed to society by those who served them, maximization of profits (rather than adherence to the highest standards) sometimes was the goal of those selling "medicinal" products. Philip J. Hilts (2003) describes the evolution of drug regulation in the United States beginning in the late nineteenth century through the end of the twentieth century. During the late nineteenth century and well into the middle twentieth century, laws governing the content and quality of medicinal products provided, by today's standards, little or no protection to an unknowledgeable and unsuspecting public. Members of a relatively uninformed society were left to their own devices in making decisions for the purchase and use of medications. Subsequently, it took the occurrence of sentinel events such as the Elixir Sulfanilamide tragedy of 1937 and the thalidomide disaster of 1962 to raise consumer ire and prompt government action aimed at protecting the public from dangerous drug products.

The evolution of the pharmacy profession in the United States from colonial times to the present is rather astounding. During this time, pharmacy made the transition from an unlicensed occupation that in many ways resembled a trade to its current status requiring a professional doctorate (Pharm.D.) degree to become eligible for licensure. At first, scant formal education and long periods of apprenticeship were required to attain full status as a pharmacist. During this period the American Pharmaceutical Association (now the American Pharmacists Association) was established in 1852. Contemporaneously, the more classic definitions of professions and professionals applied. Professionals were expected to be ethical and honest in their dealings with the public, and the pharmacy profession was largely self-regulating, with sanctions from within its ranks as the only punishment for violation of the profession's standards.

HISTORICAL OVERVIEW OF LEGAL DEVELOPMENTS IN THE REGULATION OF DRUGS, PHARMACIES, AND PHARMACISTS

This section examines some of the more pivotal pieces of legislation enacted during the last century and discusses how they have evolved to provide pharmacy with the current legal and regulatory environment for the regulation of drugs, pharmacists, and pharmacies.

Regulation of Food and Drug Safety: Standards for Foods and Drugs Sold at Retail

The authority to regulate foods and drugs sold in interstate commerce is given to the federal government by the commerce clause of the US Constitution (US Constitution, Article I, Sec. 8, Clause 3). Until the beginning of the twentieth century, the only federal law regulating drugs in the United States was the Drug Importation Act of 1848, which empowered the US Customs Service to prevent the importation of adulterated (i.e., contaminated) drugs from other countries (FDA, 2002). Beginning in the early twentieth century, a series of highly publicized dramatic events provided the impetus for changes and improvements in the regulation of food, drug, and cosmetic safety.

Pure Food and Drug Act of 1906

The Pure Food and Drug Act of 1906 (59th Congress, Session I, Chap. 3915, pp. 768–772) was prompted by increased interest in the popular press concerning food safety that culminated in the publication of Upton Sinclair's exposé, *The Jungle,* a book that highlighted filthy and unsanitary conditions in meat packing plants. As stated in the 1906 act, the purpose of the new law was "for preventing the manufacture, sale, or transportation of adulterated or misbranded or poisonous or deleterious foods, drugs, medicines, and liquors, and for regulating traffic therein." In essence, this law required that foods and drugs be hygienic and accurately labeled. Before this law was enacted, there was a lack of standards and "traveling medicine shows," "patent medicines," and other unregulated products and activities were rampant. Products such as Lydia Pinkham's Vegetable Compound were nothing more than alcohol, whereas "soothing syrups" marketed as remedies for teething babies contained undisclosed and varying amounts of opium (Hilts, 2003).

The Food, Drug and Cosmetic Act of 1938 and Amendments

Passage of the Food, Drug and Cosmetic Act of 1938 was preceded by the Elixir Sulfanilamide tragedy of 1937. The 1906 act required drugs to be pure and labeled accurately but contained no requirement that drugs be safe. As one of the first effective oral antimicrobial drugs, sulfanilamide was very popular with physicians and was used widely to treat streptococcal infections. Bitter in taste, it was not easy to administer to children. Therefore, with some difficulty, the manufacturer developed a liquid dosage form called *Elixir Sulfanilamide.* Sulfanilamide powder is not soluble in either water or alcohol. Chemists at the manufacturer settled on ethylene glycol—the same chemical used today as an automobile antifreeze/coolant. This sweet-tasting chemical is highly toxic, causing painful kidney failure and death with in a few days of ingestion.

In 1937, no safety testing was required prior to marketing a drug product, and no premarketing safety tests were performed on Elixir Sulfanilamide. Two hundred and forty gallons were shipped to physicians and pharmacies all over the country, and 107 children died after using the product. Despite the extreme danger that this product represented to the public, the only legal basis the Food and Drug Administration (FDA) had for removing it from the market was that the product label stated "elixir," whereas technically it was not an elixir because it contained no alcohol and therefore was misbranded. The danger of allowing drug products to enter the market without safety testing became obvious, and the public demanded that something be done. The result was the requirement for premarketing safety testing in the Food, Drug and Cosmetic Act of 1938.

The 1938 act was strengthened subsequently by amendments. The 1951, Durham–Humphrey Amendments created separate categories for prescription-only and over-the-counter (OTC) drugs. Prior to passage of these amendments, there was no legal prohibition against selling drugs without a prescription. These 1951 amendments transformed pharmacy in ways likely unintended by their sponsors (Senator Hubert Humphrey was a pharmacist). There was a synergy between these amendments and the increased availability of finished-dosage forms in the post-World War II pharmaceutical industry boom that transformed the professional activities of neighborhood pharmacists. This transition from compounding and selling drugs at retail to "lick, stick, count, and pour" occurred simultaneously with the creation of the prescription-only market niche—a niche that only pharmacists were allowed to fill.

Next, the early 1960s saw another tragedy related to an unsafe drug product. Thalidomide was a drug marketed in Europe as a tranquilizer and used extensively to treat morning sickness in pregnant women. Although the manufacturer was eager to market this product in the United States, the efforts of FDA pharmacologist and reviewer Dr. Frances Kelsey prevented thalidomide from reaching the US market. At the time, an FDA reviewer had 60 days either to approve or reject a new drug application (NDA) from a manufacturer. However, an FDA reviewer could request further information from the manufacturer and restart the 60-day clock—a tactic that Dr. Kelsey employed several times because she was satisfied with neither the quantity nor quality of the data she had received about thalidomide's safety.

Tragedy in the United States was averted by Dr. Kelsey's efforts. Her refusal to approve the thalidomide NDA without further proof of safety occurred just as news from Europe revealed that thalidomide was responsible for a birth defect that caused infants to be born with flipper-like limbs. This near miss in the United States led to passage of the 1962 Kefauver–Harris Amendments to the 1938 act. These amendments established requirements that testing for *both* safety and proof of drug efficacy had to be conducted in well-controlled clinical trials before an NDA could be approved and a drug allowed to reach the market (Bren, 2001).

Establishment of State Pharmacy Practice Acts and State Boards of Pharmacy

Prior to 1870, when Rhode Island became the first in the nation to enact a state pharmacy practice act, regulation of the pharmacy profession was accomplished sporadically—generally at the local level or through the regulation of the medical profession (Green, 1979). States subsequently enacted their own pharmacy practice acts over the next several decades. The establishment of state pharmacy practice acts and the state boards of pharmacy created by these acts represents a legally binding codification of society's expectations of professional performance and a delineation of legal consequences for violation of these standards. The regulation of professional behavior by the states is pursuant to the police powers granted to the individual states by the US Constitution. The establishment of state statutes and regulations governing the practice of pharmacy and operation of a pharmacy business not only provided a new layer of safety for the public but also created a real barrier to entry into the pharmacy profession. This was a significant step in increasing both the professionalism of pharmacy and the expectations that society had of pharmacists. Prior to establishment of such standards and legal requirements, practically anyone could operate a business and call it a pharmacy.

Currently, all states have some form of pharmacy practice act (a state statute) and state board of pharmacy regulations. These laws establish legally binding standards for the conduct of pharmacists and ancillary personnel, as well as standards for the physical facilities licensed as pharmacies. These statutes and regulations are not to be taken lightly. Violations can result in penalties ranging anywhere from reprimands and fines to the loss of licensure to practice the profession or maintain operation of a given pharmacy facility. Practicing pharmacy without a license is a violation of criminal law, so it is important for pharmacy managers to have a clear understanding of their responsibilities under these statutes and regulations and to communicate these responsibilities clearly to nonpharmacist management personnel involved in operation of the pharmacy. For example, consider the situation where a pharmacy is located within a larger store that is open when the pharmacy department is closed. If the nonpharmacist store manager decides to open the pharmacy to get someone's medication during hours when the store is open but the pharmacy department is closed (and, of course, there is no pharmacist on duty), this would violate the pharmacy practice act and board of pharmacy regulations in any state. A managing pharmacist has to make clear to nonpharmacist managers what they are not allowed to do under the law. Further, a pharmacist who allows such illegal practices also has committed a violation and may be subject to both sanctions from the board of pharmacy as well as criminal prosecution.

FEDERAL LAW AND THE CONDUCT OF PHARMACISTS

Omnibus Budget Reconciliation Act of 1990

Until the passage of Omnibus Budget Reconciliation Act of 1990 (OBRA 1990; Public Law 101–508), federal law in the pharmacy arena had been concerned primarily with drug product safety. OBRA 90, while not explicitly usurping the police powers of the states, required that to be eligible for federal matching dollars, states participating in the Medicaid program would have to establish standards for

- *Maintaining proper patient records.* Pharmacies must make reasonable efforts to obtain, record, and maintain at least the following patient information: patient name, address, telephone number; age and gender; individual history (where significant), including disease state or states, known allergies and/or drug reactions, and a comprehensive list of medications and relevant devices; and the pharmacist's comments about the patient's drug therapy.
- *Prospective drug use review (pro-DUR).* Prior to dispensing a prescription, a pharmacist must conduct an evaluation of a patient's medication record to detect potential therapy problems, such as therapeutic duplication, drug–disease contraindications, drug–drug reactions (including serious interactions with OTC medications), incorrect drug dosage or duration of drug treatment, drug–allergy interactions, and evidence of clinical abuse/misuse.
- *Patient counseling.* A dispensing pharmacist must offer to counsel regarding matters that are, in the pharmacist's professional judgment, significant, which include but are not limited to name and description of the mediation, route of administration, dose, dosage form, and duration of therapy. In addition, such standards require pharmacists to discuss special precautions and directions, common severe side effects or interactions, therapeutic contraindications that may be encountered (including how to avoid them and what to do if they occur), proper storage, techniques for self-monitoring of drug therapy, what to do if a dose is missed, and refill information.

Not wanting to establish two separate legal standards of care—one for Medicaid patients and another for non-Medicaid patients—states generally adopted standards to meet the OBRA 90 criteria while extending the standards to benefit all pharmacy patients, not just Medicaid patients (Catizone et al., 1993). Implications for pharmacy management include how the manager decides to structure employee duties and the organization of work in the pharmacy. It is the managing pharmacist's duty to maintain compliance with applicable state and/or federal laws by ensuring that requirements for prospective drug use review and patient counseling are followed. From a management perspective, this means organizing work in the pharmacy and staffing the pharmacy to facilitate performance of these legal duties. Individual states may have their own requirements that may be stricter—but not more lenient—than federal law.

Health Insurance Portability and Accountability Act of 1996

This statute and its rules establish, for the first time, federal standards for protecting the privacy and security of patients' protected health information (PHI). These standards include, but are not limited to, how patient PHI must be stored, under what conditions it may be released, and to whom. This law has sweeping implications for pharmacies and pharmacists alike. The Health Insurance Portability and Accountability Act (HIPAA) privacy rules are designed to strike a balance between maintaining the flow of patients' health information among persons and entities providing health care to patients while simultaneously maintaining privacy for individuals. Essentially, this combination of statute and implementing regulations increases privacy and security for private information by establishing a "need to know" basis for who may have access to someone's PHI and to what extent they may have that access. Further, it establishes requirements for security of storage and for transmission of PHI by anyone who has access to the information. The purpose of this chapter does not include an exhaustive summary and explanation of this landmark legislation; numerous resources have been devoted to the subject.[1] The rules implementing this federal statute became effective as of April 14, 2003. Suffice it to say that pharmacy managers are responsible for making sure that their staff and policies and procedures are in compliance with HIPAA.

From a pharmacy manager's perspective, it is essential to understand that HIPAA establishes transaction standards, security standards, and privacy standards for PHI. Transaction standards and security standards are concerned primarily with how data are handled and transmitted. In the day-to-day operation of pharmacy, a manager needs to understand and comply with the requirements for privacy standards. As stated in the summary of the HIPAA privacy rule:

> A major goal of the Privacy Rule is to assure that individuals' health information is properly protected while allowing the flow of health information needed to provide and promote high quality health care and to protect the public's health and well-being. The Rule strikes a balance that permits important uses of information, while protecting the privacy of people who seek care and healing. Given that the health care marketplace is diverse, the Rule is designed to be flexible and comprehensive to cover the variety of uses and disclosures that need to be addressed (DHHS, 2012b).

[1]See (1) *HIPAA Privacy Standards: A Compliance Manual for Pharmacists.* National Association of Chain Drug Stores, Inc., and Mintz, Levin, Cohn, Ferris, Glovsky, and Popeo, P.C., 2003; and (2) Fitzgerald WJ. 2003. *The NCPA HIPAA Compliance Handbook for Community Pharmacy.* Alexandria, VA: National Community Pharmacists Association.

A pharmacy manager should know the answers to the following questions regarding these privacy standards:

1. *Who is covered by the privacy rule*? The privacy rule considers health plans, health care providers, and health care clearinghouses as covered entities. "Every health care provider, regardless of size, who electronically transmits health information in connection with certain transactions, is a covered entity" (DHHS, 2012a). This definition includes pharmacies.
2. *What information is protected*? According to the Department of Health and Human Services Office of Civil Rights, The Privacy Rule protects all *individually identifiable health information* held or transmitted by a covered entity or its business associate, in any form or media, whether electronic, paper, or oral. The Privacy Rule calls this information *protected health information* (PHI). Further, the Privacy Rule states that *individually identifiable health information* is information, including demographic data, which relates to
   - the individual's past, present, or future physical or mental health or condition,
   - the provision of health care to the individual, or
   - the past, present, or future payment for the provision of health care to the individual, and that identifies the individual or for which there is a reasonable basis to believe can be used to identify the individual. Individually identifiable health information includes many common identifiers (e.g., name, address, birth date, Social Security Number) (DHHS, 2012b).
3. *What must the covered entity do to protect information*? Every covered entity must have an individual designated as the facility's "privacy officer"—a person who is charged with the responsibility of keeping the site in compliance with HIPAA. Essentially, a covered entity may not release or disclose PHI except as allowed under the privacy rule. The following subsections summarize briefly what a pharmacy manager (a person who also may be the privacy officer) must be aware of.

Employee Training

Employees of a pharmacy should be trained in HIPAA rules and procedures as a condition of employment. Newly hired personnel should receive training before being allowed to work with PHI. This training should be documented as having been completed and repeated, if necessary, for employees who do not perform up to the standard. At a minimum, the training should include making clear to employees (1) how, to whom, to what extent, and under what circumstances PHI may be released and (2) that PHI should not be included in casual conversations with others—even in conversations with other health care providers if they are not involved in the patient's care. Also, employee access to PHI should be restricted to what is necessary in the performance of their duties.

Notice of Privacy Practices

Under the HIPAA privacy rule, all covered entities are required to provide patients with a "notice of privacy practices." The covered entity must provide this notice to all patients, and it should be written in understandable language. The privacy officer, most likely the pharmacy manager, is responsible for documenting patient signatures acknowledging receipt of the notice and documenting the reasons for any patient refusals of the notice or any patient refusal to sign in acknowledgment of having received the notice. The covered entity must maintain records of these documents for 6 years. Again, the importance of maintaining well-organized and easily retrievable records cannot be overemphasized.

Business Associates

The HIPAA privacy rule definition of a business associate and requirements regarding business associates are as follows:

Business Associate Defined. In general, a business associate is a person or organization, other than a member of a covered entity's workforce, that performs certain functions or activities on behalf of, or provides certain services to, a covered entity that involve the use or disclosure of individually identifiable health information. Business associate functions or activities on behalf of a covered entity include claims processing, data analysis, utilization review, and billing. Business associate services to a covered entity are limited to legal, actuarial, accounting, consulting, data aggregation, management, administrative, accreditation, or financial services. However, persons or organizations are not considered business associates if their functions or services do not involve the use or disclosure of PHI, and where any access to PHI by such persons would be incidental, if at all. A covered entity can be the business associate of another covered entity.

Business Associate Contract. When a covered entity uses a contractor or other nonworkforce member to perform "business associate" services or activities, the Rule requires that the covered entity include certain protections for the information in a business associate agreement (in certain circumstances governmental entities may use alternative means to achieve the same protections). In the business associate contract, a covered entity must impose specified written safeguards on the individually identifiable health information used or disclosed by its business associates. Moreover, a covered entity may not contractually authorize its business associate to make any use or disclosure of PHI that would violate the Rule (DHHS, 2012b).

In general, a pharmacy manager and/or privacy officer (in consultation with legal counsel) should tailor the pharmacy's relationships with business associates via the business associate contract. The overarching goals in an appropriately constructed business associate contract are to minimize the business associate's exposure to PHI while clearly establishing what uses of the PHI are permitted by the business associate. The privacy officer should have a clear idea of what business associates plan to do with any PHI they obtain and should make sure that any subcontractors have similar agreements. The privacy officer should monitor the business associate for any violations of the contract. In fact, the contract should stipulate that it is the responsibility of the business associate to report unauthorized disclosures of PHI. Finally, the privacy officer is responsible for the disposition of any PHI released to the business associate and should make sure that after it has been used by the business associate, PHI is either returned, held securely, or destroyed.

Patient Authorization Required for Release of PHI

A pharmacy, as a covered entity, needs to obtain a patient's written authorization for any disclosure or use of PHI that is not for treatment, payment, or health care operations. This authorization cannot be used as a precondition for benefits eligibility, payment, or treatment. The authorization document must be written in plain and specific language, and it may allow use and disclosure of PHI by the covered entity. An example of a disclosure of PHI that would require a written authorization by a patient is disclosure of such information to a drug manufacturer for marketing purposes. All authorizations must specify what information may be disclosed and must identify the person(s) disclosing and receiving the information, must specify an expiration date for the authorization document, and must state that a patient has the right to revoke the authorization in writing. Patient authorization for the release of PHI is not required for circumstances where a pharmacist reports spousal abuse or child neglect, becomes involved in legitimate law enforcement situations (including compliance with workers' compensation laws), is avoiding a threat to health or safety, or is reporting an adverse drug reaction to the FDA Medwatch program.

Circumstances Where PHI May Be Released without Explicit Patient Authorization

PHI may be released without explicit patient authorization under certain circumstances defined in the law and rules. These circumstances (with examples) include treatment (e.g., when a pharmacist discusses a patient's condition with the patient's physician), payment (e.g., when a claim for payment is submitted to a third-party payer), regular health care operations (e.g., the transfer of PHI among departments within a hospital), and when the information has been "de-identified."

PHI is considered to be "de-identified" when the following data elements have been removed:

- Patient's name, Social Security Number, and telephone and/or fax numbers
- Patient's town, street address, and/or ZIP code (state of residence need not be removed)
- Any dates of service (except year)
- Medical record number, health plan number, account number, and/or prescription number
- Any vehicle identifiers (e.g., license plate number)
- Medical device identifiers and/or serial numbers
- Patient's Web site URL, computer IP address, and/or e-mail address
- Biometric identifiers (e.g., DNA, fingerprints, voice recording, body description, retinal scan, etc.)
- Photographic images (identifiable)
- Any other unique characteristic or code

Remember, though, that "de-identification" of information is not necessary between covered entities involved in a patient's care. "De-identification" is also not necessary between a covered entity and a business associate with which the covered entity has a business associate contract.

The HIPAA statute and rules have created considerable confusion for pharmacy managers who have wondered about how these changes may affect normal operations in their pharmacies. Questions arise regarding situations such as when a neighbor is picking up a prescription for a patient. (*Note:* HIPAA rules allow the pharmacist to release a prescription to a patient's neighbor and counsel that neighbor as the patient's *agent.*) In response to these sorts of questions, the U.S. Department of Health and Human Services (DHHS) Web site has a search function that finds answers to many common questions about a wide variety of health care practice situations (DHHS, 2012c).

An Amendment to the Social Security Act Enacted as part of HIPAA

When HIPAA was passed, a small but significant amendment to the Social Security Act [Section 1128A(a)(5)] was included. This amendment prohibits offering inducements (i.e., remuneration) for

Medicare or Medicaid recipients to utilize the services of any particular provider. This provision is enforced by the Office of Inspector General (OIG) within the U.S. DHHS. The OIG interpretation of the amendment permits "Medicare or Medicaid providers to offer beneficiaries inexpensive gifts (other than cash or cash equivalents) or services without violating the statute. For enforcement purposes, inexpensive gifts or services are those that have a retail value of no more than $10 individually, or no more than $50 in the aggregate annually per patient." (U.S. DHHS, 2002).

When a pharmacist manager works in setting with a nonpharmacist manager (e.g., a large community pharmacy or a pharmacy department in a discount or grocery store), the nonpharmacist may not be aware of this prohibition, and may want to include Medicare and Medicaid recipients in coupon offerings or discounts in the store, but outside of the pharmacy department, to keep the recipients' business. This situation provides a difficult, but absolutely necessary opportunity for the pharmacist to educate the nonpharmacist manager regarding compliance with federal law. Failure to comply with this provision can result in serious legal and financial consequences—". . . a person who offers or transfers to a Medicare or Medicaid beneficiary any remuneration that the person knows or should know is likely to influence the beneficiary's selection of a particular provider, practitioner, or supplier of Medicare or Medicaid payable items or services may be liable for civil money penalties (CMPs) of up to $10,000 for each wrongful act." (U.S. DHHS, 2002). So, as difficult and cumbersome as it may seem, a pharmacy engaged in offering small "gifts" to Medicare and Medicaid beneficiaries must limit individual gifts to a monetary value of $10 or less and must limit the annual total to $50 for each beneficiary. Actions that would likely be in violation of this statute include providing in-store gift cards or coupons that can be spent in the store just like cash as incentives to utilize a given pharmacy's services. For example, it is not difficult to imagine that someone who receives a $15 store coupon every time they get a Medicare/Medicaid prescription filled might be more likely to find ways to increase their prescription drug utilization.

Prescription Drug Marketing Act

Pharmacy managers must also comply with federal laws regulating other economic issues in pharmacy. The Prescription Drug Marketing Act of 1987 (PDMA) represents one area where some pharmacists have encountered considerable legal problems, resulting in large fines and/or prison sentences (Associated Press, 2000; Eiserer, 1999). In brief, the PDMA prohibits the diversion of prescription drug samples into the retail market sector. Pharmacies may not have in their stock any prescription drug samples, and pharmacies may not possess or sell any prescription drug samples. Further, the PDMA restricts the annual distribution of prescription drugs by pharmacies to other pharmacies to no more than 5 percent of the annual dollar value of prescription drug sales for the distributing pharmacy (e.g., one pharmacy providing prescription drugs to another pharmacy that has run out of stock of an item). Pharmacy managers must ensure compliance with the PDMA or be prepared to face stiff penalties. In a Nebraska case, a pharmacist violated the PDMA by colluding with a pharmaceutical manufacturer's sales representative to divert and profit from the sale of drug samples. In 1999, the pharmacist pled guilty to illegally selling prescription drug samples over a 15-year period (Eiserer, 1999). In 2000, the pharmacist was sentenced to 18 months in prison and ordered to pay nearly $147,000 in fines and restitution (Associated Press, 2000).

State Prescription Drug Monitoring Programs

In order to curb the practice of "doctor shopping" that is used by some patients to obtain controlled substances, a number of states have enacted a prescription drug monitoring program (PDMP). These PDMPs collect information on controlled substances and "drugs of concern" dispensed within the state and maintain an electronic database of the information. The agencies that administer and house these programs vary from state to state as do "drugs of concern". For example, Louisiana's 2006 Prescription Monitoring Program Act empowered the state board of pharmacy to promulgate regulations to identify "drugs of concern" in addition to drugs in Schedules II through V that are now being monitored as of September 1, 2010. The Louisiana board has identified two such drugs: (1) butalbital when in combination with at least 325 milligrams of acetaminophen per dosage unit, and (2) tramadol. A useful resource for identifying whether a state has a prescription monitoring program and drugs that are monitored is the Alliance of States with Prescription Monitoring Programs (http://www.pmpalliance.org).

Information collected by PDMPs is then distributed to individuals authorized by state law to receive such information for their professional purposes. Individuals authorized to access PDMP data vary from state to state, but usually include prescribers and pharmacists. For example, in a state with a PDMP where both prescribers and pharmacists are allowed to access PDMP data, each is able to check if their patient is obtaining prescriptions for controlled substances from other prescribers and/or other pharmacies. This sharing of information can help to deter abuse and diversion of controlled substances while identifying patients who may need to be directed to drug abuse treatment programs. Also, in cases of criminal prosecution for drug diversion via falsified prescription documents, data from prescription monitoring programs would be discoverable and could be used as evidence by prosecutors.

According to the US Drug Enforcement Administration Office of Diversion Control, 37 states had operational PDMPs with the capacity to receive and distribute controlled substance prescription information to authorized users as of March 2012 (U.S. Department of Justice, 2012). States with operational programs include:

Alabama, Arizona, California, Colorado, Connecticut, Florida, Hawaii, Idaho, Illinois, Indiana, Iowa, Kansas, Kentucky, Louisiana, Maine, Massachusetts, Michigan, Minnesota, Mississippi, Nevada, New Mexico, New York, North Carolina, North Dakota, Ohio, Oklahoma, Oregon, Pennsylvania, Rhode Island, South Carolina, Tennessee, Texas, Utah, Vermont, Virginia, West Virginia, and Wyoming.

Eleven states (Alaska, Arkansas, Delaware, Georgia, Maryland, Montana, Nebraska, New Jersey, South Dakota, Washington, and Wisconsin) and one U.S. territory (Guam) have enacted legislation to establish a PDMP, but are not fully operational as of March 2012.

Where pharmacy managers have access to PDMP data, they have a useful tool in maintaining their pharmacy in compliance with federal and state controlled substance statutes and regulations. Where PDMPs are in place and available for access by pharmacists, pharmacy managers should ensure that pharmacists practicing at their site take advantage of this resource. Failure to do so could result in board of pharmacy actions against the license of a pharmacist who did not use the PDMP tool to ascertain whether or not prescriptions for controlled substances and "drugs of concern" were valid prior to dispensing.

Civil Law and Liability Concerns

When a pharmacist or pharmacy organization is sued, the issue of negligence becomes the key to what the outcome of the lawsuit will be. Negligence theory revolves around either the failure to do something that a reasonable and prudent person *would* do, or doing something that a reasonable and prudent person *would not* do. In this case, the person is the pharmacist. The pharmacist's role has changed over time because of the evolving nature of pharmacy practice (e.g., OBRA 90 ushered in the requirement to offer patient counseling). Case law also changes pharmacy practice standards. Case law is based on precedents established by the outcomes of civil cases. For example, if the result of a lawsuit establishes that a pharmacist had a duty to warn a patient about certain dangers of a drug that was dispensed, then a new standard of behavior for pharmacists is established through case law, not by statute or regulation.

The thought of being sued for something one has done while practicing, or the thought of a pharmacy manager being sued for the actions of his or her staff, is not at all pleasant. The first thing someone might think of is, "How can I prevent that from happening to me?" This question opens the door to a field of management called *risk management* that deals with how to reduce and manage exposure to risk (see Chapter 27). Sound practice site design, consistent adherence to applicable law, and a well-organized work-flow system designed to detect errors before they reach the patient are all essential to minimizing exposure to risk. As with all laws governing the activities of pharmacists, managers are encouraged to become familiar with these important provisions.

HOW DO LEGAL STANDARDS AFFECT WHAT AN ORGANIZATION SHOULD AND/OR NEEDS TO DO?

It is important for managers to understand that statutory and regulatory standards create an environmental context for an organization, a factor critical in determining whether or not the organization prospers and grows. The manager is a person embedded within an organization that is, in turn, embedded within the environment—an environment that is constantly changing. For pharmacists and pharmacies, statutes and regulations represent society's codification of standards beyond its normative expectations—beyond the sanctions implicit in not meeting the expectations of professional peers. Statutes and regulations also provide for enforcement by way of penalties if they are violated. Regulations are standards that are derived from statutes and have legal enforcement mechanisms (i.e., potential penalties) attached to them. For example, state pharmacy practice acts create a board of pharmacy and empower that board to establish rules and/or regulations to interpret and implement the practice act. Board of pharmacy regulations carry the full force of the law and establish penalties anywhere from warnings, fines, and on to suspension and/or revocation of pharmacist's or pharmacy's licensure.

Performance Improvement versus Meeting Minimum Performance Standards

To avoid legal sanctions for practitioners and/or the pharmacy, the manager can take steps to prevent or avoid substandard practices that could lead to penalties. How should a manager approach such a task? One way some organizations approach making sure they meet minimum legal standards is by developing programs to foster performance improvement. Meeting minimum performance standards is compliance with the bare minimum legal requirement, whereas performance improvement goes beyond this and can provide additional protection in the risk prevention and risk management arenas. If a pharmacy and its pharmacists aim to establish standards for the performance of the organization that exceed the legal minimum, it is much less likely that performance quality will result in violations of the law or in performance so poor that it results in a civil lawsuit. For example, a pharmacist manager may decide to establish a policy that every patient visiting the pharmacy will receive a personal offer of counseling from a licensed pharmacist, even where state law may allow pharmacy interns or other pharmacy staff to perform this function. Further, if a lawsuit is filed against the pharmacy, it can work in a pharmacy's favor if the pharmacy has in place standards of care and policies and procedures that exceed the legal minimum and afford better protection for clients. Also, with such systems in place, it is much less likely that a pharmacy will encounter legal difficulties of either kind. Establishment of a practice environment and philosophy that are centered on doing what is best for the patient while knowing and obeying all applicable laws is essential to avoiding legal problems in either the civil or criminal realm.

Quality measurement of pharmacy professional services by groups such as the Pharmacy Quality Alliance (PQA, see http://www.pqaalliance.org/) is beginning to set standards and measures that pharmacies can use to evaluate themselves that go beyond minimum legal requirements. Other groups (including third-party payers) are also likely to develop standards to evaluate the quality of a pharmacy practice site. In the not too distant future, pharmacy managers may well need to incorporate quality measures to assure that their pharmacy is compensated for professional pharmacy services.

CONCLUSION

This chapter began by reviewing the history of and motivation for the development of standards, statutes, and regulations governing the manufacture of drugs and the practice of pharmacy. Next, within this context, some of the milestones of pharmacy and drug regulation, such as HIPAA, OBRA 90, and the PDMA, were summarized. Finally, civil law and its impact on pharmacy practice were considered. All these aspects of pharmacy and drug regulation were examined from the viewpoint of the pharmacy manager.

The chapter concludes with the following case examples for discussion of laws pertinent to the operation of a pharmacy. These cases are presented as starting points for discussion and analysis of practice-based situations a pharmacy manager is likely to encounter. Pharmacy and drug law, as well as civil law, all present managers with criteria on which to fashion their own management style in operating a pharmacy. Law, while quite explicit in its language, often can be silent on some issues and thus open to interpretation and the exercise of professional judgment. Pharmacy students reading this chapter are encouraged to work together in analyzing the situations presented here and to come up with their own plausible solutions to the problems presented.

QUESTIONS FOR FURTHER DISCUSSION

Case Examples for Discussion of Laws Pertinent to Operating a Pharmacy

Case 29.1: Why Won't the Pharmacist Just Refill My Prescription?

A FEDERAL DRUG LAW: THE CONTROLLED SUBSTANCES ACT OF 1970 Maureen Smith, R.Ph., the pharmacist manager of ABC Drugs Community Pharmacy, encounters the following situation within 10 minutes of arriving at the pharmacy on a Tuesday morning. She finds herself dealing with a complaint from a patient, Mr. Jones, about one of the staff pharmacists. Yesterday evening, Monday, at about 8:30 p.m., Mr. Jones came to the pharmacy and presented an empty prescription vial to the pharmacist on duty and asked for a refill of his acetaminophen with codeine no. 3 tablets. Acetaminophen no. 3 is a schedule III controlled substance, and the federal Controlled Substances Act limits prescriptions for such medications to a maximum of five refills within 6 months of the time they are issued. Mr. Jones had not seen the prescribing physician in about 7 months and was now experiencing pain unrelated to the reason for his visit 7 months ago. However, the label on his vial stated that he had three refills remaining, and he wanted one right away.

Sally Howard, Pharm.D., the pharmacist who was on duty Monday evening, explained to Mr. Jones that she would need further authorization from Mr. Jones' prescriber because the prescription had been written over 6 months ago and was now no longer valid for refilling. Sally tried to reach Mr. Jones's doctor to obtain authorization but was unsuccessful in reaching the prescriber before the pharmacy closed at 9:00 p.m. Therefore, she informed Mr. Jones that the pharmacy would not be able to refill the prescription until it could reach the prescriber. Mr. Jones became angry when he heard this and remains very angry as he tells Maureen about the situation.

DISCUSSION QUESTIONS

1. What are the essential legal issues involved?
2. How should the pharmacy manager handle this situation?
3. How might another manager deal with the problem presented by this difficult patient?

Case 29.2: The Grandmother Who Did Not Need an Easy-Open Prescription Vial

A FEDERAL CONSUMER PROTECTION LAW: THE POISON PREVENTION PACKAGING ACT The (federal) Poison Prevention Packaging Act requires that prescription medications (with very few exceptions, such as sublingual nitroglycerin tablets) be dispensed in child-resistant containers. Mrs. Mabel Brown, a 79-year-old great grandmother to 2-year-old Barbara Brown, is a longstanding patient at the community pharmacy where you are the manager. You have just been informed by Mrs. Brown's great grand daughter's pediatrician that little Barbara was treated at the local hospital emergency room yesterday evening. It seems that while Barbara and her parents were visiting Mabel at her house, Barbara climbed up on the kitchen counter and grabbed Mabel's prescription vial containing propranolol 80 mg long-acting capsules. Little Barbara had only been out of her mother's sight for about 2 minutes when her mother walked into the kitchen and found Barbara sitting on the kitchen counter munching away on Mabel's medicine. Although she became a bit lethargic, luckily she did not have enough time to consume a dangerous quantity and was treated and released.

After speaking with the pediatrician, you do some checking in Mabel's patient record, and you discover that all her medications have been dispensed in nonchild-resistant containers (i.e., "easy open" flip-top containers). On further investigation, you discover that there is no request on file where Mabel or her physician actually asked for easy-open containers. While discussing this with your pharmacy staff, you learn that everyone just assumed that a 79-year-old patient would want the nonchild-resistant containers but that no one had ever asked her if she wanted them.

Discussion questions

1. How would the pharmacy manager need to articulate and address the issues presented by this situation?
2. What are the key issues, and how should a pharmacy manager handle them with pharmacy staff?
3. What recommendations for change, if any, would be appropriate to assist the pharmacy in refining the pharmacy's policies and procedures?
4. What additional civil liability issues arise from situations like this one?

Case 29.3: The Super-technician

A state practice act/board of pharmacy provision Trudy Hamilton, Pharm.D., is a licensed pharmacist and is currently the manager of a hospital pharmacy department. In the state where Dr. Hamilton is licensed, nonpharmacist personnel are prohibited by both statute (the state pharmacy practice act) and state board of pharmacy regulation from engaging in activities defined as the practice of pharmacy. The specific activities that fall within the definition of the practice of pharmacy are limited to being personally performed by licensed pharmacists only. Such activities include counseling patients about their medications and responding to drug information requests from other health care professionals (e.g., physicians and nurses).

Robert Allen recently earned his certification as a certified pharmacy technician (C.Ph.T.) and has been working as a technician in the pharmacy department for the past 3 years. Robert is rightly proud of his accomplishment and recently has expressed interest in applying for admission to pharmacy school. Today, Dr. Hamilton received a phone call from Ann Brown, D.O., an attending physician at her institution. Dr. Brown was noticeably angry. Yesterday, Dr. Brown called the pharmacy with a drug-interaction question about a drug that is new to the hospital's formulary (i.e., the list of drugs that the hospital pharmacy regularly keeps in stock). She was told by the "pharmacist" who answered the phone that the pharmacy department's computer system showed no interactions. Today, Dr. Brown's patient experienced a severe interaction between the new drug and a medication that the patient was already taking.

At a recent continuing-education seminar, Dr. Hamilton and her staff pharmacists learned of the potential for a significant interaction between the two medications in question. She was puzzled as to why one of the pharmacists would have told a physician that there are no drug interaction problems with the new drug. Dr. Hamilton and the staff pharmacists are aware that the hospital information technology department has not yet updated the pharmacy department computer system to include this interaction. As she concludes her conversation with Dr. Brown, she promises to find out what happened and take corrective action.

In Dr. Hamilton's investigation, she discovers that technician Robert Allen in fact took the phone call and answered Dr. Brown's question. Dr. Hamilton calls a meeting of the pharmacists to discuss how to prevent such problems from occurring in the future. During the meeting, she discovers that a few of the staff pharmacists have, on occasion, observed Robert stepping outside his technician role because he was trying to be helpful. They tell her that they have attempted to correct his behavior but have had little success. This is the first time Dr. Hamilton has heard of the problem.

Discussion questions

1. How should Dr. Hamilton address this situation?
2. Are there problems with the way the department is functioning as a unit?
3. Is this situation simply a "personnel" issue confined to Robert's behavior?
4. Are there other issues or combinations of issues that should be addressed?

Case 29.4: A Recently Hired Pharmacist and the Nonpharmacist Store Manager

FEDERAL STATUTES (SOCIAL SECURITY ACT AND HIPAA) Pauline Rodgers, Pharm.D., recently started working as a staff pharmacist at Big Box Stores, Inc. right after she passed her board examinations and became licensed as a pharmacist. The pharmacy manager, Len Roberts, R.Ph., has been working for Big Box for about 20 years and has a fairly cordial relationship with Don Smith, the store manager. Mr. Smith, a business school graduate, is very pro-pharmacy and wants to do all he can to help the pharmacy department increase its business through various marketing promotions. After working at the store for a few weeks, Pauline notices that Len makes a practice of giving in-store coupons to patients who are Medicare and Medicaid beneficiaries. These coupons, each worth $10, can be used toward the purchase groceries, DVDs, clothing, and so on. Realizing that she will soon likely encounter a situation where a Medicare or Medicaid beneficiary will expect to receive a coupon from her, Pauline asks Len what recordkeeping system is in use for tracking the total annual value of coupons given to each beneficiary. Len responds with a puzzled look on his face and asks: "Why would we do that? Mr. Smith wants us to keep handing out these coupons to increase our business. When it comes to running the business, I do what Mr. Smith wants and I don't ask questions."

Discussion questions

1. How should Pauline respond to Len?
2. What do you think are the important legal and managerial issues here?
3. How should Pauline respond to a request for a coupon from a Medicaid beneficiary?
4. Describe how you would handle this situation if you were Pauline.

Case 29.5: The Poorly Written Prescription and the Hurried Pharmacist

Civil liability (tort law) Stuart Johnson, R.Ph., is manager of Johnson's Apothecary, a community pharmacy. When he arrived at the pharmacy today, there was a frantic voice-mail message left for him in the middle of the night while the pharmacy was closed. It seems that a staff pharmacist, Dave, made a dispensing error yesterday, and Suzie Jones, a 3-year-old child, was taken unconscious by ambulance to the local community hospital emergency room at 2:00 a.m. Suzie and her family had just moved to town about 2 weeks ago, and yesterday was their first visit to Johnson's Apothecary.

In the process of both calling the hospital and interviewing Dave, the staff pharmacist, Stuart learns the following: Somehow Dave misinterpreted a poorly written prescription that was supposed to be for glycerin suppositories (Directions: "Use as directed") as a prescription for Glynase 5-mg tablets (a drug used to treat diabetes in adults). As a result of this error, Suzie's blood sugar dropped to dangerously low levels, and she is now in a coma. Dave was very busy when the error occurred and did not determine that the patient, Susan Jones, was in fact a 3-year-old child. He also did not speak to Suzie's mother, who brought in the prescription. Because he was very busy, he quickly checked a pharmacy technician's work and let her dispense the prescription to Mrs. Jones, an uninsured cash-paying customer. The sad truth is that the doctor had not even intended this written note to be a prescription (glycerin suppositories are available without a prescription); it just looked like one because it was on one of the doctor's prescription blanks.

Discussion questions

1. From this case, describe violations of both state and federal law and the tort law implications (i.e., potential for being sued).
2. What is the manager's role in determining what happened internally that was out of conformance with standards, with external regulatory bodies, and

with professional performance standards beyond the letter of the law?

3. How can all these be brought to bear on the pharmacy?
4. How should Stuart as the manager respond when the local TV station and newspaper want interviews?

REFERENCES

Abood RR. 2010. *Pharmacy Practice and the Law*, 6th edn. Boston: Jones and Bartlett.

Associated Press. 2000. Drug Representative, Pharmacist Sentenced. *Omaha World-Herald*, Feb. 12, 2000, p. 16.

Bledstein BJ. 1976. *The Culture of Professionalism*. New York: Norton, p. 78.

Bren L. 2001. Frances Oldham Kelsey: FDA medical reviewer leaves her mark on history. *FDA Consumer Magazine*, 35(2):24–29.

Catizone CA, Teplitz J, Clark BE (eds.). 1993. *NABP Survey of Pharmacy Law*. Park Ridge, IL: National Association of Boards of Pharmacy.

Draper R. 2003. The Toxic Pharmacist. *New York Times Magazine*, June 8, 2003, A83.

Eiserer T. 1999. 2 Plead Guilty in Fraudulent Drug Sale Case. *Omaha World-Herald*, October 9, 1999, p. 34.

Green MW. 1979. Epilogue, Prologue. In *From the Past Comes the Future—The First 75 Years of the National Association of Boards of Pharmacy*. Chicago: National Association of Boards of Pharmacy.

Hilts PJ. 2003. *Protecting America's Health: The FDA, Business and One Hundred Years of Regulation*. New York: Knopf.

May WF. 1988. Code and covenant or philanthropy and contract: Hastings Center report 1975. In Callahan JC (ed.) *Ethical Issues in Professional Life*. New York: Oxford University Press, p. 93.

Stafford M. 2002. *Ex-Pharmacist Gets 30 Years for Diluting Cancer Drugs*. Omaha World Herald, December 5, 2002, p. 1.

U.S. Department of Health and Human Services (DHHS). 2002. Office of Inspector General (OIG) Special Advisory Bulleting, Offering Gifts and Other Inducements to Beneficiaries. Available at http://oig.hhs.gov/fraud/docs/alertsandbulletins/SABGiftsandInducements.pdf; accessed on May 27, 2011.

U.S. Department of Health and Human Services (DHHS). 2012a. Covered Entity Decision Tools, Centers for Medicare and Medicaid Services. Available at http://www.cms.gov/HIPAAGenInfo/06_AreYouaCovered Entity.asp; accessed March 20, 2012.

U.S. Department of Health and Human Services (DHHS). 2012b. Office of Civil Rights (OCR) Privacy Brief: Summary of the HIPAA Privacy Rule, available at www.hhs.gov/ocr/privacy/hipaa/understanding/summary/privacysummary.pdf; accessed March 20, 2012.

U.S. Department of Health and Human Services (DHHS). 2012c. HIPAA Questions and Answers. Available at www.cms.gov/MMIS/Downloads/smd40402.pdf; accessed March 20, 2012.

U.S. Department of Justice (DOJ), Drug Enforcement Administration (DEA), Office of Diversion Control. 2012. State Prescription Drug Monitoring Programs, updated July 2010. Available at http://www.deadiversion.usdoj.gov/faq/rx_monitor.htm; accessed on March 20, 2012.

U.S. Food and Drug Administration (FDA). 2002. FDA Backgrounder: Milestones in U.S. Food and Drug Law History, updated August 5, 2002. Available at www.fda.gov/opacom/backgrounders/miles.html; accessed on March 21, 2003.

Webster's Online Dictionary. 2012. Available at http://www.merriam-webster.com/dictionary/standard accessed on March 20, 2012.

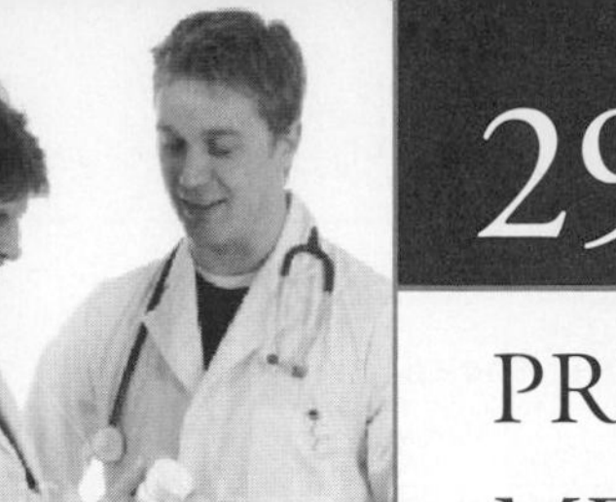

29

PREVENTING AND MANAGING MEDICATION ERRORS: THE PHARMACIST'S ROLE

Matthew Grissinger and Michael Cohen

About the Authors: Matthew Grissinger, R.Ph., FISMP, FASCP is the Director of Error Reporting Programs at the Institute for Safe Medication Practices (ISMP). Prior to joining ISMP, he served as a home care and long-term care pharmacy surveyor for the Joint Commission (TJC). Mr. Grissinger has published numerous articles in the pharmacy literature, including regular columns in *P&T* and the *Patient Safety Advisory* (PSA). He serves on the National Quality Form (NQF) Common Formats Expert Panel, the Faculty Advisory Board for the Pharmacy Learning Network (PLN), and the Publications Advisory Board for Davis's *Drug Guide for Nurses.* He is an adjunct assistant professor for Temple University School of Pharmacy and clinical assistant professor for the University of the Sciences in Philadelphia. Mr. Grissinger received a B.S. in Pharmacy from the Philadelphia College of Pharmacy and Science and is a fellow of the ISMP as well as the American Society of Consultant Pharmacists.

Michael Cohen, R.Ph., M.S., Sc.D., is president of the ISMP. He is editor of the textbook *Medication Errors* and serves as coeditor of the *ISMP Medication Safety Alert!,* publications that reach over 2 million health professionals and consumers in the United States and in over 30 countries. Dr. Cohen is a member of the Sentinel Event Advisory Group for TJC and recently served as a member on the Committee on Identifying and Preventing Medication Errors for the Institute of Medicine (IOM). In 2005, he was recognized as a MacArthur Fellow by the John D. and Catherine T. MacArthur Foundation. In 2008, Dr. Cohen was honored by The National Quality Forum (NQF) and The Joint Commission (TJC) with the John M. Eisenberg Patient Safety and Quality Award in recognition of his lifelong professional commitment to promoting safe medication use and a safe medication delivery system.

LEARNING OBJECTIVES

After completing this chapter, readers should be able to

1. Discuss the role of the pharmacist in preventing medication errors.
2. Define latent and active failures and the role each plays when a medication error occurs.

3. Define the types of medication errors that can occur during the ordering and dispensing process.
4. List some commonly used drugs that can result in medication error-related deaths.
5. Describe what changes are needed at the risk management level to better address medication safety issues, including the use of failure mode and effects analysis to reduce the potential for errors.
6. Identify specific problems in our approach to error prevention and what needs to be changed to ensure patient safety.
7. Describe a variety of methods that can be used to identify risk and provide meaningful data on the relative safety of their facility's medication use process.
8. Select high-leverage error reduction strategies based on sound safety principles.

SCENARIO

This scenario is based on a true story that demonstrates the multiple breakdowns that can occur during the medication use process.

An infant was born to a mother with a prior history of syphilis. Despite having incomplete patient information about the mother's past treatment for syphilis and the current health status of both the mother and the child, *a decision was made to treat the infant for congenital syphilis.* After phone consultation with infectious disease specialists and the health department, an order was written for one dose of "benzathine penicillin G 150,000 units IM."

The physicians, nurses, and pharmacists, unfamiliar with the treatment of congenital syphilis, also had limited knowledge about this medication. The pharmacist consulted *Drug Facts and Comparisons* to determine the usual dose of penicillin G benzathine for an infant. However, *she misread the dose* as 500,000 units/kg, a typical adult dose, instead of 50,000 units/kg. Consequently, the pharmacist also *incorrectly read and prepared the order as 1,500,000 units, a 10-fold overdose.* Owing to the lack of a consistent pharmacy procedure for independent double checking, *the error was not detected.* The pharmacy *dispensed the 10-fold overdose in a plastic bag containing two full syringes of Permapen® (the brand name of penicillin G benzathine) 1.2 million units/2 mL each,* with green stickers on the plungers to "note dosage strength." A pharmacy label on the bag indicated that 2.5 mL of medication was to be administered intramuscularly to equal a dose of 1,500,000 units. After glancing at the medication sent from the pharmacy, the infant's primary care nurse expressed concern to her colleagues about the number of injections required to give the infant the medication (since there a maximum of 0.5 mL per intramuscular injection allowed in infants, the dose would require five injections).

Anxious to prevent unnecessary pain to the infant, the two nurses *decided to investigate the possibility of administering the medication intravenously instead of intramuscularly.* The monograph on penicillin G did not specifically mention penicillin G benzathine; instead, it noted the treatment for congenital syphilis with aqueous crystalline penicillin G slow intravenous push or penicillin G procaine intramuscularly. Nowhere in the two-page monograph was penicillin G *benzathine* mentioned, and no specific warnings regarding "IM use only" for penicillin G procaine and penicillin G benzathine were present. Unfamiliar with the various forms of penicillin G, a nurse practitioner *believed that "benzathine" was a brand name for penicillin G* and concluded that the drug could be administered safely intravenously. While preparing for drug administration, *neither nurse noticed the 10-fold overdose, and neither noticed that the syringe was labeled by the manufacturer, "IM use only."* The nurses *began to administer the first syringe of Permapen as a slow intravenous push.* After about 1.8 mL was administered, the infant became unresponsive, and resuscitation efforts were unsuccessful (ISMP, 1998).

The three nurses involved in this case were indicted for criminally negligent homicide in the death of the baby. Over 50 different system failures allowed this error to occur, go undetected, and ultimately, reach a healthy newborn child, causing his death. Had even just one of these failures not occurred, either the accident would not have happened, or the error would have been detected and corrected before reaching the infant.

CHAPTER QUESTIONS

1. At what stages of the medication use process do medication errors occur?
2. What types of contributing factors lead to medication errors during the ordering process?
3. What procedures should be followed when taking a verbal order?
4. What steps should be followed during the prescription-filling process to prevent medication errors?
5. What three important factors play a role in any patient interface?
6. Which types of patients are more at risk for noncompliance?

INTRODUCTION

Patient safety has become a major concern since the November 1999 release of the Institute of Medicine's (IOM) report *To Err Is Human.* Health care practitioners may have been surprised to learn from this report that errors involving prescription medications kill up to 7,000 Americans a year (Kohn et al., 1999). The IOM released a report in 2006 entitled *Preventing Medication Errors* and indicated that medication errors are among the most common medical errors, harming at least 1.5 million people every year. The reports concluded that 400,000 preventable drug-related injuries occur each year in hospitals. Another 800,000 occur in long-term care settings, and roughly 530,000 occur just among Medicare recipients in outpatient clinics. Assuming conservatively, an annual incidence of 400,000 in-hospital preventable adverse drug events (ADEs) yields an annual cost of $3.5 billion in 2006. The report noted that these are likely underestimates because the data excluded errors of omission such as the failure to prescribe medications for which there is an evidence base for the ability to reduce morbidity and morbidity (Aspden et al., 2006).

With this increased attention to medication errors, concern has intensified in both the public and health care sectors. Research demonstrates that injuries resulting from medication errors generally are not the fault of individual health care professionals, but rather represent failures in a complex health care system. Medication error prevention starts with recognizing that errors are multifactorial and are faults of the system as a whole rather than results of the acts or omissions of the people in the system. Even when an error can be traced directly to a specific individual (e.g., the pharmacist dispensing or nurse administering the wrong medication), further investigation often determines that a number of factors, such as poor order communication between the physician and pharmacist, dangerous storage practices in pharmacies, and look-alike labeling may have played a role in the error. Protecting patients from inappropriate administration of medications has become an important focus for pharmacists and technicians, including those in ambulatory, acute care, long-term care, home care, and managed-care settings.

Pharmacists and technicians play a pivotal role in assuring medication safety. After summarizing several studies performed in hospitals and long-term care facilities, Allan and Barker (1990) estimated that medication errors occur at a rate of about 1 per patient per day. In a more recent study performed in ambulatory pharmacies, they found an overall dispensing accuracy rate for prescription medications of 98.3 percent (Allan et al., 2003). Although most of these errors probably have minimal clinical relevance and do not affect patients adversely, many experts believe that medication error rates may be higher in the ambulatory care setting because errors may not always be evident to the health professionals who work there. For example, medication errors can occur when a patient purchases nonprescription medications without speaking with the pharmacist about any potential interactions with his or her prescription medications, or if patients fail to verify the appropriate dose of the over-the-counter (OTC) medication.

This chapter focuses on system enhancements and the checks and balances needed to proactively prevent medication errors as pharmacists and technicians prepare, dispense, and monitor the effects of medications in all practice settings. In addition, focus is placed on the importance of determining latent failures that contribute to medication errors by developing effective reporting programs to discover how latent failures occur and how they can be prevented.

BACKGROUND

Many organizations take an ineffective approach to preventing medication errors. Investigations tend to focus on the *front end* or *active end* of the error (e.g., the front-line practitioner, such as the pharmacist dispensing the medication). When an error occurs, human nature needs to assign blame to someone or something. In addition, health care practitioners work in an environment where they strive for perfection. Individuals involved in the commission of an error may be considered inattentive, incompetent, lazy, and uncaring. They are often subject to punitive action such as disciplinary action, public or private reprimands, remedial education, suspensions, or termination. As a result, the practitioner develops feelings of inadequacy, denial, and embarrassment.

Effective approaches, on the other hand, consider factors that contribute to medication errors that occur at the organizational level, known as the *latent end* or *blunt end* of an error. Latent failures are weaknesses in organizational structure, such as faulty information management or ineffective personnel training, that may have resulted from decisions made by upper management (Reason, 1990). Latent failures can also stem from incomplete patient information, such as missing allergy or diagnosis information, unclear communication of a drug order, lack of an independent double check before dispensing, lack of computer warnings, ambiguous drug references, drug storage issues, and look-alike/sound-alike medications. These latent failures are properties of the medication use system. To prevent medications errors, we must change and improve the *system* and not rely on changing people and their behaviors.

ISMP has identified 10 key elements that have the greatest influence on medication-use system. System-based causes of medication errors can be directly traced to weaknesses or failures in these key elements:

- Patient information
- Drug information
- Communication of drug information
- Drug packaging, labeling, and nomenclature
- Drug device acquisition and use
- Drug storage, stock, and distribution
- Environmental factors
- Staff competency and education
- Patient education
- Quality processes; and risk management (Cohen, 2007).

By themselves, latent failures often are subtle and may not cause problems directly. The potential consequences are often hidden, becoming apparent only when they occur in a certain sequence and combine with the active failures of an individual.

Medication use is a complex process that consists of subprocesses such as the ordering, preparing, dispensing, administration, and the provision of patient education. Because failed communication of medication orders is at the heart of many errors, pharmacists must be aware of the types of breakdowns that can occur during the ordering process that can lead to medication errors.

ORDERING MEDICATIONS

Physicians or their designees—pharmacists, nurse practitioners, physician assistants, and nurses—initiate the drug dispensing and administration process through a medication order or prescription. While computerized prescriber order entry (CPOE) and electronic prescribing (e-prescribing) systems, each with clinical decision-support tools, are being implemented in more settings, as of 2011 most pharmacists still dispense from handwritten medication orders. Illegible, ambiguous, or incomplete handwritten prescriptions or medication orders contribute to many errors made by nurses, pharmacists, pharmacy technicians, and other health care workers.

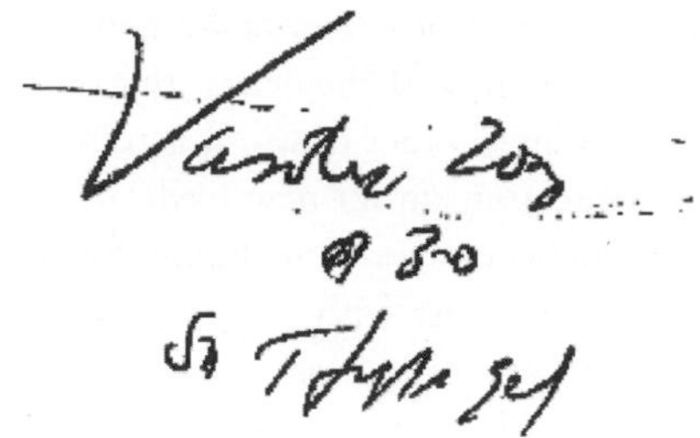

Figure 29-1. Order for Vantin 200 mg misread as Vasotec 20 mg.

Illegible Handwriting

To minimize the chance of misinterpretation due to illegibly handwritten orders, encourage physicians with poor handwriting to print prescriptions and medication orders in block letters. In the institutional setting, have physicians review orders with the nursing staff before leaving the patient care area. More importantly, ask physicians to include the purpose of the medication as part of the prescription or medication order to help readers distinguish drug names when handwriting legibility is less than ideal. Preprinted orders, dictation, and direct order entry into the computer by physicians are other solutions for poor handwriting.

Because even skilled individuals can misread good handwriting, a system of independent double checks for order/prescription transcription should be in place in which several individuals interpret and transcribe an order. In many hospitals, each order is read by a unit secretary and reviewed by a nurse. At the same time, an exact copy of the order is sent to the pharmacy either directly, scanned, or by facsimile. In the pharmacy, pharmacists and technicians have a number of opportunities to check the order, including a double check against labels, printouts, and the drug containers. A technician often screens the order and sometimes enters it into the computer. After data entry, a label is printed, and a pharmacist should interpret the original order/prescription and verifies the technician's computer entry by comparing it with the label. Later, the order and label will be read again by technicians and pharmacists as doses are prepared and dispensed. In the outpatient setting, this system should include a final check when providing counseling to the patient. In no case should pharmacy technicians interpret orders on their own because this process does not offer enough checks to prevent an error. In addition, orders must not be filled only from computer-generated labels. Rather, the original order should accompany the label to serve as another check.

Look-Alike Drug Names

Medications with names that are spelled similarly can be easily misread for one another. Pharmacists and technicians must be alert to this problem and should never guess about a prescriber's intent.

Study the handwriting in Figs. 29-1 and 29-2. These are actual examples of handwritten orders in both the inpatient and outpatient settings, each of which led to medication errors. The problem was not uncertainty. On the contrary, each order was misread from the start. No consideration was ever given to the alternative drug because in each case the pharmacy staff members thought they were reading the order correctly.

When pharmacists and technicians interpret prescriptions and medication orders, newly marketed

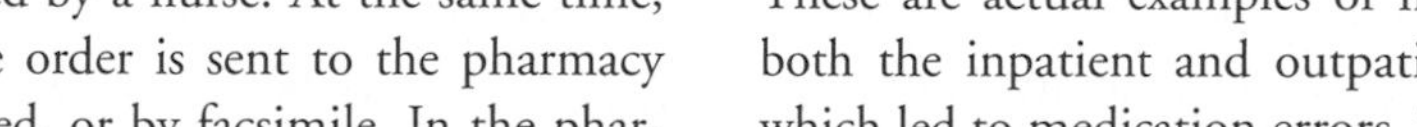

Figure 29-2. Order for Avandia 4 mg misread as Coumadin 4 mg.

drugs are a particular problem. Staff members are not as familiar with names of the drugs, and they tend to misinterpret them as older drugs. It is important that up-to-date education on all new medications is provided to the pharmacy staff, including any potential for error that may exist with these new products. In the ambulatory care setting, physicians can write both the generic and trade names legibly on the prescription, and they can add the intended purpose of the medication to further alert pharmacy staff to the correct medication name. Many medications have look-alike names, but very few name pairs that are spelled similarly are used for similar purposes.

Sound-Alike Names

Drug orders communicated orally are often misheard, misunderstood, misinterpreted, or transcribed incorrectly. Celebrex® and Cerebyx® sound alike, as do Celexa® and Zyprexa®, alprazolam and lorazepam, Flomax® and Volmax®, and hundreds of other name pairs. Each of these drugs has been confused for the other, resulting in patients receiving incorrect medications. In many cases, serious injuries have occurred because of misinterpreted verbal orders. This is a good reason for health care facilities such as hospitals and long-term care facilities to establish policies that prohibit verbal requests for medication without pharmacy review of a hard copy of the order. Sound-alike drug names present many of the same problems as look alikes. Obviously, when uncertainties exist, the pharmacist must contact the prescriber for clarification.

To decrease the opportunity for misunderstanding, health care facilities and community pharmacies should discourage verbal orders. TJC, a national accrediting agency for health care organizations, requires in its standards that accredited organizations improve the effectiveness of communication among caregivers by implementing a process for taking verbal or telephone orders that mandates that a verbal order to be transcribed and then "read back" completely by the person receiving the order (TJC, 2011).

Greater use of computerized order entry, scanning technology and facsimile machines among hospital areas, medical offices, pharmacies, and nursing units will help improve communication of medication orders. When verbal communication is unavoidable, strict adherence to these procedures can minimize errors:

- In acute care settings, spoken orders should be limited to true emergencies or circumstances in which the prescriber is physically unable to write or electronically transmit orders (e.g., the prescriber is working in a sterile field).
- Prohibit spoken orders for selected high-alert medications (e.g., chemotherapy, IV insulin for neonates) because of their complexity and potential for serious errors.
- Verbal orders should be taken only by authorized personnel.
- If possible, a second person should listen while the prescription is being given.
- The order should be written down and then read back, repeating exactly what has been ordered, sometimes spelling the drug name for verification and the strength by using a digit-by-digit technique for the dose (1–5, not 15).
- In the acute care setting, record the verbal order directly onto an order sheet in the patient's chart whenever possible. Transcription from a scrap of paper to the chart introduces another opportunity for error.
- Obtain the prescriber's phone number in case it is necessary for follow-up questions.
- The prescribed agent must make sense for the patient's clinical situation. (Cohen, 2007a)

To prevent sound-alike and look-alike errors, physicians must be encouraged to include complete directions, strengths, route of administration, and indication (purpose) for use. With this information, pharmacists and other skilled health care professionals can judge whether the drug ordered makes sense for the patient in the context in which it is written. For example, knowing that the patient has a diagnosis of diabetes would be important in determining that Avandia® is intended by the medication order in Fig. 29-2. Diagnostic procedures along with orders could also provide important information. This is why it is important for pharmacists to verify all orders processed by

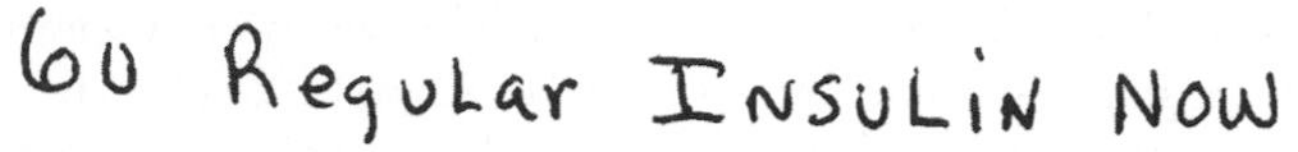

60 Regular Insulin Now

Figure 29-3. Misinterpretation of 6 units (U) of Humalog insulin for 60 units.

technicians. When in doubt, technicians should check with the pharmacist, who can contact the prescriber for clarification if the intent is not completely clear.

Abbreviations to Avoid

Certain abbreviations are easily misinterpreted. Controlling dangerous abbreviations can reduce communication errors. Although many health care facilities have lists of abbreviations that are approved for use by professional staff, it would be far safer if each hospital also developed a list of abbreviations that should never be used. TJC has recommended that accredited organizations standardize abbreviations, acronyms, and symbols used throughout their facilities, including a list of abbreviations, acronyms, and symbols not to use.

The ISMP has developed a list that contains several easily misinterpreted abbreviations from actual medication errors, some of which resulted in patient harm (ISMP, 2010). These abbreviations should never be used in medication orders, on pharmacy labels, in newsletters, or in other communications that originate in a pharmacy or pharmacy computer systems. Examples of some of the most problematic abbreviations used to communicate orders include:

- *The abbreviation* U *for units.* Errors have occurred when the letter *U* was mistaken for the numerals 0, 4, 6, and 7, and even cc, resulting in disastrous drug overdoses of insulin, heparin, penicillin, and other medications whose doses sometimes are expressed in units. For example, an order written as "Humalog 6U" has been misinterpreted as "60 units." (see Fig. 29-3).
- *Q for "every," as well as other abbreviations with this letter (QD, QID, and QOD; or qd, qid, and qod).* QD for "daily" can result in fourfold overdosages if seen as QID (q.i.d.) for "four times daily," or subtherapeutic doses if seen as QOD for "every other day." Errors associated with QD and QOD have been reported to PA Patient Safety Authority (PSA) [Pennsylvania Patient Safety Authority (PSA, 2005)]. In one case, an order for Zithromax® (azithromycin) 500 mg written as QD was misinterpreted as QID. In another report, an order was written for digoxin 0.125 mg po QOD (every other day), but the medication was given QD (every day).
- *D/C.* It has been written to mean either "discontinue" or "discharge," sometimes resulting in premature stoppage of a patient's medications. In Fig. 29-4, the "d/c" order was incorrectly interpreted as "discontinuation" of an antibiotic that the patient had never even received. In reality, the "d/c" is really "OK," meaning that the drug was approved for use by the infectious disease physician. Drug names also should not be abbreviated.

Abbreviating drug names have led to frequent medication errors, including:

- *Magnesium sulfate (MgSO4 or simply Mg) and morphine sulfate (MSO4 or simply MS).* In one example, a prescriber used an abbreviation for magnesium sulfate and wrote "MgSo4 2g IV × 1 dose" for a 45-year-old female patient. However, the unit clerk and nurse misinterpreted the order as morphine sulfate (MSO4) "2 mg IV × 1 dose." The patient received a 2 mg dose of morphine sulfate. Contributing to this error was the fact that the patient was having pain, so morphine seemed reasonable [Pennsylvania Patient Safety Authority (PSA, 2005)].

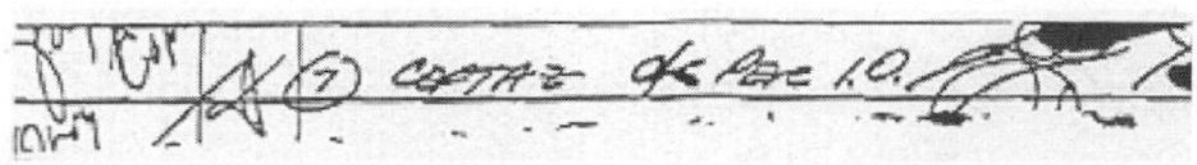

Figure 29-4. Ceftazidime "OK" per ID misread as ceftazidime "d/c" per ID.

- *MTX.* This means "methotrexate" to some health professionals, but others understand it as "mitoxantrone."
- *AZT.* This has been misunderstood as "azathioprine" (Imuran®) when "zidovudine" (Retrovir®) was intended. In one case, this misinterpretation led to a patient with AIDS receiving azathioprine, an immunosuppressant, instead of the intended antiretroviral agent. The patient's immune system worsened, and he developed an overwhelming infection.
- *HCT and HCTZ.* Orders for "HCTZ50 mg" (hydrochlorothiazide) can be mistaken for "HCT 250 mg" (hydrocortisone).

Ambiguous Orders

Errors can result when ambiguous orders are interpreted in a manner other than what the prescriber intended. Proper expression of doses is vital in a drug order. Pharmacists should be able to recognize improper expressions of doses and their potential for error. When the order is not clear, the pharmacist must contact the prescriber for clarification. Pharmacists and technicians should avoid using dangerous expressions of doses as they process orders, type labels, and communicate with others. The following examples include several improperly expressed orders that were reported to the ISMP:

- *Zeros and decimal points.* When listing drug doses on labels or in other communications, never follow a whole number with a decimal and a zero. For example, "Coumadin 1.0 mg" is a very dangerous way to express this dose. If the decimal point were not seen, the dose would be misinterpreted as "10 mg," and a 10-fold overdose would result. The same could happen when "Dilaudid 1.0 mg" is written. The proper way to express these orders would be "Coumadin 1 mg" and "Dilaudid 1 mg."
- *Leading zeros.* Always place a leading zero before a decimal point when the dose is smaller than 1. For example, "Vincristine .4 mg" was seen as "Vincristine 4 mg" due to a poor impression of the decimal, as is common on faxes or copies of orders. Avoid using decimal expressions when recognizable alternatives exist because whole numbers are easier to work with. For example, "Digoxin 0.125 mg" is acceptable, but "Digoxin 125 mcg" is a better alternative. So too would be to indicate a dose as "500 mg" instead of "0.5 g."
- *Tablet strengths.* Orders specifying both strength and number of tablets are confusing when more than one tablet strength exists. For example, "Metoprolol 1/2 (one-half) tablet 25 mg once daily" appears clear enough. However, when you realize that this product is available in both 25- and 50-mg tablets, the ambiguity of this order becomes apparent. What is the intended dose, 25 or 12.5 mg? Orders are clearer if the dose is specified regardless of the strengths available (e.g., "Metoprolol 12.5 mg once daily"). For doses that require several tablets or capsules, the pharmacy label should note the exact number of dosage units needed. For example, the label on an 800-mg dose of Asacol® (mesalamine), which is available only in 400-mg tablets, should read "2 × 400-mg tablets = 800 mg." For a 6.25-mg dose of captopril, which is available in 12.5-mg tablets, the label should read one-half (1/2) × 12.5-mg tablet = 6.25 mg." Fractions should be displayed in fraction format and not as 1 slash 2 (1/2) (ISMP, 2011). The same type of notation should be used on computer-generated medication administration records (MARs) for nurses.
- *Liquid dosage forms.* Expressing the dose for liquid dosage forms in only milliliters or teaspoonfuls is dangerous. For example, acetaminophen elixir is available in many strengths, including 80, 120, and 160 mg per 5 mL. If the prescriber wrote "5 mL," the intended number of milligrams would be unclear. However, an order of "80 mg" states the appropriate dose. The amount of drug by metric weight, as well as the volume, should always be included on the pharmacy label (e.g., "Acetaminophen elixir 80 mg/5 mL"). Further, the patient dose should also be included. For a 320-mg dose, the label should read, "320 mg = 20 mL." The same holds true for unit dose and bulk labels.
- *Injectable medications.* The same rules apply for injectable drugs. Because solution concentrations can

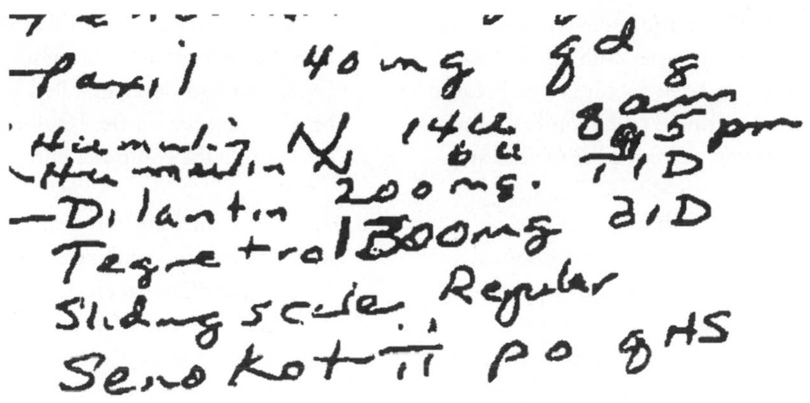

Figure 29-5. Order for Tegretol misread as 1300 mg instead of 300 mg.

vary, list the metric weight of the dose, or the metric weight and volume of the dose, but never the volume alone. An example of this error occurred at a hospital where hepatitis B vaccines were being administered. A preprinted physician's order form was used to prescribe the vaccine, listing only the volume to be given. When the clinic switched to another brand of vaccine, containing a different concentration of vaccine, the same preprinted forms continued to be used. This resulted in the underdosing of hundreds of children until the error was discovered. This could have been avoided had the amount of vaccine been prescribed in micrograms rather than just the volume in milliliters.

- *Variable amounts.* A drug dose should never be ordered solely by number of tablets, capsules, ampules, or vials because the amounts contained in these dosage forms vary. Drug doses should be ordered with proper unit expression (e.g., "20 mEq potassium chloride"). A patient whose doctor orders "an amp" of potassium chloride might get 10, 20, 30, 40, 60, or 90 mEq. Under certain circumstances, the higher doses of this drug could be lethal.
- *Spacing.* Overdoses have been reported because a lowercase *l* (ell) was the final letter in a drug name and was misread as the number 1. In one case, an order for 300 mg Tegretol® (carbamazepine) twice daily appeared as "Tegretol 300 mg bid" and was misinterpreted as "1300 mg bid" (see Fig. 29-5). In another case, a nurse misread an order for 2 mg Amaryl® (glimepiride) as 12 mg because there was insufficient space between the last letter in the drug name and the numerical dose. In addition, when labels are printed, make sure that there is a space after the drug name, the dose, and the unit of measurement.
- *Apothecary system.* Use the metric system exclusively. The apothecary system (grains, drams, minims, and ounces) has been found to be very inaccurate. For example, symbols for dram have been misread as "3," and minim has been misread as "55." Orders for phenobarbital 0.5 gr (30 mg) have been mistaken as "0.5 gram (500 mg)." Use of the apothecary system is no longer officially recognized by the United States Pharmacopeia (USP).

PREPARING AND DISPENSING MEDICATIONS

An important safety enhancement for preventing dispensing errors is the development of a system of redundant checks from the time a prescription order first is written in the physician's office or on the nursing unit to receipt in the pharmacy and through dispensing and administration. The more "looks" an order receives (while efficient workflow is maintained), the better. Health professionals can review orders at several checkpoints and thereby maximize the chances of errors being discovered. Pharmacies with computerized drug distribution systems have an advantage because labels and reports can be printed so that order interpretation and order entry can be verified at various steps.

Steps in Prescription Filling

It is important that all health care professionals, including prescribers, nurses, and pharmacy personnel, work together when filling prescriptions so that the lines of communication are kept open if questions should arise. It is also important that pharmacy personnel understand the processes involved in the communication of orders in their particular practice setting so that breakdowns can be addressed and improvements can be made to improve both efficiency and safety.

Community Pharmacy

1. The prescriber sees the patient; performs an assessment; determines the appropriate medication, dose, route, and frequency; and writes the order or communicates the order verbally to nursing personnel or the pharmacy.
2. A direct copy of the order is transported by the patient, faxed/scanned to the pharmacy, or the prescriber's computer entry system (ePrescribing) directly reaches the pharmacy order entry system.
3. The pharmacist or pharmacy technician reads the order and enters it in the pharmacy computer system.
   a. If the technician finds a duplicate order, incorrect dose, drug allergy or other problem, it is documented and called to the attention of the pharmacist during the clinical screening.
4. A pharmacist reviews the prescriber's or pharmacy technician's computer entry, compares it with the original prescription (handwritten or electronic), and performs a clinical screening of the prescription with respect to the need for the drug, allergies or other contraindications, proper dose, and proper route of administration.
5. A label and/or medication profile is printed. It is important that a copy of the original prescription or medication order continues to accompany the label or medication profile while the order is filled. Orders should never be filled solely on the basis of what appears on the label or medication profile because the computer entry may have been in error.
6. To choose an item for dispensing, a technician reviews both the label and the medication order for possible discrepancies.
7. A pharmacist checks the technician's work, reviewing the label against the medication order and the dose that has been prepared. The drug is labeled and dispensed.
8. The pharmacist uses the patient counseling session to further assess that the correct medication is being dispensed and that the patient has a condition treatable with the product being provided.
   a. Pharmacists should not simply ask patients if they have any questions about their medication, but confirm their understanding of the medication and its proper use.
   b. For refills and medications patients have received in the past, patients should be encouraged to ask the pharmacist about any changes in the appearance of the product.
   c. If patients or caregivers are provided with administration device, such as an oral syringe or inhaler, pharmacists must ensure that the patient or caregiver understands how to use the device properly. Demonstrate for patients how to use the device, and follow with a return demonstration by the user.
9. Patients in the community setting should be educated about the common adverse effects of medications they are taking and understand what clinical signs to watch for and report to health professionals.
10. The final step in the process is the assurance of adherence to medication therapy. If the patient is taking too much medication or is not taking the drug as frequently as prescribed, the pharmacist should speak with the patient to determine the reasons for and address the variation. In addition, patients should be asked about common

adverse effects and about signs of serious drug toxicities.

Hospital Pharmacy

1. The prescriber sees the patient; performs an assessment; determines the appropriate medication(s), dose(s), route(s), and frequency(ies); and writes orders or communicates the orders verbally to nursing personnel or the pharmacy.
2. A unit secretary reads and transcribes the order onto the MAR. A nurse checks the unit secretary's transcription for accuracy. This step is unnecessary in hospitals where computers generate an electronic medical record (eMAR), where prescribers can enter orders directly into a computerize physician-order entry system (CPOE) or pharmacy prints MARs for the nursing staff.
3. A direct copy of the order is transported, faxed/scanned to the pharmacy, or the prescriber's computer entry system (CPOE) reaches the pharmacy order entry system. The pharmacist or pharmacy technician reads the order and enters it in the pharmacy computer system. If the technician finds a duplicate order, incorrect dose, drug allergy or other problem, it is documented and called to the attention of the pharmacist during the clinical screening.
4. A pharmacist reviews the prescriber's or pharmacy technician's computer entry, compares it with the original prescription (handwritten or electronic), and performs a clinical screening of the prescription with respect to the need for the drug, allergies or other contraindications, proper dose, and proper route of administration.
5. The pharmacy label is printed. A copy of the medication order(s) continues to accompany the label while the order is filled. Orders should *never* be filled solely on the basis of what appears on the label because the computer entry may have been in error.
6. To choose an item for dispensing, a technician reviews both the label and the medication order for possible discrepancies and obtains the product from its storage area.
7. A pharmacist checks the technician's work, reviewing the label against the medication order and the dose that has been prepared. The drug is labeled and dispensed.
8. The medications are delivered to the patient's care area. Medications are stored in a variety of areas that include individual patient cassettes/bins or automated dispensing cabinets (ADCs).
9. The nurse obtains the drug and compares the medication and pharmacy label against the copy of the physician's order, as well as the MAR/eMAR.
10. The nurse administers the dose, giving the drug's name, explaining the drug's purpose and potential adverse effects, and answering questions and concerns raised by the patient.

Selecting Medications

The importance of reading the product label while selecting medications and filling prescriptions cannot be overemphasized. Too often the wrong drug, strength or concentration is dispensed. Such errors often stem from failure to read the label thoroughly. During drug preparation and dispensing, the label should be read three times:

1. When the product is selected
2. When the medication is prepared
3. When either the partially used medication is disposed of (or restored to stock) or product preparation is complete

Selecting the correct item from the shelf, drawer, or bin can be complicated by many factors. Similar labeling and packaging, as well as look-alike names, are common traps that lead to medication errors (see Figs. 29-6 and 29-7). Restocking errors are common and can lead to repeated medication errors before being detected.

ADCs (e.g., Pyxis, Omnicell) have become common on nursing units in many hospitals. The nurse must enter a security code and a password into the dispensing device, along with the name of the patient and the name of the medication, before the machine

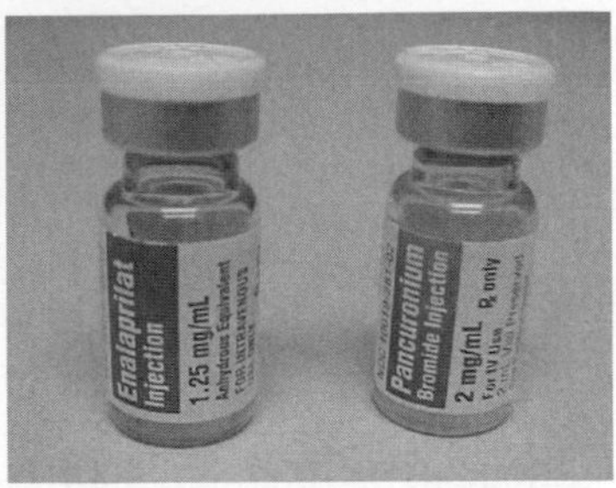

Figure 29-6. Similar packaging might lead to medication errors.

will allow access to remove the medication. This system allows better control of items kept on the nursing unit and serves as a check for the nurse who retrieves the medication. One important feature that should be included in these dispensing units is online communication with the pharmacy system that allows a pharmacist to review medication orders before nursing accesses the medication.

ADCs create several situations that can result in errors. While these machines are routinely restocked, the wrong drug still can be placed into the wrong bin during this process. Devices that have multiple medications in each drawer and/or that do not require pharmacist review of orders before access have drawbacks that are identical to the flaws in traditional floor-stock systems:

- The pharmacy can replenish the system with an incorrect medication.

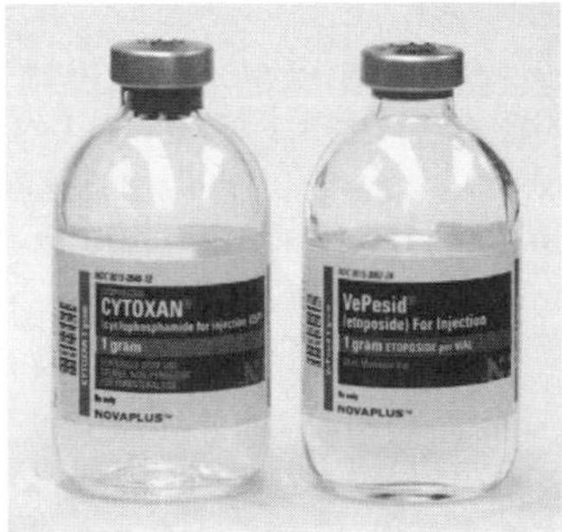

Figure 29-7. Another example of packaging that might lead to medication error.

- The nurse can retrieve either the wrong item or additional items to use for other patients.
- Lack of pharmacist double checking and screening orders before a nurse withdraws a medication from the cabinet allows prescribing errors, wrong dosages, incorrect routes of administration, and other clinical errors to occur.

The term *confirmation bias* is used to describe the phenomenon that when choosing an item, people see what they are looking for, and once they think they have found it, they stop looking any further. Often health professionals choose a medication container based on a mental picture of the item. Staff members may be looking for some characteristic of the drug label, the shape and size or color of the container, or the location of the item on a shelf, in a drawer, or in a storage bin instead of reading the name of the drug itself. Consequently, they may fail to realize that they have the wrong item in hand.

A number of approaches can be used to minimize the possibility of such errors in the pharmacy, care areas, and in automated dispensing machines. Physically separating drugs with look-alike labels and packaging reduces the potential for error. Some pharmacies also separate drugs with similar names and overlapping strengths, especially those labeled and packaged by the same manufacturer. For example, chlorpromazine 100-mg tablets and chlorpropamide 100-mg tablets, both from the same unit-dose packager (see Fig. 29-8), might pose a problem. So might tramadol 50 mg and trazodone 50 mg or metformin 500 mg and metronidazole 500 mg. Another strategy would be to change the appearance of look-alike product names on computer screens, pharmacy shelf labels and bins, and pharmacy product labels by highlighting, through boldface, color, or the use of "tall man" letters, the parts of the names that are different (e.g., hydrOXYzine and hydrALAzine). In fact, the Food and Drug Administration (FDA) Office of Generic Drugs requested that the manufacturers of 16 look-alike name-pair drug products voluntarily revise the appearance of their established names to minimize medication

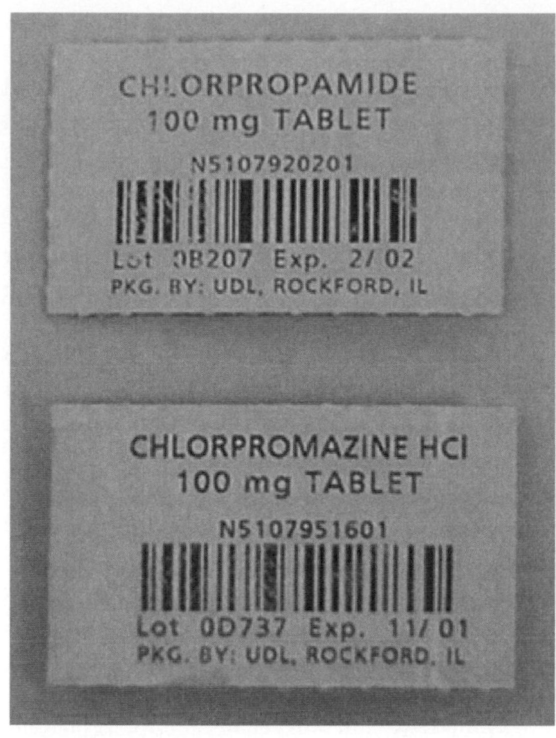

Figure 29-8. Similarity in labeling of two different medications.

errors resulting from look-alike confusion. Manufacturers were encouraged to differentiate their established names visually with the use of "tall man" letters. Examples of established names involved include chlorproMAZINE and chlorproPAMIDE, vinBLASTINE and vinCRISTINE, and NICARdipine and NIFEdipine.

In institutional and community pharmacies with several staff members, everyone should have input in deciding how and where drugs are available, how doses are prepared, who is responsible for preparing them, the appearance of the storage containers, and how they are labeled. In addition, staff members should be encouraged to use a technique known as *failure mode and effects analysis* (FMEA) to examine the use of new products to determine points of potential failures and their effects *before any error actually happens* (see Chapter 8). In this regard, FMEA differs from *root-cause analysis* (RCA). RCA is a reactive process, employed after an error occurs, to identify its underlying causes. In contrast, FMEA is a proactive process used to carefully and systematically evaluate vulnerable areas or processes. FMEA can be employed before the purchase and implementation of new products to identify potential failure modes so that steps can be taken to avoid errors before they occur [Institute for Safe Medication Practices (ISMP), 2011a, 2011b]. Procedures to ensure safe medication use must be written, and the importance of adhering to the guidelines must be shared by all involved pharmacy, medical, and nursing personnel.

Selecting Auxiliary Labels

To help prevent errors and improve patient outcomes, pharmacists and technicians should apply auxiliary labels in certain circumstances, especially in the community setting. For example, amoxicillin oral suspension is available in dropper bottles for pediatric use. When the suspension is used for an ear infection, some parents have been known to place the suspension in the child's ear rather than to give it properly (orally). An auxiliary label, "For oral use only," would help to prevent this administration error. However, this practice can be unsafe if the patient is unable to understand the warning. The application of an auxiliary label should not be done in lieu of speaking with the patient. A study that appeared in the *American Journal of Health-System Pharmacy* showed that there is a high level of misunderstanding of auxiliary labels among adults with low literacy, defined as a reading level at or below the sixth-grade level (Wolf et al., 2006). The rate of correct interpretation of these labels ranged from 0 to 78.7 percent. With the exception of the label "Take with food," less than half of all patients were able to provide adequate interpretations of the warning labels' messages. In fact, no one was able to correctly interpret the label, "Do not take dairy products, antacids, or iron preparations within 1 hour of this medication." Studies also have shown that a combination of a verbal description of a warning along with visual symbols improves the overall comprehension of the warning (Lesch, 2003).

STERILE ADMIXTURE PREPARATION

In preparing fluids for injectable administration, the potential for grave errors is increased for several reasons. First, patients often are sicker when they need intravenous drugs, so the medications used have more dramatic effects on the body's function and physiology. Further, most injectable solutions are clear, colorless, water-based fluids that look alike, regardless of what drug and how much of it are actually in the fluid.

A five-hospital observational study on the accuracy of preparing small- and large-volume injectables, chemotherapy solutions, and parenteral nutrition showed a mean error rate of 9%, meaning almost 1 in 10 products was prepared incorrectly and then dispensed (Flynn et al., 1997). Error rates for complex solutions such as parenteral nutrition were especially high—37% for manual preparation and 22% for preparations that were partly automated. More recently, a 2009 State of Pharmacy Compounding Survey showed that 30% of hospitals have experienced a patient event involving a compounding error in the past 5 years (Pharmacy Purchasing & Products, 2009). In 2006, an infant received a lethal dose of zinc stemming from an error that occurred during the order entry and compounding of a total parenteral nutrition (TPN) solution. TPN was prescribed for a preterm infant born at 26 weeks gestation. On the day of the event, the physician's TPN order included directions to add zinc in a concentration of 330 mcg/100 mL. Because the automated compounder used for TPN required entry of zinc in a mcg/kg dose, the pharmacist converted the mcg/mL dose to a mcg/kg dose. She performed this calculation correctly, but accidentally entered the zinc dose in the pharmacy computer in mg, not mcg. This resulted in a final concentration of 330 mg/100 mL—a 1,000-fold overdose (ISMP, 2007).

In the sterile admixture preparation setting, dosage miscalculations and measurement errors must be minimized by systems designed with procedures that require independent double checks by two staff members. In many pharmacies, independent double checks are required for all calculations or measurements, whereas others may require it only for calculations falling in special categories, such as dosage calculations for admixture compounding for any child under age 12, critical care drug infusions requiring a dose in micrograms per kilogram per minute, insulin infusions, chemotherapy, and patient-controlled analgesia. Calculators and computer programs may improve accuracy, but they do not eliminate the need for a second person to review the calculations and solution concentrations used.

Another important way to minimize calculation errors is to avoid the need for calculations in the first place. This can be accomplished by using the unit-dose system exclusively as follows:

- Using commercially available unit-dose systems such as premixed critical care parenteral products.
- Standardizing doses and concentrations, especially of critical care drugs such as heparin, insulin, dobutamine, dopamine, and morphine.

Similar steps can be taken in community pharmacies that provide sterile admixtures to physician offices, home care programs and patients, long-term care facilities, and other clients.

The use of standard dosage charts on nursing units in institutions and standard formulations in the pharmacy minimizes the possibility of error and makes calculations much easier. For example, in critical care units, physicians need to order only the amount of drug they want infused and list any titration parameters. No one has to perform any calculations because dosage charts can be readily available for choosing appropriate flow rates by patient weight (in kilograms) and dose ordered.

Standard concentrations for frequently prepared formulations should be recorded and be readily accessible for reference in the admixture preparation area of the pharmacy. Of course, all calculations must be double-checked and documented by the pharmacist. Diluents as well as active drugs must be checked before they are added to the base solution. The stock container of each additive with its accompanying syringe should be lined up in the order it appears on the container label to facilitate the checking procedure. When compounding TPN solutions, at least three verification processes should occur in the pharmacy: after initial order entry of TPN; before manually injecting additives into the TPN; and once the TPN has been compounded. Each verification should require a pharmacist to compare the actual prescriber's order to the printed labels, and the printed labels to the additives and final product, as appropriate. Verification of manual additives should include inspection of the actual vials and syringes that contain the additives. The final verification of the compounded TPN should include a comprehensive review of the TPN order, the label on the product, and the work label.

In many hospitals and home infusion pharmacies, automated compounding equipment is being used for admixing both large- and small-volume parenterals. While automated equipment improves the accuracy of compounding parenterals, it is not perfect and has been known to occasionally fail. Also, accidents can occur when solutions are placed in the wrong additive channel. These can result in serious medication errors. Therefore, it is important that the pharmacy have an ongoing quality assurance program for the use of automated compounding equipment. This program should include double checks and documentation of solution placement within the compounder, final weighing or refractometer testing of the solution to ensure that proper concentrations have been compounded, and ongoing sampling of electrolyte concentrations. Pharmacists who prepare special parenteral solutions in batches (e.g., TPN base solutions or cardioplegic solutions) should have additional quality assurance procedures in place, including sterility testing and quarantine until confirmation.

PATIENT COUNSELING AND EDUCATION

The patient is the last individual involved in the medication use process. The pharmacist–patient interface can play a significant role in catching medication errors before they occur. Unfortunately, many health care organizations do not take advantage of this key interaction. Three important factors play a role in any patient interface and often determine the outcome of error-prevention efforts. These include direct patient education, health care literacy, and patient compliance.

Community pharmacies in the United States filled 3.6 billion prescriptions in 2009, and prescription volumes continue to increase at a rate of approximately 3% per year (StateHealthFacts, 2011). This increase in prescription volume often results in a decrease in the amount of time available for direct pharmacist involvement in patient education. A 1999 study involving community pharmacies in eight states revealed that 87 percent of all patients received written information with their prescriptions. However, only 35 percent of pharmacists made any reference to the written leaflet, and only 8 percent actually reviewed it with the patient (Svarstad, 2000). Contributing to this gap in patient education is the failure to provide patients with understandable written instructions.

The second factor is patient literacy, which includes general literacy levels and health care literacy. Many people have difficulty understanding their illness or disease, proper management of disease, and their role in maintaining their health. Whether limited by knowledge, socioeconomic factors, emotional or clinical state, or cultural background, patients' level of health literacy (i.e., the ability to read, understand, and act on health care information) often is much lower than many health care providers appreciate. Examples of patients who have had difficulty reading and understanding medication directions are plentiful. For example, an elderly patient could not tell the difference between his bottle of Coumadin® (warfarin) and Celebrex® (celecoxib). A mother, who after reading the label on a bottle of acetaminophen, could not accurately state her child's dose. And a teenager who misunderstood directions for contraceptive jelly and ate it on toast every morning to prevent pregnancy.

According a report published by the American Medical Association Ad Hoc Committee on Health Literacy, more than 40 percent of patients with chronic illnesses are functionally illiterate, and almost a quarter of all adult Americans read at or below a fifth grade level. Unfortunately, medical information leaflets typically are written at or above a tenth grade reading level. Further contributing to the dilemma is the fact that an estimated three-quarters of patients throw out the medication leaflet stapled to the prescription bag without reading it, and only one-half of all patients take their medications as directed (AMA, 1999).

One reason for this lack of understanding may be that people who have difficulty reading or understanding health information are too embarrassed or ashamed to acknowledge their deficits. Instead, they are hesistant to ask questions of their health professionals and often pretend to understand instructions. In addition, low literacy is not obvious. Researchers have reported poor reading skills in some of the most poised and articulate patients (ISMP, 2011a).

Compliance is the third patient-related factor contributing to medication errors. One study found a 76 percent difference between medications patients actually are taking when compared with those recorded in their charts as prescribed. Two factors that contribute to this high rate of discrepancy include confusion that may accompany advancing age and the increase in the number of prescribed medications (Bedell et al., 2000). Another study demonstrated that patient noncompliance played a role in 33 percent of hospital admissions (McDonnell et al., 2002).

Noncompliance may be exhibited by patients in many ways, such as not having a prescription filled initially or refilled, dose omissions, taking the wrong dose, stopping a medication without the physician's advice, taking a medication incorrectly or at the wrong time, taking someone else's medication, and financial inability to purchase their medications. Patients at risk for being noncompliant include those taking more than one drug, those with a chronic condition who are on complex drug regimens that may result in bothersome side effects, those who take a drug more than once daily, and those who have a condition that produces no overt symptoms or physical impairment such as hypertension or diabetes (National Council on Patient Information and Education (NCPIE), 2002). In addition, elderly patients are more at risk owing to factors such as decrease in mental acuity and increased confusion, lack of family or caregiver support, decreased coordination and dexterity, and impaired vision (Lombardi and Kennicutt, 2001). Pharmacy managers must consider these factors in developing and providing patient education tools or methodologies.

A New Model of Accountability

Despite a growing awareness of the system-based causes of errors, many in health care are still struggling to come to terms with the role of individual accountability. Even when we seem to understand the system-based causes of errors, it's still hard to let individuals "off the hook." We ask, "How can we hold individuals accountable for their actions without punishment?" Some have suggested that a nonpunitive approach to error reduction leads to increased carelessness as people learn that they will not be punished for their mistakes. However, another perspective is that staff awareness of safety issues, as well as their enthusiasm for changing systems and practices associated with errors, actually grows in a nonpunitive system. A nonpunitive, system-based approach to error reduction does not diminish accountability; it redefines it and directs it in a more productive manner by focusing on the most manageable component of the error: the medication-use system itself.

Typically when an error happens, only those individuals at the "sharp end" of an error (for example, pharmacists and pharmacy technicians) are held accountable. But, we must shift from this thinking and realize that accountability must be shared among all health care stakeholders. In the new patient safety model, each individual becomes accountable, not for zero errors (which is an unrealistic and unattainable expectation for any human), but for making patient safety a part of every aspect of their job. In addition, all become accountable for identifying safety problems, implementing system-based solutions, and inspiring and embracing a culture of safety.

Because we are not capable of practicing without making errors, health care practitioners should be held accountable for speaking out about patient safety issues, voluntarily reporting potential and actual errors as well as hazardous situations, and sharing personal knowledge of what went wrong when an error occurs. Also, practitioners must be empowered to ask for help when needed, consistently provide patient education, and be willing to change their practices to enhance safety.

Management should be held equally accountable for making it safe and rewarding for practitioners to openly discuss errors and patient safety issues. They must hold regular safety briefings with staff to learn about improvement needs, discuss strategic plans, and identify new potential sources of error. When practitioners recommend error prevention strategies, leaders must support them and provide the means necessary within a reasonable timeframe to implement system enhancements to improve efficiency and safety. Leaders should be held accountable for understanding and addressing barriers to safe practice such as distractions and unsafe workloads. Leaders should incorporate patient safety as a value in the organization's mission and engage the community and staff in proactive continuous quality improvement (CQI) efforts, including an annual self-assessment of patient safety. All health care personnel should be held accountable for working together as a team, not as autonomous individuals. Finally, leaders and staff alike need to review and share safety literature frequently and offer visible support to their colleagues who have been involved in errors.

This model of shared accountability spreads far beyond the walls of individual health care settings to encompass licensing, regulatory, and accrediting bodies; institutions that educate and train students and health care professionals; professional associations; governments and public policy makers; the pharmaceutical industry; medical device and technology vendors; and even the public at large. These often-overlooked participants share equal accountability for doing their part to make health care safer. For example, licensing, regulatory, and accrediting bodies should be held accountable for adopting standards related to error reduction recommendations that arise from expert analysis of adverse events and scientific research. Educators should seek out patient safety information and use it in curriculum design. Professional organizations should support local and national reporting systems and disseminate important patient safety information to their members. Companies that produce medical devices, pharmaceutical products, health care computers and software, and other health-related products should be held accountable for pre- and postmarket evaluation, continuous improvement in the design of devices and products as well as labels and packages. Purchasers of health care should provide incentives and rewards for patient safety initiatives. And all health care professionals, including pharmacists, should encourage the public to ask questions and stay informed about their care and ways to avoid errors.

The system-based model of accountability requires that all who interact with the health care system help to define its weaknesses and find ways to make it stronger. Organizational leaders and other stakeholders who simply hold the workforce accountable when an error happens are inappropriately delegating their own responsibility for patient safety. Managers must stop blaming and punishing those closest to an error, and instead accept a model of shared accountability to collectively translate our sincere concern for patient safety into effective system-based error solutions. Implementing such solutions and inspiring and embracing a culture of change to reach the goal of safety may not be easy, but is certainly necessary.

Effective Risk-Reduction Strategies

Selecting the best error-prevention strategies is not an easy task. Often, the most effective action is not obvious, and the best error prevention tools to use in each situation are not clear, even when system-based causes have been identified. In addition, pharmacists should focus their efforts on medications that may lead to harm if involved in an error. Although most medications have a wide margin of safety, a few drugs have a high risk of causing patient injury or death if they are misused. Special precautions are needed to reduce the risk of error with these "high-alert" medications. Errors with these drugs may not be more common than with other medications, but their consequences can be more devastating (ISMP, 2008).

Listed below are examples of error-prevention strategies for creating lasting system changes for safe

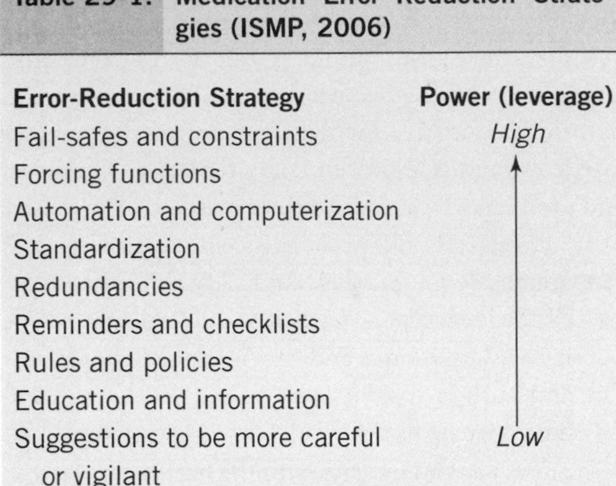

Table 29-1. Medication Error Reduction Strategies (ISMP, 2006)

Error-Reduction Strategy	Power (leverage)
Fail-safes and constraints	*High*
Forcing functions	↑
Automation and computerization	
Standardization	
Redundancies	
Reminders and checklists	
Rules and policies	
Education and information	
Suggestions to be more careful or vigilant	*Low*

medication use (See Table 29-1). Those listed first are considered to be "high leverage" strategies, such as constraints and forcing functions, are more powerful because they focus on changes to the system in which individuals operate. As the list descends, strategies that target system changes but rely in some part on human vigilance and memory, considered to be "low leverage" strategies, such as education and information, are presented. Strategies toward the end are familiar and often easy to implement, but rely entirely on human vigilance (ISMP, 1999; ISMP, 2006).

- Fail-safes and constraints are among the most powerful and effective error-prevention strategies. They involve true system changes in the design of products or how individuals interact within the system. In the hospital setting, one example includes removing concentrated potassium chloride for injection from all patient care areas. In this situation, a nurse could not accidentally administer this medication because it would not be available to select from stock. Another acute care example includes eliminating nursing access to the pharmacy when it is closed by establishing a carefully selected nighttime formulary and dispensing cabinet. At a community pharmacy where the pharmacy computer system is integrated with the cash register, a fail-safe would prevent the clerk from "ringing up" the prescription unless final verification by a pharmacist was noted in the system.
- Forcing functions are procedures that create a "hard stop" during a process to help ensure that important information is provided before proceeding; often referred to as a "lock and key" design. Examples outside of health care would include the inability to drive your car unless you first place your foot on the brake before shifting the car into "drive." For example, a pharmacy order entry system that requires a weight to be entered for each patient receiving an order for a weight-based medication (e.g., heparin, enoxaparin) before it is processed, or a bar-code scanning system that does not allow final verification of a product without a positive match between the selected product and the profiled medication.
- Automation and computerization of medication-use processes and tasks can lessen human fallibility by limiting reliance solely on vigilance or memory. Examples include use of electronic prescribing software that includes clinical decision support; pharmacy computer systems that can receive prescriptions sent electronically from a prescriber's hand-held device or computer and thus eliminate transcriptions and misinterpretations; robotic prescription preparation and dispensing technology; and computer systems that provide accurate warnings related to allergies, significant drug interactions, and excessive doses.
- Standardization creates a uniform model to adhere to when performing various functions and it tends to reduce the complexity and variation of a specific process. For example, standardized processes could be created to guide the pharmacist's final verification of a medication or to enhance the safety of giving or receiving a telephoned medication order. Prescriber use of carefully designed preprinted prescription blanks or standardized order forms that contain commonly used protocols (e.g., steroid tapers, insulin regimens, weight-based heparin) or frequently prescribed medications can reduce problems with confusing or missing instructions and illegible handwriting. On its own, standardization relies on human vigilance to ensure that a process is

followed; therefore, it is less effective than the strategies mentioned previously.

- Redundancies incorporate duplicate steps or add another individual to a process to force additional checks in the system. Involving two individuals in a process reduces the likelihood that both will make the same error with the same medication for the same patient. However, the potential for error still exists since the redundant step may be omitted or ignored. Examples of redundancies include use of both brand and generic names when communicating medication information or requiring independent double checks of high-alert medications before dispensing. Patient counseling is often an underutilized redundancy that can detect many errors.
- Reminders and checklists help make important information readily available. For example, using auxiliary labels to distinguish products; building look- and sound-alike alerts into order entry systems; and using preprinted prescription blanks that include prompts for important information (e.g., medication indication, allergies, patient birth date).
- Rules and policies are useful and necessary in organizations. Effective rules and policies should guide staff toward an intended positive outcome. However, some may add unnecessary complexity and may be met with resistance, even rightfully so, especially when implemented in response to an error. Because their use relies on memory, they should be used as a foundation to support more effective strategies that target system issues.
- Education and information are important tactics when combined with other strategies that strengthen the medication-use system. But, the effectiveness of these tactics relies totally on an individual's ability to remember what has been presented. Thus, on their own, they offer little leverage to prevent errors.

While each tool mentioned above can play an important role in error prevention, beware of those that, on the surface, seem to provide the easiest and fastest solution. While strategies at the bottom of the list may be used initially, we must realize that they will not be effective for long-lasting error prevention when used alone. In order to do a better job at preventing errors, we need to employ a variety of strategies that focus on the medication-use system issues and address human factors issues for those who work within that system. Since people cannot be expected to compensate for weak systems, managers should routinely evaluate the error-prevention strategies being used in their organizations. Consider if there are more powerful strategies that could be implemented to enhance medication safety.

Risk Identification Methods

All drug-dispensing procedures should be examined regularly, both proactively and retrospectively, and the potential problems as well as causes of system breakdowns must be discovered so that prevention measures can be designed. Pharmacy staff needs to communicate clearly to managers what it takes to do the job correctly in terms of personnel, training programs, facilities design, equipment, drug procedures and supplies, computer systems, and quality assurance programs. In addition, reducing medication errors requires using a number of effective risk identification methods including a nonpunitive environment and a voluntary medication error reporting system.

Currently, many pharmacies have an ineffective approach to error reduction. Often their primary means of identifying risk involves investigations that occur during the error reporting process. These investigations tend to focus their attention on the front end or active end of the error, such as the front-line practitioner. Human nature tends to assign blame to these front-line practitioners involved in medication errors. It is easier and in our nature to blame individuals and resort to familiar solutions: disciplinary action, individual remedial education, placing error information into personnel files, or developing new rules. While these actions may not seem outwardly punitive, these forms of reprimand lead to underreporting of errors. In fact, punishing individuals for errors actually can be dangerous to an organization. It inhibits open discussion about errors, creates a defensive and reactive environment, and hinders careful and unbiased consideration of the system-based root causes of errors.

Pharmacies are weakened further by punitive actions, especially if the sole responsibility for safe medication practices rests on individuals rather than on strong systems that make it difficult for practitioners to make errors.

The goal of patient safety is best served with a nonpunitive environment that places more value on a variety of risk identification methods, in addition to reporting problems so that they can be remedied, rather than on pursuing the unprofitable path of disciplining employees for errors. Methods to proactively identify the potential for problems in an organization include performing FMEAs to see where breakdowns may occur, using self-assesssment tools, and using external sources of information such as reviewing the literature for errors that have taken place in other organiztions and applying the "lessons learned" and determine if your organization could experience the same problems.

Self-assessments can help organizations assess the safety of medication practices throughout the facility, identify opportunities for improvement, and possibly compare their experiences with the aggregate experiences of demographically similar hospitals (ISMP, 2011b). One key consideration when undergoing this type of process is the establishment of an interdisciplinary team that should consist of representatives from all aspects of an organization, ranging from leadership (CEO, CMO, and nurse executives), directors of pharmacy as well as front line staff including nursing, pharmacists and physicians.

It is also important for pharmacy staff not just to focus on their own internal errors but also to look at other pharmacies' errors and methods of prevention and to learn from them. Organizations such as the ISMP, TJC, and many others provide ongoing features to facilitate these reviews in publications such as *Hospital Pharmacy, Pharmacy Today*, and *Pharmacy and Therapeutics* or newsletters that report on current medication safety issues and offer recommendations for changes.

The direct observation technique, in which a trained observer accompanies the person giving medications and witnesses the preparation and administration of each dose, was developed by Barker and McConnell (1962). The observer writes down in detail what the subject does when preparing and administering the drug (Barker et al., 2002). The notes are then compared with the prescriber's orders. An error is counted if the subject did not carry out the order accurately. The error rate is the percentage of doses administered in error, and the accuracy rate is the percentage of doses accurately administered. This method has many advantages. For example, it is not affected by lack of awareness of errors, lack of willingness to report errors, faulty memory, poor communication skills, or selective perception of the subject observed. Its reliability has been established through replication over many years. A large quantity of data can be accumulated at a rate 24 times that of chart review and 456 times that of incident reports. It can detect more errors and more types of error per unit of time than other methods, and it can identify clues about the causes so that future errors can be prevented (Cohen, 2007b).

A retrospective, voluntary, confidential reporting program provides pharmacists and pharmacy technicians with the opportunity to tell the complete story without fear of retribution. The depth of information contained in these stories is critical to understanding the error. This information is critical to identification of system deficiencies that can be corrected to prevent future errors. However, successful and sustained improvement of error-prone processes cannot occur if there is little information available about factors that contribute to an error.

Many organizational factors inhibit the reporting of medication errors. Examples include inconsistent definitions of a medication error within an organization, a punitive approach to medication errors, failure to improve the medication system or address reported problems reported by staff, lack of feedback to staff, over concern with medication error rates when reporting of an error may increase a facilities "error rate", complex reporting processes, a perception that reporting is a low priority andconcern for personal liability. A voluntary program encourages practitioners to report hazardous situations and errors that have the potential to cause serious patient harm. A confidential reporting system where everyone understands that errors will not be linked to performance appraisals is critical. Many pharmacy organizations have regular meetings where medication errors are addressed. The results of these meetings often are not shared with the front-line staff, therefore giving the impression that "nothing is being done" when errors are reported. In addition, busy practitioners tend to avoid reporting errors owing to the cumbersome nature of their organizations' reporting forms and processes. It is important to make error reporting easy, reward error reporting, and provide timely feedback to show what is being done to address problems. Consistently applying a nonpunitive approach to errors is important. If even one person is disciplined for an error, mistakes will be hidden. Employees should not be evaluated based on errors or lack of making mistakes but on positive measures that evaluate an employee's overall contribution to the organization. Armed with these tools, pharmacists can become aware of the deficiencies in their organizations and make performance-improvement changes. Without them, pharmacies can only address errors when they surface rather than at the root cause.

To be successful, medication error-reduction efforts must result in system improvements that are identified through a four-pronged analysis of errors. The first two prongs, both reactive in nature, include analysis of organization-specific errors that have caused some degree of patient harm and analysis of aggregate medication error data (e.g., trends by drugs or location of drugs involved in errors). Equally important, the other two prongs, both proactive in nature, include analysis of "close calls" (errors that have the potential to cause patient harm) and analysis of errors that have occurred in other organizations. Each prong contains valuable information about weaknesses in the system that, collectively, can lead to effective error-reduction strategies. Yet many organizations focus primarily on the first two prongs of error analysis and action. Most often proactive efforts are not given high priority. As a result, organizations may be busy "fighting fires" rather than preventing them. A "close call" should be clear evidence that a tragic event could occur. Unfortunately, too often this wakeup call is not heard. Little attention is focused on thorough analysis of errors that, fortunately, do not cause actual patient harm, especially if organizations identify errors that require analysis by a severity rating that is based on actual patient outcome. For example, a serious overdose detected before administration may not be given the same priority and analysis as a similar error that actually reached and possibly harmed the patient. Worse, some organizations fail to use errors that have occurred elsewhere as a road map for improvement in their own organization. Staff will be more comfortable discussing a serious external error than one that has occurred within its own organization. Because blame is not an issue, defensive posturing and other obstacles to effective discussion will not be present. Staff can identify possible system-based causes of the error more easily and the likelihood of a similar error in their facility and make suggestions for improvement. As improvements are made, enthusiasm builds for identifying, reporting, and analyzing errors that are actually occurring within the organization. In the end, discussion about external errors leads to more effective analysis of internal errors.

Multidisciplinary educational programs should be developed for health care personnel about medication error prevention. Because many errors happen when procedures are not followed, this is one area on which to focus through newsletters, discussions during staff meetings, and in-service training.

Lastly, organizations should report medication errors externally so that the lessons learned from these events can be shared with others to prevent future occurances in their facilities. In 1999, the IOM issued a landmark report entitled, "To Err is Human: Building a Safer Health System" that highlighted critical areas of research and activities needed to improve the safety and quality of health care delivery. One critical area of the IOM report addressed the reporting and analysis of data on adverse events.

The IOM report and its findings spotlighted a serious need to capture information that would help to improve quality and reduce harm to patients. Addressing this need, Congress passed The Patient Safety and Quality Improvement Act of 2005 (Patient Safety Act). To implement the Patient Safety Act, the Department

MEDI-CATION ERRORS REPORTING PROGRAM

The National Medication Errors Reporting Program (ISMP MERP)

Operated by the Institute for Safe Medication Practices, a federally certified Patient Safety Organization and an FDA MedWatch partner

Do not provide any identifiable health information, including names of practitioners, patients, healthcare facilities, or dates of birth.

Date and time of event:

Please describe the error. Include description/sequence of events, type of staff involved, and work environment (e.g., code situation, change of shift, no 24-hour pharmacy, floor stock). If more space is needed, please attach a separate page.

Did the error reach the patient? ☐Yes ☐No

Was the incorrect medication, dose, or dosage form administered to or taken by the patient? ☐Yes ☐No

Circle the appropriate Error Outcome Category (select one—see back for details): A B C D E F G H I

Describe the direct result of the error on the patient (e.g., death, type of harm, additional patient monitoring).

Indicate the possible error cause(s) and contributing factor(s) (e.g., abbreviation, similar names, distractions).

Indicate the location of the error (e.g., hospital, community pharmacy, clinic, nursing home, patient's home).

What type of staff or healthcare practitioner made the initial error?

Indicate if other practitioner(s) were also involved in the error (type of staff perpetuating error).

What type of staff or healthcare practitioner discovered the error or recognized the potential for error?

How was the error (or potential for error) discovered/intercepted?

If available, provide patient age, gender, diagnosis. Do not provide any patient identifiers.

Please complete the following for the product(s) involved. (If more space is needed for additional products, please attach a separate page.)

	Product #1	**Product #2**
Brand/Product Name (If Applicable)		
Generic Name		
Manufacturer		
Labeler		
Dosage Form		
Strength/Concentration		
Type and Size of Container		

Reports are most useful when relevant materials such as product label, copy of prescription/order, etc., can be reviewed.

Can these materials be provided? ☐Yes ☐No Please specify:

Suggest any recommendations to prevent recurrence of this error, or describe policies or procedures you instituted or plan to institute to prevent future similar errors.

Name and Title/Profession | Telephone Number ( ) | Fax Number ( )

Facility/Address and Zip | E-mail

Address/Zip (where correspondence should be sent)

Please check the box that applies: ☐Consumer ☐Licensed Healthcare Practitioner ☐Student/Technician

Copies of reports, without any identifying information, will be sent to third parties such as the manufacturer/labeler and to the Food and Drug Administration (FDA). You have the option of including your name on these copies.

ISMP may release my identity to these third parties as follows (check boxes that apply):

☐FDA ☐The manufacturer and/or labeler as listed above ☐Anonymous to all third parties

Signature | Date

Submit via the web at: **www.ismp.org/merp** Email: **merp@ismp.org**

Mail: ISMP, 200 Lakeside Dr., Ste. 200, Horsham, PA 19044 Phone: 800-Fail-Saf(e) (800-324-5723) Fax: 215-914-1492

Figure 29-9. Used with permission, Form used in reporting medication errors, preventable adverse drug reactions, close calls, or hazardous conditions to the National Medication Errors Reporting Program (ISMP MERP), operated by the Institute for Safe Medication Practices. You may submit reports to the ISMP MERP via the Internet at: www.ismp.org/merp.

of Health and Human Services issued the Patient Safety and Quality Improvement final rule. The Patient Safety Act and the Patient Safety Rule authorize the creation of Patient Safety Organizatoins (PSOs) to improve quality and safety through the collection and analysis of data on patient events [Agency for Healthcare Research and Quality (AHRQ), 2011].

PSOs are organizations that share the goal of improving the quality and safety of health care delivery. Organizations that are eligible to become PSOs include: public or private entities, profit or not-for-profit entities, provider entities such as hospital chains, and other entities that establish special components to serve as PSOs. By providing both privilege and confidentiality, PSOs create a secure environment where clinicians and health care organizations can collect, aggregate, and analyze data, thereby improving quality by identifying and reducing the risks and hazards associated with patient care. ISMP is certified as a Patient Safety Organization (PSO) by the Agency for Health care Research and Quality, which offers the highest level of legal protection and confidentiality for medication error reporting and analysis

Reporting errors to organizations like ISMP can also inform pharmaceutical companies of labeling and packaging problems. Many pharmaceutical companies have responded to suggestions made by technicians and pharmacists. Health professionals can report all of the aforementioned close calls and actual medication errors by using the ISMP Medication Error Reporting Program (MERP). Reports are forwarded to the individual pharmaceutical company and the FDA, and ISMP provides follow-up when appropriate. Call 1-800-FAILSAFE, visit ISMP's Web site at www.ismp.org, or complete an ISMP MERP report (see Fig. 29-9).

CONCLUSION

Pharmacists play a key role in the drug use process throughout any health care organization. Pharmacists and other members of the pharmacy department should lead a multidisciplinary effort to examine where errors arise in this process. Pharmacy department administrators should encourage their staff to collaborate in designing quality assurance programs to obtain information that helps to establish priorities and make changes. For example, joint reviews of the accuracy of unit-dose cart fills are of great help in detecting reasons for missing or inaccurate doses and changing the drug-dispensing system accordingly. Programs can be established to monitor the accuracy of order entry into computers in the pharmacy. Quality assurance efforts that include a review of medication error reports help to develop a better understanding of the kinds of systemic or behavioral defects being experienced so that necessary corrections can be identified. The medication error problem will never be eliminated completely, but pharmacy managers, working together with their staffs and other health care providers, can use their expertise to address issues of safety and thus ensure best outcomes in the safest environment possible.

QUESTIONS FOR FURTHER DISCUSSION

1. Have you witnessed or been involved in a medication error, and what actions did you take to prevent any future errors?
2. Have you counseled a patient whom you know did not understand his or her doctor's instructions? What steps did you take to ensure that the patient thoroughly knew his or her medication, directions, and indication for use?
3. Will you include medication error prevention strategies in the orientation process for new employees and ongoing education for pharmacy staff?
4. Do you think that you will be involved in reporting medication errors both internally within your organization and externally to reporting agencies such as the ISMP or the FDA? Do you think this will make a difference in your pharmacy practice setting?

REFERENCES

Agency for Healthcare Research and Quality (AHRQ). 2011. Patient Safety Organizations. Available at: http://www.pso.ahrq.gov/psos/overview.htm; accessed on June 9, 2011.

Allan EL, Barker KN. 1990. Fundamentals of medication error research. *Am J Hosp Pharm* 47:555.

Allan EL, Barker KN, Carnahan BJ. 2003. National observational study of prescription dispensing accuracy and safety in 50 pharmacies. *J Am Pharm Assoc* 43:191.

American Medical Association (AMA), Ad Hoc Committee on Health Literacy for the Council on Scientific Affairs. 1999. Health literacy: Report of the Council on Scientific Affairs. *JAMA* 281:552.

Aspden P, Wolcott JA, Bootman L, Cronenwett LR (eds.). 2006. *Preventing Medication Errors: Quality Chasm Series.* Washington, DC: The National Academies Press.

Barker KN, Flynn EA, Pepper GA. 2002. Observation method of detecting medication errors. *Am J Health Syst Pharm* 59(23):2314–6.

Barker KN, McConnell WE. 1962. The problems of detecting medication errors in hospitals. *Am J Hosp Pharm* 19:360–9.

Bedell SE, Jabbour S, Goldberg R, et al. 2000. Discrepancies in the use of medications: Their extent and predictors in an outpatient practice. *Arch Intern Med* 160:2129.

Cohen MR (ed.). 2007. *Medication Errors,* 2nd edn. Washington, DC: American Pharmacists Association, p. 56.

Cohen MR (ed.). 2007a. *Medication Errors,* 2nd edn. Washington, DC: American Pharmacists Association, pp. 192–3.

Cohen MR (ed.). 2007b. *Medication Errors,* 2nd edn. Washington, DC: American Pharmacists Association, p. 27.

Flynn EA, Pearson RE, Barker KN. 1997. Observational study of accuracy in compounding IV admixtures at five hospitals. *Amer J Health-System Pharm* 54:904–12.

Institute for Safe Medication Practices (ISMP). 1998. *ISMP Medication Safety Alert!* Washington, DC: ISMP, p. 3.

Institute for Safe Medication Practices (ISMP). 2007. Fatal 1,000-fold overdoses can occur, particularly to neonates, by transposing mcg and mg. 12(18). 1–2.

Institute for Safe Medication Practices (ISMP). 2008. ISMP's List of High-Alert Medications. Available at http://www.ismp.org/Tools/highalertmedications.pdf; accessed on September 19, 2011.

Institute for Safe Medication Practices (ISMP). 2010. *ISMP's* List of Error-Prone Abbreviations, Symbols, and Dose Designations. Available at http://www.ismp.org/Tools/errorproneabbreviations.pdf; accessed on May 18, 2011.

Institute for Safe Medication Practices (ISMP). 2011a. Principles of Designing a Medication Label for Oral Solids for Patient Specific, Inpatient Use. Available at http://www.ismp.org/Tools/guidelines/labelFormats/solids.asp; accessed on May 18, 2011.

Institute for Safe Medication Practices (ISMP). 2011b. 2011 ISMP Medication Safety Self Assessment for Hospitals. Available at http://www.ismp.org/selfassessments/Hospital/2011/Default.asp; accessed on June 20, 2011.

ISMP. 1999. Medication error prevention "toolbox." *ISMP Medication Safety Alert!* 4(11):1.

ISMP. 2006. Selecting the best error-prevention "tools" for the job. *ISMP Medication Safety Alert!* Community/Ambulatory Care Edition. 5(2):1–2.

Kohn LT, Corrigan JM, Donaldson MS (eds.). 1999. To Err Is Human: Building a Safer Health System, Institute of Medicine Report, November 29. Available at http://bob.nap.edu/html/to_err_is_human/; accessed on March 18, 2003.

Lesch MF. 2003. Comprehension and memory for warning symbols: Age-related differences and impact of training. *J Safety Res* 34:495.

Lombardi TP, Kennicutt JD. 2001. Promotion of a safe medication environment: Focus on the elderly and residents of long-term care facilities. Available at www.medscape.com/; accessed on May 14, 2001.

McDonnell PJ, Jacobs MR, McDonnell PJ. 2002. Hospital admissions resulting from preventable adverse drug reactions. *Pharmacotherapy* 36:1331.

National Council on Patient Information and Education. 2002. Avaliable at www.talkaboutrx.org/compliance.html; accessed on October 30, 2002.

National Medication Errors Reporting Program (ISMP MERP). Institute for Safe Medication Practices. www.ismp.org/merp; accessed on April 23, 2012.

Pennsylvania Patient Safety Authority. 2005. Abbreviations: A shortcut to medication errors. *PA-PSRS Patient Safety Advisory.*2(1):19–21. Available at http://www.patientsafetyauthority.org/ADVISORIES/Advisory Library/2005/Mar2(1)/Pages/19.aspx; accessed May 19, 2011.

Pharmacy Purchasing & Products. 2009. State of pharmacy compounding 2009: survey findings. *Pharmacy Purchasing & Products* 6(4):4–20.

Reason J. 1990. The contribution of latent human failures to the breakdown of complex systems. *Philos Trans R Soc Lond B Biol Sci* 327:475–84.

StateHealthFacts. 2011. Total number of retail prescription drugs filled at pharmacies, 2009. Available at http://www.statehealthfacts.org/comparemaptable.jsp?ind=265&cat=5; accessed June 3, 2011.

Svarstad B. 2000. FDA-Commissioned Research, University of Wisconsin–Madison. Presented February 2000, Rockville, MD, and June 2000, Kuopio, FL.

The Joint Commission (TJC). 2011. Available at www.jcaho.org/accredited + organizations/patient + safety/npsg/npsg_03.htm; accessed on April 30, 2003.

Wolf MS, Davis TC, Tilson HH, Bass PF 3rd, Parker RM. 2006. Misunderstanding of prescription drug warning labels among patients with low literacy. *Am J Health Syst Pharm* 63:1048.

SECTION VIII

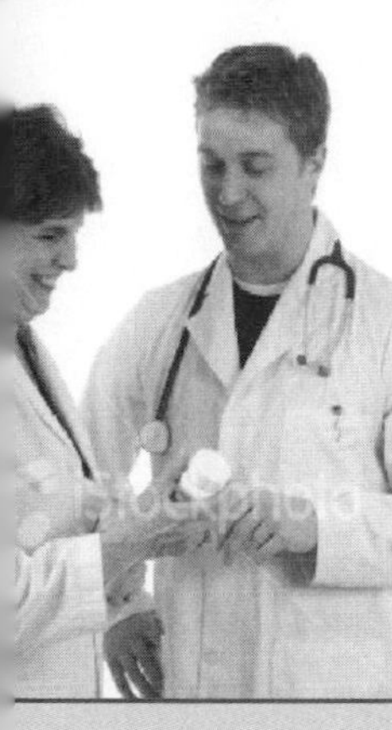

MANAGEMENT APPLICATIONS IN SPECIFIC PHARMACY PRACTICE SETTINGS

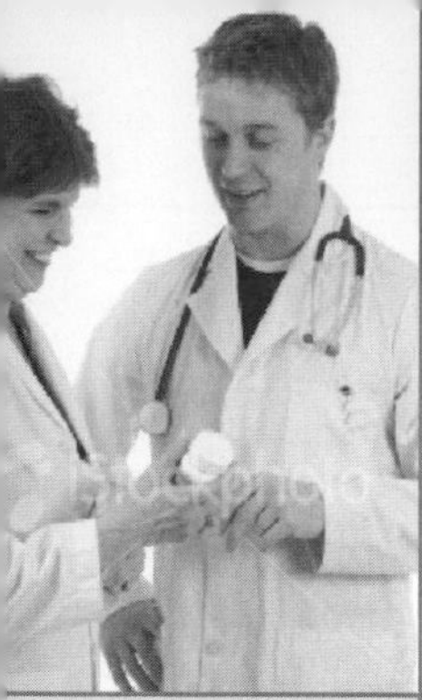

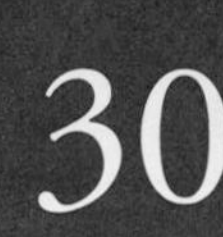

30

ENTREPRENEURSHIP AND INNOVATION

Bradley Tice

"The practice has to move in the direction where more and more pharmacists think outside the box and think about better ways to deliver their professional skills."

Clayton McWhorter
Pharmacist and Entrepreneur

About the Author: Dr. Tice is Chief Clinical Officer of PharmMD Solutions, LLC. PharmMD is an early-stage medication therapy management (MTM) delivery company based in Nashville, Tennessee. Dr. Tice learned a B.S. and a Pharm.D. from the University of Kansas and is currently in the Executive MBA program at Vanderbilt University's Owen School of Management. Prior to his current position, Dr. Tice was an Associate Professor at the Drake University College of Pharmacy & Health Sciences. His work has focused primarily on the development, implementation, and evaluation of innovative pharmacy services and has evolved into entrepreneurship. Dr. Tice attended the Experiential Classroom for Entrepreneurship Educators at Syracuse University and the Executive Management Program for Pharmacy Leaders at the Wharton School of Business and was a leader in the development of the DELTA (Drake Entrepreneurial Leadership Tools for Advancement) Rx Institute at Drake University. Dr. Tice defined and introduced the concept of *entrepreneurial leadership* in pharmacy through his presentation and accompanying publication and was awarded the Alfred B. Prescott Leadership Award in 2005. He has been an advocate of the integration of entrepreneurship principles into pharmacy education. He has also developed a software product to enable pharmacists to deliver and document their services and subsequently started a company, RXInterventions, LLC. He has also served on numerous committees and in elected positions with the Iowa Pharmacy Association, the American Pharmacists Association, and the American Association of Colleges of Pharmacy.

LEARNING OBJECTIVES

After completing this chapter, readers should be able to

1. Define *entrepreneurship.*
2. Discuss characteristics and types of entrepreneurs.
3. Discuss the applicability of entrepreneurship principles in the profession of pharmacy.
4. Given an "opportunity concept," apply the process of entrepreneurship to evaluate, pursue, execute, and harvest the venture.

CHAPTER QUESTIONS

1. What are three common characteristics of entrepreneurs?
2. What are the four types of entrepreneur personalities, which one do you most identify with, and what leads you to identify yourself with this characterization?
3. Why is the understanding and use of the "process" of entrepreneurship an important component in the establishment of entrepreneurship as its own body of knowledge?
4. Why is it important for an entrepreneur to be able to clearly and succinctly communicate the business concept?

SCENARIO

Pharmacist John Adams works for a chain pharmacy in a large city with a population of over 1 million people. He has been out of school for several years and has worked through such positions as staff pharmacist and pharmacy manager. In the last year, he has started focusing his work on patients with diabetes. He has incorporated a complete diabetes program into his practice that includes classes on blood glucose monitoring, sick-day management, insulin administration, meal planning and healthy eating for patients with diabetes, and a general overview of diabetes. He also has one-on-one counseling sessions that he offers in these areas. During the course of delivering these sessions, John has discovered that a recurring problem patients have is not getting enough blood for a measurement when they stick their fingers to check their blood sugar. In addition, patients often find this painful and do not do this as often as they should. One day John develops a device that is very effective at getting the necessary blood sample from patients and is nearly pain free. The device is very popular among his patients, and he starts to get referrals for the device.

While the high salary as a pharmacist was attractive to John at first, he now is starting to feel more confident in his abilities and would like a new challenge and opportunity. He wonders if this lancet device he has developed could be worth something. He did not take any business classes in pharmacy school; however, when he was growing up, his father ran the hardware store in their small town, so he has some exposure to running a business. He thought that his father might be interested in helping him out. John has developed a number of relationships with businesspeople through his involvement in the community and thinks that he might elicit their advice, too.

Some questions running through his mind are

- Should he pursue developing this idea into a product?
- If he does, should he do this through the company that he is currently with or on his own?
- If he chooses to do this on his own, would he need to completely quit what he is currently doing?
- How much money will he need, and is he really ready to commit his money to this?

BACKGROUND

Entrepreneurship has been a longstanding component of the profession of pharmacy, going back to the earliest days of the corner drugstore. Coca-Cola (Coca-Cola, 2007) and Dr. Pepper (Dr. Pepper, 2007) are two examples of products that arose from some of the earliest days of that practice setting. In an era when industrialized medicinal products did not exist, pharmacists were in the position of creating new recipes and formulations to meet physicians' orders and treat patients. As the industry evolved and more standardized and large-scale methods were developed, the profession of pharmacy evolved with it. Traditionally, independently owned pharmacies were started and run usually with one pharmacist opening up the store as an owner-operator. Some pharmacists saw opportunities beyond single-store ownership and pursued and developed multiple stores. This led to the development of what is now referred to as *chain store pharmacies.* These pharmacies often are thought of as not being entrepreneurial for pharmacists who enter as employees; however, chain pharmacy itself is an example of entrepreneurship, and as will be discussed later, there are opportunities for entrepreneurship within large companies. Within the hospital setting, clinical pharmacy was developed in the 1960s and eventually made its way into the community pharmacy practice setting. In the last 15 to 20 years, the concept of *pharmaceutical care* was established and transitioned into medication therapy management (MTM), which has led to many entrepreneurial activities and endeavors in disease management, immunization delivery, and other new businesses.

To date, the entrepreneurial endeavors within the profession have been undertaken largely without formal training in entrepreneurship within the pharmacy curriculum. It is likely that formal training in entrepreneurship can increase the success rate of these entrepreneurial endeavors. The ability to integrate this formal training is increasing because the field of entrepreneurship is a growing rapidly. In 1975, 104 colleges and universities offered courses in entrepreneurship (Kauffman Foundation, 2006). By 1990, this had increased to 370, and by 2005, the number of schools offering courses in entrepreneurship had exploded to 2,662 (1,194 two-year schools and 1,468 four-year schools). There are now over 895 programs in entrepreneurship for business students, 126 programs for undergraduate minors, and 463 programs for nonbusiness students.

WHAT IS ENTREPRENEURSHIP?

The word *entrepreneurship* has come to have many definitions. One commonly used definition is "the process by which individuals pursue opportunities without regard to resources they currently control." One of the key aspects of this definition is that entrepreneurship is a process. This has several implications. First of all, a process is something that can be taught and is something that is repeatable. It also implies characteristics of passion and perseverance. In pursuing opportunities without regard to resources currently controlled, the entrepreneur must believe in and have a passion to succeed that will carry him or her through difficult times. The end goal is achieving the vision. As Michael Morris, Witting Chair of Entrepreneurship at Syracuse University, states and teaches, entrepreneurship is a "philosophy of life" (Morris, 1998). It is a way of approaching life to identify problems and proactively turning them into opportunities to improve the situation, whether that is society, individual life, or the profession.

Pharmacists work with patients every day to help solve their problems in managing their medications and health. Because of this, pharmacists are in an ideal position to identify opportunities that may be viable business opportunities.

WHO IS AN ENTREPRENEUR?

There are often misperceptions about *who* an entrepreneur is (Kuratko, 2004). Some common stereotypes are that an entrepreneur is someone who is lucky, highly charismatic, and greedy and often that they

Table 30-1. Types of Entrepreneurs

Personal Achievers	Super Sales People
Need for feedback	Capacity to understand others, empathize
Need for achievement	Belief that social processes are important
Strong commitment	Good at external relationship building
Internal locus of control	Belief in sales force
Expert Idea Generators	**Real Managers**
Build venture around new products	Desire to take charge, compete, be decisive, stand out
Involved with high-tech companies	Desire to be corporate leader, desire for power
Desire to innovate	Positive attitude toward authority
Intelligence as source of competitive advantage	

are just "born." The definition given earlier helps to debunk these misperceptions. The process orientation and ability to teach the process shows that entrepreneurship is not something a person is just born with or that just depends on luck.

Likely because of the misperceptions, the area of identifying who is an entrepreneur is one of the most heavily researched areas in the field. Some of the common characteristics of entrepreneurs include a high level of achievement motivation, an internal locus of control, and a tolerance for ambiguity. John Miner, is his book, *The Four Routes to Entrepreneurial Success* (Miner, 1996), identifies four types of entrepreneurs (Table 30-1). Each of these types has unique characteristics that can help to break through the stereotypes. For instance, the "super sales person" is the more charismatic individual typical of some stereotypes, but the other three types help to identify where less charismatic people fit as entrepreneurs. In addition, "real managers" identifies the type of entrepreneur that can fit into corporate entrepreneurship. One characteristic that is not present in the descriptions of entrepreneurs is "high-risk gamblers." Entrepreneurs have been found to have a tolerance for ambiguity but not to be inclined to take unnecessary risk and even have been found to be more risk averse than people who are not entrepreneurs (Xu and Ruef, 2004).

An important aspect of entrepreneurs to recognize is that they are not necessarily experts in all areas of business (e.g., finance, accounting, marketing, operations, etc.). It is not possible for one person to be an expert in every area necessary to start, grow, and run a business. Entrepreneurs typically are very good at establishing networks of people who can help them in areas that are not their strengths. An example of this is Henry Ford (Hill, 1960). During World War I, a Chicago newspaper called Mr. Ford an "ignorant pacifist." Mr. Ford did not like this and took the paper to court. When Mr. Ford was on the witness stand, the attorney drilled him with questions to test his knowledge with the intent of showing that Mr. Ford was unable to answer the questions and was indeed "ignorant." After getting frustrated with the line of questioning, Mr. Ford stated that if he really wanted to know the answer to any question, he had a row of electronic buttons on his desk. By pushing the right buttons, he could summon to his aid someone who could answer any question he could think to ask, so why should he clutter up his mind with this knowledge. The attorney was stumped, and Mr. Ford showed that he was not an "ignorant" man. Knowing how to get access to the people and information needed and not being afraid to ask are important characteristics of entrepreneurs.

Another important characteristic of entrepreneurs is *passion.* Passion is important because the entrepreneurial road is often not easy. There are often peaks and valleys the entrepreneur must navigate to bring the business idea to fruition. There likely will be times of challenges on cash flow, challenges on bringing the product or service to market, and challenges with hiring, to name a few. Passion for the business concept is required to provide the perseverance to make it through challenging times. Investors and key hires also look for this trait. Investors want to know the person they are investing their money with has the fortitude to make it through challenging times. Key hires also want to know they are going to be with someone who is steadfast in their commitment to help pull them through demanding circumstances. Specific to pharmacy, the profession needs passionate professionals who are motivated to improve the profession without regard to resources they feel are under their control.

THE ENTREPRENEURIAL PROCESS

Understanding the process of entrepreneurship and its application is one of the most important aspects of "learning" entrepreneurship because it provides a structured approach that can repeated, analyzed, and improved on. For these reasons, integrating the process of entrepreneurship into pharmacy practice is likely to provide a methodology that can increase the success of entrepreneurial activities.

Identifying an Opportunity

Ideas can come in many different forms and from many different places. Table 30-2 lists categories where ideas can come from. While this table was not created specifically to address pharmacy, there are many opportunities in each category on the list that exist within pharmacy. Once trained to look at life through the lens of an entrepreneur, an individual likely will generate many ideas (e.g., the "expert idea generator" type) and see opportunity where others do not. McGrath and MacMillan (2000), in their book, *The Entrepreneurial Mindset*, indicate that entrepreneurs often generate and maintain an *opportunity register*. This is an ongoing list of ideas for opportunities. The entrepreneur then chooses which one to pursue and maintains the list to go back to when he or she is ready to move to the next opportunity. It is impossible to pursue every idea. The entrepreneur must be disciplined in the selection of opportunities to pursue because resources likely will be limited and pursuit of an opportunity requires focus, perseverance, and dedication.

Developing the Concept

As the opportunities are identified, the next step is to develop the concept further and determine where the best market opportunity lies. Most ideas have multiple ways that they can be implemented. Table 30-2 lists some of the possible options. Determining which idea to pursue and how to execute the opportunity are key decisions for the entrepreneur to make. To guide these decisions, the entrepreneur often will perform a *feasibility analysis* (Barringer and Ireland, 2006).

In the feasibility analysis, extensive research is performed on the product/service, industry, market, organizational feasibility, and financial feasibility of the opportunity. This is an extremely important component of the decision to pursue or not pursue opportunities and speaks to the risk-averse nature of entrepreneurs. Much of this research will go into the building of a business plan (see Chapter 5).

When pursuing opportunities within a corporation, the feasibility analysis can be used to weigh opportunities, or projects, against each other. This type of entrepreneurship is called *corporate entrepreneurship, or intrapreneurship* (Morris and Kuratko, 2002).

One might argue that pharmacist John in the scenario has demonstrated perhaps as much intrapreneurship as entrepreneurship. The device he developed might be shared with management and corporate executives, and they might be able to help determine how this device might better position the company, or how John might leverage this innovation to the best possible benefit to both him and to patients/society. Intrapreneurship, like entrepreneurship, has its potential pitfalls, including potential envy among coworkers, potential piracy of ideas, and being taken advantage of. However, an intrapreneurial spirit is one of the more sought after qualities in organizations, and often positions someone to ascend high and quickly up the organizational chart. Intrapreneurism is actually a necessary component of today's ever-changing

Table 30-2. The Entrepreneurial Process

Identify an opportunity	Changing demographics Emergence of new market segments Process needs New technologies Incongruities Regulatory change Social change	**Acquire the necessary resources**	Debt Equity Leveraging Outsourcing Leasing Contract labor Temporary staff Supplier financing Joint ventures Partnerships Barter Gifts
Develop the Concept	New products New services New processes New markets New organizational structure/forms New technologies New sales or distribution channels	**Implement and manage**	Implementation of concept Monitoring of performance Payback of resource providers Reinvestment Expansion Achievement of performance goals
Determine the required resources	Skilled employees General management expertise Marketing and sales expertise Technical expertise Financing Distribution channels Sources of supply Production facilities Licenses, patents, and legal protection	**Harvest the venture**	Absorption of new concept into mainstream operations Licensing of rights Family succession Sell venture Go public Shut down the venture

Source: Used with permission from Morris MH, Kuratko DF, Schindehutte M. 2001. Towards integration: Understanding entrepreneurship through frameworks. *International Journal of Entrepreneurship and Innovation*, Volume 2, No 1, February 2001.

health care environment; and from a management perspective, should be encouraged among your employees without fear of retaliation or other repercussions. Innovative ideas that propel an organization forward are often borne from innovative pursuits of intrapreneurs. From the employee perspective, being an intrapreneur can provide significant advantages to you and the organization while providing a safety net of steady employment. A culture of intrapreneurism allows someone to unlock their creative juices, thus increasing their own work satisfaction, before they might eventually decide to go off into a more "nontraditional" path, such as starting up their own company and becoming more *entrepreneurial*.

Determining the Required Resources

As the definition at the beginning of the chapter describes, entrepreneurs typically will not have all the resources needed to pursue the identified opportunity. This step in the process, which can be a part of the feasibility analysis, will help to identify what resources are needed and help to determine if the entrepreneur can obtain those needed resources. The list in Table 30-2 identifies at least some of the areas to be included in the analysis. This is an especially important point for pharmacists to evaluate because pharmacists have a specialized body of knowledge and are often not diverse in their training in business, management, marketing, finance, and other areas important to pursuing an entrepreneurial venture. It is important to realize that this does not have to be a limiting factor but rather a factor that can and needs to be managed.

This step in the process also will help to identify the extent to which financial resources need to be acquired and at what stage in the business-development timeline they are needed. In general, when outside financial resources are needed, they are not all acquired at the same time. To maintain an equity position for those starting the business, rounds of funding are established that enable the business to develop, having enough capital to operate but not an overabundant amount of money as to be wasteful. Acquiring capital from investors results in awarding those investors with shares of the business. The investors who are in at the earliest time are subject to the most risk and therefore get more shares for less money. Conversely, this early money is costing the business owner more equity for the dollars he or she is getting. Acquiring the money in stages lets the owner maintain a larger equity position in the business. It should be noted that one of the biggest mistakes entrepreneurs make is not being willing to give up equity to fund their venture. While it can be important to be smart about how and when to give up equity, one analogy in entrepreneurship compares equity to manure (yes, manure). The more manure is piled up, the more it smells, but the more it is spread around (on a field), the more it helps things to grow.

Acquiring the Necessary Resources

Once the entrepreneurial idea and venture have been well defined and researched through the feasibility analysis, resources are acquired to pursue the idea. Table 30-2 lists some of the ways to acquire resources. Usually, to help get others to invest, the entrepreneur will have to put some of his or her own money into the development. This is referred to as having "skin in the game." Entrepreneurs can get very creative in how to get their businesses started. Grants and small business loans are used often, but grants can take longer to acquire than other methods. The benefit of not having to pay back the financing or to give up equity in the company can be very attractive. A lot of "sweat equity" (time put into developing the business without receiving payment for the time put in) is usually also required, and this typically does not translate into actual dollar equity. If the entrepreneur cannot identify enough resources himself or herself, identifying an *angel investor* may be the next best alternative. An angel investor is someone who can supply the money himself or herself. This person also often helps to mentor the entrepreneur to ensure success.

It can also be beneficial to go after *strategic money*. Once someone provides capital to the business, he or she is likely to have a vested interest in seeing the business succeed. Money from individuals who can help make connections to potential customers and other stakeholders can be an important part of getting the business established. Joint ventures and partnering also can help to speed up the adoption process and get buy-in to the business.

Financial resources are not the only types of resources that will need to be acquired. One of the most important resources to be acquired is a management team. Finding key people who can drive the business idea forward is an essential component of the success of the business. As implied earlier in the example of Henry Ford, having a strong network is an extremely powerful characteristic of an entrepreneur. Entrepreneurs who are able to identify key individuals and make connections through the people they know can get the right people to work for them, obtain funding, and get work done (e.g., marketing and business development/client recruitment) without having to spend as much money on regular outsourcing.

Implement and Manage

Implementation and management of the startup, growth, and ongoing operations are also critical components of the entrepreneurial process. The skills needed for this level of the process can be self-taught or learned in more formal training. Entire business degrees focus on the different areas where expertise is needed to run a business. Still, there are many successful business owners who do not have a formal degree in business. Decision-making abilities and experience are two of the most important attributes for success in this process. While some people may seem "born" with natural abilities in these areas, both decision-making ability and experience often are learned over time and can be learned within the profession of pharmacy after licensure. Pharmacists are put in many decision-making positions in professional practice. This experience, along with others that can be gained in managing a pharmacy, growing a practice, or working in a business unit of a large company, can serve as training and provide confidence to pharmacists to decide later in their career to pursue an opportunity. These same attributes can be acquired outside the profession and earlier as well.

Any exposure to running a business or decision-making positions can help to provide training that is beneficial to developing entrepreneurial abilities. The 5 + 5 + 5 Bernelli Entrepreneurial Learning (BEL) Method (Table 30-3) was developed by a pharmacist, Cynthia Ianerelli, now president of Bernelli University, who left the profession to help with the family business. In pursuing more formal training to run the business, she realized that many of the decisions in business school were easier for her than for others. She attributes this to her growing up around the family business and the subtle experiences she had in doing so. Her research has focused in this area and developed this method of teaching entrepreneurship that focuses on experiential learning, even starting as early as preschool, to train for entrepreneurship. As is seen in Table 30-3, the BEL Method identifies five stages of development and provides initially for exposure and hands-on experience. Once the individual has this, he or she can grow into broader experiences. It is not until after the person has these earlier experiences that he or she builds into formal entry and leadership stages. Research and reports (Hise, 2007) also support the value of experience in developing entrepreneurial thinking.

For any business, the key to implementing and managing the opportunity will center on cash flow. First, acquiring capital to get the business started, as discussed earlier, and then, once the business is started, balancing the expenditure of money with the need to obtain more to keep the business going. Businesses often fail because they do not have enough cash when they start. It is recommended that a business have enough cash to support it for 3 years when it is started. However, this is often difficult to obtain. Additionally, in opportunities where the business is obtaining funding through investors and venture capital and is giving up equity, it is typical for the business to pursue rounds of funding. The reason for this is that investors at the earlier stages get more equity for the money they put in because it is a riskier stage of the business. As the business develops and can demonstrate success, funding is not as risky and requires less equity to be given up.

Balancing the use of cash to operate the business with the need for funds to grow the business is delicate. Typically, the business is using funds to acquire supplies

Table 30-3. The 5 + 5 + 5 Bernelli Entrepreneurial Learning Method

Five Stages of Development	Five Skills to Teach at Each Stage	Five Steps How to Transmit the Information Effectively
Exposure	Self-starting skills	Continuity
Hands-on	People skills	Problem solution
Broadening experience	Marketing skills	Meet and greet
Formal entry	Money skills	Create networks
Leadership	Leadership skills	Recap

and resources to support the product. If the business is not paid expediently when sales are made, it can be difficult to replenish the supplies and resources for the next round of sales, and this can cause difficulty for the business in paying its bills on time.

Harvest the Venture

Harvesting the venture refers to how the entrepreneur will reap the rewards of the endeavor. There are many ways that an entrepreneur can "exit" the business. Some of these include selling the business to someone else, passing the business on to someone in the family, licensing the rights of the intellectual property developed in the business, going public with the business, or simply shutting the business down. To maximize the reward of the opportunity, it is important to develop the *exit strategy* or list of potential exit strategies early on in the concept-development process. Often, the best time to cash in on a venture will be when the venture blossoming. This can be a difficult time to part with the venture unless a strategy is mapped out in advance. Having the exit strategy(ies) mapped out in advance can help in business planning and execution and in identifying opportunities to maximize reward.

MENTORSHIP FOR INTRAPRENEURS/ ENTRAPRENEURS

Mentorship is important for breaking down barriers to entrepreneurship. As noted above in the BEL method, having the opportunity for exposure to entrepreneurship is an important key to developing entrepreneurial abilities. Having a mentor provides someone with experience to troubleshoot ideas, provide guidance on important decisions, and to shepherd the less experienced entrepreneur through the journey. There will be many decisions to make, and there will be many opportunities for missteps that a mentor can help steer through. Young entrepreneurs and pharmacists should pay close attention to whom they choose to work with early in their careers, as this can shape and mold them for future opportunities and career growth. Mentorship is critical to success in many ways, and many pharmacy organizations, community programs, and Fortune 500 programs have initiated mentorship programs that focus on the mentee's quality of work life and whole-life actualization, while having the mentor hone the mentee's skills to navigate political minefields and become more savvy about communicating their ideas of innovation for greater acceptance by important stakeholders.

APPLICATION WITHIN PHARMACY

Work has been done to understand the characteristics of entrepreneurship within the pharmacy profession. Research examining practice change that considers both the environment and characteristics of individuals and practices related to implementing patient care services has been performed. This research reinforces the work previously mentioned specific to the field of entrepreneurship. Doucette and Jambulingham (1999) described a PHARMacist Entrepreneurial Orientation (PHARMEO), which is a multidimensional model for measuring market entry to practice change and "refers to the processes, practices, and decision-making activities that lead to market entry." In this model, six dimensions are identified that can indicate a pharmacy's entrepreneurial orientation. These include proactiveness, innovativeness, risk-taking, autonomy, competitive aggressiveness, and work ethic. Four antecedents, or factors leading to a pharmacists entrepreneurial orientation were identified. These include dynamism—the degree to which new products and services are being introduced in the market, environmental munificence—the extent to which an organization can support sustained growth, pharmacy type—being an independently owned pharmacy or small chain, and organicity of the pharmacy structure—the degree to which the policies and structure are less rigid, lending to more of an entrepreneurial orientation.

Willink and Isetts (2005) also examine the characteristics of pharmacists implementing advanced patient care activities. They identify essential components, including profession-related aspects such as philosophy of practice and clinical knowledge, in addition to patient care process and environmental aspects of the practice. A group of highly successful, entrepreneurial pharmacists all reported on being empathic toward patients, giving back to the community, emphasized relationship building, and fostered climates of innovation in their pharmacies. Nimmo and Holland (1999) identified a "three-ring circus" of required elements to achieve practice change to include having the appropriate practice environment, having appropriate training, and the presence of appropriate motivational strategies.

Mapping the work done in the pharmacy literature to the previously discussed process of entrepreneurship provides insights into pharmacy entrepreneurship. Most of what has been identified focuses on characteristics of identifying new opportunities and developing the concept to be introduced to the market. Going back to the definition introduced earlier in this chapter of an entrepreneur pursuing opportunities without regard to resources currently controlled, these models mostly suggest that the environment has to be appropriate for entrepreneurship in pharmacy to occur. Opportunities for further inquiry would be to identify if entrepreneurs self-select into environments where they can see their ideas being more easily implemented, or if the environmental factors help to prompt the entrepreneurial spirit.

The opportunities for intrapreneurism and entrepreneurism in pharmacy are virtually endless. Many pharmacists have developed alternative dosage forms or repackaged prefabricated products in a way that meets a consumer demand; developed software that helps clinical pharmacists document and bill for MTM services; used their expertise in compounding to create new products sold at the local or national level; begun to niche into the handling and storage of specialty pharmaceuticals (see Chapter 34); identified opportunities for particular target markets, such as veterinary pharmacy; and began consulting firms to provide insight on more effective buying of pharmaceutical goods and/or developing care management plans, just to name a few.

■ INTELLECTUAL PROPERTY

One of the most important aspects of entrepreneurship is protecting the idea, referred to as *intellectual property*. Intellectual property can take many forms, from logos, to products, to business processes, as some examples. Types of protection include copyrights, trademarks, and patents (Allen, 2003).

Copyright protection is the easiest and least costly to acquire. However, it also generally provides the least amount of protection. This protection does not protect the ideas, processes, or methods of the intellectual property. It only protects the form, or original work, which is the end result of the ideas, processes or methods. Copyrights can be obtained officially through the U.S. Copyright Office for as little as $30.

Trademarks are used to protect names, brands, logos, and other marketing devices that are distinctive. Trademarks are somewhat more expensive. They generally can be filed for $750. It is also possible to do a trademark search on your own on the Internet through the US Patent and Trademark Office Web site (www.uspto.gov). It is also possible to pay attorneys to do the search for you.

Patents offer the highest level of protection. They take the most time and money to acquire, usually taking at least 2 years and $4,000 to file. It is generally necessary to hire intellectual property attorneys to assist with the filing and defense of the patent. Patents protect the idea, method, and design of products and businesses. (For a full description of patents and the filing process, go to www.uspto.gov.) It is important to research the timelines for filing—generally within 1 year of use—and to decide if you need only a patent in the United States or a patent filed in other countries as well (and there are specific timelines on when this needs to be done).

■ INCUBATORS

A useful concept for entrepreneurs that may be especially applicable to pharmacist entrepreneurs is the *incubator*. This term describes an entity that exists to help get new businesses started. As stated earlier, entrepreneurs cannot be experts in every area required of entrepreneurship. Incubators bring all or many of the necessary areas together (e.g., accounting, business plan development, legal, capital acquisition, etc.) to help entrepreneurs bring their ideas to market. As discussed previously, investment early in the idea development process costs the most. Incubators usually take significant equity of the business to get started. The entrepreneur must assess how much is really needed and how much the incubator is really going to contribute before signing on. Incubators are often found connected to academic institutions, especially those with entrepreneurship programs. They can also exist within an area's business community and can serve as a method for local investors to formalize or outsource their investment process. For example, a person wishing to invest in new opportunities can use the incubator to screen opportunities and provide structure to the opportunities to lessen the risk of the investment. Locating an incubator can also be done by searching on the Internet.

TIMING AND COMPETITION

One of the most important aspects of bringing an idea to market is timing. No matter how good the idea is, if the market is not prepared for it, it will not reach its full potential. First-movers, the first person to bring a concept to market, can have what is called *first-mover advantage,* allowing them to gain the rewards of early entry into a market. At other times, the second person into the market can gain the advantage because the first-mover has had to go to all the effort to train and educate the market about the concept. Deciding exactly when an opportunity is ripe is one of the most important decisions an entrepreneur must make. Research, focus groups, forecasting, and competitive analysis can go a long way toward identifying when the timing is right. However, many companies spend enormous resources to identify when the timing is right and exactly what the product should be only to see their product fall flat or short of expectations. As is described by Zaltman (2002), people cannot tell in advance of a product offering what their true reaction to the product will be. Zaltman's research showed that 95 percent of people's thinking occurs in their subconscious mind, so while they may even desire to help, their true reaction can be seen only with exposure to the product and all the parallel decisions accompanying it. One often counterintuitive factor that can help to identify a product's success is whether or not a similar product offering exists. Competition, in general, can be a positive sign that the market is ready for the concept and can serve to bring down the costs of bringing the product to market. The competition's presence and marketing can serve to validate the need for the product, increase awareness of the need for the product, and help tear down walls of resistance to the new product.

SELLING THE CONCEPT

To sell the opportunity effectively, the entrepreneur must be able to quickly communicate the value proposition associated with the product, service, or business. In entrepreneurship circles, this is referred to as the *elevator pitch.* The elevator pitch refers to the ability to pitch the concept to a potential investor in the amount of time it takes to get on an elevator and then get off. The idea behind this is for the entrepreneur to be ready to pitch the concept clearly and concisely at any time. This skill actually fits in well for pharmacists because it is similar to how pharmacists often must counsel patients and make drug therapy recommendations to prescribers. One method of getting additional training in doing this effectively is the book, *How to Get Your Point Across in 30 Seconds or Less* (Frank, 1986). Three key questions that may be helpful to address are the following:

1. What is the benefit?
2. How is the opportunity new and different?
3. What is the reason to believe?

One common mistake that is made by inexperienced entrepreneurs and pharmacists in "selling" their product or service is to focus on its *features.* They describe these features or aspects of the product or service but do not relate to the customer or how the features provide benefit or value. Benefits relate directly to how the product or service will make buyers' lives better. Investors are looking for an obvious value proposition and preferably one that is recurring or leads to multiple selling opportunities.

ADDITIONAL RESOURCES

There are many resources for entrepreneurs. Searching the Internet can easily identify a number of resources.

Networking in the community with business owners also can identify mentors who can be a vital resource as well. Some recommended resources include:

- *The DELTA Rx* Institute (www.deltarx.com). The DELTA Rx Institute is based at the Drake University College of Pharmacy & Health Sciences. DELTA stands for "Drake Entrepreneurial Leadership Tools for Advancement." The Web site provides resources on entrepreneurship, profiles pharmacy entrepreneurial leaders, and provides tools and courses that can help to get pharmacists started on the path to entrepreneurship.
- *The Stanford Technology Venture Program* (http://stvp.stanford.edu/). This is a Web site through the Stanford University School of Engineering that is "dedicated to accelerating high-technology entrepreneurship research and education to engineers and scientists." The Web site has many resources and podcasts from entrepreneurs, including many from successful entrepreneurs in Silicon Valley that can provide great insights.
- *The Entrepreneurship and Emerging Enterprises Program at Syracuse University* (http://whitman.syr.edu/eee/). This Web site also has many resources that can assist in growing entrepreneurial capabilities and links to other sites targeted to entrepreneur-ship.

REVISITING THE SCENARIO

John Adams decides that the time is right to pursue this opportunity. He decides that to really give this opportunity the chance for success that it needs, he will focus his attention by fully researching the opportunity, identifying a mentor, and setting everything in place. Once that is accomplished (under a planned timeline), he will turn to this as a full-time opportunity, leaving his current employment. "Traditional pharmacist positions are easy to get back into, and I can probably get a sign-on bonus somewhere if I needed it, so why not?" John is wisely pursuing his intrapreneurial goal and keeping the shelter of his current employment until a greater amount of time must be dedicated to his venture and becoming an entrepreneur. John also is willing to take some risks, given that in the event his venture does not reach the goals he had hoped for, he can always return to his position as a full-time staff pharmacist, with some valuable experience under his belt that can propel him forward in any setting/organization for which he might come back to work.

CONCLUSION

Entrepreneurship has strong roots in the pharmacy profession. The specialized knowledge, skills, and practice of pharmacy provide a solid foundation for identifying and pursuing entrepreneurial endeavors. While stereotypes often portray entrepreneurs as charismatic, high-risk gamblers, evidence suggests that people can be successful entrepreneurs with a variety of personal characteristics. Passion for the profession and business concept are important aspects of building the opportunity. Relationship building, empathy, understanding internal/external forces, and performing hard work and due diligence are also paramount. Importantly, identifying that entrepreneurship is a formal process that can be repeated and taught shows that it is not simply a trait individuals are "born with." Applying the described process of entrepreneurship can provide a framework for success and for quality improvement through refinement of the process. Financing the entrepreneurial endeavor requires a skillful balance of managing cash flow and equity to bring the opportunity to market successfully. Throughout pharmacy's history, entrepreneurship has been a strong component of the profession that has helped it to adapt and strengthen itself over the years. With the explosive growth of entrepreneurship education and the rapid change in today's world, there is no doubt that it will be just as vital in moving the profession forward. Young pharmacists should look for a mentor early in their career and choose who they work with carefully, as this can both shape them and provide opportunities to build their career.

QUESTIONS FOR FURTHER DISCUSSION

1. Describe the importance of networking for entrepreneurs, and identify methods of networking in the profession, community, and business world.
2. What, in your opinion, is the most difficult step in the process of entrepreneurship? Describe and explain why?
3. Describe an approach to financing an entrepreneurial venture. Include a discussion of the pros and cons of debt acquisition, using personal and "friends and family" funds, and venture capital.
4. After identifying an opportunity, develop a 30-second elevator pitch that clearly communicates the value of the concept.
5. Which category from Table 30-1 do you most readily identify with, and how would you see this leading toward your own individual entrepreneurship?

REFERENCES

Allen KR. 2003. *Launching New Ventures: An Entrepreneurial Approach,* 3rd edn. Boston: Houghton Mifflin.

Barringer BR, Ireland RD. 2006. *Entrepreneurship: Successfully Launching New Ventures.* Upper Saddle River, NJ: Pearson Prentice-Hall.

Coca-Cola. 2007. The chronicle of Coca-Cola. Available at www.thecoca-colacompany.com/heritage/chronicle_birth_refreshing_idea.html; accessed on October 7, 2007.

Doucette DR, Jambulingham T. 1999. Pharmacy entrepreneurial orientation: Antecedents and its effect on the provision of innovative pharmacys services. *J Soc Adm Pharm* 16:26–37.

Dr. Pepper. 2007. A history of Dr. Pepper, the world's oldest major soft drink. Available at www.drpeppermuseum.com/dr-pepper-facts.html#history; accessed on October 7, 2007.

Frank MO. 1986. *How to Get Your Point Across in 30 Seconds or Less.* New York: Pocket Books.

Hill N. 1960. *Think and Grow Rich.* New York: Ballantine Publishing Group.

Hise P. 2007. A chance to prove my worth. *Fortune Small Business* 17:1.

Kauffman Foundation. 2006. *Kauffman Panel on Entrepreneurship Curriculum in Higher Education.* Report I on Research Projects. Kansas City, MO: Kauffman Foundation.

Kuratko DF, Hodgetts RM. 2004. *Entrepreneurship: Theory, Process, Practice,* 6th edn. Mason, OH: Thomson Learning.

McGrath RG, MacMillan I. 2000. *The Entrepreneurial Mindset.* Boston: Harvard Business School Press.

Miner JB. 1996. *The Four Routes to Entrepreneurial Success.* San Francisco: Berrett-Koehler.

Morris MH. 1998. *Entrepreneurial Intensity: Sustainable Advantages for Individuals, Organizations, and Societies.* Westport, CT: Quorum Books.

Morris MH, Kuratko DF, Schindehutte M. 2001. Towards integration: Understanding entrepreneurship through frameworks. *International Journal of Entrepreneurship and Innovation* 2(1):35–49.

Morris MH, Kuratko DF. 2002. *Corporate Entrepreneurship.* Orlando, FL: Harcourt College.

Nimmo CM, Holland RW. 1999. Transitions in pharmacy practice, part 3: Effecting change – the three-ring circus. *Am J Health Sys Pharm* 56:2235–41.

Willink DP, Isetts BJ. 2005. Becoming 'indispensable': Developing innovative community pharmacy practices. *J Am Pharm Assoc* 45:376–89.

Xu H, Ruef M. 2004. The myth of the risk-tolerant entrepreneur. *Strategic Organization* 2:331.

Zaltman G. 2002. *How Customers Think: Essential Insights into the Mind of the Market.* Boston: Harvard Business School Press.

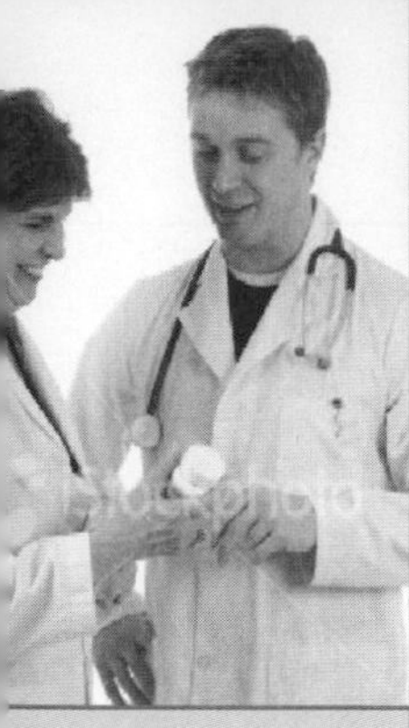

31

APPLICATIONS IN INDEPENDENT COMMUNITY PHARMACY

Joseph Bonnarens

About the Author: Dr. Bonnarens is currently associate dean for student affairs and associate professor in pharmaceutical science and pharmacy administration at Manchester College School of Pharmacy in Fort Wayne, Indiana. He received a B.S. in general science and a B.S. in pharmacy from Oregon State University in 1990. He worked as a pharmacist in several practice settings, including independent, chain, and hospital pharmacies. In 1992, he completed the American Society of Health-System Pharmacists Executive Residency, followed by his employment with the National Community Pharmacists Association in Alexandria, Virginia, until 1996. Dr. Bonnarens pursued graduate education, earning an M.S. in 1999 and a Ph.D. in 2003 in pharmacy administration from the University of Mississippi. Dr. Bonnarens began his academic career as at the University of Wisconsin School of Pharmacy, where we worked from 2003 to 2007. In 2007, Dr. Bonnarens joined Pacific University School of Pharmacy, serving as assistant dean for student and alumni affairs prior to joining Manchester College in 2011. His research interests include leadership, entrepreneurship, patient care service development, workforce issues, and management issues facing pharmacy practitioners in various practice settings.

LEARNING OBJECTIVES

After completing this chapter, readers should be able to

1. Identify evolutionary changes leading to current independent community pharmacy practice.
2. Identify the characteristics of entrepreneurship and describe the opportunities that exist within independent community pharmacy practice.
3. Compare and contrast starting up a new independent community pharmacy versus purchasing an established pharmacy.
4. List and describe the steps necessary for starting an independent community pharmacy.

5. Identify methods of purchasing an established pharmacy.
6. List and discuss various issues facing independent community pharmacy practice.

SCENARIO 1

As Sue Franklin was completing her last Advanced Pharmacy Practice Experience (APPE) rotation during her final year of pharmacy school, she began to think about where she wanted to work after graduation. As part of her required and elective APPE rotations, Sue gained experience in a number of practice settings. She really enjoyed the critical care rotation at University Medical Center. However, she knew that a residency probably would be required to land a clinical position there. Sue had completed a rotation with the Indian Health Service and had thoroughly enjoyed her experience caring for a Native American population in New Mexico. She also had gained experience working at a chain pharmacy and then a supermarket pharmacy during holidays and vacations throughout pharmacy school. "What am I going to do?" thought Sue. She had so many great experiences and in some ways too many employment options. She had already received job offers from the chain and supermarket pharmacies, each paying a very good salary. She also had received an offer from Professional Pharmacy, a local independent community pharmacy in which she completed two rotations, community and administrative. Sue was surprised by the offer, because she had spent only 10 weeks in the pharmacy. Prior to her rotations, Sue had never considered working in an independent community pharmacy. One of her favorite APPE projects was the development of an immunization program for Professional Pharmacy. Sue loved the ability to create new programs and offer specialty services to patients in need. Darrel Burke, the owner of Professional Pharmacy, was very enthusiastic about the ideas Sue had shared with him regarding the development of other patient care specialty services. As Sue thought back about her experience, she was also impressed with Mr. Burke's management style. She remembered that the workflow was very organized and that the employees enjoyed taking care of patients and took pride in their jobs. Mr. Burke took great care of the entire staff. He was the only manager that Sue had worked with to hold brief staff meetings every couple of weeks to find out how things were going and to take action on issues raised during the meetings. Sue was also amazed at how much the patients cared for Mr. Burke and the staff, and vice versa. She could not remember receiving cookies from a patient whom she had helped on any other rotation. While the salary offered by Professional Pharmacy was slightly lower than those offered by other prospective employers, Sue realized how unique Professional Pharmacy is and began to see the value of working in a place that accepted and even encouraged its employees to seek creative strategies for enhancing customer service.

CHAPTER QUESTIONS

1. What is independent community pharmacy? From a practitioner's perspective? From a patient's perspective?
2. Historically, independent community pharmacies and the pharmacists owning them have been criticized as being "only in it for the money." How would you dispel this myth?
3. How can an independent community pharmacy owner of 15 years keep the entrepreneurial spirit alive in the pharmacy?
4. What are the advantages and disadvantages of starting a new pharmacy versus purchasing an existing one?

INTRODUCTION

As stated in Chapter 1, "The managerial sciences of accounting, finance, economics, human resources management, marketing, and operations management are indispensable tools for today's practitioner." Each of the tools referred to is critical to all pharmacy practitioners in varying degrees. This statement could not be more accurate when discussing independent community pharmacists. An independent community pharmacist works in an environment that demands a unique level of understanding of the proper use of each tool in providing patient care, in addition to running a respected business in a community. While a discussion of managing an independent community pharmacy practice could incorporate most of the concepts from this book, the goal here is to provide a cursory overview and discuss the application of management tools critical to this environment.

WHAT IS INDEPENDENT COMMUNITY PHARMACY?

What comes to mind when the word *pharmacy* is mentioned? Depending on your age, hometown size and location, personal health history, and experiences shared by family and friends, a number of examples might appear. While the descriptions would vary regarding the name and even the practice setting, many would envision a privately owned business that not only filled prescriptions but also took care of patients and their families. This type of pharmacy has been described in many ways: a "mom and pop" shop, a drugstore, a chemist's shop, an apothecary, a prescription shop, or hundreds of brand names ranging from Abe's Drug to Zimmerman's Pharmacy. The business that is described by most is an independent community pharmacy.

A stereotypic description of an independent community pharmacy might include the existence of a small business with a prescription counter operated by the owner and located in the back of the store. The front of the store might contain a wide variety of offerings that could range from a small section of over-the-counter (OTC) medications, vitamins, and other health-related products to an expanded OTC area with additional offerings, such as greeting cards, candy, gifts, and health and beauty products. In general, one might find a relatively small but very helpful and friendly staff that know their customers by name and provide great service.

Historical Perspective

Pharmacy practice in the United States was founded on the shoulders of independent community pharmacy owners. Beginning with the earliest apothecary shops in colonial America, independent practices manufactured most medications that were provided to customers. In the early 1800s, apothecaries and drugstores became more prominent in cities and towns (Higby, 2003). Reasons surrounding this growth include the evolution of medicine and pharmacy into separate professions and the growing need for medications as the country and its population continued to expand. The drugstore became recognized as the place to purchase medicine. These practices diversified and began to offer additional products and services to their respective communities.

In the late 1800s, the pharmacy began to stock and sell more products that were being created by pharmaceutical manufacturers. With this change, pharmacies needed less space for compounding products. The prescription department moved to the back of the store, with the front opening up for salable goods and creation of the soda fountain. Since the pharmacist had a background in chemistry and experience with mixing and flavoring, the soda fountain was a perfect fit for the pharmacy. While the soda fountain attracted customers, events such as the prohibition movement greatly increased its popularity. A unique combination of prescription department, general store, and soda fountain established the drugstore as a cultural icon (Higby, 2003).

Independent community pharmacy practice evolved with the rest of the profession through the education reform of the early 1900s, increased competition from the development of chain and mass-merchandiser pharmacies, and the decreased need for practitioners compounding coinciding with the increased availability of mass-produced medications. The 1950s ushered in the "count and pour" era of pharmacy practice: a momentous surge in antibiotics and other medications coming to market, increases in the number of prescriptions dispensed, limited roles of pharmacists in patient care, and boom times for pharmacy businesses (Higby, 2003).

The 1960s witnessed a new era that dramatically changed the face of independent community pharmacy practice. Legislation created the Medicare and Medicaid programs and, with that, the birth of public pharmaceutical benefit programs (Williams, 1998). These events drastically changed the economics of independent pharmacy practice by introducing greater influence from government and private payers. Also during this time, the profession was beginning to embrace the concept of clinical pharmacy. Eugene White, an independent pharmacist, was advocating patient-oriented professional pharmacy practices, by example, with the development of a patient drug profile and an office-based practice (Ukens, 1994). The public, which had been viewed only as customers, now was recognized as patients (Higby, 2003).

Through the 1980s, community pharmacists began carving out their own niche in health care as drug information experts by expanding their scope of practice into patient care areas such as consulting, home health care, and long-term care. Independent community pharmacists began to accept this expanded role and fostered the pharmacist–patient relationship by continuing to provide high-quality, personalized service to all patients.

The dawn of clinical pharmacy provided the groundwork for the shift to the pharmaceutical care era. With significant changes in the areas of law (e.g., the Omnibus Budget Reconciliation Act of 1990 and the Health Insurance Portability and Accountability Act of 1996), health care reimbursement (e.g., the rise of managed care), and scope of practice (e.g., disease-state management programs, wellness programs, and collaborative practice agreements between pharmacists and physicians), independent practice has had to diversify and change to meet the needs of the various players in this environment. In addition, the independent community pharmacist has had to become a better manager in order to survive in such a competitive marketplace.

The 2000s brought major changes to health care and pharmacy in particular. In 2003, the Medicare Prescription Drug, Improvement and Modernization Act was passed that provided prescription drug coverage through Medicare Part D. With its implementation at the beginning of 2006, the nation's community pharmacies bore the burden of this new program by experiencing increased prescription volume and major delays in reimbursements (Kostick, 2006). Most recently, health care reform has taken center stage as a major national issue. Year 2010 provided the venue for President Obama to sign into law the first health care reform legislation in decades (APhA, 2011). The two laws that make up the Affordable Care Act—the Patient Protection and Affordable Care Act and Health Care and Education Reconciliation Act of 2010—include pharmacy-related provisions regarding medication therapy management (see Chapter 19), recognizing the pharmacist's role in medication use, and improving patient access to medications and service (APhA, 2011). Independent community pharmacists continue to be very active participants in these areas to improve the care of their patients (Hoey, 2011).

Today's Independent Community Pharmacy

According to various agencies, a strict definition of *independent community pharmacy* means that no more than three pharmacies are owned and operated by one person (Smith, 1986). Even with this established definition, other organizations have expanded the number of pharmacies that can be owned to as many as 11. A better sense of what independent community pharmacy is can be gained from the views of various stakeholders.

What do patients think? Beginning in 1976, Gallup has conducted a survey of Americans to rate the honesty and ethical standards of a variety of professions (Jones, 2010). Since 1981, pharmacists have consistently been rated one of the most trusted and respected professions identified in the Gallup survey (NCPA, 2010b). In recent years, *Consumer Reports* has been conducting a survey of their readers and asking them to rate drugstores. In 2003, over 85 percent of customers were very satisfied or completely satisfied with their experience at independent community pharmacies. This highlights the fact that customers found independent pharmacists to be accessible, approachable, and easy to talk to while also being very knowledgeable about prescription and nonprescription medications (Consumer Reports, 2003). In the May 2011 issue, 94 percent of readers shared that they were highly satisfied with their experiences at independent community pharmacies, which sustained their reputation in areas of pharmacists' knowledge, helpfulness, personal service, and approachability (Consumer Reports, 2011). Independent community pharmacies also were recognized for offering additional patient care services, such as disease-state management education, health screenings, and specialty services such as compounding. In the fourth annual U.S. National Pharmacy Study conducted by J.D. Power and Associates, independent community pharmacies received the highest rankings for customer satisfaction (J.D. Power and Associates, 2010).

While these examples provide a look at patient perceptions, it is important to get a sense of what independent community practitioners think. One of the principal advantages of this type of practice frequently pertains to personal control. Referred to in various ways, such as "being my own boss," "wanting to do things my way," and "besides my patients, I answer to no one but myself," the issue of personal control is a driving force for individuals to become owners. Other factors, such as involvement and recognition in the community and personal motivations, are also considered to be advantages of this practice setting (Smith, 1986). One of the predominant disadvantages of independent community pharmacy relates to the increased responsibilities assumed by the owner: financial, legal, and professional. Because the pharmacy is a business, in some sense everyone (e.g., customers, employees, payers, and regulators) is the "boss" of the independent (Smith, 1986). An additional disadvantage that also might be included are the long hours typically put in by the owner, especially during the business's formative years (Smith, 1986).

THE ENVIRONMENTS OF INDEPENDENT COMMUNITY PHARMACY

Overall Health Care Environment

Pharmacy continues to assume a larger portion of the health care dollar. Spending for prescription drugs accelerated in 2009 to $249.9 billion, representing 5.3 percent growth from the previous year (Centers for Medicare and Medicaid Services, 2009). Spending for drugs is expected to reach nearly $500 billion by 2016 (Poisal et al., 2007).

Through 2003, Medicaid reimbursement had remained one of the best-paying third-party programs for independent community pharmacies. In addition, Medicaid programs had been the active "laboratories" for pilot projects paying community pharmacists fees for managing the therapy of select groups of patients based on their disease state, such as diabetes and asthma (English, 1998). As the costs of each state's Medicaid program continued to grow, additional changes were looming on the horizon that would affect the revenue stream of independent community pharmacies dramatically.

The Medicare Modernization Act (MMA) of 2003 (CMS, 2005) introduced a major change to the entire health care environment, with millions of beneficiaries eligible for this new program. This influx of individuals with an opportunity for prescription drug coverage can be shown by examining the changes in prescription drug spending by payer from 2005 through 2006 (Fig. 31-1) (CMS, 2005; Poisal et al., 2007). Medicare, as a payer, jumped from 2 to 22 percent in spending for prescription drugs, whereas Medicaid and out-of-pocket expenditures decreased. Although it has been suggested that Medicare Part D might not have much impact on the future prescription drug growth rate, the immediate impact in a variety areas has been significant and will be long lasting (Poisal et al., 2007).

Independent community pharmacies/pharmacists were the front-line professionals dealing with the issues leading up to and far after January 2, 2006—the

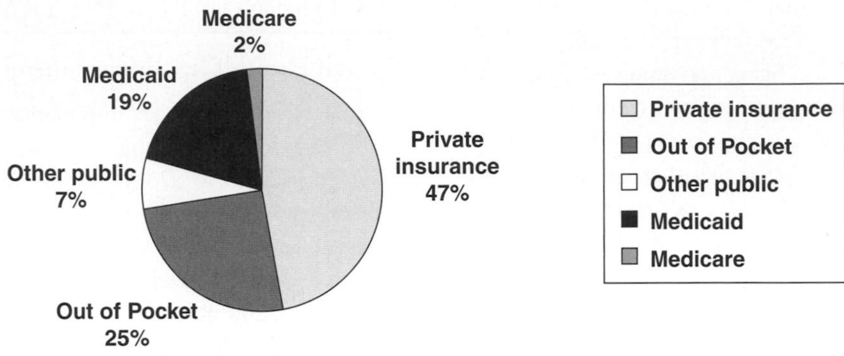

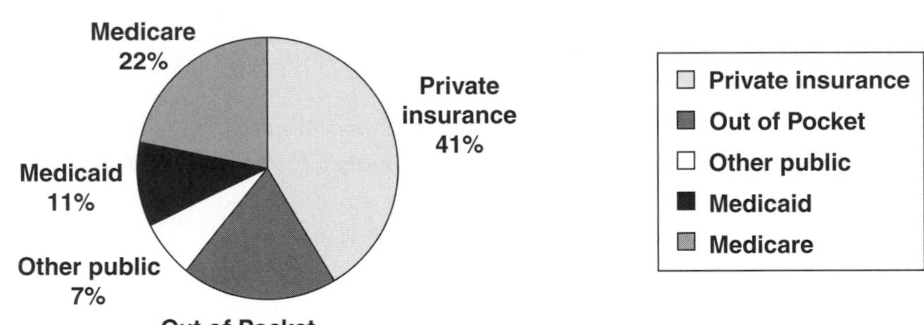

Figure 31-1. Changes in payers with implementation of Medicare Part D.

first day of Part D. Such major change in the payment structure for prescription drugs has significant repercussions. Leading up to "Part D Day," there was great concern regarding the profitability of pharmacies with the shift in payers and subsequent reimbursement rates (Ukens, 2006). A July 2006 survey of over 500 independent community pharmacists revealed that 89 percent of respondents reported a worsening of cash flow, 55 percent reported that they had to obtain outside financing to supplement their cash flow, and 33 percent admitted to considering closing their pharmacy (Edmondson, 2007). A major factor relating to the cash-flow issues was the slow reimbursement rates related to the Part D program. A 2007 study confirmed the slow reimbursement rates to pharmacies (Medical News Today, 2007). The researchers found that 50 percent of community pharmacy claims were being paid more than 30 days after adjudication and that over 17 percent experienced delays over 60 days (Sheppard et al., 2007). These delays are critical considering that pharmacies must pay their wholesalers/supplies every 2 weeks to receive added benefits and within 30 days to avoid penalties.

Internal Pharmacy Environment

A unique publication provides financial benchmarks for independent community pharmacies. The *NCPA*

Table 31-1. Characteristics of a Typical Independent Community Pharmacy

	2009[a]	2008[b]
Total pharmacy size	4,623 sq ft	3,342 sq ft
Prescription area	1,275 sq ft	970 sq ft
Prescription volume (annually)	64,635 Rxs	62,379 Rxs
New	28,813 (45%)	28,412 (46%)
Refills	35,822 (55%)	33,967 (54%)
Third-party prescription coverage	89%	87.8%
Medicaid	14%	14.5%
Medicare Part D	30%	29.6%
Other third-party programs	45%	43.7%
Hours and days/week open	55 hours 6 days	55 hours 6 days
Total sales (100.0%)	$4,026,097	$3,880,802
Prescription sales	93.3%	93.3%
Gross margin	23.8%	23.2%
Total expenses	20.5%	20.0%
Net profit (before taxes)	3.3%	3.2%
Cost of dispensing	$11.97	$11.01

[a]Based on 2010 NCPA Digest.
[b]Based on 2009 NCPA Digest.

Digest, sponsored by Cardinal Health, is an annual survey that compiles and summarizes financial data from independent pharmacies nationwide (NCPA, 2011). Data from the past 2 years of the *NCPA Digest* are used as a benchmark to describe the typical independent community pharmacy, as shown in Table 31-1. In general, the typical independent community pharmacy has a total sales volume of just over $4 million, of which 93 percent is derived directly from prescription sales. Over 64,000 prescriptions are filled annually, with 89 percent of those prescriptions being paid for by a third party: 14 percent by Medicaid, 30 percent by Medicare Part D, and 45 percent by other third-party payers.

Independent community pharmacies have incorporated various elements of technology into the practice setting, including specialized software that checks for medication errors, fills and labels each prescription, and even processes the sales transaction. Additional uses have grown to include automated dispensing machines, specialized compounding and intravenous mixing equipment, and customized software that can be used in the management of patients with particular disease states such as diabetes. One of the major technological growth areas is electronic prescribing. These capabilities refer to the connectivity between a prescribing physician and a community pharmacy, allowing for the electronic transmission of a patient's prescription from the physician to the patient's pharmacy of choice. This trend is relatively new, occurring within the past 3 to 5 years. The 2010 *NCPA Digest* reported that 92 percent of participating pharmacies were connected and capable of receiving electronic prescriptions, with 12.2 percent of prescriptions received electronically (NCPA, 2010).

A typical *NCPA Digest* pharmacy offers patients a number of specialized services, including but not limited to delivery, patient charge accounts, compounding, health screenings, hospice, and durable medical goods, as well as scheduling of patient appointments and speaking to local organizations (NCPA, 2010). The trend to offer disease-state specialty services in independent community pharmacies continues to increase. Based on a survey conducted by the National Institute for Pharmacist Care Outcomes (NIPCO), nearly 15,000 community pharmacists have completed disease management programs accredited by NIPCO since its formation in 1995 (NCPA, 2003b). In the latest *Digest*, disease management service offerings continue to increase in frequency. The most frequently offered programs are immunizations, diabetes training, and blood pressure monitoring (NCPA, 2010).

In addition to patient care services, another area that has been expanded by Medicare Part D has been medication therapy management (MTM) services and programs. MTM programs are designed to improve medication use, enhance patient safety, and increase patient adherence to their medication regimens (NCPA, 2007). Many of these initial MTM programs offered in independent community pharmacies do not include the service of a pharmacist; however, this trend is changing. The 2007 *NCPA-Pfizer Digest* reported that over 46 percent of independent community pharmacies offer MTM services, with an average charge of $40, and that 48 percent of the pharmacies are receiving reimbursement under Medicare Part D. The most recent *Digest* reported an increase in pharmacies offering MTM services to 68 percent, with a corresponding increase in the number of pharmacies receiving reimbursement to 59 percent (NCPA, 2010).

CHARACTERISTICS OF THE INDEPENDENT COMMUNITY PHARMACIST

Independent community pharmacy provides a unique venue for an individual pharmacist. Opportunities exist to be an owner and run the pharmacy, a part-time employee interested in staying in touch with community pharmacy practice, an entrepreneur with ideas for creating new service offerings for patients, or an employee working for the owner/manager. In this venue, the individual is limited only by his or her imagination. Thus, with this in mind, who chooses a career path in independent community pharmacy?

Whether one is interested in ownership or not, one of the key characteristics for a pharmacist in this practice setting is the importance of interacting with people. The independent community pharmacy provides pharmacists with a great opportunity to help patients. Problem-solving skills are critical as a pharmacist, and this setting provides constant challenges that require those skills. Other characteristics that are fostered by the independent setting are the ability to embrace change, deal with risk, and adapt to an ever-changing environment.

It is important that stereotypes sharing a negative connotation of independent community pharmacists be addressed. In some cases, pharmacists who are business oriented have been viewed in a negative light. In addition, many individuals interested in independent community pharmacy practice have been falsely accused of generalities such as "They are only going into business for the money," "They are not very clinical," and "They have a lack of professionalism."

Based on the descriptions of independent community pharmacy practice and the characteristics of the individuals who pursue this career path, several points must be made. First, independent pharmacists are placed in a difficult situation because of their need to possess expertise in pharmacy practice and business. All pharmacy organizations must stay in business so that they may provide goods, services, and care to patients. Second, independent community pharmacy practice represents one of the most accessible health care venues for patients. Because of this, there exist numerous clinical opportunities for pharmacists in the provision of quality patient care and positive patient outcomes. Third, independent community pharmacists contribute to the overall health of any community not only in the care provided but also in contributions to the economic and civic health of the community. As a health care provider, the pharmacy adds a stable business to any town's economic structure. In addition, through involvement of the owner and other staff members in civic organizations, these individuals serve as volunteer leaders in activities ranging from school and hospital boards to elected offices.

Today's Independent

In visiting one of over 23,000 independent community pharmacies across the country, one might find the following two individuals. The first individual is the younger of the two. This pharmacist received a doctor of pharmacy (Pharm.D.) degree from an accredited program. There is a chance that this individual completed an MBA in conjunction with the pharmacy degree or at least had the chance to take some business courses. During his or her professional education, this individual took the required courses that introduced issues such as management, marketing, and economics into pharmacy practice. If available at the alma mater, any electives focusing on subjects ranging from pharmacy management and economics to entrepreneurship and ownership also would have been taken. While not a requirement, this individual probably was active in pharmacy school organizations. After graduation, this individual may have gained work experience at various practice settings or may have completed a community pharmacy residency. The individual has gained a variety of experiences from the practice settings work that ranged from one independent pharmacy to a variety of jobs that included experiences in hospital, chain, and other specialty practice areas, such as long-term care, home infusion therapy, or compounding pharmacy. This individual is in the process or has already established a specialty patient care service, such as an immunization program or disease-specific monitoring program in diabetes or asthma. The individual, along with other staff members, has received certification in these various specialty areas.

The second individual has been an owner for over 15 years. This individual received a bachelor of science degree. More than likely, this individual also completed course work pertaining to management and ownership. This individual may even have taken a class or two from the business school. This individual has a vast background of practice experience, often focused in community practice. This individual may have spent time working in a chain, a hospital clinic, or even another independent before pursuing ownership of his or her own practice. This individual manages a staff of pharmacists, technicians, clerks, delivery personnel, and other individuals, such as bookkeepers, accountants, part-time help, and contract employees. The owner has been a preceptor and has provided a recognized rotation site for the state's college or school of pharmacy since opening the store. This individual has always felt that the students provide the pharmacy with as much as the pharmacy gives to them. This individual may also have additional training experiences available, such as an administrative rotation or a community residency program. In addition, this individual is an active member of several civic groups in the community, such as Rotary and the Chamber of Commerce. The owner is politically active, knowing the state and federal senators and representatives and voicing concerns to them regarding issues related to independent pharmacy practice. The owner supports various activities of the local schools, such as speaking at career days and sponsoring various programs. The pharmacy may sponsor a little league team in the summer and a basketball team in the winter. The owner knows his or her patients and is now taking care of several generations of families. He or she continues to participate in various certificate-training programs and has implemented a variety of specialty services.

It is clear that both individuals enjoy their jobs from a professional, clinical, and personal perspective. They value the freedom to care for their patients through the variety of services they provide. Their career choice provides them with a salary that can support them individually and their families if appropriate. They are constantly learning and growing as practitioners, managers, and businesspeople. For both individuals, management plays an important role in their lives. The application of management tools is critical to the success of these individuals, as well as to the success of the independent community pharmacy.

SCENARIO 2

Sue has been on staff at Professional Pharmacy for 6 months. She is beginning to feel comfortable with the employees, customers, and flow of the business. The immunization program that she helped institute while a student has continued to grow, now offering vaccinations year round for influenza, diphtheria, and tetanus, in addition to miscellaneous travel and childhood vaccinations.

Sue began to realize that a large portion of Professional Pharmacy's patient population was diabetic. As she learned more by participating in diabetes-related continuing-education programs, Sue started to see opportunities for enhanced patient services that could be provided to this specific population of patients. In one of the continuing-education programs that she attended, Sue learned how to create a business plan (see Chapter 5) for the development of a diabetes care center. Sue created a business plan for a service that would help patients identify whether they were diabetic, as well as to help educate and train those with diabetes to care for themselves and enhance their quality of life.

ENTREPRENEURSHIP/ INTRAPRENEURSHIP

In Scenario 2, Sue has formulated an idea, developed the idea through education and analysis, and created a business plan to test the strength of the idea. The process that Sue progressed through and the steps she took to develop her idea implicate her as a potential entrepreneur (see Chapter 30).

It is easy to see why most small-business owners, including independent community pharmacy owners, are categorized as entrepreneurs. There is more to being an entrepreneur, however, than just setting up a business. Entrepreneurs typically demonstrate the effective application of a number of enterprising attributes such as creativity; initiative; risk-taking, problem-solving ability; and autonomy and often will risk their own capital to set up a business (Bloomsbury Publishing, 2002).

Prior to a more descriptive discussion regarding the characteristics of an entrepreneur, Scenario 2 must be reexamined. Although it was suggested that Sue may be a potential entrepreneur, she is not really starting a business. She is an employee of Professional Pharmacy, and Sue's idea will provide a new business opportunity for the pharmacy and Mr. Burke, the owner. A more accurate definition of Sue in this scenario is as an intrapreneur. An *intrapreneur* is an employee who uses the approach of an entrepreneur within an organization (Bloomsbury Publishing, 2002). As a business ages and grows, the original entrepreneurial spirit can diminish. Intrapreneurs are critical to any established business in that they question the establishment and provide the internal spark to pursue innovation and new opportunities.

Characteristics of Entrepreneurs

Entrepreneurship is a growing area of research. A major area of interest is in identifying that magic combination of characteristics that makes a successful entrepreneur. Over 40 traits believed to be associated with entrepreneurship have been identified. Five of the more frequently identified characteristics include the following (Daft, 1994; Gartner, 1985):

- *Internal locus of control.* A belief by individuals that they are in control of their future and that other external forces will have little or no influence.
- *Need to achieve.* A human quality in which people are motivated to excel, so they pick situations in which they will be challenged but where success is likely.
- *Tolerance for ambiguity.* The psychological characteristic that allows a person to be untroubled by disorder and uncertainty.
- *Risk-taking propensity.* The likelihood of being a risk taker no matter the circumstance.
- *Demographics factors.* These factors focus on a number of characteristics, including past work experience (experience in independent settings supports entrepreneurial tendencies), entrepreneurial parents (more likely to be entrepreneurial when parents have been as well), and age (most businesses are launched between the ages of 25 and 40).

ENTREPRENEURIAL OPPORTUNITIES IN INDEPENDENT COMMUNITY PHARMACY

The history of independent community pharmacy provides a wealth of examples of entrepreneurship. Independent practitioners were some of the first to provide and use (Gumbhir, 1996)

- Complete patient medication profiles.
- Total parenteral nutrition.
- Delivery of products and care to prisons and long-term care facilities.
- Home infusion services.
- Veterinary pharmacy.
- Specialty compounding services.

In today's marketplace, entrepreneurial opportunities are everywhere. Individuals are limited only by their imagination in developing new services or other innovations. The biggest concern for any business is the ability to keep the entrepreneurial spirit alive. To continue that spirit, the owner/manager must create a climate that will support and foster the entrepreneurs and intrapreneurs in the pharmacy. Some rules that can be used in creating that climate in the pharmacy include (1) encourage action, (2) tolerate failure and use as a learning example, (3) be persistent in getting an idea to market, (4) use informal meetings to provide opportunities to share ideas, (5) provide challenges with the staff to help problem-solve given situations, and (6) reward and/or promote innovative personnel (Daft, 1994).

SCENARIO 3

Sue loves her job. In the 3 years that she has been at Professional Pharmacy, she has developed patient care services in such areas as immunizations and osteoporosis, created a disease management program in diabetes, and successfully marketed the pharmacy's services to other health care providers in town. She has a great relationship with Mr. Burke, the owner, and thoroughly enjoys the people she works with and the patients she cares for in the community. While she is pleased with her accomplishments, she is beginning to detect the emergence of several obstacles. Mr. Burke has been very supportive of her ideas, and even when he has disagreed, he has carefully explained his position against an idea. Over the past year, Sue has become more involved in the area of specialty compounding. A new dermatologist recently moved to the area, and during one of Sue's "detailing" visits to the Midtown Physicians Group, she struck up a conversation that has evolved into a steady stream of prescriptions for his "special" ointments and creams. Mr. Burke, although appreciative of the new business, is not interested in any expansion of the pharmacy to incorporate additional technology for use in compounding specialty items. Sue has been thinking so much about the potential for such a service that she sketched out a rough business plan one night when she could not sleep. Sue believes that this is a major local market that is going untapped; however, she knows that Mr. Burke wants no part in this venture. If she were her own boss, she could direct the business in the direction she saw fit. "Hmmm," she thought, "should the idea be shelved for a while, or is it time to look at the potential for owning her own business?"

INDEPENDENT COMMUNITY PHARMACY OWNERSHIP

While working for an independent owner can be a very fulfilling experience for many, one of the most attractive aspects of the independent setting is the opportunity to own a pharmacy. Interest in ownership has peaked and waned over the past 30 years. A significant decline in the number of independent community pharmacies occurred between 1990 and 1997 (NACDS, 2003). From the late 1990s to 2006, the number of independent practices has hovered around 24,000 sites (NCPA, 2007). From 2006 through 2009, the trend marked a decline of independent community pharmacies, reaching a first-time low of 22,728.

However, 2010 marked a reversal to this trend, with the total number of independent pharmacies returning to just over 23,000 (NCPA, 2010). This number of pharmacies represents a significant portion of pharmacies in the United States (NCPA, 2010).

Some of the top reasons for wanting to go into business include self-management, creative freedom, and financial independence. Other reasons include (1) not having to answer to others regarding the focus of the pharmacy, (2) being recognized and playing an important role in the business and health care needs of the community, (3) achieving a level of self-fulfillment and pride, and (4) continuing the legacy of pharmacy ownership established by family and/or mentors (Smith, 1986, 1996). Each individual who pursues ownership is driven by his or her own reasons. Once the decision of pharmacy ownership is made, the prospective owner must do the following: identify available pharmacies for sale or suitable locations for a new pharmacy, determine a satisfactory purchase price, evaluate and determine capital needs, and investigate and select the best source of capital (Gagnon, 1996). He or she must determine whether to start a new independent practice or purchase an established pharmacy.

Option 1: Starting from Scratch

Sue is determined to pursue her idea of creating a compounding specialty service. After her discussions with Mr. Burke confirmed his lack of interest, she realized that she has two options: Find another pharmacy that would be interested in pursuing this specialty service or start her own business. Sue decides that despite how well things have been for her at Professional Pharmacy, the time is right to start her own business.

The act of starting a new independent community pharmacy practice in a given community follows a long and rich history. As mentioned previously, a new pharmacy appears for various reasons, ranging from support of unmet health care needs for a particular patient population to taking advantage of a potentially lucrative business opportunity. Starting a new pharmacy, as with any business, requires considerable planning.

A number of distinct advantages are available to an owner opening a new independent community pharmacy. The opportunity to select and purchase each item of this new venture, such as fixtures, equipment, and inventory, is a great advantage. Also, hiring your own personnel, finding a great location, creating sound policies and procedures, and avoiding paying for intangible assets are additional advantages.

One of the intangible assets that requires further attention is goodwill. By definition, goodwill is an intangible asset of a company that includes factors such as reputation, continued patronage, and expertise, for which a buyer of the company may have to pay a premium (Bloomsbury Publishing, 2002). For an independent community pharmacy, specific factors that contribute to goodwill include the prescription files and accounts receivable (Smith, 1996). Since goodwill is related to the profitability of the pharmacy, the most frequently used method to estimate goodwill is some multiple of the annual net profit. The most recent year's net profit generally is considered the minimum price for goodwill, whereas a common value for goodwill is estimated at 1 to 2 years of net profit (Jackson, 2002; Smith, 1996).

If the venture is not planned carefully, the advantages of opening a new pharmacy can turn into disadvantages. There is a greater amount of risk that must be assumed by the owner and an increased chance of experiencing unforeseen events. For one, the lag time between startup and profit tends to be longer. Moreover, the challenge to secure capital is a formidable one.

How to Get Started

An individual interested in starting a new business can find a great number of books on the topic. While there are few books that specifically relate to the opening of a pharmacy, the general topics covered in the new business development literature are pertinent to any business type. This section offers a list of steps that can be followed on the path toward independent community pharmacy ownership:

1. Decide on the type of pharmacy.
2. Assess the potential market.
3. Develop a detailed business plan.
4. Determine the organization's structure.

5. Identify financing options.
6. Select a location.
7. Obtain licenses, permits, and insurance.
8. Develop a marketing and promotion plan.
9. Establish the management philosophy of the business.

Decide on the Type of Pharmacy

This question can only be answered by the potential owner. While it seems a very simple question, the answer requires considerable contemplation. As in Sue's case, most individuals have a general idea of what type of business they want to start. For Sue, a compounding specialty pharmacy is her wish. Now Sue must begin to evaluate her idea thoroughly by resolving such questions as

- What products and services will I sell?
- From what base will I derive my customers?
- What skills do I bring to this business?
- Where should I be located?
- Will I have any competition?

Assess the Potential Market

Based on her evaluation of the type of pharmacy she would like to open, Sue has decided that she will start a compounding prescription business in the community where she currently lives. She has had a great deal of specialized training in this area and believes that there is a need for this type of pharmacy in the community. Now she must assess the potential market.

As described in the Chapter 22, Sue must undertake a complete market assessment of the area in which she plans to locate. Some of the questions to resolve include

- What is the potential customer base?
- How many physicians are in the community? Specialists?
- What is the competition? Other pharmacies? Other businesses?

Develop a Detailed Business Plan

It is important that the plan is well thought out and that due diligence is paid to eliminate as much uncertainty as possible when starting a new pharmacy (see Chapter 5).

Determine the Business Structure of the Pharmacy

A decision regarding the legal structure of the pharmacy must be made fairly early in the business development phase. Deciding on the legal structure of the pharmacy is critical to the overall success of the business. Each business venture is unique, and there is no one single ownership structure that suits every situation. The prospective owner should consult with an accountant and an attorney to help select the ownership structure that will best meet her needs.

In general, three legal structures are available to pharmacy owners: sole proprietorship, partnership, and corporation. Table 31-2 identifies some of the unique characteristics of each legal structure (SBA, 2011a, 2011b, 2011c, 2011d; Spadaccini, 2009; Tootelian and Gaedeke, 1993).

Sole proprietorship This is the simplest ownership form because the business is owned by one individual. The sole proprietor owns all the assets, receives all profits, and is responsible for all aspects of the business. While the owner receives all the profits generated from the business, there is also no legal distinction between the business and the owner, making the owner completely responsible for any liabilities and debts. This form of ownership is ideal for starting a business (Spadaccini, 2009). However, as a business grows, there are other ownership forms that provide more security to the owner and the business.

Partnership By definition under the Uniform Partnership Act, a partnership is an association of two or more persons to carry on as co-owners of a business for profit (Tootelian and Gaedeke, 1993). While seemingly straightforward, partnerships have the potential to be complex. Because of this, it is strongly recommended that a written legal agreement between the partners be executed. The agreement, also referred to as *articles of partnership,* should outline issues including, but not limited to, profit-sharing, business decisions, resolving disputes, adding additional partners, and dissolving the partnership.

Table 31-2. Comparisons Between Business Structures

	Sole Proprietor	Partnership	S Corp	C Corp	LLC
Number of owners	One	Two or more	No more than 75 shareholders	Unlimited	No maximum, 1 person LLC permitted in most states
Level of liability	Unlimited, personal liability	Unlimited, all partners jointly liable for actions of other partners	Limits personal liability to the amount invested to the limit of assets of the company	Limits personal liability to the amount invested to the limit of assets of the company	Limits personal liability to the amount invested
Tax issues	Owner pays tax on personal returns	Profits divided among partners; individuals must pay taxes	Profits flow to shareholders; individual pays taxes	Corporation pays tax on profit; shareholders pay on dividends	Flexibility, Profits flow to members; individual pays taxes
Can deduct losses on personal tax returns?	Yes	Yes	Yes	No	Yes
Ability to tranfer ownership	Totally transferable	May need consent of other parties	May be limited in order to preserve S status	Totally transferable	Generally need consent of all owners

Sources: SBA, 2011a, 2011b, 2011c, 2011d; Spadaccini, 2009. Tootelian and Gaedeke, 1993.

There are two types of partnership for consideration: general and limited. A *general partnership* entails all partners to divide the responsibility for management and liability, as well as profit or loss (Tootelian and Gaedeke, 1993). In addition, partners are jointly and individually liable for the actions of one another. While this is usually considered the least favorable form of ownership, a partnership can be less complicated than a corporation. For example, a payroll is not required for the partners in this relationship, and this provides for less paperwork and similar tax benefits to a sole proprietor (Spadaccini, 2009). A *limited partnership* consists of at least one general partner and one or more "limited" partners (Tootelian and Gaedeke, 1993). *Limited partners* are individuals who provide capital to the business but are held liable only for the amount of their investment. These same individuals are not involved in any of the management decisions or operational issues of the business.

CORPORATION A *corporation* is a business that is chartered by the state and legally operates as a separate entity from its owners. The Supreme Court defined the corporation in 1819 as "an artificial being, invisible,

Table 31-3. Summary of Corporation Types

Type of Corporation	Advantages	Disadvantages
S corporation	• Limited personal liability • Corporate losses can pass through to shareholders • No corporate taxes • Shareholders and employees do not pay Medicare or FICA on profits/dividends	• Shareholder restrictions • Employee benefit expenses are included in gross income • All shareholders must agree to the election of S corporation status
C corporation	• Deduct 100% of health insurance paid for employees • Deduct fringe benefits such as qualified education costs, portion of life insurance, and employer-provided transportation for work • Profits up to $50,000 annually are taxed at lower rate if left in corporation rather than pay higher personal income tax rate	• If corporation loses money, owners cannot deduct on personal income tax • Corporate taxes on profit • If profits distributed to shareholders, they must pay personal income tax on dividends • More complicated and requires close monitoring
LLC	• Owners are protected from personal liability as with corporation • As with partnership, income or losses are reported on member's individual tax return • In general, fewer restrictions and more flexibility	• Owners experience same self-employment tax treatment as partners and sole proprietors • States may differ in tax treatment • Newer corporation form - less precedents

Source: SBA, 2011a, 2011b, 2011d; Spadaccini, 2009.

intangible, and existing only in contemplation of the laws" (Tootelian and Gaedeke, 1993). This means that a corporation can be sued, taxed, own property, and enter into contractual agreements, whereas the owners of the corporation, the stockholders, are protected from liability. The stockholders elect a board of directors to oversee the entity and adopt bylaws to govern the corporation during its existence.

While incorporating a business seems like good move with regard to the limited personal liability experienced by the owners, there are challenges to consider. The complexity of corporations requires a great deal of time and money for the setup and running of such an organization. Based on this structure, operating in accordance with local, state, and federal governments may result in higher taxation and require additional resources.

There are three forms of corporations that most businesses use the S corporation, the C corporation, and the limited-liability corporation (LLC) (Table 31-3). Over 82 percent of "average" *NCPA Digest* pharmacies identified their structure as a corporation, with one-fourth of those 82% further identifying themselves as C corporations (NCPA, 2010). Overall, the trend toward LLCs is recent because this corporate form is relatively new.

Identify Financing Options

Once the business plan has been outlined and the organizational structure has been selected, the next step for the soon-to-be owner is financing the pharmacy. Some questions that must be resolved include

- What are the financial needs for this venture?
- What type of financing will be best for the given situation?
- Where does one go to obtain capital for such a venture?

FINANCIAL NEEDS Every business has financial needs. These needs vary with the type and individualistic nature of each business. A pharmacy located in an urban area will have different financial needs than one located in a rural area. The buyer must understand the needs of the business venture. These financial needs refer to capital. *Capital* is wealth, in the form of cash, equipment, property, or a combination of these factors, that can be used in the production or creation of income (Kelly, 1996).

There are three areas of capital need: setup capital, startup capital, and operating capital (Tootelian and Gaedeke, 1993). Each area represents a period of time in the life of a business during which particular activities that require capital are conducted.

Establishing a pharmacy, whether starting new or making changes to an existing business, often requires a considerable amount of capital. The activities that represent the largest initial capital expenditure focus on the physical aspects of the business. The remodeling and renovation of the pharmacy, purchasing of fixtures and equipment, finalizing the building's lease deposit if it is not owned directly, and purchasing the beginning inventory, prescription and nonprescription merchandise, are the major sources of capital expenditure. Most of the other activities in the area of startup relate more to paperwork and attention to detail. Such activities include prepaying insurance and utilities, obtaining the appropriate licenses and permits, and covering the professional fees of hired advisors (e.g., attorneys and accountants).

TYPES OF FINANCING Having identified a number of financial needs that come with the purchase of a pharmacy, the next step is to identify the type of funding available. Three main types of financing will be discussed: personal, debt, and equity.

Personal financing is just what it sounds like, the use of personal funds to finance the purchase of the pharmacy. It is no different from saving money for that first bicycle, car, or even one's retirement; personal savings is an important type of funding. This type of funding provides the buyer with the best possible funding source because there is no cost or payback terms, the amount can be unlimited, and it is relatively easy to use, whereas the only detractor is that there is a risk of loss (SBA, 2011e). However, in most cases, the buyer will need additional funds for the purchase, setup, startup, or operation of the pharmacy.

A common type of funding for a pharmacy is debt financing. *Debt financing* can be defined as something of value such as money that is borrowed at interest for a specified period of time (Kelly, 1996). Debt financing provides a buyer with an advantage by allowing him or her to borrow the needed capital without having to share any of the profits with the lender and to keep control of the management of the pharmacy. The disadvantages of debt financing highlight the fact that if something is borrowed, it must be returned. Loans must be repaid, with some measure of interest, over a defined period of time. In addition, the amount of debt incurred is limited by the value of assets and earning record of the borrower (Tootelian and Gaedeke, 1993). Debt financing can consist of either/or a combination of short- and long-term strategies (see Chapter 18).

Used less frequently, *equity financing* results in the buyer sharing ownership with investors who contribute funds. This level of investor ownership brings with it varying degrees of involvement in management of the business. Depending on the structure of the pharmacy, investors could be recognized as anything from a partner to a stockholder in the business. An advantage to equity financing is the chance to reduce the debt that must be repaid on a particular scale. Depending on the fiscal health of the business, partners or stockholders may or may not receive paid dividends. A significant

Table 31-4. Potential Capital Sources for Financing a New or Established Pharmacy Business

Source	Type	Positive	Negative
Personal savings	Personal	Easy, cheap	Risk of loss
Family	Personal, debt, or equity	Flexible	Can cause problems
Friends	Personal, debt, or equity	Flexible, usually good rate	Problems
Granting agencies	Personal	Cash awarded	Few, competitive, restricted regarding use
Credit cards	Debt	Easy to qualify, no collateral	Small amounts, high interest
Banks/savings & loans	Debt	Most common debt source	Hardest to qualify for
Commercial finance companies	Debt	More flexible alternative to banks	More expensive, collateral more important
Consumer finance companies	Debt	Personal loan, not loan to business; no restrictions on use of funds	High interest, personal collateral, not business
Wholesalers/suppliers	Debt	Line of credit, sometimes loans	Terms and conditions, requirements for use as wholesaler/supplier
Small business association	Debt	Longest payback time	Complex and competitive process
Venture capitalists	Equity	Can be large amounts	Hard to find, share ownership

Sources: SBA, 2011e; Kelly, 1996; Tootelian and Gaedeke, 1993.

disadvantage is that ownership of the pharmacy is spread among a larger group of individuals, thus reducing the owner's decision-making abilities (Tootelian and Gaedeke, 1993). Most small businesses, such as a pharmacy, are unable to attract much funding in this manner owing to the risk of small business survivals.

Sources of financing Banks are not the only source for obtaining capital. In fact, establishing an entirely new independent community pharmacy may not be appealing to a bank. Banks view the purchase of an established pharmacy as less risky, but there is no guarantee of obtaining a loan.

The choice of a funding source is critical to the future of a business venture and should be made carefully. The buyer must thoroughly weigh the options regarding the types of financing and the specific requirements provided for by each funding source. Table 31-4 provides a brief list of potential lenders (Kelly, 1996; SBA, 2011e; Tootelian and Gaedeke, 1993).

Select a Location

The familiar mantra Sue hears consists of three words: Location! Location! Location! The selection of the trade area, as well as the actual physical site of the pharmacy, is a primary factor in determining the success of the business. Sue has already incorporated the idea of location into her planning process by deciding on the type of pharmacy she wants to start and in conducting a market analysis.

Sue must evaluate the location of her pharmacy thoroughly with regard to population, potential customers, competition, physician availability, and community trends ranging from general health to economic issues (Kelly, 1996). To help Sue in accomplishing this task, a number of information resources are available to help analyze her pharmacy's location, including, but not limited to, public libraries; realty companies; utility companies; local, state, and federal documents and Web sites; state and national small business administration (SBA) offices; and individually conducted or contracted surveys, interviews, or traffic counts. Sue is also reminded continuously that this is a process that will be time-consuming and take hard work. She should not depend solely on what the computer provides in the way of information. By putting in the work on the front end, the next steps will be smoother.

Obtain Licenses, Permits, and Insurance

As the owner of this new pharmacy, Sue will need to obtain specific licenses and permits to operate. While local zoning laws, building permits, and standards set by health, fire, and police are requirements that must be met by all businesses in a given community, Sue also must ensure compliance with a variety of state and federal regulations that pertain specifically to pharmacy (NABP, 2011; Tootelian and Gaedeke, 1993). Insurance is of critical importance to a pharmacy. Sue will need to find an insurance agent to help with creating a comprehensive insurance plan that covers events ranging from natural disasters and physical accidents to employee health and workers' compensation. In addition, Sue must examine and acquire professional liability insurance for herself, professional staff members, and the business.

Develop a Marketing and Promotion Plan

How will Sue inform the community of her new pharmacy and the innovative services that she will be offering? Using the techniques and tools provided in Chapter 22, Sue will be able to develop a specific marketing plan to educate the community. Through the use of the local media outlets, such as newspapers, radio, television, and local Web site sponsorship, Sue will be able to execute a specific promotion plan for the new pharmacy. Sue should not focus all her marketing and promotional efforts on potential customers. A critical area for her specialty pharmacy will be the community of health care professionals, ranging from physicians and nurse practitioners to specialty practices such as dermatologists and veterinarians.

Establish the Management Philosophy of the Business

The owner of an independent community pharmacy sets the tone for the business. The owner has been involved in virtually every aspect of the business, from conceptualization and planning to development and completion. As the new owner, Sue will be involved in all aspects of the business. In addition to the potential tools available in print, the experience that she has gained from working in an independent community pharmacy will be even more valuable to the dissemination of her management philosophy.

Option 2: "Why Reinvent the Wheel?"—Purchasing an Established Pharmacy

Sue has worked for Professional Pharmacy for 3 years. As she was closing up the pharmacy one night, Mr. Burke, the owner, brings up the idea that he is starting to think about retirement. He and his wife Helen eventually would like to move into a beachfront property. There they could take out their boat and have a place for their kids and grandchildren to visit. Sue is shocked by this sudden revelation. Mr. Burke reassures her that retirement is in the near future, but he wants to chat about her future career goals and whether those goals might include pharmacy ownership.

For a potential buyer, looking for the right pharmacy may seem like a daunting task. There are a number of places to begin a search. In many cases, the potential buyer already may have identified several businesses either through research or as a result of his or her current job. Local and state pharmacy associations are excellent resources for initial listings and referrals. A common section in the flagship publications of these organizations is a "pharmacy for sale" listing. The journals of most national pharmacy organizations have similar pharmacy listings. In addition, professional brokers who deal on the business side of the real estate market can be contacted and hired. There also exist specialty services provided by organizations. One example of this is the Independent Pharmacy Matching Service (IPMS), found on www.PharmacyMatching.com that is coordinated by the National Community Pharmacists Association (NCPA). The IPMS helps match prospective buyers and sellers on various criteria, including geographic location.

Once a potential pharmacy is identified, an important question to ask is, "Why is this pharmacy for sale?" (Cotton, 1984). Is the owner retiring? Has the neighborhood changed owing to increased competition or economic changes to "sour" the location? Is the pharmacy on the verge of bankruptcy? These are just a few of the many questions that should be asked regarding the pharmacy. These questions reinforce the importance of researching the business and obtaining advice from various sources.

Purchasing an established pharmacy can provide an excellent opportunity to a potential buyer. Identifying the advantages and disadvantages of this ownership alternative will provide valuable insight into an individual's decision-making process regarding ownership (Smith, 1986, 1996; Tootelian and Gaedeke, 1993).

Table 31-5. Advantages and Disadvantages of Purchasing an Established Pharmacy

Advantages
Lower level of risk for the buyer
No additional competition added to the current marketplace
Reduced startup costs/less risk
Less time required to show a profit
Buyer receives established goodwill
Business has an established clientele
Business provides buyer with trained employees, inventory, physical facilities, and established relationships area health care providers
Disadvantages
Inadequate facilities
Old/outdated fixtures and equipment
Inventory that is too large and/or unsalable
Established policies and procedures do not match with new ownership's philosophy
Inflated sale price
Problems with the location
Undesirable established leases

Advantages and Disadvantages

According to many in the pharmacy and business literature, there are a number of advantages to purchasing an established pharmacy (Table 31-5). An established pharmacy already has eliminated a number of the unknowns that face the startup of a new pharmacy. There is a lower level of risk on the buyer's part because the pharmacy has an established history. Pending thorough research and assessment, the buyer should have fewer uncertainties regarding the pharmacy, ranging from the physical facility, inventory, and equipment to the personnel and patient base of the pharmacy. Based on this transfer of ownership, the pharmacy obtains new management while not adding another business to a competitive marketplace. Another advantage is that an established pharmacy provides the buyer with great potential for reducing startup costs and decreasing the length of time between startup and profitability. In addition, the buyer receives the goodwill and reputation of the pharmacy.

The advantages related to this method of ownership can just as easily become disadvantages. The established assets, such as facilities and equipment, may be outdated or inadequate to meet the needs of the interested parties. The inventory of the business in question could consist of a large amount of out-of-date and unsalable items or even be too large for the pharmacy to support. The previously established policies and procedures could be in direct conflict with what the potential owner has in mind, thus creating potential human resources management problems. In addition, the pharmacy's location may not be optimal, and the purchase price may be overinflated by goodwill.

During the negotiation of such a transfer of ownership, the careful review of all leases is a critical factor that is often overlooked. A *lease* refers to a long-term agreement to use or rent a fixture, a piece of equipment, the physical structure in which the pharmacy is located, or the land the business occupies (Gagnon, 1996).

Value Assessment and Price Determination

Once the decision has been made to purchase an established pharmacy and a specific property has been identified, the next step is to determine the value of the business. Prior to a value assessment, the future owner should conduct a thorough review of the external environment of the business; that is, the community in which the business is located.

The predominant method of determining the value of a business is through financial analysis. Chapter 17 discussed the basic principles of financial analysis. In determining the fiscal health of the business, its financial records (income statements and balance sheets) from at least the past 3 to 5 years should be reviewed. From these data, the various facets of financial analysis—solvency, liquidity, efficiency, and profitability—can be determined for the business, and trends can be projected based on the time frame analyzed. A number of financial formulas are used to provide a range of values that serve as a guide for either the buyer or seller to begin the negotiation process (Jackson, 2002). It is important to note that while there is no single formula that must be used, each formula determines the value of the business from various perspectives, providing a range of values that can be used to determine an initial buying or selling price.

Based on the preceding discussion, it should be obvious that determining the value of a business is not an exact science. While a number of established techniques may be used, each business is unique. In fact, the value of a business ultimately is determined through negotiation between the buyer and the seller (Jackson, 2002). The agreed-on price usually will lie somewhere between the initial price of the seller and the initial offer of the buyer. The valuation of a business is based on the assessment of facts about the business, informed judgment, and some common sense (Jackson, 2002).

Purchasing Methods

The next step for the prospective owner is to finance the cost of purchasing the pharmacy.

Financing

As was done during the preceding discussion regarding the financing of a new pharmacy, similar questions regarding the needs of the business, the type of financing, and the sources of capital must be addressed for the purchase of an established pharmacy. Whether purchasing an established pharmacy or starting one from scratch, a significant amount of capital will be needed to cover the cost of the venture. In this case, the buyer has a significant advantage over someone starting a new business because the established pharmacy will have lower startup costs and should take less time to begin making a profit.

From a buyer's perspective, various types of financing are available for purchase of a pharmacy. While personal, debt, and equity financing are examples available to the buyer, the main question that must be determined is will the pharmacy be bought outright, or will there need to be some financial arrangement made for purchasing over a period of time. In most cases, an individual buyer would have great difficulty in securing financing to buy a pharmacy outright. With this in mind, the following discussion illustrates a transfer of ownership that provides a win-win scenario for both the buyer and the seller.

Junior Partnership

A junior partnership provides an opportunity for a buyer to purchase a pharmacy with little or no initial capital and a seller to ease out of ownership and keep the legacy of the independent pharmacy alive in the community (Jackson, 2002). Instead of trying to figure out a way to sell the pharmacy when the owner is ready for retirement, this option allows the current owner to transfer ownership to a buyer, continue to have an income, and prepare for retirement.

The advantages of a junior partnership range from less risk and less initial capital needed by the potential buyer to the continued presence of an independent pharmacy to the economic and health care needs of the community. A junior partnership has disadvantages that are similar to those of any partnership arrangement. However, in this situation, because of the established relationship, the chance for both parties to determine compatibility, and the detailed nature of the agreement, a junior partnership proves beneficial.

SCENARIO 4

It has been 4 years since Sue entered into a junior partnership with Mr. Burke, and at the end of next year, she will be majority owner of Professional Pharmacy. While the time has just flown by, Sue marvels at all she has learned about pharmacy practice from both the business and professional sides. Sue came to this realization shortly after her first scheduled meeting with this year's community pharmacy resident, Cindy Ryan. After laughingly explaining to Cindy that there is no such thing as a typical day when you are in the business of caring for patients, Sue offered the following description:

> As the owner, I am responsible for the 40-member staff that makes up Professional Pharmacy, Incorporated. This includes the main pharmacy, Professional Pharmacy West, and the compounding/home infusion pharmacy, Professional Pharmacy East. My day usually begins at East, where I check in with Jerry, the manager, to review the workload for the day and take care of any problems, usually human resources issues. I am usually at East for most of the morning, taking care of e-mail, mail, and so on. I usually spend the afternoons at West. There I meet with Lois, the store manager, to go over things for the day and take care of problems. In each facility, on a weekly basis, an all-staff meeting is conducted to update staff regarding procedure changes and new third-party coverage, address employee concerns, and check in with everyone. The meeting can last up to 20 minutes. As the owner, I have had to spend more time managing the business and less working with the compounding center and the diabetes care program that we established several years ago. While I miss the time with patients, I have come to realize that becoming the best manager I can be helps to ensure that the patients we serve receive the best possible care.

CURRENT ISSUES/ OPPORTUNITIES FACING INDEPENDENT PHARMACY PRACTICE

The life of an independent community pharmacy owner provides numerous challenges and can be highly rewarding. As Sue pointed out, most of her responsibilities have evolved into a management role. As a manager, the success or failure of the business is that individual's responsibility, and that success is dictated by the decisions made and actions taken.

The owner must balance a number of issues and ideas related to the pharmacy. Today's owner must be able to evaluate the issues, determine the feasibility of ideas, and take action. The following is a list of four issues that require a great deal of attention by an owner of an independent community pharmacy: competition, third parties, patient care service development, and niche development.

Competition

Independent community pharmacy practices operate in one of the most dynamic and competitive marketplaces. Most competition is readily apparent, such as traditional chain drugstores, supermarket pharmacies, and mass merchandisers. Independent community pharmacies also have experienced competition from other less obvious entities. This additional group of competitors consists of mail-order pharmacies, managed-care pharmacies, hospital ambulatory clinics and pharmacies, and even Internet pharmacies. While the total number of retail pharmacies has remained relatively steady, the marketplace portrait has changed. Independents have experienced a decline in total numbers, whereas chains, defined as outlets including traditional chain drugstores, supermarket pharmacies, and mass merchandisers, have become more prolific. One contributing factor to this role reversal has been competition in the prescription market. A number of independents that closed were unable to compete in certain markets for reasons ranging from third-party reimbursement rates that were too low to individuals being unable to embrace the changes that were taking place in the market. Those remaining continue to compete successfully.

Third-Party Issues

For an independent community pharmacy, addressing third-party issues is critical not only to the success of the business but also to its very survival. Addressed previously in this chapter, the average *NCPA Digest* pharmacy reported that 89 percent of prescriptions filled were paid for by a third party (NCPA, 2010). This relationship identifies the importance of understanding third-party issues for owners and managers.

Third-party issues are wide ranging. One of the most prominent issues from this arena focuses on the reimbursement rates for prescription medications that are received by independent community pharmacies from third parties (see Chapter 19). It is a constant struggle between third parties, who want to lower costs by lowering reimbursement rates to pharmacies, and independent practitioners, who must monitor the rates constantly to ensure that the pharmacy will be able to cover costs and have some profit margin.

Again, Medicare Part D has added an additional issue to an already complex topic. While some of the problems have been improved, the difficulties for independent community pharmacy still remain (Chi and Paul, 2006). The issues of prompt payment and reimbursement rates will continue to contribute to an already complex and stressful environment, keeping everyone's focus on the continued evolution of the Medicare Part D program.

Patient Care Service Development

Independent community pharmacies have a rich tradition of service to patients. This tradition has evolved into a number of identifiable patient care services that are offered in many pharmacies. Patient care services can range from home delivery and patient charge accounts to specialized patient care such as disease-state management programs focusing on diabetes or asthma. The development of such services usually is based on the fact that patients needed to be cared for and the pharmacist began stocking the product and creating the service to help their patients. In areas such as herbal medicine, homeopathy, and nutrition, patients not only obtain specific products but also receive valuable information and learn that the pharmacist is a valuable information resource. As a complement to this continued development of patient care services comes the MTM programs and services (NCPA, 2007). All of pharmacy is striving to develop quality and cost-effective services that will continue to provide their patients with exceptional customer service while also helping to further secure the means to receive compensation directly for such services. Only through continued political and professional pressure will pharmacy earn the right to bill for the patient care services provided, as well as the evershrinking compensation for the medication itself.

Niche Development

The nature of independent community pharmacies and pharmacists is to develop and offer patient care services. In specific cases, certain services may be developed to fill a niche in the community. In Scenario 4, Sue identified and developed a niche with the creation of her compounding specialty business. The specialty service was created and succeeded because there was an unmet need for compounding services in the community. As was discussed in the entrepreneurship section of this chapter, independent community pharmacies provide a wealth of opportunities to develop specialty services based on an idea, such as patient monitoring programs focusing on anticoagulation therapy, AIDS services, or anticoagulation therapy. The development of niches provides the pharmacy and its staff with new challenges and opportunities for additional business success through the introduction of potential revenue streams.

CONCLUSION

Independent community pharmacy practice provides a vast array of opportunities for professional development and personal satisfaction. This venue accommodates all types of practitioners, ranging from allowing entrepreneurs and intrapreneurs the freedom to develop their ideas into actual goods or services to offering individuals interested in "being their own boss" the chance to start their own pharmacy and pursue unique practice niches. The independent community pharmacy continues to evolve from its earliest appearance in the United States to the technologically advanced patient care service entities of the twenty-first century. Independent pharmacists will continue to deal with unique issues facing their practices, and yet they will continue to innovate and provide quality patient care.

QUESTIONS FOR FURTHER DISCUSSION

1. Do you consider yourself to be entrepreneurial? Intrapreneurial? Why or why not? Can you identify another individual as being entrepreneurial and/or intrapreneurial? Explain why you selected that person.
2. After reading this chapter, what interests (or what does not interest) you about a career in independent community pharmacy practice?
3. Imagine that you are the owner of a new independent community pharmacy. If money were no object, where would you be located? What patient care services would you offer? Would you have a general or specialized practice?
4. What is the most difficult management responsibility for the owner of an independent community pharmacy?
5. In your opinion, what is the future of independent community pharmacy? What are the largest challenges facing independent practice this year? In 5 years? In 10 years?

REFERENCES

American Pharmacists Association (APhA). 2011. APhA Legislative and Regulatory Update – 2010 Year-End Review. Available at http://www.pharmacist.com/AM/Template.cfm?Section=Health_Care_Reform& TEMPLATE=/CM/ContentDisplay.cfm& CONTENTID=25702; accessed on June 8, 2011.

Bloomsbury Publishing (ed.). 2002. *Business: The Ultimate Resource*. Cambridge, MA: Perseus Publishing.

Centers for Medicare and Medicaid Services (CMS). 2005. Available at www.cms.hhs.gov

Centers for Medicare and Medicaid Services (CMS). 2009. Available at www.cms.hhs.gov

Chi J, Paul R. 2006. NCPA: Independents are down, but don't count them out. *Drug Topics* 150(21):10.

Consumer Reports. 2003. Time to switch drugstores? *Consum Rep* 68:30.

Consumer Reports. 2011. Consumer Reports' drugstore ratings: 94% of shoppers "highly satisfied" with independents. Consumer Reports.org Press Room. Available at: http://pressroom.consumerreports.org/pressroom/2011/04/consumer-reports-drugstore-ratings-94-of-shoppers-highly-satisfied-with-independents.html; accessed on July 20, 2011.

Cotton HA. 1984. Pharmacy for sale: How to arrive at a fair price. *Curr Concepts Retail Pharm Manag* 2:2.

Daft RL. 1994. *Management*. Fort Worth, TX: Dryden Press.

Edmondson M. 2007. Viewpoint: Three ways to fight reduced reimbursement. *Drug Topics* 151(3):92.

English T. 1998. Mississippi Medicaid will pay for pharmacy services. *Pharm Today* 4:17.

Gagnon JP. 1996. Establishing and financing a community pharmacy. In Huffman DC Jr (ed.) *Effective Pharmacy Management*. Alexandria, VA: National Association of Retail Druggists, p. 87.

Gartner WB. 1985. A conceptual framework for describing the phenomenon of new venture creation. *Acad Manage Rev* 10:696.

Gumbhir AK. 1996. Entrepreneurship. In Huffman DC Jr (ed.) *Effective Pharmacy Management*. Alexandria, VA: National Association of Retail Druggists, p. 1.

Higby GJ. 2003. From compounding to caring: An abridged history of American pharmacy. In Knowlton CH, Penna RP (eds.) *Pharmaceutical Care*. Bethesda, MD: American Society of Health-System Pharmacists, p. 19.

Hoey BD. 2011. Community pharmacists can help improve health outcomes. The Hill's Congress Blog. Available at: http://thehill.com/blogs/congress-blog/healthcare/

162603-community-pharmacists-can-help-improve-health-outcomes; accessed on July 20, 2011.

Jackson RA. 2002. Maintaining our independents. *America's Pharmacist* 124:54.

J.D. Power and Associates Reports. 2010. As Consumers Shoulder More Healthcare Expenses, Cost Increasingly Drives Overall Customer Satisfaction with Pharmacies. Westlake Village, CA: J.D. Power and Associates. Available at: http://businesscenter.jdpower.com/news/pressrelease.aspx?ID=2010187; accessed on May 12, 2011.

Jones JM. 2010. Nurses top honesty and ethics list for 11th year. Available at: http://www.gallup.com/poll/145043/Nurses-Top-Honesty-Ethics-List-11-Year.aspx

Kelly ET III. 1996. Location analysis and lease evaluation. In Huffman DC Jr (ed.) *Effective Pharmacy Management.* Alexandria, VA: National Association of Retail Druggists, p. 29.

Kostick JH. 2006. Medicare Part D: A financial drain for pharmacies? Mediscape pharmacists. Available at: http://www.medscape.com/viewarticle/537279; accessed on May 12, 2011.

Medical News Today. 2007. University of Texas Study details lengthy payment delays for Medicare Part D prescription drug claims, confirming need for legislative fix. *Medical News Today,* September 8; Available at www.medicalnewstoday.com/articles/81802.php; accessed on May 12, 2011.

National Association of Boards of Pharmacy (NABP). 2011. *Survey of Pharmacy Law.* Mount Prospect. IL: National Association of Boards of Pharmacy.

National Association of Chain Drug Stores (NACDS). 2003. Industry Statistics. Available at www.nacds.org/wmspage.cfm?parm1=507; accessed on July 20, 2011.

National Community Pharmacists Association (NCPA). 2007. *NCPA-Pfizer Digest.* Alexandria, VA: National Community Pharmacists Association.

National Community Pharmacists Association (NCPA). 2009. *NCPA-Pfizer Digest.* Alexandria, VA: National Community Pharmacists Association.

National Community Pharmacists Association (NCPA). 2010b. Pharmacists Among Most Trusted Professions in Gallup's 2010 Honesty and Ethics Survey. Alexandria, VA: National Community Pharmacists Association. Available at: http://www.ncpanet.org/index.php/news-releases/2010-news-releases/833-ncpa-pharmacists-among-most-trusted-professions-in-gallups-2010-honesty-and-ethics-survey; accessed on July 20, 2011.

National Community Pharmacists Association (NCPA). 2011. Independent Pharmacies Garner Top Ratings from Consumer Reports Readers. Alexandria, VA: National Community Pharmacists Association. Available at: http://www.ncpanet.org/index.php/news-releases/959-independent-pharmacies-garner-top-ratings-from-consumer-reports-readers; accessed on July 20, 2011.

Poisal JA, Truffer C, Smith S, et al. 2007. Health spending projections through 2016: Modest changes obscure Part D's impact. *Health Aff (Millwood)* 26:W242 (published online February 21, 2007).

Sheppard M, Richards K, Winegar A. 2007. Prescription drug payment times by Medicare Part D Plans: Executive summary. Available at www.ncpanet.org/pdf/leg/ut_study_exec_sum_090607.pdf; accessed on November 1, 2007.

Small Business Association (SBA). 2011a. Starting and Managing a Business. Starting a Business. Incorporating & Registering Your Business. Corporation. Available at http://www.sba.gov/content/corporation; accessed on July 20, 2011.

Small Business Association (SBA). 2011b. Starting and managing a business. Starting a business. Incorporating & registering your business. Limited liability company (LLC). Available at http://www.sba.gov/content/limited-liability-company-llc; accessed on July 20, 2011.

Small Business Association (SBA). 2011c. Starting and managing a business. Starting a business. Incorporating & registering your business. Partnership. Available at http://www.sba.gov/content/partnership; accessed on July 20, 2011.

Small Business Association (SBA). 2011d. Starting and managing a business. Starting a business. Incorporating & registering your business. S corporation. Available at http://www.sba.gov/content/s-corporation; accessed on July 20, 2011.

Small Business Association (SBA). 2011e. Starting and managing a business. Starting a business. Loans, grants & funding. Finding loans & grants. Search for business loans, grants and financing. Available at http://www.sba.gov/content/search-business-loans-grants-and-financing; accessed on July 20, 2011.

Smith HA. 1986. *Principles and Methods of Pharmacy Management.* Philadelphia: Lea & Febiger.

Smith HA. 1996. Purchasing an established pharmacy. In Huffman DC Jr (ed.) *Effective Pharmacy Management.* Alexandria, VA: National Association of Retail Druggists, p. 57.

Spadaccini M. 2009. The basics of business structrure. *Entrepreneur*. Available at http://www.entrepreneur.com/startingabusiness/startupbasics/article200516.html; accessed on May 12, 2011.

Tootelian DH, Gaedeke RM. 1993. *Essentials of Pharmacy Management*. St. Louis, MO: Mosby Year Book.

Ukens C. 1994. Whatever happened to pharmaceutical care? *Drug Top* 138:38.

Ukens C. 2006. Medicare part D off to rocky start. *Drug Top* 150(2):12.

Williams CF. 1998. *A Century of Service and Beyond*. Alexandria, VA: National Community Pharmacists Association.

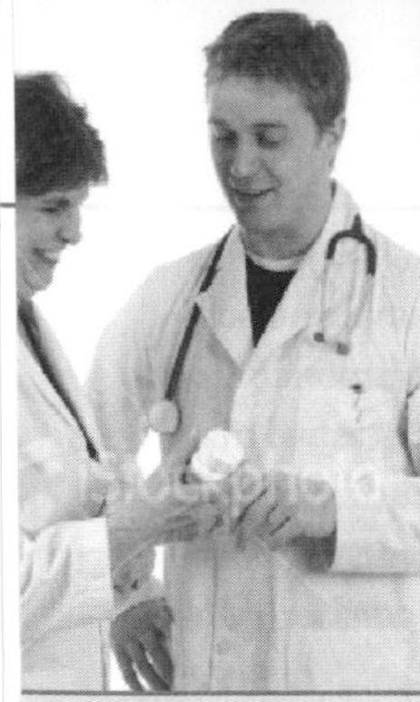

32

APPLICATIONS IN CHAIN COMMUNITY PHARMACY

Michele Belsey

About the Author: Ms Belsey is vice president of college relations and professional recruitment for Rite Aid Corporation. Michele received a B.S. in pharmacy from Duquesne University in 1992. She has been with Rite Aid Corporation since that time and has been involved with the company's development training and recruitment since 1998. Her department specializes in talent acquisition throughout the company. Ms. Belsey has served on 13 colleges/schools of pharmacy advisory boards.

LEARNING OBJECTIVES

After completing this chapter, readers should be able to

1. Describe the career paths a chain community pharmacy can create and implement based on new pharmacy practices.
2. Evaluate contemporary management culture and how it can apply or applies to chain community practice.
3. Define the competencies chain community management prefers for their pharmacists.
4. List the steps in identifying and creating management positions for pharmacists in chain community practice.
5. Identify unique opportunities for pharmacists in chain community practice.

SCENARIO—EXPANDING ROLES OF THE PHARMACIST IN CHAIN COMMUNITY PRACTICE

Pharmacist Judy Davis was working in the local chain pharmacy, Remedies, when a patient approached the counter and asked the pharmacy technician if they were giving pneumonia immunizations. The technician replied, "Yes, we are giving immunizations today, and we provide them everyday, so would you like to have one today? We can take care of you here." Smiling, the patient, John, quickly replied, "Yes, I would like to have one today."

multiple factors to consider when selecting a new employee instead of just filling a position.

It can be difficult to predict who the best candidate is going to be, especially when there are many well-qualified candidates who have applied for the position. It is those candidates who also appropriately work through the interview process with the employer with flexibility in schedule, positive attitude, timely correspondence, and respectful response to telephone calls or e-mails which can give a clear indication of how the person is going to be to work with in the future.

Additional questions employers may ask a candidate is to see where they would like to be in their careers within the next 1, 3 and 5 years? Employers are looking for leaders who are willing to grow with the organization and take on additional duties that are not currently part of the position they are seeking. The candidate who can thoughtfully present growing the position and also how they themselves will grow in the position are what most employers are looking for and is difficult to find.

There are some key action steps to take to continuously stay engaged in a career search, such as

- Attend career fairs and engage in three interviews at a minimum
- Search on-line regularly
- Signup for Internet alerts to your e-mail about relative positions
- Search for a recruiter to represent your portfolio
- Work on reflective exercises to be prepared for an interview when the time arises

Positions in a corporation are determined by their importance and responsibility in fulfilling the business objectives of the corporation. For instance, if the executives in the company determine that the company's focus is going to be within the marketing department, the company will determine how to dedicate resources to fulfilling that focus. Resources can be defined as anything from providing greater budgetary priority for supplies and new materials to creating an entirely new department with multiple positions in order to complete the company's business goals.

Once the goals of the company have been determined and the corporation has made a decision as to where to dedicate its resources, actual position descriptions should be developed. It is important to note that the company's size and cultural objectives can determine the importance a pharmacist has within the company. For example, if the pharmacy department in an organization represents 70 percent of the company's total gross profit, this company would be more sensitive to recognizing and developing its pharmacists compared with an organization in which pharmacy represents only 10 percent of the company's total gross profit. The actual description of a position is called a *job description* (see Chapter 12). Table 32-1 illustrates components of a job description.

Additional items may be added to a job description based on the characteristics of the corporation and

Table 32-1. Components of a Job Description

Title of Position
Reporting lines
Location
Job number
Work status
Level of supervision received
Work pace
Internal customer contact
External customer contact
Creation/revision date
Job description summary
Essential duties and responsibilities
Supervisory responsibilities
Qualification requirements
Education and/or experience
Language skills
Mathematical skills
Reasoning ability
Other skills, abilities, and/or training
Certificates, licenses, and/or registrations
Physical demands
Work environment

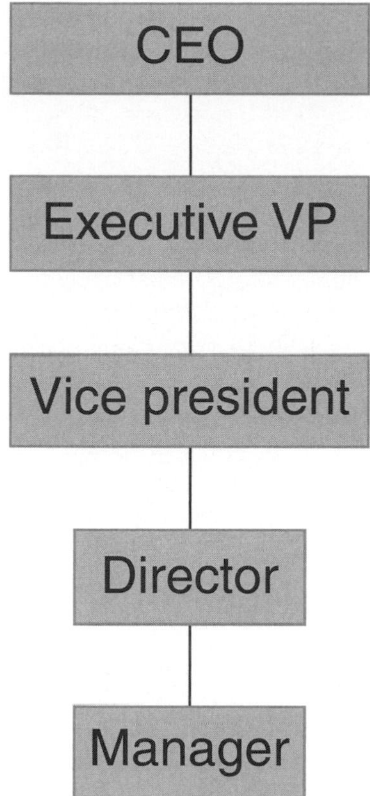

Figure 32-1. An abbreviated organizational chart.

the specific needs that determine a position. For instance, a corporation that has multiple jobs in areas of distribution, marketing, and operations will have job descriptions that vary considerably based on the work performed.

The hierarchy in a corporation is also defined by position titles. Figure 32-1 is a "typical" abbreviated organizational chart within a corporation.

Positions may have prefixes added to them that can alter their significance within the organization. For example, the word *assistant* may be added to the beginning of the title *manager* to make it *assistant manager,* which would rank below the actual manager. In contrast, placing the word *senior* before the manager title results in *senior manager,* which would rank above the actual manager. This technique can be used for any position within the organization. Once a title is changed, the job description for that position likewise should comply with the hierarchy. If the position created has a higher rank within the organization, the job description should reflect the additional responsibilities over the previous position, and vice versa.

Organizational charts become more complex as the organization grows (Fig. 32-2). Departments may be created based on the organization's needs and goals for the fiscal year. Many organizations typically operate on the calendar year January 1 to December 31 as their fiscal year. Some organizations, however, owing to the nature of their business or possibly when they went public (issued public stock), may operate on an alternative schedule.

Some departments, such as marketing, accounting, distribution, human resources, information systems, legal, and operations, are common to almost any organization. Each of these departments should have a department head who oversees its direction. The department head then reports to the chief executive officer (CEO) or another person at the top of the organization, such as a chief operating officer (COO) or president.

The board of directors defines the overall operating guidelines of the corporation. The board of directors is the governing body, consisting of various representatives who are either internal or external to the company. The board of directors is responsible for taking a strict look at the operating functions of the business without being immersed in its day-to-day operations. Boards typically meet quarterly but may meet more frequently. There may be emergency meetings called to vote on more urgent issues. Boards have a senior representative, the chairman of the board, who is elected by the board members. When working with a public company, it is very important to recognize that the board of directors is responsible to government organizations such as the Securities and Exchange Commission (SEC).

The Case of Retail Chain Pharmacy

What about the career path for a pharmacist? Which positions can a pharmacist aspire to within a chain

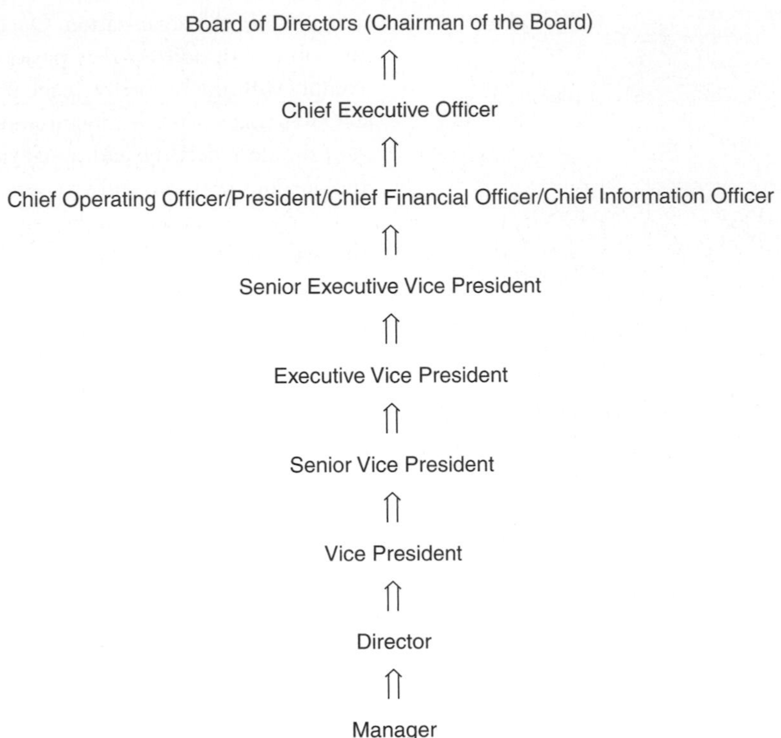

Figure 32-2. Basic organizational chart of publicly held company.

pharmacy? A lot of this depends on the company, its operating culture and changes in the marketplace. Is the company focused on pharmacy, and does it promote internally? If both these answers are "Yes," then there is a very good chance that a pharmacist can rise to almost any position within the company.

Pharmacists have significant upward mobility prospects in many chain pharmacy organizations. For example, a pharmacy development manager (PDM) oversees the operation of about 25 pharmacies in an area. A district manager (DM) is a field management position; however, unlike a PDM, a DM oversees the operation of merchandising of the products in the front of the store. It is not a requirement to be a pharmacist to secure a DM position, but some district managers are pharmacists. The DM works closely with the merchandising department and vendors who have products represented in the DM's specific operating area. The PDM and the DM positions have specific job descriptions, but job descriptions and position requirements change as titles change. For example, the title *vice president* does not have a department focus until the department is added to the title, such as *vice president, pharmacy operations.* With the changes occurring in health care reform, many new opportunities are emerging in areas such as regulatory law, government affairs, compliance positions, managed care, and clinical services.

Based on the preceding example, there are a number of positions within retail chain pharmacy to which pharmacists may aspire. Figure 32-3 shows how a degree in pharmacy can grow into multiple career opportunities within an organization. The key to all these positions is to begin a career as an intern or as a graduate intern for the organization. These positions lend themselves to the candidate learning more about the organization and the characteristics,

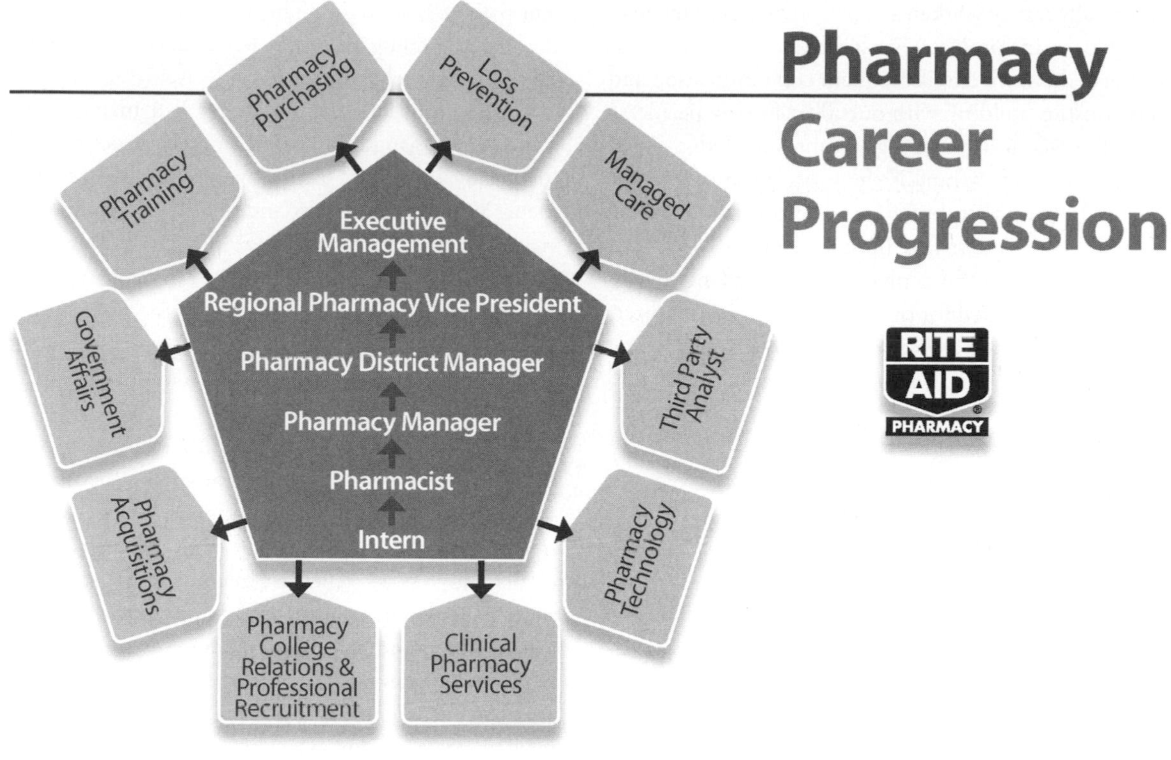

Figure 32-3. Pharmacy career progression chart.

responsibilities, and behaviors required to make the organization successful.

Once an intern has graduated from pharmacy school and becomes a graduate pharmacy intern, the next hurdle is to take and pass the national licensure examination plus any additional examinations required to practice in a particular state. Once verification of licensure has been made, the former intern now can practice as a pharmacist. For a pharmacist to move to the next level within the corporation, such as to pharmacy manager, or for the pharmacy manager to move to a pharmacy development manager level, a series of evaluations takes place. Many organizations in pharmacy are emphasizing annual performance appraisals of associates. An appraisal may be scheduled more frequently than once per year as well. Reviews may be scheduled at 3, 6, or 9 months if the employee requires guidance or if he or she desires promotion within the organization. One of the best contemporary appraisal systems is one that contains three parts, such as

1. The performance appraisal from the supervisor
2. A self-appraisal from the associate who is being evaluated
3. A performance appraisal addendum that contains action plans for training and education for the candidate

Appraisals are not always performed by an associate's supervisor alone. Appraisals can be performed by a second superior with whom the candidate works with but does not report to, by peers of the associate (especially if they work in an environment that involves constant team projects), or a vendor or outside customer if the work entails frequent communication and relationship building with outside company partners.

The acquisition of significant knowledge about drugs and drug therapy is the expectation of a newly licensed pharmacist, but it is the demonstration of excellent management and human resources skills that is often necessary for a pharmacist to become recognized and evaluated for promotion. Important aspects in the operation of a chain community pharmacy that are reviewed during an associate evaluation are

- Customer satisfaction
- Containment of costs—profit and loss statements, more commonly referred to as P&Ls
- Personnel management

Customer satisfaction is different from customer service. Customer service is an aspect of customer satisfaction. Satisfying a customer involves anticipation of the items a customer is looking to buy, inventory of the product, location of the product in the store, availability of personnel to service the customer in a timely and friendly manner, convenience, and price of the product.

Chain pharmacy practice is challenging because of the diverse needs of various patients. One of the best ways to rate patient satisfaction is to continuously survey patients through electronic surveys, comment cards, or a Web site where patients can voice their opinions about pharmacy personnel. Once the comment cards have been received at a destination for evaluation, entering the results into a computer database for quick analysis can provide a platform for the pharmacy to determine how it can improve its patient satisfaction skills and how it will schedule the training for associates.

For example, at least one national pharmacy chain has a satisfaction training program for associates. Pharmacy managers are responsible for all new associates and for the experienced associates to participate in the training. There is a rewards program wherein associates are given company gift cards when they provide excellent patient satisfaction. This is an example of "catching" people doing the right behavior and rewarding them for that behavior.

The profit-and-loss statement is a management tool used to gauge how the company is performing financially. Each store has its own profit-and-loss statement. When a pharmacist and pharmacy manager are visited by the pharmacy development manager, the profit and loss statement is reviewed to make sure that the company is on or within plan. If the pharmacy is not operating to plan, the area of concern is evaluated, an action plan is developed, and then it is put into play to achieve the desired results.

Personnel management is the third factor when evaluating a pharmacy for performance. When an associate is going through the appraisal process, it is not uncommon for his or her peers to evaluate his or her progress as well. Part of this evaluation is designed to encourage team leadership and interaction skills. Companies have become more inclined to offer management development courses to associates who aspire to become promoted. For example, live training may be provided for associates to understand about how important communication skills are to working in pharmacy. Courses delivered through CD-ROM, the Internet, or self-directed study offer a number of options for associates to design their development. If a supervisor or peer feels that an associate who is being evaluated could benefit from one of the courses, a recommendation can be made on the associate's evaluation, or a supervisor could suggest the course options to the associates so as to focus him or her on such development.

The beginning of a new career can be very exciting but can also be confusing if the pharmacist is not aware of the potential career path. A typical human resources benchmark for determining if someone has become a professional is if he or she remains in a position for about 3 years. The first 3 years in a career can set the tone of success or struggle. In human resources, it is recognized that a person's best performance is typically within the first year he or she is in a position. Performance can be accomplished in a short amount of time (known as the "quick win"). If the candidate continues to exceed the operating goals in years 2 and 3, he or she is ready to take on more business responsibility, such as the financial and other aspects of managing a store.

Once the pharmacist has become a pharmacy manager, he or she has the responsibility to maintain the manager's position based on pharmacy state law and the organization's expectations. Once the pharmacy manager has proven that he or she can comply with and then exceed expectations, then he or she can become a candidate for promotion. In the organizational chart shown in Fig. 32-3, the pharmacy manager has the opportunity to move into the corporate office or to move up into a field operations position. The more typical career path for a pharmacy manager is into the field operator position, but once in a while a corporate position will open up for a pharmacy manager. The field operator position may have multiple bosses, and the lines describe the reporting responsibility one has to those higher up. A straight reporting line means that the position reports directly to the position above it, and a dotted reporting line means that the position has some reporting responsibility to the position above it, but that the position is not a direct boss. When the corporate position is available, there are many points to take into consideration, such as possible relocation, variable work hours, a salaried position (work until you accomplish your project goals regardless of how many hours it takes to complete), politics, and overall increased responsibility.

A career path is a combination of self-management, fiscal management, and operations management. When all three of these are accomplished, the candidate has the potential for a great career. Quite frequently executives are asked, "How do I move up in your organization?" The following are some helpful suggestions:

- Read a newspaper every day.
- Read a current business management book.
- Read a current-events magazine each week.
- Become involved in pharmacy organizations.
- Become involved in charitable organizations.
- Learn multiple languages.
- Become a mentor to a pharmacy intern, technician, or high school student.
- Enroll in a management class or take a certificate course in a pharmacy specialty.
- Prepare/update a current résumé—be very careful of any spelling errors.
- Enroll in a business etiquette course.

In addition to self-development, there are some common pitfalls to avoid:

- *Never be late for work.* Always report to work at least 10 minutes before you are scheduled and stay until the work is cleaned up from your shift. This will create the impression that you are a responsible partner in the work environment, and your partner will not walk into a mess the following morning.
- *Always leave a place in better condition* (cleaner, more organized) than how it was when you arrived.
- *Never bite the hands that feed you.* This includes not only your boss's hand but also your department head's hand and, most important, the company that signs your paycheck.
- When you are required to turn in a project for your supervisor, *turn it in before the deadline.*
- Always remember to *ask your coworkers how you can help them* instead of not extending help.
- *Be courteous when working with printers, staplers, and other office equipment.* For example, do not leave printers without paper, a copier without paper, or if you used the last staple, refill the stapler.
- *Always follow company dress code policy and represent yourself as the professional you are or going to be in the future.* This includes appropriate name badge or identification.
- *Always make sure that you are properly groomed as a professional.* Hygiene is recognized not only by coworkers and supervisors but also by customers/patients.
- *Always greet your coworkers every morning and say "good night" when leaving work* regardless of the position they hold within the company. You never know who tomorrow's next boss is going to be, so be nice to everyone.

- *Do not gossip about other people.* It is unprofessional and can damage their reputation. Remember that the old axiom "What comes around goes around" could not be more truthful in the corporate world.
- *Keep personal information personal.* Do not discuss your issues at work or with coworkers. This includes the amount of pay you receive and additional benefits.

REVISITING THE SCENARIOS

This chapter has provided a glimpse of the new services being offered and career opportunities in chain community pharmacy. Revisiting each scenario one more time might help reinforce concepts about this swiftly changing practice environment.

Scenario I

Pharmacist Judy continues throughout the day to provide various types of immunizations to her patients when her supervisor comes to the pharmacy for a regular visit. The supervisor tells Judy what a great job she is doing and how can he provide additional support to her for this initiative. Judy replies "We are scheduling a lot of immunizations, so I am going to need help coordinate the intern schedules to optimize support for this program. Is there anything else we can do?" Judy and her supervisor brainstorm to coordinate a float team of technicians throughout the district for immunization processing.

Scenario II

Career pathing continues to evolve as community pharmacy practice continues to change. New opportunities at all levels of an organization are developing from the expanding roles. Emily, who works in the pharmacy, contemplates career opportunities and approaches her district supervisor on the possibilities. Elizabeth, the pharmacy supervisor also approaches Perry, the pharmacy manager, about his success and if he has an interest in being promoted. It is important to work with talented aspiring associates who are looking for career progression to develop new opportunities in the profession and, as a supervisor, create a plan to develop staff.

QUESTIONS FOR FURTHER DISCUSSION

1. What would you find the most challenging aspect of creating a culture that reflects each associate's point of view?
2. Which opportunities in community chain practice would you be most interested in?
3. Could you see yourself moving up the corporate ladder in a chain pharmacy organization? Why or why not? If not, what could you do to make yourself a more suitable candidate to do so?

REFERENCES

Blanchard K. 2002. *Whale Done!—The Power of Positive Relationships.* New York: Free Press, p. 40 and 42.

Blanchard K, Muchnick M. 2003. *The Leadership Pill—The Missing Ingredient in Motivating People Today.* New York. Free Press.

Bossidy L, Charan R. 2002. *Execution—The Discipline of Getting Things Done.* New York: Crown Business, pp. 85–6, 109–13.

Chowdhury S. 2001. *The Power of Six Sigma.* Chicago: Dearborn Trade, pp. 19, 22, 24–5.

Lyles D. 2000. *Winning Ways–4 Secrets for Getting Great Results by Working Well with People.* New York: Putnam, pp. 48, 62, 75, 86.

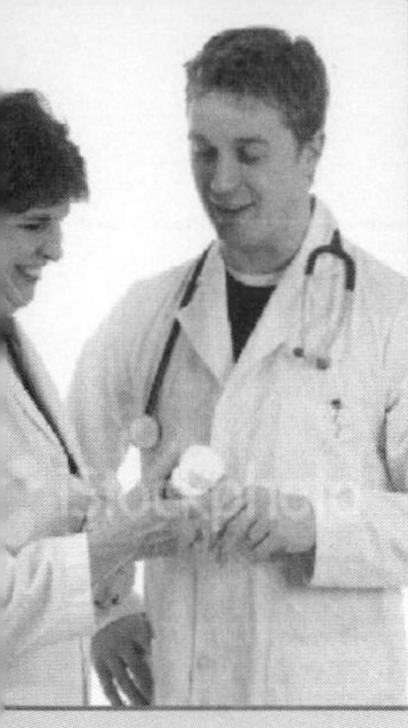

33

APPLICATIONS IN HOSPITAL PHARMACY PRACTICE

Frank Massaro and William A. Gouveia

About the Authors: Frank Massaro is pharmacy practice manager at Tufts Medical Center. Dr. Massaro manages clinical programs for the Department of Pharmacy and is responsible for the professional development of the pharmacist staff. He is a member of the General Internal Medicine patient care team and an active member of several interdepartmental performance improvement committees. Dr. Massaro received both a B.S. in pharmacy and a Pharm.D. from the Philadelphia College of Pharmacy and Science. He completed a residency in hospital pharmacy at New England Medical Center. Dr. Massaro's current faculty appointments include Tufts University School of Medicine and Northeastern University's Bouvé College of Health Sciences.

William A. Gouveia retired in 2008 after serving for 36 years as Director of Pharmacy at Tufts Medical Center. Mr. Gouveia has served the American Journal of Health-System Pharmacists (AJHP) in a number of editorial positions, most recently as Contributing Editor, Pharmacy Practice Management. Mr. Gouveia received his Master of Science Degree in Hospital Pharmacy and Bachelor of Pharmacy Degree from Northeastern University College of Pharmacy. He has been Chairman of the American Society of Health-System Pharmacists Commission on Goals and was named ASHP Fellow in 1993. He received the ASHP Research and Education Foundation Award for Achievement for Sustained Contributions to the Literature and the Outstanding Alumni Award in Health Sciences from Northeastern University. Mr. Gouveia also served on the ASHP Board of Directors from 1986 to 1989. He received The Harvey A. K. Whitney Lecture Award, health-system pharmacy's highest honor, from the ASHP in 1999. Mr. Gouveia's faculty appointments include Tufts University School of Medicine, and Northeastern University's Bouve College of Health Sciences. In 2001, Mr. Gouveia was appointed to the L'Academie National de Pharmacie in Paris, France. He also received the American Pharmacists Association Academy of Pharmacy Practice and Management Distinguished Achievement Award in Hospital and Institutional Practice in 2005. Mr. Gouveia received an honorary Doctor of Humane Letters Degree from Western University of Health Sciences, Pomona, California in May 2006. Gouveia was appointed Inaugural Chair, International Commission Accreditation Council for Pharmacy Education in 2011.

LEARNING OBJECTIVES

After completing this chapter, readers should be able to

1. Describe a typical organizational chart, management structure, and flow of information for a hospital and a hospital's pharmacy department.
2. Describe the integration of clinical and managerial roles assumed by pharmacists in the hospital setting.
3. Identify and describe models for managing clinical pharmacist services in a hospital.
4. Describe budgetary issues confronting a hospital's pharmacy department. Identify strategies undertaken by the department's director and staff pharmacists to reduce operating costs without compromising patient care.
5. Identify strategies for managing personnel, including clinical pharmacists, in a hospital pharmacy.

INTRODUCTION

Every hospital pharmacist is a manager. Every pharmacist must acquire, maintain, and constantly update a unique and specialized body of knowledge. Every pharmacist must learn to direct, support, persuade, discipline, and collaborate with others. Every pharmacist is expected to understand and use the principles of accounting, finance, economics, marketing, and informatics. Indeed, optimal patient care depends on a pharmacist's ability to thoughtfully apply the science of therapeutics and on his or her ability to manage people and information.

In many situations, a pharmacist with excellent management skills and average clinical knowledge is more effective than a pharmacist with poor management skills and an excellent knowledge base. Consider the clinical pharmacist who appears to approach and solve problems with ease compared with the pharmacist who has difficulty gathering even basic information to make an informed decision. This paradox has led some to ascribe this skill in managing to "experience" or "judgment." To be sure, the ability to manage improves with study and experience. However, managing a budget or a group of individuals is not a mysterious process. It is a method that parallels the clinical problem-solving process. It is a method that can be both taught and learned. It requires both knowledge and skill. And these skills can be refined only through practice.

SCENARIO 1

As a critical care clinical pharmacist for 10 years, Ken had performed all the functions of a hospital pharmacist. He had provided pharmacy care to individual patients, worked in a satellite pharmacy, served as a preceptor for pharmacy students and residents, taught the critical care section of a course at a school of pharmacy, and published journal articles. He was a successful clinician and was highly regarded by his peers, by the medical community, and by nursing staff. At some point Ken decided that it was time for a change. While he still enjoyed caring for individuals, he yearned for the chance to influence a larger number of patients. He wanted to make a contribution to the broader context of the health system. Thus, when the opportunity arose to develop a hospital-wide antimicrobial management program, Ken gladly accepted the challenge.

After only a year in his new position, Ken was able to show improvements in the appropriate use of anti-infective drugs while reducing drug costs and to describe a comprehensive plan for the future. He was able to engender the support of the hospital's senior managers, physicians, and pharmacists. He was able to document a positive impact on patient outcomes. The quality of pharmacy services provided and the hospital's financial position improved. How was all this possible in such a short time?

THE HOSPITAL ENVIRONMENT

The pharmacist in Scenario 1 is, like many practitioners, a skilled clinician. His successes as a critical care pharmacist were supported by his formal education and his close working relationship with the medical and surgical staffs. His successes as the leader of a hospital-wide program are no more surprising. Ken simply applied the same skills he used in caring for patients to the development of a new clinical service. He worked to identify the types of information he needed to make informed decisions. He generated a list of clearly articulated goals and gathered the necessary resources to reach the stated goals. His first step, however, was to understand how the hospital is organized.

Figure 33-1 shows a typical hospital organizational chart. The chart shows the reporting structure and formal lines of communication within the institution. It is important to realize that the position of the pharmacy department and the administrator to whom the director of pharmacy reports can significantly affect how senior managers and others view the pharmacy. If, for example, the director of pharmacy reports to an ancillary services administrator along with housekeeping, maintenance and security, pharmacy is more likely to be viewed as a service department; one not directly involved in patient care. On the other hand, if the pharmacy falls under the patient care division along with radiology, the clinical laboratory, and the emergency department, then the pharmacy is more likely to be viewed as a participant in direct patient care. Figure 33-2 shows an organizational chart for a typical department of pharmacy. The chart hints at the

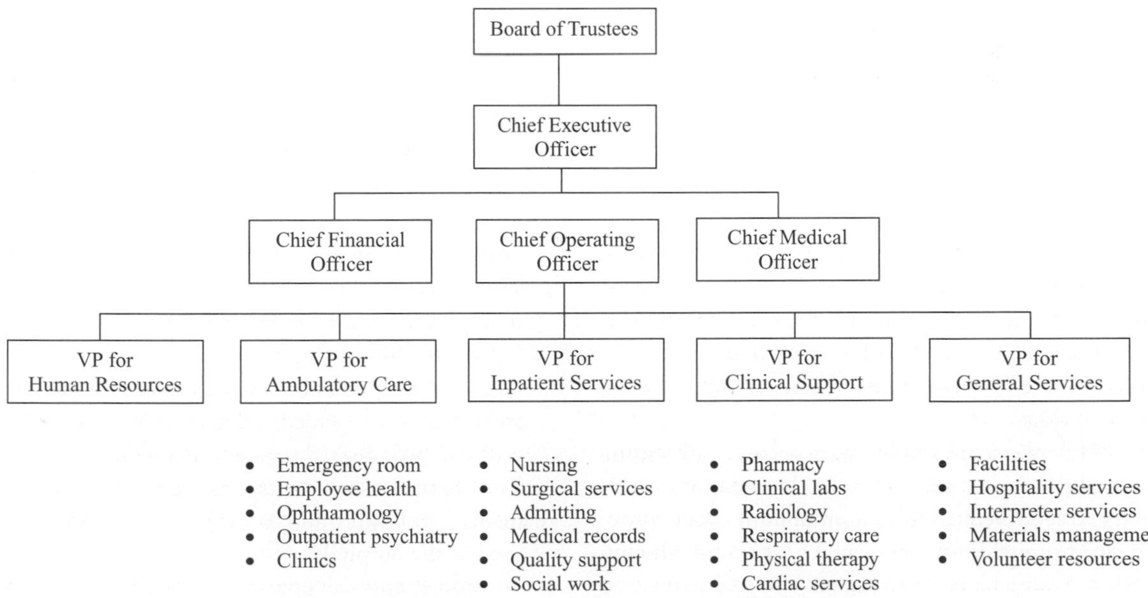

Figure 33-1. Hospital organizational chart.

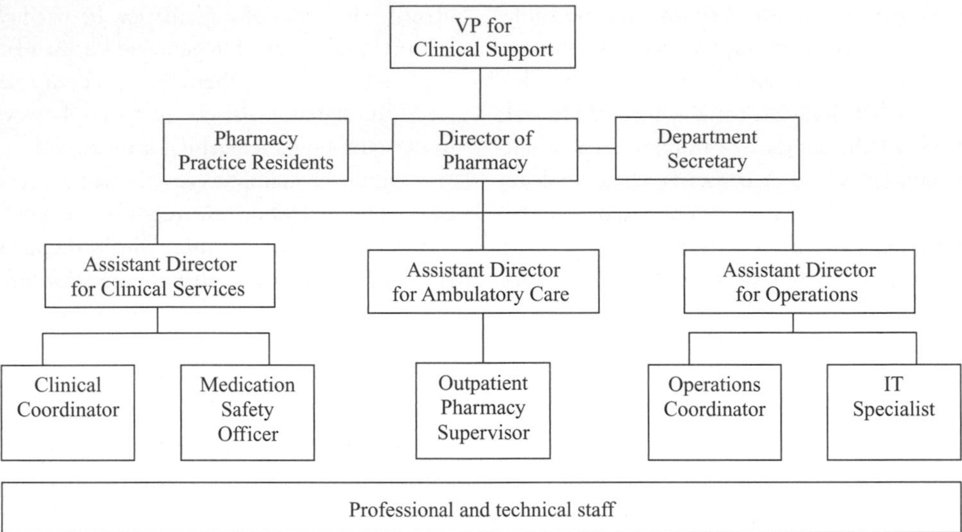

Figure 33-2. Department of pharmacy organizational chart.

information-, product-, and outcome-oriented nature of the profession. It also gives some indication of a key goal of the pharmacy, that is, to control the acquisition and use of drugs. This focus helps ensure that a patient's drug therapy is appropriate, safe, and cost effective and achieves the proper outcome.

When a pharmacist accepts his or her first job in a hospital, it is important that he or she fully understand the structure of the drug control system. Control implies accountability, not for its own sake, but to promote safety, effectiveness, and fiscal responsibility. This accountability for drug therapy can be achieved through a variety of pharmacy functions. Pharmacists decide how drugs are selected and obtained, how drugs are ordered for individual patients, and how drugs are prepared for administration. Pharmacists monitor the therapeutic benefit or possible harm that may result from the use of drugs and the costs associated with these services.

While the scope of pharmacy services varies from hospital to hospital depending on the needs of the patients served, there are certain minimum standards to which a hospital must conform. These published standards provide a basis for evaluation and goal setting for the hospital pharmacy director. The American Society for Health-System Pharmacists (ASHP) has developed a list of practice standards that define acceptable professional practices (American Society of Health-System Pharmacists, 2009a, p. 379). The six basic standards are

1. The pharmacy shall be managed by a professionally competent, legally qualified pharmacist. The director of pharmacy service must be thoroughly knowledgeable about hospital pharmacy practice and management.
2. The pharmacist shall provide patient-specific drug information and accurate and comprehensive information about drugs to other pharmacists, other health professionals, and patients as appropriate.
3. The pharmacist, in concert with the medical and nursing staffs, must develop policies and procedures for ensuring the quality of medication therapy. This must include processes designed to ensure the safe and effective use of medications and to increase the probability of desired patient outcomes.
4. The pharmacy shall be responsible for the procurement, distribution, and control of *all* drug products used in the hospital.
5. To ensure optimal operational performance and quality patient care, adequate space, equipment,

and supplies shall be available for all professional and administrative functions relating to medication use.

6. The pharmacist should initiate, participate in, and support medical and pharmaceutical research appropriate to the goals, objectives, and resources of the specific hospital.

State boards of pharmacy and departments of public health also influence hospital pharmacy practice. The state boards serve as licensing bodies for both the location of pharmacies and those individuals able to practice. The primary duty of the department of public health (DPH) is to uphold the public interest in quality pharmacy service within the laws and regulations of the state. In fulfilling these obligations through an evaluation of the pharmacy, the board of pharmacy and the DPH assure the public that minimum standards of practice are met. These regulatory bodies also review citizens' complaints and investigate reports of drug loss and diversion.

The major nongovernmental regulatory body to which many hospitals must conform is The Joint Commission. The Joint Commission is an independent, not-for-profit organization governed by a board that includes physicians, nurses and consumers. The Joint Commission sets the standards by which health care quality is measured. A team of Joint Commission surveyors usually visit acute care hospitals once every 3 years. The surveyors compare a department's performance to a set of published standards in the context of the larger hospital organization (Joint Commission, 2010). The purpose of the review is to evaluate a hospital's performance and to improve the safety and quality of care provided to the public through health care accreditation.

The hospital organization, external regulatory bodies, and standards of pharmacy practice define the formal structure within which a pharmacy manager must operate. However, the real hospital environment is much more complicated. The skilled manager also recognizes the informal relationships within the hospital and works to develop a good rapport with influential clinicians, key hospital administrators, and physician leadership. Pharmacy managers who display a genuine concern for patients and can work effectively with the hospital's professional staffs will achieve the pharmacy's mission more easily. The development of such relationships should be a priority for every pharmacist. One way to demonstrate knowledge and to cultivate strong bonds with other professionals is to participate in a variety of patient care committees (Table 33-1). In Scenario 1, the pharmacist's success was due in part to his ability to develop relationships with members of the hospital's pharmacy and therapeutics committee, the medication safety committee, and the antibiotic control committee.

Table 33-1. Patient Care Committees with Pharmacist Involvement in Many Hospitals
Antibimicrobial Stewardship
Cancer Care
Human Investigation Review Board
Infection Control
Patient Safety and Quality
Pharmacy and Therapeutics

Committees dealing with patient care always include members of the medical staff. To conduct its business, the medical staff, with approval of the board of trustees, elects officers and organizes itself into various groups, as outlined in its bylaws. The hospital usually has two kinds of committees, standing and special, or ad hoc, committees. Standing committees are permanent and cannot be dissolved without changing the bylaws. Such committees usually have ongoing business to conduct throughout the year and therefore must meet regularly. Examples include the hospital's committee on credentialing and the pharmacy and therapeutics committee. Ad hoc committees are chartered as needed to solve special problems and then are dissolved when the task is completed. All committees of the medical staff report their activity and make recommendations to the medical board or executive committee.

Most medical staff bylaws call for a pharmacy and therapeutics (P&T) committee consisting of physicians, nurses, pharmacists, and administrators. The primary purposes of the P&T committee are (American Society of Health-System Pharmacists, 2009b, p. 126)

1. *Policy development.* The committee formulates policies regarding evaluation, selection, and therapeutic use of drugs and related devices.
2. *Education.* The committee recommends or assists in the formulation of programs designed to meet the needs of the professional staff (i.e., physicians, nurses, pharmacists, and other health care practitioners) for complete current knowledge on matters related to drugs and drug use.
3. *Formulary management.* The committee develops a list formulary of medications accepted for use in the hospital. The formulary is a continually revised compilation of drug products that reflects the current clinical judgment of the medical and pharmacy staffs. The selection of items in the formulary is based on an extensive literature review and evaluation. The written monographs presented to the committee for analysis include the relative therapeutic merits of a drug, its safety, and its cost. The committee tries to minimize duplication of basic drug types, drug entities, or drug products. Limiting the number of drug products available from the pharmacy can produce substantial patient care and financial benefits. These benefits are increased greatly through use of generic equivalents (drug products considered to be identical with respect to their active components, e.g., two brands of amoxicillin capsules) and *therapeutic equivalents* (drug products differing in composition that are considered to have very similar pharmacologic and therapeutic activities, e.g., two different first-generation oral cephalosporins). The P&T committee must make clear the policies and procedures governing the dispensing of generic and therapeutic equivalents. The pharmacy department, working through the P&T committee, must make certain that the medical and nursing staffs are informed about the existence of the formulary system and the policies and procedures governing its operation.

The safety of the medication system is the primary concern of every hospital pharmacist. Numerous published reports of the incidence, causes, and cost of injury resulting from medication errors have led many hospitals to critically evaluate their quality assurance systems (Bates et al., 1996, 1997; Classen et al., 1997; Kohn et al., 1999; Leape et al., 1991, 1995; Poon et al., 2006; Stelfox et al., 2006). Written incident reports were once the standard for gathering information about medication misadventures. This method is now believed to lack sufficient completeness and reliability for identifying weaknesses in a medication system (Classen et al., 1991; Cullen et al., 1995; Leape, 1994, 2002; Leape et al., 1995).

Medication safety is now widely considered under the auspices of many continuous quality improvement (CQI) initiatives by the entire hospital, with pharmacy playing an integral role with other health care professionals aimed at maximizing therapeutic outcomes, reducing errors, and complying with increasingly stringent standards from various regulatory agencies. Doing so is good for patients and also good for the hospital's and pharmacy's bottom line (see Chapter 8).

Deficiencies in reporting errors have spawned the formation of new standing committees in many hospitals. Medication safety committees are charged with developing processes to identify and quantify medication errors and adverse drug reactions. Pharmacists, physicians, nurses, risk management personnel, legal counsel, administrators, and patients work together to implement specific changes to improve the medication system. Most programs are designed to gather information about *potential errors* (i.e., mistakes that are detected and corrected *before* actual administration to the patient) and *actual errors* (i.e., mistakes identified *after* the drugs are administered or failure to administer a scheduled drug).

Well-designed systems can (1) describe the stage in the medication process where the error occurred (i.e., prescribing, transcription, pharmacy computer entry error, dispensing, and administration), (2) the nature of the error within each stage of the process, and (3) the therapeutic category of the drug involved. Such systems provide meaningful data about medication errors and adverse drug reactions and allow for the development of strategies to prevent recurrences. For example, early in the development of the infection control program described in Scenario 1, the pharmacist noticed a trend in prescribing errors reported through the medication safety committee. Physicians consistently chose the correct antibiotic to treat a suspected or known infection, but the prescribed dose was often inappropriate. Physicians often failed to consider the site of the infection, the likely virulence of the pathogen, possible antibiotic resistance, and the patient's organ function. The pharmacist used the information to focus his educational efforts to improve patient care and to demonstrate his clinical expertise. The pharmacist's active involvement in the medication safety committee served to promote safe and effective drug therapy, and served to enhance the image of the pharmacy department.

SCENARIO 2

Suburban General is a 350-bed community hospital located just outside a major metropolitan area. The department of pharmacy at Suburban General is well respected within the institution for its financially efficient operation and its use of cutting-edge technology. It was the first community hospital in the state to install automated dispensing machines in all patient care areas. Decentralized pharmacists use radiofrequency laptop computers to enter medication orders into the pharmacy computer system, and nurses rely on the pharmacists to accurately manage an electronic medication administration record for every patient.

The department of pharmacy is directed by a visionary with the ability to get others to look into the future with her. Interestingly, her vision of the future includes helping to raise her many grandchildren. Thus, after 27 years of service, the director of pharmacy decided to retire. Before leaving Suburban General, the outgoing director convinced senior management that the new director should be someone who could bring a level of clinical sophistication to the department that could match its operational efficiency. The incoming director of pharmacy was charged with maintaining the current level of operational efficiency while developing and implementing clinical pharmacy services.

MANAGING CLINICAL PRACTICE

The new director in Scenario 2 is presented with a significant challenge. The director must expand the mission of the department to include services that maximize the department's contributions to the clinical outcomes of patients. This is not a new idea. Three major conferences sponsored by the ASHP and numerous publications over the past 30 years have firmly established the importance of hospital pharmacists' participation in clinical decision making (American Society of Health-System Pharmacists, 2011; Bond et al., 2000; Bond et al., 2002; Bond and Raehl, 2006; Hepler and Strand, 1990; Zelmer, 1986). The challenge is to design a practice model that best serves the patients and the hospital.

Vermeulen and colleagues (2007) designed a strategic approach to improving the medication use process in hospitals by using a framework for setting priorities on the basis of feasibility, the potential for financial return, and the effect on quality and safety. They identified seven dimensions of high-performance hospital pharmacy practice: medication preparation and delivery, patient care services, medication safety, medication-use policy, financial performance, human resources, and education. Their work is intended to be a tool for pharmacy departments to assess current performance, make plans for improvement and identify relevant references and standards. Publications such as this are a great place for the director in Scenario 2 to begin planning for an expanded clinical role for pharmacists.

Two models, the *generalist model* and the *specialist model*, can describe traditional approaches to the organization of clinical pharmacy services in a hospital. The generalist model evolved as a result of the decentralization of hospital pharmacy practice that began in the 1960s. Decentralization relocated many pharmacists from the basement to patient care areas. This model maintains that for the pharmacist to affect the care of patients it is necessary to be present when and where drug therapy decisions are made. The defining feature of the generalist model is that pharmacists are responsible for both clinical and drug distribution services. For this model to work, some of the pharmacist's activities must be supported by the use of qualified pharmacy technicians and the optimal use of technology.

Some pharmacy departments use the *specialist model* in which a distinction is made between clinical pharmacists and staff pharmacists. The specialists are responsible for providing clinical pharmacy services throughout the hospital. Staff pharmacists oversee drug distribution. In this model, it is not always possible to provide comprehensive clinical care to all patients. The only patients who receive clinical pharmacy services are those who conform to specialty categories (e.g., critical care, oncology, or pediatrics) defined by the clinical manager. The clinical care a patient receives may depend on the patient care area to which the patient was admitted, the practice in which the pharmacist is most interested, and whether a specific pharmacist is scheduled on a particular day.

The generalist and the specialist models have been successful in many hospitals, provided that there has been a systematic approach to the development, implementation, and evaluation of the clinical services provided. Full integration of clinical practice into drug distribution services optimizes the chances for success. In 2010, ASHP launched a practice model initiative to help develop a future practice model that is responsive to health care reform and the health system of the future (American Society of Health-System Pharmacists, 2010). ASHP has a long-standing policy supporting an integrated, team-based approach to patient-centered care (American Society of Health-System Pharmacists, 2011).

The first priority in any clinical service must be to achieve desired patient outcomes; that is, to promote health and prevent disease by ensuring rational drug therapy. The second priority is efficient procurement, preparation, and distribution of drug products for the purpose of supporting the clinical service. The successful integration of patient-specific clinical pharmacy services with an efficient drug distribution operation will result in the best care possible.

■ SCENARIO 3

Hospitals are big business. And like many privately owned companies, final responsibility for the fiscal integrity of a private not-for-profit hospital rests with the board of trustees. Bayside Medical Center (BMC) is no different.

BMC has been in business for more than 100 years. Its financial success is due in part to strong leadership by the chief executive and a very active board of trustees. Until recently, BMC has generated enough revenue to meet operating expenses and to expand services to outlying communities. Unfortunately, in the past 3 years, dramatic decreases in investment income and reductions in reimbursement from third-party payers have almost eliminated the cash available for expansion. If the trend continues, there will be a shortage of operating capital within the next 2 years.

Ever vigilant, the board of trustees identified the problem early. To better understand the cost of providing care, the board hired a health care consulting firm. The consultants are charged with meeting with key hospital department heads to identify opportunities for reducing the cost of doing business. Of course, the director of pharmacy and his staff are on the list.

■ BUDGETING AND FINANCE

Financial control of a hospital is of utmost importance in maintaining the institution's solvency. The hospital will not survive unless there is adequate income to cover operating expenses and capital improvements. This survival requires that every senior administrator and every department director be highly skilled financial managers. What is unique about the department of pharmacy is the disproportionate cost of supplies (e.g., drugs) versus wages compared with other hospital departments. Typically, 90 percent of a pharmacy's budget is for drugs, whereas less than 10 percent is for employee wages. The reverse is true for most other departments. The overall cost of medications and the proportion of the drug expenditures that are under the influence of each clinical pharmacist require that every hospital pharmacist understands the principles of financial management. A review of the usual financial administrative structure within a hospital, the budget process, and the difference between cost and charge may be helpful.

As described in Scenario 3, the board of trustees is ultimately responsible for the fiscal health of a private not-for-profit hospital. It has a financial responsibility to the public. The board typically delegates all routine responsibilities to the chief executive officer (CEO) of the institution. The board also appoints a finance committee of the board to advise the CEO on overall financial management. The finance committee is responsible for overseeing the financial position of the hospital to ensure that there is adequate operating and long-term capital available. The committee advises the board of trustees on all fiscal and investment matters.

While the board delegates day-to-day financial matters to the CEO, it is impossible for one person to supervise all aspects of the hospital's operations. The number of internal and external demands that require the CEO's personal attention and the highly technical nature of operations require the CEO to delegate many tasks to the hospital's senior managers and department directors. Financial management is a principal function delegated to all administrators and managers.

An important and fundamental part of financial control is budgeting. Each hospital department will have an annual budget. A good department manager will be able to anticipate revenue and predict expenses for the coming year. To estimate next year's budget, it is useful to review carefully the current budget and the budget for the past 2 or 3 years. By observing the trends in cost for major items (e.g., intravenous solutions and specific therapeutic categories of drugs), it is easier to forecast future expenses. Experienced directors of pharmacy also gather information from two additional sources to predict the future: published reports and clinical pharmacy specialists.

Published reports in the lay press and in health care journals continue to predict increasing drug expenditures. Financial analysts speculate in the *Wall Street Journal* on sales of soon-to-be marketed drug products. Group purchasing organizations (GPOs) publish annual drug price forecasts for use by their members to plan for the coming year. And national professional organizations such as ASHP support the development and publication of estimates of future drug prices (Doloresco et al., 2011). The astute pharmacy manager gathers predictive data from a variety of sources and applies the information to the development of the department's drug budget. An understanding of market forces gathered by scanning the literature helps the manager to be prepared for the future and to educate hospital senior management about drug costs.

Clinical pharmacists working in the hospital are an often-underutilized source of information about future trends in drug expense. They care for patients and participate in drug therapy discussions with staff physicians every day. They see first hand the effects of investigational drug products and of marketed drugs used in novel ways. They keep up with the scientific literature. The pharmacy director and the clinical pharmacy staff should share information frequently to get a better look into the future. For example, in many hospitals, pharmacy managers and clinicians were able to predict the economic impact of a new drug to help manage sepsis before the drug was on the market. They were also able to develop widely accepted guidelines for use to ensure appropriate prescribing and reasonable expenditures. As a result, costs were managed, and only those patients who would benefit from the drug received it.

The budget process begins with a directive from the board of trustees regarding the general policies and goals for the next year. These policies may include changes to the physical plant or capital equipment or approval to provide new services. Next, the budget department outlines departmental guidelines consistent with the directives from the board of trustees. Basic operating statistics such as patient days, anticipated admissions, and the impact of inflation, are prepared. Target expenses and revenues are identified for each department and are rolled up into the hospital's

Table 33-2. Six-month Financial Analysis

	YTD Actual	YTD Budget	Variance
Expenses			
Regular salary and wages	1,122,272	1,105,155	(17,117)
Overtime	14,150	35,669	21,519
Holiday pay	16,265	19,227	2,962
Weekend premium	8,756	10,708	1,953
Evening differential	9,668	12,338	2,670
Night differential	4,974	4,548	426
Contract labor	77,854	33,857	(43,997)
Total salary and wages	**1,243,939**	**1,221,502**	**(31,584)**
Drugs	10,194,429	10,409,290	214,861
Service contracts	0	24,000	24,000
Dues/subscriptions/books	5,996	4,305	(1,691)
Software contracts	17,731	65,016	47,285
Med/surg supplies	40,717	47,767	7,050
Drug packaging supplies	23,865	45,745	21,880
Office supplies	18,138	6,380	(11,758)
Repairs	0	2,500	2,500
Telephone	12,863	9,295	(3,568)
Equipment rental	59,878	63,275	3,397
Printing	4,883	5,684	801
Total non-labor expenses	**10,378,500**	**10,683,357**	**304,857**
Revenue			
Inpatient revenue	18,958,395	19,824,126	(968,846)
Outpatient revenue	11,860,376	13,260,055	(1,399,679)
Miscellaneous revenue	6,995	0	6,995
Total revenue	**30,825,766**	**33,084,181**	**(2,258,415)**
Net operating income (loss)	**20,447,266**	**22,400,824**	**(1,953,558)**

consolidated budget. The third step is for each department to prepare its budget based on the budget guidelines. Next, a final review is conducted. The department budget is compared with the established targets, and senior management conducts negotiations of the final figures. A final roll-up of actual budgets is then prepared and submitted to the board of trustees for approval or modification.

Most hospital pharmacy budgets contain three major components: (1) salary and wage expense; (2) drugs, supplies, and equipment expense; and (3) revenue. Every hospital will have its own format of financial reporting and budgetary summary. Table 33-2 is a hypothetical income and expense report compared with a budget for a 6-month period.

- *Salary and wage expense.* This includes payroll expense for regularly scheduled hours and for salaried employees. The salary subsection also includes a budgeted amount for overtime, sick, vacation, and holiday pay. It should be noted that sick, vacation, and holiday pay represent nonproductive expenses. While most department budgets do not represent benefits (e.g., health insurance, disability insurance, etc.), the hospital's overall budget will. Benefits generally are 20 to 30 percent of total salary and wage costs.

- *Supplies and equipment expense.* This nonsalary section of the budget usually is sufficiently detailed so that the manager can monitor it by category. The supplies and equipment budget may include expense categories such as drugs, office supplies, and maintenance contracts (see Table 33-2). Many pharmacy directors subdivide the drug expense category into therapeutic classes to better monitor new services or trends in therapy. For example, the economic impact of a newly marketed drug to treat pancreatic cancer is easier to track if the expense is shown in the antineoplastic category of the drug section of the expense budget.
- *Revenue.* Revenue is sometimes used interchangeably with charges. In general, a department's charges must cover its expenses. However, in some hospitals, pharmacy department charges are used to subsidize non-revenue-producing departments. This component of the budget differs widely among hospitals. The pharmacy may be a cost center or a revenue center, or a mixture of both. The department manager must clearly understand the mechanism for establishing pharmacy charges, whether by a fee structure or a percent markup, so that revenue can be reported and compared with the various expense categories in the expense budget.

The system for establishing pharmacy charges must be fair, economically sound, and explainable to patients and third-party payers. Some hospitals use a simple *percent markup* on drug cost strategy. The charge for a drug is the product of the acquisition cost and the markup. Higher-cost drugs theoretically yield a higher return. The *professional fee* concept is based on the fact that a prescription medication is not an article of trade capable of being bought and sold by anyone and that the cost of dispensing, including the skill and knowledge involved, is not related to the cost of the ingredients used. A professional fee may be applied to doses dispensed or on a per-diem or per-patient basis. This approach has particular merit for nondistributive clinical services. Hospitals may choose a combination of approaches, using a percent markup for drugs dispensed and a professional fee for services, such as drug information or patient education, which are not necessarily related to a specific drug product.

Most important to this discussion on hospital revenue is the fact that the true economic cost of a medical service seldom is reflected by its charge. Because hospital accounting in the United States has been designed for the purposes of maximizing third-party payment and thus hospital reimbursement, the charge for a service may be very different from the true costs of the resources that are actually consumed in providing it. Hospital overhead and other shared expenses usually are allocated systematically and are not necessarily allocated according to the way the overhead is actually used.

In Scenario 3, it is likely that the external consultants will be asked to evaluate the potential cost savings and the reduction in revenue that would result from eliminating a patient care service. Since charges do not accurately reflect the average cost of providing a service, the expenses would not necessarily be saved if the service were not provided. The only costs that would be saved if the service were not given to a particular patient are the costs that are incurred by providing that one additional unit of service. For example, a clinical laboratory in a hospital that reduces the number of laboratory tests it performs will save only the portion of its expenses that would have been added by each additional test (e.g., the cost of the reagents). The laboratory will not save expenses that are incurred independent of the number of tests performed (e.g., purchasing expensive pieces of equipment) if only a few tests are eliminated. These costs are described as *variable costs* because they vary with the volume of services provided. In contrast to variable costs, another set of costs is incurred regardless of the volume of services. These are described as *fixed costs.* The expensive equipment that a clinical laboratory might purchase, such as a multichannel autoanalyzer, are examples of fixed costs. The elimination of a few laboratory tests will not reduce the expense that was incurred in buying the equipment.

In calculating the savings that a hospital might enjoy if it were able to reduce the frequency with which a drug is given, fixed and variable costs should be distinguished. Only the variable costs will be avoided. For example, a laminar flow ventilation hood is required in the pharmacy for sterile product preparation whether a few or many units of a particular drug are dispensed. The cost of the hood is independent of volume and, therefore, can be described as a fixed cost. Other costs may be incurred as a result of the initiation of a new program (e.g., hiring new pharmacy technicians to prepare and deliver sterile products) but remain independent of the volume of activity once the program has been set up (within limits, of course). A very large increase in the number of patients requiring parenteral drugs might require hiring another technician. Other costs of drug administration may be variable, such as the number of intravenous piggyback bags that contain a dose of an antibiotic. The more doses that are administered, the larger will be the number of bags used. Other costs are not so simply variable. If the number of doses that need to be prepared is decreased, will the pharmacy be able to employ fewer people? Because reductions in costs such as personnel require relatively large decreases in volume, they are often described as *stepped-variable* costs. In reviewing the economic impact of any service, it is important to be sure that the assumptions of certain costs as variable and others as fixed costs are acceptable.

SCENARIO 4

Joan has been serving as the clinical coordinator for the department of pharmacy in a 500-bed hospital for more than 9 years. She provides clinical services to patients admitted to the general medicine service, manages clinical programs for the department, and is responsible for the continued professional development of 12 clinical pharmacists. Joan is a member of the pharmacy and therapeutics committee, the nutrition support committee, and an ad hoc committee to improve the patient discharge process. She also chairs the hospital's smoking-cessation campaign.

This morning Joan began her day like every other. She got to the office early to review her scheduled appointments:

7:00–8:30 a.m.	Patient care rounds
9:00–9:30 a.m.	Meet with architect to review pharmacy office renovation
11:00–12:00 noon	Pharmacy leadership meeting
12:15–1:00 p.m.	Third-year medical student lecture
2:00–2:30 p.m.	Meet with vendor to discuss TPN deliveries
3:00–4:00 p.m.	Mark's performance review

TPN, Total parenteral nutrition.

MANAGING HUMAN CAPITAL

The role of any hospital pharmacy manager is complicated by his or her broad span of responsibility. Managers are expected to allocate hospital resources, supervise professionals and nonprofessionals, control drug distribution, and influence prescribing. These middle managers accomplish their goals by cultivating relationships in multiple dimensions. They relate to superiors as a subordinate: They take orders. They relate to their team as a superior: They direct. And they relate to peers in the organization as their equal: They cooperate. Pierpaoli (1987) contends that hospital pharmacy managers must be "bilingual." He believes that managers must effectively relate to two major (and at times competing) organizational constituencies within the hospital: the hospital's corporate administration (for day-to-day management) and the medical staff and patients (for issues related to drug use and control). The "bilingual" manager must be able to span the boundaries of professional ideology and bureaucratic necessity. The successful pharmacy manager must participate in multiple pairs of "bilingual" communication every day to ensure that the department meets its goals while maintaining its flexibility.

Effective hospital pharmacy managers are, above all, good leaders. Shortell (1985) described a new management paradigm for high-performing health care organizations that puts the focus on leadership through the development of one's subordinates. He maintains that hospitals should be organized to maximize learning, that is, to push information down to the lowest possible level. He suggests that organizations should exhibit a loose coherence, where members are allowed considerable autonomy while coordinating individual contributions. He believes that employees must be held to the overall goals and mission of the organization while they are allowed to experiment and try novel approaches to solving problems.

Pharmacy clinicians and managers must develop sound leadership qualities if they are to succeed in today's hospital environment. Good leaders are intelligent, flexible, creative, enthusiastic, socially and psychologically mature, willing to take risks, and good communicators (Bennis, 2003). While most hospitals do not have formal educational programs for those interested in becoming department heads, well-managed departments do include leadership training in their staff development plans. A department's success depends ultimately on the motivation and competence of its employees. And it is the responsibility of the department managers to ensure their competence.

Today's workforce is the best educated and best informed in history. Many of these graduates are investing another year or two in residency or fellowship programs or both. Young people who have devoted so much time and effort to preparing for a career will not be satisfied with assigned jobs with narrow responsibilities that are performed under close supervision. What they want is to have a positive influence on the outcomes of patient care in an environment that values quality and continued learning. The worry is that the pharmacist workforce will not expand fast enough to meet patients' needs (Knapp 2002). Successful departments of pharmacy are able to attract and retain competent personnel and to use those staff members to respond creatively to the needs of patient care.

The primary duties and responsibilities of clinical pharmacists vary among hospitals. A representative job description is included in Fig. 33-3. Most hospital pharmacists are responsible for supervising drug distribution, providing patient-specific clinical services, educating students and residents, conducting research, and administering the programs of the department. While pharmacists will continue to have ultimate responsibility for drug distribution and drug control activities, certified pharmacy technicians should carry out as many of these functions as is permitted by law. This will free the major portion of pharmacists' time for clinical services. Further, drug distribution should be automated and mechanized to as great an extent as possible.

Pharmacy managers should consider the mission of the department to determine the composition of the workforce needed. This human resources plan usually allows for (1) identification of the right number of people with the proper skills that will be needed, (2) acquiring or training and developing the people who will be needed, and (3) motivating them to achieve their highest level of performance and become long-term employees. Pharmacy managers should consider that clinical services become more specialized as they expand. A mature clinical program requires pharmacists with more advanced and specialized training or experience or both.

One of the most important duties of a manager is to work with employees to develop them in such a way that they better meet the needs of the department while fulfilling their own desires and ambitions. Periodic written evaluations of an employee's skills and accomplishments should be performed. Employees should be encouraged to make self-assessments of their assets and to develop a career plan. Through discussions between the employee and manager, a development plan can be devised to help the department accomplish its

JOB TITLE:	**Clinical Pharmacist**	**GRADE:**
DEPARTMENT:	**Pharmacy**	**JOB CODE:**
FLSA:	**Exempt**	**DATE:**
REPORTS TO:	**Pharmacy Practice Manager**	**APPROVED BY:**

I. GENERAL SUMMARY:

Clinical pharmacists (CPs) work closely with other health practitioners to meet the various needs of patients. They improve the health of patients by providing pharmaceutical care to individual patients and by serving as a resource to physicians, nurses, and other health professionals. Clinical pharmacists provide leadership by facilitating the development, implementation, and maintenance of hospital and departmental systems that promote desirable patient outcomes. They educate students, interns, residents, nurses and patients , and they participate in drug therapy research. Pharmacists review and approve medication orders, monitor drug therapies, and provide drug information. Pharmacists supervise and direct support personnel. In the absence of the pharmacy manager, a clinical pharmacy specialist may be required to assume the essential responsibilities and perform the duties of the pharmacy manager.

II. PRINCIPAL DUTIES AND FUNCT IONS:

A. Education, Training and Development

1. Provide continuing education for the hospital's professional staffs (e.g., pharmacists, physicians, nurses).
2. Serve as preceptor for co-operative education students and pharmacy interns.
3. Serve as a preceptor for Doctor of Pharmacy students.
4. Educate other health care providers by publishing drug information articles in the pharmacy newsletter.

B. Policy and Procedure Development and Maintenance

1. Identify the need for, and create new policies and procedures.

C. Formulary Review and Maintenance

1. Participate in periodic reviews of therapeutic classes of drugs and present findings to the Pharmacy and Therapeutics Committee and others.
2. Prepare and present to the appropriate committees evidence-based reviews of drugs requested for formulary addition.
3. Initiate and facilitate completion of drug use evaluations.

Figure 33-3. Clinical pharmacist job description.

D. Guideline Development and Implementation

1. Participate in the development and implementation of treatment guidelines, protocols and clinical pathways.
2. Monitor compliance with treatment guidelines, protocols and clinical pathways and present findings to the appropriate committees.

E. Ensure Optimal Drug Therapy

1. Participate in the development of departmental drug-specific and population-specific initiatives.
2. Detect and report medication errors and adverse drug reactions in a timely manner.
3. Provide clinical consultation to physicians, nurses and pharmacists.
4. Provide accurate, adequate and timely drug information to the hospital's professional staff.
5. Conduct medication history interviews, reconcile patients' medication therapies and provide drug information to patients and their families.
6. Document in the medical record patient evaluations and recommendations, medication reconciliation and medication histories.
7. Document pharmacist interventions according to established policies.

F. Drug Cost Management

1. Identify changes in drug usage (volume and patterns) based on published literature and hospital practices.

G. Department of Pharmacy Operational Support

1. Collaborate with other pharmacists to provide service to every patient covered by a pharmacist team. This includes weekend, holiday, evening, night and on-call coverage as described in departmental policies and procedures.

H. Department of Pharmacy Quality Programs

1. Participate by gathering and reporting data from one or more than one of the following Department of Pharmacy Quality Programs that relate to:

   i. People
   ii. Clinical excellence
   iii. Operational excellence
   iv. Financial performance and growth
   v. Safety and quality
   vi. Research

III. <u>JOB REQUIREMENTS:</u>

Clinical pharmacists must be able to work independently with minimal direct supervision. They must be able to handle frequent interruptions and adapt to changes in workload and work schedule. They must be able to set priorities, make critical decisions, and respond quickly to emergency requests. Clinical pharmacists must be able to provide a high level of service to patients in a specialty practice.

Figure 33-3. *(Continued)*

To perform this job successfully, an individual must be able to execute each duty satisfactorily and be able to use various computer systems proficiently. The candidate must be able to communicate effectively in English (orally and in writing).

IV. CREDENTIALS:

Must be a graduate of an accredited college or university with a BS in Pharmacy or a PharmD degree. The ideal candidate has a PharmD degree and has two years of related practice experience. Board certification is not required but is encouraged.

V. LICENSURE:

Licensed to practice pharmacy in the state.

VI. WORK SCHEDULE:

Full-time employment is 40 hours per week. Includes evenings, nights, weekends, and holidays as necessary.

VII. WORKING CONDITIONS:

Repetitive use of hand and fingers (e.g., use of computer keyboard). May required lifting and carrying light loads, including boxes, equipment, and stooping or kneeling. Must be able to physically operate equipment used for the job.

AMERICANS WITH DISABILITIES STATEMENT:

Must be able to perform all essential functions of this position with reasonable accommodation if disabled.

THE PROCEEDING DATA ARE INTENDED TO CONVEY INFORMATION ESSENTIAL TO MAKING FAIR PAY DECISIONS ABOUT THE JOB, AND ARE NOT EXHAUSTIVE LISTS OF THE SKILLS, EFFORTS, DUTIES, RESPONSIBLITIES OR WORKING CONDITIONS ASSOCIATED WITH IT.

Figure 33-3. *(Continued)*

business goals and the employee to grow professionally. For example, in Scenario 4, the pharmacy manager is scheduled to meet with a clinical pharmacy specialist to finalize his yearly performance evaluation. The manager and the employee recognize the need for the clinician to gain more experience speaking in public. Since the hospital is planning to institute new sedation guidelines for use in the adult intensive care unit, and since the clinical pharmacist practices in the adult ICU, the perfect opportunity exists for several goals to be met. The pharmacist agrees to present a lecture to the pharmacy and nursing staffs about conscious sedation and the new sedation guidelines.

CONCLUSION

The fundamental purpose of pharmaceutical services in a hospital is to ensure the safe and appropriate use of drugs. Fulfillment of this responsibility is enhanced through the pharmacist's involvement in all aspects of the use of drugs. These goals will be met only if the pharmacy is well organized and is staffed by professionals, all of whom work to manage the department. This chapter describes how the environment, professional relationships, regulatory agencies, practice standards, finances, and human resources influence the effectiveness of hospital pharmacy managers.

QUESTIONS FOR FURTHER DISCUSSION

1. How might some of the roles and responsibilities of hospital pharmacists identified in the chapter differ from what you envisioned or experienced thus far?
2. Do you think that you have or will acquire the skills necessary to effectively manage clinical pharmacist services in a hospital?
3. What contributions can you make toward effective patient care while holding operating budgets in check?
4. The chapter mentions issues such as the acquisition of capital and loss of various opportunities resulting from poor investment income. From what sources might a hospital acquire capital, and why is capital so important to a hospital's solvency? How can declines in investment income affect a hospital's operations and indirectly affect patient care?
5. What sorts of skills, knowledge sets, and experiences are necessary to become the manager of a hospital pharmacy department? Is this something you can see yourself doing, someday?

REFERENCES

American Society of Health-System Pharmacists (ASHP). 2009a. ASHP guidelines: Minimum standard for pharmacies in hospitals. In *Best Practices for Hospital and Health-System Pharmacy*. Bethesda, MD: American Society of Health-System Pharmacists, p. 379.

American Society of Health-System Pharmacists (ASHP). 2009b. ASHP statement on the pharmacy and therapeutics committee. In *Best Practices for Hospital and Health-System Pharmacy*. Bethesda, MD: American Society of Health-System Pharmacists, p. 126.

American Society of Health-System Pharmacists. 2011. Pharmacy practice model initiative. Available at www.ashp.org/PPMI/PPMISummit.aspx; accessed on April 25, 2011.

Barker KN, Flynn EA, Pepper AG, et al. 2002. Medication errors in 36 health care facilities. *Arch Intern Med* 162:1897.

Bates DW, Cullen DJ, Laird N, et al; the ADE Prevention Study Group. 1996. Incidence of adverse drug events and potential adverse drug events. *JAMA* 274:29.

Bates DW, Spell N, Cullen DJ, et al; the Adverse Drug Events Prevention Study Group. 1997. The costs of adverse drug events in hospitalized patients. *JAMA* 222: 307.

Bennis W. 2003. *On Becoming a Leader.* Cambridge, MA: Perseus Publishing.

Bond CA, Raehl CL, Franke T. 2000. Clinical pharmacy services, pharmacy staffing, and the total cost of care in Untied States hospitals. *Pharmacotherapy* 20: 609.

Bond CA, Raehl CL, Franke T. 2002. Clinical pharmacy services, pharmacy staffing, and medication errors in Untied States hospitals. *Pharmacotherapy* 22:134.

Bond CA, Raehl CL. 2006. Clinical pharmacy services, pharmacy staffing, and adverse drug reactions in Untied States hospitals. *Pharmacotherapy* 26:735.

Classen DC, Pestonik SL, Evans RS, et al. 1991. Computerized surveillance of adverse drug events in hospitalized patients. *JAMA* 266:2847.

Classen DC, Pestotnik SL, Evans RS, et al. 1997. Adverse drug events in hospitalized patients: Excess length of stay, extra costs, and attributable mortality. *JAMA* 277:301.

Cullen DJ, Bates DW, Small SD, et al. 1995. The incident reporting system does not detect adverse events. *Jt Comm J Qual Improv* 21:541.

Doloresco F, Fominaya C, Schumock GT, et al. 2011. Projecting future drug expenditures – 2011. *Am J Health Syst Pharm* 68:e1.

Hepler CD, Strand LM. 1990. Opportunities and responsibilities in pharmaceutical care. *Am J Hosp Pharm* 47:533.

Knapp DA. 2002. Professionally determined need for pharmacy services in 2020. *Am J Pharm Educ* 66:421.

Kohn LT, Corrigan JM, Donaldson MS. 1999. *To Err Is Human: Building a Safer Helath System.* Washington, DC: Institute of Medicine.

Leape LL. 1994. Error in medicine. *JAMA* 272:1851.

Leape LL. 2002. Reporting of adverse events. *N Engl J Med* 347:1633.

Leape LL, Brenan TA, Laird N, et al. 1991. The nature of adverse events in hospitalized patients: Results of the Harvard medial practice study II. *N Engl J Med* 324: 377.

Leape LL, Bates DW, Cullen DJ, et al; the ADE Prevention Study Group. 1995. Systems analysis of adverse drug events. *JAMA* 274:35.

Pierpaoli PG. 1987. Management diplomacy: Myths and methods. *Am J Hosp Pharm* 44:297.

Poon EG, Cina JL, Churchill W, et al. 2006. Medication dispensing errors and potential adverse drug events before and after implementing bar code technology in the pharmacy. *Ann Intern Med* 145:426.

Shortell SM. 1985. High-performing health care organizations: Guidelines for the pursuit of excellence. *Hosp Health Serv Adm* 30:8.

Stelfox HT, Palmisani S, Scurlock C, et al. 2006. The "To Err is Human" report and the patient safety literature. *Qual Saf Health Care* 15:174.

Strand LM, Guerrero RM, Nickman NA, Morley PC. 1990. Integrated patient-specific model of pharmacy practice. *Am J Hosp Pharm* 47:550.

The Joint Commission. 2010. *2011 Comprehensive Accreditation Manual for Hospitals (CAMH): The Official Handbook.* Oakbrook Terrace, IL: Joint Commission Resources.

Vermeulen LC, Rough SS, Thielhe TS, et al. 2007. Strategic approach for improving the medication-use process in health-systems: The high-performance pharmacy practice framework. *Am J Health Syst Pharm* 64:1699.

Zelmer WA. 1986. Perspectives on Hilton Head. *Am J Hosp Pharm* 43:1439.

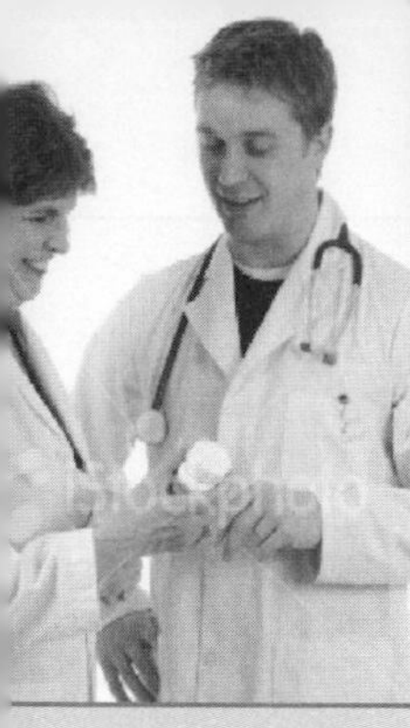

34

APPLICATIONS IN MANAGED AND SPECIALTY ENVIRONMENTS

Mark Siracuse

About the Authors: Dr. Siracuse is Associate Professor, Department of Pharmacy Sciences, School of Pharmacy and Health Professions, Creighton University. He received a BS in pharmacy for the University of Connecticut, a Pharm.D. from the University of Michigan, and an M.S. and Ph.D. in Social and Administrative Pharmacy from the University of Minnesota. Dr. Siracuse completed a fellowship in pharmacoeconomics with the PRIME Institute at the University of Minnesota, Hoechst Marion Roussel, and Aetna Pharmacy Management. Dr. Siracuse teaches courses in U.S. health care systems, pharmacy practice management, and pharmacoeconomics. His research interests include economic and public policy issues related to pharmaceuticals, patient safety, health information technology, pharmacy student issues and medication therapy management. Dr. Siracuse won the school's scholarly achievement award in 2008 and is a member of Creighton University's Institutional Review Board. In 2011–2012, he participated in the Academic Leadership Fellows Program of the American Association of Colleges of Pharmacy.

LEARNING OBJECTIVES

After completing this chapter, readers should be able to

1. Discuss the basic functions of a pharmacy benefit manager (PBM).
2. Discuss financial relationships between PBMs and various stakeholders.
3. Identify and discuss the various roles of pharmacists working for a PBM.
4. List and discuss management and business skills required to be successful in the PBM industry.
5. Discuss specialty pharmaceutical products and the unique characteristics of specialty pharmacy providers.

SCENARIO

The following employment opportunity was recently posted on a national employment Web site for insurance companies and pharmacy benefit managers (PBMs):

Position: Manager of Clinical Pharmacy for a national managed care company

Description: This person will be responsible for leading and mentoring a formulary management team staff, managing daily formulary maintenance, and the development and maintenance of commercial and Medicare Part D formularies. The position will focus on commercial employers and set team directions, resolve problems, provide feedback and guidance to members of the team, and adopt departmental plans and priorities to address business and operational challenges. The individual will work internally with the clinical team and cross-functional business areas in the development, maintenance, and implementation of formularies. This will generally be a self-directed environment with minimal guidance. Strong analytical and communication skills are required.

Position function is researching, developing, and monitoring clinical pharmacy programs such as drug utilization review (DUR), prior authorization, health outcomes, disease state management, and specialty pharmacy programs. You will lead research for new prescription drugs or new indications for existing drugs. You are responsible for preparing drug review information for the medical director. Education and qualifications:

- Pharmacist with current license and minimum of 5 to 7 years of pharmacy experience
- Three to five years of PBM experience
- Two years working with commercial employer based contracts
- Formulary management experience preferred
- M.B.A. and/or Pharm.D. preferred

To perform the previously described job successfully, the following competencies must be demonstrated:

- Customer service: Demonstrate a commitment to responsive, high-quality service all the time by exhibiting an attitude of excellent service, ability to identify customer needs, and the use of thoughtful communication and the ability to resolve conflicts.
- Management skills: Manage workload and resources by planning, organizing, and delegating to meet deadlines and accomplish objectives while maintaining quality standards.
- Adaptability: Ability to embrace change as a necessary and desirable opportunity; flexible in dealing with different viewpoints and people with diverse backgrounds.
- Problem solving/decision making: Ability to solve problems and carry out job duties. Be able to weigh alternatives and determine a course of action.
- Communication: Ability to express thoughts and ideas both orally and in writing.
- Dependability: Demonstrate reliability and instill confidence in the ability to carry out job duties.
- Teamwork/interprofessional skills: Build and maintain working relationships with employees and customers. Cooperate to achieve common goals while demonstrating core values.

John and Susan are pharmacists considering whether to apply for this position. John graduated from pharmacy school last year and is nearing the end of a managed care residency. John believes his Pharm.D. training and the fact that he was in a unique managed care residency program make him very qualified for this position. John plans to pursue an MBA after he starts a new position with a PBM. Susan has been working in the managed care industry for 7 years and just completed her MBA at a local university. She meets or will soon meet all the education and qualification criteria and has really been reflecting on her personal strengths that are primarily superior communication skills and the ability to adapt to an everchanging business environment.

CHAPTER QUESTIONS

1. What is a PBM? Specifically, what is the function of a pharmacy benefit manager?

2. What tasks do PBMs perform?
3. How do PBMs pay pharmacies for brand name drugs and generic drugs?
4. What career options do pharmacists have in managed care and PBMs?
5. What management skills are required for a pharmacist to be successful in the managed care industry?
6. What are some specialty pharmacy products? Why are specialty pharmacy products garnering increased attention from payers and end users? What can managed care pharmacists do to optimize use and control expenditures of specialty products?

INTRODUCTION

Opportunities for pharmacists in managed care have existed for more than 30 years. Beginning in the late 1980s and early 1990s, opportunities and roles have expanded greatly, as the pharmacy benefit management (PBM) industry established itself. Today, prescription drug benefits are highly coveted and utilized by private commercial plan sponsors, as well as both major government sponsored programs, Medicare and Medicaid. A major boost to the use of PBMs occurred in 2006 with the start of Medicare Part D. Consequently, the percentage of drug expenditures now paid by a third-party entity now approaches 90 percent (West-Strum, 2009). Management of prescription drugs has become a key component of many high-cost and high-prevalence medical conditions including diabetes, hypertension, hyperlipidemia, cancer, migraine headaches, allergic rhinitis, depression, psychosis, seizure disorders, and many more. The emergence of specialty drugs (typically defined as injectable or infusible drugs used to treat chronic diseases) makes the current challenges even more acute.

BASICS OF THE PHARMACY BENEFIT MANAGER

Pharmacy benefit managers process the majority of all prescriptions claims filled in the United States. Because of their efficiencies and the highly specialized nature of pharmacy claims, PBMs process these claims for insurance companies/managed care organizations (MCOs), and the government. The pharmacy benefit is typically "carved out" to PBMs, which means they are hired as a separate service provider to perform the pharmacy benefit function in an otherwise self-contained benefit. In processing a prescription claim, PBMs must perform multiple tasks that include confirming member eligibility, checking the price of the drug billed, surveying the patient's records for potential clinical problems, and accounting for the drug transaction for both the buyer (the plan sponsor) and the seller (the pharmacy). PBMs often are paid a fee for the service they provide based on a charge for each prescription processed or a flat fee based on the number of members in the prescription plan. Other times PBMs can be paid via differentially contracting a higher price from the payer than the price paid to the pharmacy.

PBM Clients

The clients that hire a PBM are known as sponsors, or plan sponsors. In general, there are three principle PBM clients: traditional insurance companies/health plans, the government, and private employers.

Insurance Company

The traditional insurance company or managed care organization (MCO) may have a contract with a large group of employees, and that group needs medical coverage and a pharmacy benefit. Pharmacy benefit managers are, in most cases, more efficient in processing prescription claims than these entities, especially if they do not own a PBM. Pharmacy benefit managers quite often take the job of pharmacy claims administration in a "carve out" arrangement. The concept of a carved out service is common in health care and is simply a provider hired to do a highly specialized job in a comprehensive health care benefit. Other areas commonly carved out in the health care benefit include the dental, vision, and behavioral health benefits.

The Government

The government is a very large and important PBM client. This can include local, state, or federal governments. For example, a city may need pharmacy benefit coverage for its employees (e.g., employees at City Hall, the elected officials and/or law enforcement, etc.). In addition, state governments employ large numbers of persons such as state agency personnel and public officials. The federal government is a plan sponsor when a PBM is hired to provide pharmacy claims administration for a program such as the Department of Defense, which has approximately 1.6 million employees (US Office of Personnel Management, 2011).

In addition to government employees, both Medicare Part D and Medicaid beneficiaries are large users of PBM services. In 2009, nearly 45 percent of all prescriptions filled were covered under either a Medicaid program or Medicare Part D (West-Strum, 2009). Most state Medicaid plans contract with a PBM to provide services that are commonly seen with PBMs, including, but not limited to, claims adjudication, formulary management, and prior authorization. In 2007, there were over 58 million people enrolled in a state Medicaid program (KFF, 2007), and as of February 2010, approximately 60 percent of eligible Medicare beneficiaries (≈27.7 million people) were enrolled in a Medicare Part D plan administered by a PBM (KFF, 2010).

Employers

Employers run the spectrum of size from the owner of a three-employee business up to the largest public companies that employ hundreds of thousands of persons. In general, smaller employers with fewer than one or two hundred employees will go to an insurance company and the insurance company will provide for all the small business' health coverage in exchange for a regular premium payment. Many times that insurance company will subcontract with a PBM to administer the pharmacy benefit. In the case of larger sponsors, companies may go directly to a PBM and contract on their own behalf.

PBM Tasks

Pharmacy benefit managers have the infrastructure necessary to make pharmacy benefit cards work. While PBMs perform many functions, the core competency is clearly claims processing, or more precisely, claims adjudication. In addition to claims adjudication, the following PBM tasks will be described here: (1) contracting with pharmacy providers; (2) formulary development; (3) drug utilization review; and (4) communication with sponsor, plan members, and pharmacies.

Claims Adjudication

Claims adjudication entails the transmission of electronic claims from the pharmacy filling the prescription to a PBM and back again. The pharmacy filling the prescription transmits the claim to the PBM processor where the claim is verified as belonging to an eligible member. In addition, an algorithm determines whether the drug is eligible on the member's plan. A PBM's software determines the drug price consistent with the sponsor's contract. Clinical checks are made, such as allergies and drug–drug interactions. The processor also checks other rules specified in the sponsor's contract, such as the allowed days supply of the drug being dispensed and allowed time between refills (e.g., is the controlled substance lasting as long as the directions specify?). A PBM will transmit the prescription approval back to the pharmacy, complete with the amount the PBM has approved to pay the pharmacy and the co-payment to collect from the member at the pharmacy counter. If there is a problem (e.g., early refill or member ineligible), the PBM will transmit to the pharmacy what is wrong with the claim. Finally, PBMs record and charge the prescription to the correct sponsor and record the amount of payment due to the pharmacy.

Contracting with Pharmacy Providers

Pharmacy benefit managers also must assemble a network of pharmacies across the nation to provide pharmacy service throughout a PBM's trade area. In general, most PBMs operate on a national scope and have contracts with most of the over 60,000 retail pharmacies in America (NACDS, 2010). Keep in mind that PBMs contract with pharmacies for a reimbursement rate that may be different from the rate that is charged to the plan sponsor.

Formulary Development

Another important job in the pharmacy benefit is developing a list of drugs approved for use by the plan members and their physicians. This list of approved drugs is known as a formulary. Because of the need to accommodate a wide range of medical conditions, the formulary must be quite extensive. Therefore, a PBM's formulary will have drugs from nearly every therapeutic category.

Drug Utilization Review

As mentioned in the claims adjudication paragraph, PBMs monitor prescription claims for clinical appropriateness. This process is known as drug utilization review (DUR), which can add significant value to the pharmacy benefit by alerting the pharmacist to potential problems. A PBM's computer program checks for potential drug allergies, potential interactions between a new prescription and drugs a patient might be taking, and health problems that might be exacerbated when a patient takes an inappropriate drug (e.g., a decongestant in a patient with hypertension). There are also checks to guard against patients taking duplicate drugs in a therapeutic class (e.g., two angiotensin receptor-blockers) that may occur when a patient receives prescriptions from both their cardiologist and internist. Further, if the patient is "doctor-shopping" and using the prescription card for questionable purposes, a PBM might send the pharmacy a warning such as "opiates from multiple prescribers."

Communication with Sponsors, Plan Members and Pharmacies

Pharmacy benefit managers are the central point of communication for stakeholders. PBMs maintain the eligibility file and make updates based on the authorization of the sponsor (or their agent). PBMs usually have online tools for conveying general information and to help members select drugs on the approved drug list and find convenient pharmacies. In addition, PBMs have secure sites for plan-specific information. For example, the sponsor's designee may log in to a site to confirm that changes in the eligibility files were made in a timely fashion.

Billing and payment information also flows through a PBM to the sponsor and pharmacy providers. A PBM will bill the sponsor, usually every 10 to 14 days, by sending notice of the amount of the bank draft that will be going from the sponsor to a PBM for claims filled in that pay period. After a PBM receives the sponsor's payment, they then pay the pharmacies and send an itemization of the claims paid to each pharmacy. The pharmacies can then reconcile the itemized list, commonly called the remittance advice, to determine any discrepancies.

Plan members frequently receive communication from PBMs. A correspondence might suggest that the patient talk with their physician about a generic alternative to their current therapy. In addition, promotional material may encourage the member to use a PBM-owned, mail-order pharmacy for maintenance prescriptions. Finally, PBMs may send letters to physicians as well as the member encouraging a medication change to a generic or preferred brand name.

Compensation to PBMs

Compensation for this service provided by PBMs varies depending on the revenue model. In many cases, PBMs charge a specified per-transaction fee. This fee can range from approximately \$1.00–\$5.00/Rx, depending on the provider PBM. In other cases, PBMs might want to avoid the perception that they are incentivized to do as many transactions as possible; in this case, the PBM will bill the sponsor a fee based on a per-employee-per-month (PEPM) basis. So, if the sponsor had 1000 employees in the plan, there would be a regular charge to the sponsor by the PBM each month to compensate the PBM for the services provided. If each employee household had on average 2.3 persons, that monthly charge would cover the PBM service to adjudicate prescriptions for all covered dependents in each household. Another payment mechanism is a per-member-per-month (PMPM) fee in which PBMs collect a regular monthly fee for each employee and dependent. So in the example of 1000 employee households with 2.3 covered members per household the PBM would collect the fee times 2300 (1000 households × 2.3 persons/household/month).

Some sponsors feel that a fixed regular fee, whether the per-prescription fee, the PEPM, or PMPM, is too expensive. These sponsors tend to prefer the "traditional" PBM compensation arrangement. The traditional model is one in which a PBM contracts differentially and makes a positive margin between the amount they pay the pharmacies that fill the prescriptions and the amount that the sponsor is charged. The sponsor does escape a regular and expensive PBM administration charge. However, the sponsor is now in a situation in which they know a PBM is making a positive albeit unknown margin. The positive margin between what the pharmacy is paid and the sponsor is billed is known as spread pricing (Garis and Clark, 2004; Siracuse et al., 2008). This is a very significant issue in the pharmacy benefit, and it is the source of considerable controversy.

Payments from PBMs to Pharmacies—Brand Name Drugs

A PBM contracts with the sponsors needing the prescription benefit and makes separate contracts with the pharmacies that supply the service. Typically, PBM payment to pharmacies is in two components: (1) reimbursement for the ingredient cost of the drug dispensed and (2) the pharmacy dispensing fee. These payment terms are depicted as follows:

Cost of the drug dispensed + Pharmacy dispensing fee = Total pharmacy reimbursement

If a pharmacist dispenses a brand name prescription and the reimbursement for the drug ingredient is \$84 and the pharmacy dispensing fee (or professional fee) is \$2, then total reimbursement to the pharmacy is \$86:

Cost of the brand drug dispensed + Pharmacy dispensing fee = Total pharmacy reimbursement
\$84 + \$2 = \$86

There is variation in the prices that pharmacies pay for the drugs they purchase because there are many drug wholesalers and many different sized pharmacy operations—some with the volume of thousands of stores and others with single pharmacy units. The likelihood of every pharmacist paying the exact amount for any given drug is not very high. Therefore, if every pharmacy turned their actual acquisition cost (AAC) for every drug submitted for reimbursement, a PBM's ability to check a price for acceptability against the sponsor contract would be difficult and not easily automated. For this reason, PBMs have instead used a discount off the drug average wholesale price (AWP) to determine the pharmacist reimbursement for brand name drugs. The AWP prices are widely available in commercial drug pricing databases. The electronic availability of the AWP data allows ingredient cost reimbursement to be automated. PBMs select a discount off AWP that is acceptable to pharmacists and reasonably approximates the AAC.

AWP is considered very much like an automobile "sticker" price for drugs that is reported by manufacturers and published in commercial print and electronic databases by data vendors First DataBank, Medi-Span and Redbook. Almost all pharmacists contracting with a PBM will be offered a contract of, perhaps, AWP 6 percent for brand-name drug reimbursement. So, in the example, AWP for the drug dispensed was \$100 less a 16 percent discount made the ingredient cost reimbursement \$84 (\$100 ×0.84).

Cost of the brand drug dispensed + Pharmacy dispensing fee = Total pharmacy reimbursement
\$84 + \$2 = \$86
Drug AWP \$100

Estimated acquisition cost (EAC) contract terms:
AWP 16 percent
\$100 − 16 percent = \$84

A PBM determines through market research and contracting experience with pharmacies that the pharmacist will, in most cases, accept terms of AWP-16 percent.

Since PBMs estimate terms to serve as a proxy for actual ingredient cost, the terms are frequently called the estimated acquisition cost, or EAC. The EAC should provide the pharmacist with full reimbursement and a small amount of profit. So, if a pharmacy is able to buy the product for AWP-17 percent, the pharmacy would make 1 percent of AWP = \$100 or \$1. The difference between the EAC, and the pharmacy's AAC is called the "AWP differential" or "earned discount."

Table 34-1. Atenolol 50 mg Pricing

AWP	$0.84/tablet
Pharmacist AAC (est.)	$0.025/tablet
MAC price by PBM	$0.10/tablet
Profit per tablet (est.)	$0.075/tablet

Payments from PBMs to Pharmacies—Generic Drugs

Instead of paying pharmacies a discount off AWP price for generics, PBMs pay a maximum allowable cost (MAC) for generic drugs. This schedule of generic drug prices is commonly called the MAC list. MAC lists are used by PBMs, MCOs, and State Medicaid Departments to put a cap on the amount that will be paid for generic drugs with three or more distributors. The MAC prices are developed by PBMs and are intended to be the lowest price that the pharmacy will, in most cases, accept.

In Table 34-1, the AWP for atenolol 50 mg is $0.84 per tablet; however, the pharmacist can buy the drug for approximately 2–3 cents per tablet. A PBM sets the MAC price very close to the actual acquisition price with just enough over the cost to get pharmacy participation. In this case, the PBM will pay the pharmacist approximately 10 cents a tablet. This will allow the pharmacist to make 7 to 8 cents on each tablet dispensed.

No matter what distributor a pharmacy uses or how much a product costs the pharmacist, they will only be paid 10 cents per tablet, unless the physician had explicitly written "Brand Name Necessary" or "Dispense as Written" on the prescription. MAC pricing list is clearly a strong incentive for the pharmacist to use generic drugs whenever available and to be careful and shrewd purchasers of generic drugs, seeking the lowest priced-goods from reputable generic drug manufacturers.

CAREER OPTIONS IN PBMs

Clinical Pharmacy Services

Pharmacists with strong clinical abilities and the ability to communicate effectively would likely find positions in the clinical pharmacy services area of a PBM to be best matched to their skills and training. Specific clinical areas or departments include formulary development and management, drug information, prior authorization of expensive and specialty drugs, drug utilization review, and disease management. Formulary development and management requires a pharmacist to constantly be informed about the latest drug therapies and the ability to compare these recent discoveries with currently available products. Comparison of products is done first and foremost with a clinical focus in mind. If a new drug product is deemed clinically superior to existing products, the costs of these drugs is compared along with the clinical outcomes in a cost-effectiveness analysis (Bootman et al., 2005, p. 83). In these types of analyses, the cost of therapy is divided by the clinical effect of that therapy (e.g., percent decrease in LDL cholesterol) to determine the most cost-effective therapy. A key function of the formulary committee is to evaluate literature where cost-effectiveness analyses have been undertaken. Pharmacists who are members of formulary committees must possess or acquire the skills to evaluate drug cost-effectiveness literature. The official name for the formulary committee is the Pharmacy and Therapeutics (P&T) Committee. The P&T Committee is comprised of several pharmacists from the PBM, plan administrators, and a physician medical director. Pharmacist members of the P&T Committee are responsible for researching new products, performing cost-effectiveness analyses on new products compared to existing products, and attending P&T Committee meetings to discuss their findings and determine the impact of those findings on which tier to place a product and whether its coverage will require prior authorization. Pharmacists also develop prior authorization protocols for drugs that are typically approved by the P&T Committee or by the medical director.

Additional activities with which pharmacists are involved include DUR and developing disease management protocols. DURs are conducted both prospectively and retrospectively. Prospective DUR involves setting up parameters such as dosing too high or drug–drug interactions that are sent to the dispensing pharmacist at the time and point of service at the moment of dispensing to alert the pharmacists of a potential problem. Retrospective DUR is performed by the clinical pharmacist reviewing claims of patients several weeks or months following dispensing of medication to track clinical problems and excess use of high cost medications. Disease management opportunities are often identified by the PBM pharmacist who might then send educational materials to certain patients.

Network Development, Contracting, and Management

Another potential area of employment for a pharmacist with the PBM industry is in the area of network development and management. PBMs form relationships with various stakeholders involved in medical and pharmacy benefits. Figure 34-1 shows the relationships and flow of money among these various stakeholders. If one follows the money trail they will be able to identify

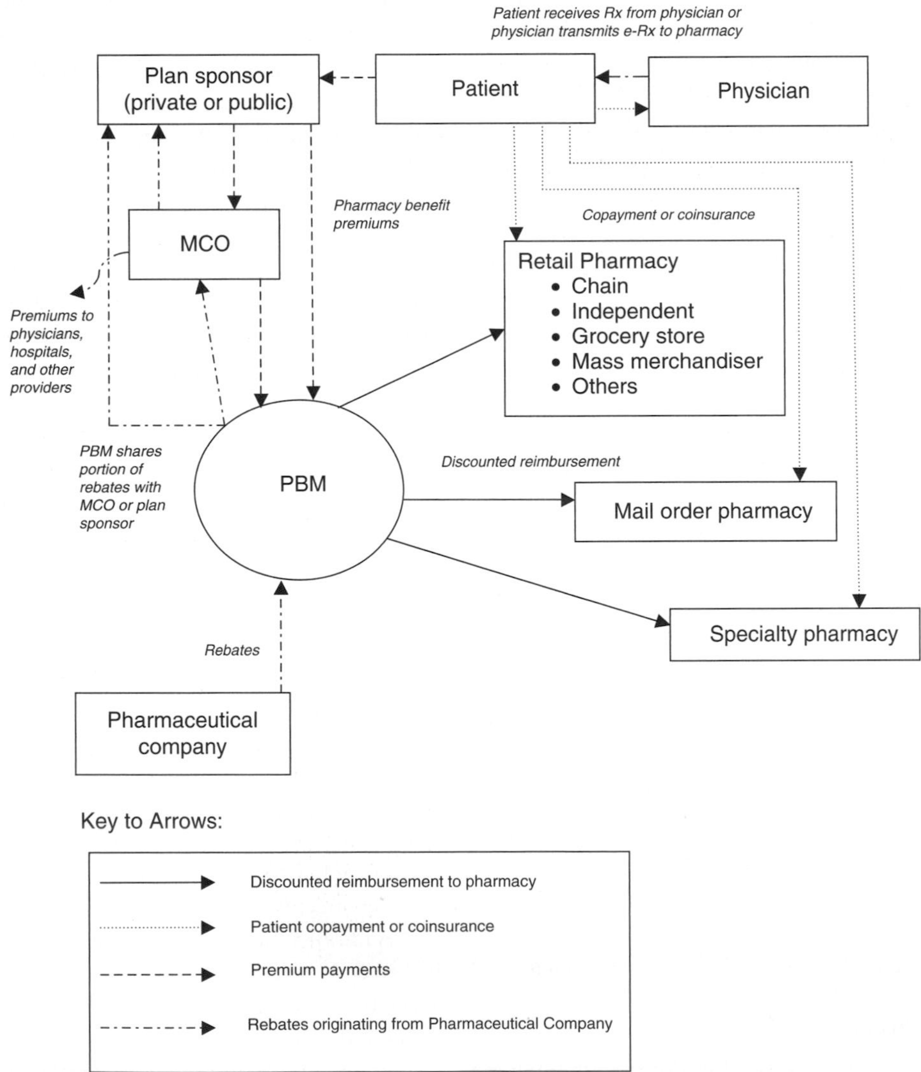

Figure 34-1. Financial relationships in managed prescription drug benefits.

entities that influence supply and demand in these markets. In the diagram, pharmacy benefit delivery is emphasized. PBMs primarily interact with plan sponsors (either public, such as Medicare, or private), dispensing pharmacies and the various pharmaceutical companies. To a lesser extent, PBMs also have interactions with patients, physicians, and other prescribers. Pharmacy network contracting and management often is overseen by a pharmacist within the PBM. In general, 85–90 percent of outpatient prescription claims adjudicated by PBMs are dispensed in community pharmacies that include traditional chains (e.g., Walgreens and CVS), supermarket pharmacies (e.g., Kroger and Supervalue), mass merchandisers (e.g., Target and Walmart), independent pharmacies, and clinic pharmacies (NACDS, 2010). The remaining prescriptions are dispensed through mail service pharmacies, most of which are associated with or owned by a PBM or one of the large chain pharmacies (Fig. 34-2). A small percentage of prescriptions are dispensed through physicians' offices. Sales of drugs at all corporate pharmacy entities (this includes traditional chain, mass merchandisers, and grocery stores) combined represented over 60 percent of the total sales in this category. As a result of this, the base for a PBM's network begins with the chain pharmacies and is supplemented with other types of pharmacies. Pharmacists at a PBM responsible for network contracting work with various pharmacies to contract for dispensing services for drugs prescribed by physicians and other prescribers to eligible members. Pharmacists contracting with PBMs must use online real time point-of-service (POS) computer systems to verify patient eligibility, drug coverage, dispensing limits or quantity limits, dispensing requirements (such as step care protocols), obtain co-payment information, and receive reimbursement information from the PBM. Pharmacies are bound by contract to dispense prescriptions in accordance with the benefit and policy coverage issues of members along with drug formulary and dispensing requirements. Pharmacy-PBM contracts will also dictate reimbursement terms based on a discount off the drug AWP for brand name drugs and MAC for generic drugs. As mentioned previously, the brand name drug's discounted AWP (often 15 percent–18 percent) approximates the actual acquisition cost by the pharmacy. A dispensing fee is usually added to calculated brand name or generic ingredient cost.

Finally, network management pharmacists are involved with provider performance issues. This usually includes audits of pharmacies to look for patterns of fraudulent billing of dispensed drugs. Fraudulent billing problems include billing for products that are not dispensed and billing for a brand name drug while dispensing the generic version. Billing for very high-priced drugs, typically thousands of dollars, may also trigger a pharmacy audit by a PBM. Audits typically

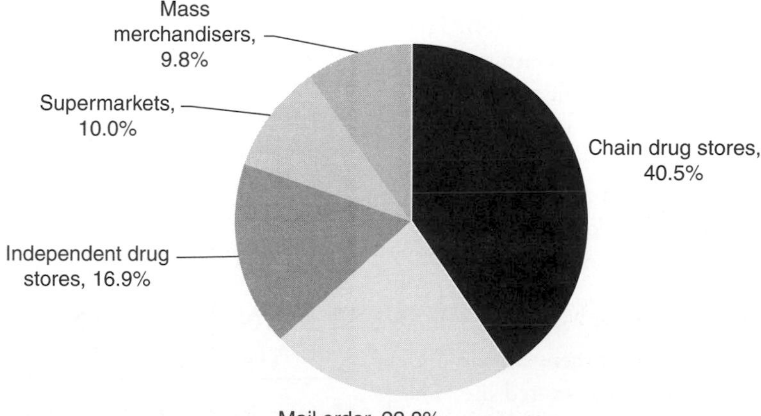

Figure 34-2. Retail pharmacy prescription drug sales, $269.9 billion in 2009 by type of store. (*Source:* NACDS 2010–2011 Chain Industry Profile.)

are carried out using computer algorithms to detect improper billing patterns. Audits also may be conducted by a PBM's audit team (often headed by a pharmacist) in the actual pharmacy being audited.

Sales and Marketing

Sales and marketing is a third area in which pharmacists are hired to work. In this situation, the PBM is trying to market and sell its pharmacy benefit package to prospective plan sponsors, including employers, government entities, MCOs, and government-sponsored programs. When marketing pharmacy benefits to potential plan sponsors, pharmacists working in a PBM must have a sophisticated understanding of drug prices, marketing channels, promotion, and the increasing use of technology including Web sites, the Internet, and blogs (Navarro, 2009, p. 58).

As plan sponsors have become more knowledgeable about drug pricing, they are looking for PBMs to tell them specific information about how the drug is priced. They will look for information on how the AWP is calculated and whether or not the lowest possible MAC rate is being applied for generic drugs. Sponsors will want to know if there is spread pricing, or if everything gets passed through to the pharmacy (Garis et al., 2004; Garis and Clark 2004; Siracuse et al., 2008). *Spread pricing* has been defined as "the difference between the amount billed to the employer by the PBM and the amount paid to the dispensing pharmacy for the same line item" (Garis and Clark, 2004). This can occur when a PBM contracts with pharmacies at a lower price than was negotiated with the plan sponsor. Savvy employers will insist that this type of arrangement is not occurring and that all discounts and cost savings that PBMs negotiate with the pharmacies be passed along to the employer. Employers also will want to know the percentage of rebate dollars that PBMs share with plan sponsors (Garis et al., 2004). Employers also should be asking PBMs what other sources of revenue it has and whether or not there are administrative fees either per claim or per covered life. The more competitive the market for pharmacy benefits, the more challenging it is to market a PBM benefit package to a plan sponsor.

Advertising for a PBM may be complex. Trade magazines that target executives in human resource positions offer a marketing avenue to a wide audience of decision makers, so it is common to see PBM advertisements in these publications. Another marketing avenue is employer-focused meetings and conferences. Pharmacists working in sales and marketing for PBMs may have the opportunity to give formal presentations at these national meetings. These meetings provide a PBM pharmacist an opportunity to promote their PBM in a way that shows a focus on real world solutions to pharmacy benefit costs that always seem to be escalating.

Pharmacists' Roles in PBM Marketing

In recent years, many pharmacists have obtained advanced degrees in business administration, which enhances their ability to be involved in various marketing aspects (Navarro, 2009, p. 69). The combination of advanced clinical knowledge regarding drug therapy with business acumen allows a PBM pharmacist to become subject matter experts to sales and marketing personnel. The managed care pharmacist may be involved in providing strategic analysis of market pricing a PBM's services, developing market-competitive pharmacy programs, developing marketing materials, joining the marketing team on sales calls to potential or existing clients, leading a marketing team, and participating in the contract negotiation process with new and existing clients. Pharmacists in a marketing position at a PBM need to have or develop skill sets that are generally not emphasized during their pharmacy education. In these highly competitive situations, strong speaking and writing skills are essential for success. Strong business and analytical skills are also important for pharmacists to be able to discuss the advantages and disadvantages of various benefit options.

MANAGING IN A MANAGED CARE ENVIRONMENT

Human Resource Management

Pharmacists working in managed care environments (e.g., PBMs) who possess the right skills are often promoted to management positions in charge of others in the company, including pharmacists and other personnel. Therefore, knowledge and ability to implement various aspects of human resource management is essential. Many of these topics have been discussed in detail in other chapters in this book. This section briefly will cover recruitment, training and development, performance appraisals, and pay decisions from the perspective of a PBM or similar organization.

Recruitment for various positions can either be external or internal (Bateman and Snell, 1996, p. 291; Longest and Darr, 2008, p. 448). As demonstrated in the chapter scenario, recruitment for professional and high-level positions often conducted through an external search process. External recruitment brings new thoughts and ideas into a company, which may inspire innovation. Internal recruitment encourages employees to remain with the company, work hard, and aspire to reach higher-level positions.

Training and development efforts are essential to ensure that employee skills in PBMs are continually upgraded (Bateman and Snell, 1996, p. 300; Longest and Darr, 2008, p. 450). PBMs should look to provide their employees training based upon their current skill level as compared to desired skills. The type of training that may be necessary includes development of management skills, communication skills, supervisory skills, customer service relation skills, sales skills, and basic computer skills. Examples of training include role-playing, lectures, business simulation, conferences, and job rotation. Role-playing is a great way for employees to learn interviewing skills, customer service or telephone training, leadership skills, and multicultural awareness. Business simulations require the participant to be actively involved in their learning, the notion being that if you physically do something, then you are more likely to remember it. Business simulations help individuals and groups develop problem-solving skills. Lectures and conferences are a great way to transfer a large amount of information to a large number of employees. The problem is that most lectures and conferences are not active learning, and consequently, the material that is presented in the lecture is not retained by the employee. All types of learners retain more material when they are involved in active learning activities. Job rotation is great for management succession planning. Job rotation allows the employee to gain a broad perspective of the organization and gets employees thinking about the prospect of job promotion. Job rotation is also a good way to provide stimulation for a burned out employee.

Performance appraisal and feedback is an essential part of any manager's job. An MBO system is seen often in managed care environments. A reward system (e.g., pay raises) is necessary to motivate and retain people (Bateman and Snell, 1996, p. 304). The manager of a PBM can determine pay raises by starting with the results of an employee's MBO evaluation. In a merit-based pay system, those employees who perform at the highest level should expect the largest pay increase (Fried and Fottler, 2008, p. 298).

Motivation

If a pharmacist wants to succeed in the PBM industry, it is important to develop leadership skills to motivate people in their department or company (Bateman and Snell, 1996, p. 356; Longest and Darr, 2008, p. 533). First, it is important to recognize that a leader influences others to attain goals. Leaders generally have the following traits or skills: drive or endeavor, integrity or character, great communication skills, great people skills, and finally, an inner self-confidence. Leaders who transform their department or organizations are able to do this through charisma, providing individual attention to followers, intellectual stimulation, forming and communicating their vision, and having positive self-regard.

Managing Teams

In the PBM environment, pharmacists often are working in a team or group environment. As in the scenario pharmacists may be asked to manage or lead a group of people. These teams often consist of other professionals (e.g., pharmacists and nurses), and they may also be working with nonhealth care professionals who have degrees and training in business and other fields. Managing in a team environment has its set of challenges. Pharmacists are generally trained and have the mindset of individualism, so for many, the team environment is likely an adjustment in work philosophy. Teams that thrive usually require participatory leadership styles (Bateman and Snell, 1996, p. 410). Teams also require their members to complement one another, so the leader needs to understand this and form teams that will ultimately be effective in reaching the organization's goals. Members of effective teams are committed to performance goals, committed to a common purpose and approach to the work that needs to be done, and hold themselves accountable to one another.

Whether you are managing a team of clinical pharmacists or a team of sales and marketing people in a PBM, it is essential to create a team with a high performance focus and a common purpose that is intrinsically motivating. The common purpose of the sales and marketing team is to attract new clients with many members. Team members could share strategies they use to effectively win new contracts. Providing rewards based on team performance is a good way to reward teams that work well together and are productive (Fried and Fottler, 2008, p. 264). The team leader should work toward a common understanding of how the team will accomplish its tasks, making it very clear that everyone must work hard and contribute in a tangible way. Team member selection should ensure that appropriate people are selected for the team. For the team member to fully contribute to the effort, training may be necessary. The team approach requires inward and outward management. When conflicts arise within a team, the leader and members should understand five basic interpersonal approaches to managing it: avoidance, accommodation, compromise, forcing, and collaboration. Conflicts are natural products of group dynamics that arise for many reasons, including ambiguity, competition for scarce resources, differing perspectives, and time horizons that are not congruent. The good team leader needs to recognize these interpersonal situations and use one of the approaches mentioned, depending on the situation.

Communication

PBMs likely employ hundreds or even thousands of people with a variety of backgrounds and experiences. The need for a pharmacist in a management or leadership position to communicate effectively, both verbally and in writing, is essential (Longest and Darr, 2008, p. 571). A clinical pharmacy manager often has inward communication issues with other professionals and outward communication issues that may be with health care professionals as well as other constituents. Pharmacists who want to be successful in this environment need to work at being a better speaker and writer. If public speaking is not one's strength, then it is imperative that training occurs. When preparing and practicing a presentation, consider your audience, your credibility, and the best way to get your message across. Practice writing, be critical of your writing, and do not be afraid to revise if necessary. Realize that communication occurs in all directions. Make sure that your message is relevant for your audience and is not overwhelming (in other words, avoid information overload). Some tips for communicating include (Phillips, 1992, p. 154, 161, 169):

- Realize that extemporaneous speaking is your avenue to the public.
- Prepare yourself thoroughly for your public speaking engagements.
- When appropriate, it is okay to be repetitive for emphasis or clarity.
- Try to couple written or electronic documents with verbal discussions, thereby catching the idea with two senses rather than just one. It is likely that you and everyone involved will remember the issues better.
- Speak in simple and familiar strains with people, without any pretension of superiority. Leave people with the feeling that they have known you all their lives.
- Do not forget that judicieus use of humor is a major component of your ability to persuade people.

- Remember that people are more easily influenced through the medium of a broad and humorous illustration than in any other way.
- Loyalty is more often won through private conservation than in any other way.
- Provide a clear, concise statement of the direction of your department or organization, and justify the action you take.
- Effective visions cannot be forced on your department or organization. Rather, you must set them in motion by means of persuasion.

Finally, informed communication can be a very effective way to manage departments. Many managers use managing by walking around (MBWA) as a way to informally interact and influence members of their department or division. By using MBWA, your subordinates know you come among them without fear, and it also shows them that you are seeking casual contact with them to get their input. Getting to know people and telling them interesting and insightful stories is a very effective form of communication in organizations such as PBMs.

SPECIALTY PHARMACY GOODS AND SERVICES

Specialty pharmacy products have become noticed in recent years as sophisticated, high-cost drug therapy for patients with rare or chronic conditions that result in significant morbidity. Characteristics of specialty pharmacy products include (Navarro, 2009, p. 151):

- High cost, in the range of $1,200–$1,500 per month
- Chronic disease target: cancer, multiple sclerosis, hepatitis C, hemophilia, and so on
- Reimbursement complexities—PBMs have special coverage limits for these items
- Customized dosing
- Few patients take these drugs, making it more efficient for specialized mail-order pharmacies to dispense and deliver them
- Complex delivery methods, including intramuscular and subcutaneous
- Medications that require refrigeration
- Clinical support being necessary for effective outcome of treatment regimen

One of the more difficult aspects of working with specialty pharmaceuticals is reimbursement issues. Payment can occur through either the medical benefit or the pharmacy benefit. As stated earlier, many of these products are injectable. When they are provider-administered in the physician's office, the medical benefit typically pays for them. Most self-administered injectables are paid through the pharmacy benefit. The characteristics of specialty pharmaceuticals present many challenges for community pharmacies. Consequently, specialty pharmacies and distributors emerged during the 1990s and currently serve a small but growing niche in the pharmacy marketplace.

Specialty pharmacy products began having a quiet impact on the market in the 1980s (Vanscoy, 2000). More recently, specialty drugs have been one of the fastest growing segments under the pharmacy benefit (Stern and Reissman, 2006). The reason for the growth of specialty pharmacy was mainly because these new biological agents required expensive and hard-to-manage inventory control procedures that were beyond the capability of most retail pharmacies (Adams, 2006). In 2007, the average treatment cost per patient per year for specialty drugs was about $18,000, with additional growth expected (Miller et al., 2007). Specialty drugs often are categorized into two distinct categories based on the site and administration method (Stern and Reissman, 2006). One category is self-administered injectables (SAIs) that can be administered by the patient or their caregiver. These products include Humira for rheumatoid arthritis and Nutropin for growth disorders (Stern and Reissman, 2006). The other category is commonly referred to as office administered injectables (OAIs). These products must be administered by physicians or other health care providers and include products such as Remicade for rheumatoid arthritis and Amevive for psoriasis.

Insurance payment for these products differs in that SAIs are included in the pharmacy benefit and adjudicated with a unique 11-digit number called the National Drug Code (NDC) that specifies drug manufacturer, strength, dosage form, and package size. On the other hand, OAIs are typically included in the medical benefit by most insurance payers. When drugs are billed under medical claims by physicians' offices, a Healthcare Common Procedure Coding System (HCPS) "J" code is used. "J" codes usually only identify the chemical name of the drug, not the manufacturer, strength, or package size. These billing differences can create challenges for insurers, pharmacies, and medical practices (Stern and Reissman, 2006).

Specialty pharmacy provides a unique opportunity for pharmacists who can effectively deal with medical specialists and effectively communicate with patients, providers, payers, and manufacturers. Some industry experts believe that specialty pharmaceuticals will account for the majority of drug spend by 2014 (Edlin, 2010). For example, several very costly specialty pharmaceuticals were approved in 2010, with annual therapy costs ranging from $93,000 to $200,000. (Johnson, 2010). As a result of these trends, the management of specialty pharmaceuticals products and services has become especially important (PSG, 2010). The term "specialty pharmacy management" is defined as a comprehensive and coordinated system of pharmacological care in which patients with chronic illness and complex medical conditions receive expert therapy management services tailored to meet their needs. Pharmacists in managed care settings play a key role in this area by ensuring that the goals of specialty pharmacy management programs are achieved for payers. These goals include (PSG, 2010):

1. Equalize benefits between pharmacy and medical care to avoid members choosing type of service rendered based only on coverage.
2. Optimize cost management by receiving the lowest unit cost from pharmacies and the maximum amount of rebates from manufacturers.
3. Ensure appropriate use by employing clinical guidelines and criteria, prior authorization, and formulary programs.
4. Improve clinical management by assessing and intervening on adherence, patient care services, therapy and case management, and demonstrating improved outcomes.
5. Expertly craft contracts to account for changes in the specialty pharmaceutical industry, including potentially emerging generic products.

REVISITING THE SCENARIO

The chapter's scenario is a compilation of positions that were recently posted to the AMCP Web site. Even though John does not have the years of experience that the job requires, he is very confident in his abilities and decides to apply. John is especially confident of his clinical abilities because he was a top student in his Pharm.D. class, winning several awards during his final year. John has never had any supervisory experience, and consequently, many of the necessary skills would have to be learned on the job if he were to succeed in this position. Susan has decided she needs a change to a new company to grow in her career. While Susan has been out of pharmacy school for about 12 years, her communication and people skills have allowed her to excel in the managed care arena. During her 7 years in the industry, Susan has had extensive experience in formulary management, both at the local level and nationally. She has never worked with any private employers, so this position would be a new experience for her. However, she feels that given her background and education, she is up for the challenge. The PBM decides to hire Susan based on her educational qualifications, management skills, and years of experience in the industry.

CONCLUSION

The managed care industry offers pharmacists with the right skill set an excellent opportunity to use their knowledge of drug therapy and apply it in an indirect patient care environment. Management and business skills described in this chapter are critical for a pharmacist to possess if he/she wants to be successful working for a PBM or other managed care company. Pharmacists working for a PBM are involved in many facets of these companies, including formulary development, DUR, disease state management, network contracting and management, and marketing and sales. Given that nearly 90 percent of all prescriptions are covered under some type of third party (either private or public), PBMs have a major impact on the financing and fiscal success of community retail pharmacies. Finally, specialty pharmacies have had a significant impact on the pharmaceutical market in recent years. This has created numerous opportunities for pharmacists who possess the necessary clinical abilities and can communicate well with all stakeholders involved with specialty pharmacy products.

QUESTIONS FOR FURTHER DISCUSSION

1. Given the information in the scenario regarding the requirements one needs for a position in managed care pharmacy, what steps would you take in your career to become qualified to work in this area?
2. Take a moment to envision a "typical day" for pharmacists working in a managed care environment. What do you think it would be like? How does this differ from traditional pharmacy practice in a community retail pharmacy or in a hospital pharmacy?
3. Assume you are a pharmacist working for a PBM and are asked to go with the sales and marketing team to a prospective new client that has over 100,000 potential members. Given your background as a clinical pharmacist, what value does your PBM offer this prospective new client that would give your PBM a competitive advantage over other PBMs?
4. How would you explain the pricing of brand name pharmaceuticals to a prospective PBM client? What about generic drugs?
5. How do you reconcile the unique skills needed to manage specialty medication use and managing people and other resources in a PBM environment? What are the differences and similarities? What characteristics do you have that would enable or raise concerns about your ability to work in this area?

REFERENCES

Adams KT. 2006. Specialty pharmacy. *Biotechnology Healthcare* 3:24–31.

Bateman TS, Snell SA. 1996. *Management: Building Competitive Advantage*. Chicago, IL: Times Mirror Higher Education Group.

Bootman JL, Townsend RJ, McGhan WF. 2005. *Principles of Pharmacoeconomics*. Cincinnati, OH: Harvey Whitney Books Company.

Department of Defense, Civilian Personnel Management Service. Information Sheet—Federal Employees Health Benefit (FEHB) Program & Uniformed Services TRICARE Health Benefits Programs. Available at http://www.cpms.osd.mil/ASSETS/441D94BF09EC4D109E3B6C813A39F8EF/272_is.pdf; accessed on May 2, 2011.

Edlin M. 2010. Traditional tools can be applied to specialty pharmacy management—the trick is balancing access with cost control. *Managed Healthcare Executive* 21: 34–37.

Fried BJ, Fottler MD. 2008. *Human Resources in Healthcare*. Chicago, IL: Health Administration Press.

Garis RI, Clark BE. 2004. The spread: pilot study of an undocumented source of pharmacy benefit manager revenue. *J Am Pharm Assoc* 44:15–21.

Garis RI, Clark BE, Siracuse MV, Makoid M. 2004. Examination of the value of pharmacy benefit managers. *Am J Health Syst Pharm* 61:81–5.

Johnson KA. 2010. *ICORE Healthcare Medical Injectables and Oncology Trend Report*, 1st edn. Available at http://www.icorehealthcare.com/trends.aspx; accessed on June 21, 2011.

Kaiser Family Foundation (KFF). 2007. State Medicaid Fact Sheets. Available at http://www.statehealthfacts.org/medicaid.jsp; accessed on May 4, 2011.

Kaiser Family Foundation (KFF). 2010. The Medicare Prescription Drug Benefit Fact Sheet. Available at http://www.kff.org/medicare/upload/7044–11.pdf; accessed on May 4, 2011.

Longest BB, Darr K. 2008. *Managing Health Services Organizations and Systems.* Baltimore, MD: Health Professions Press.

Miller SB, Hoffman TA, Houts JC, Miller JL, Pim BL, Behm A. 2007. The rise of specialty pharmacy costs. *Dis Manage Health Outcomes* 15(2):83–9.

National Association of Chain Drug Stores (NACDS). 2010. *NACDS Chain Pharmacy Industry Profile: 2010–11.* Alexandria, VA: National Association of Chain Drug Stores.

Navarro RP. 2009. *Managed Care Pharmacy Practice.* Sudbury, MA: Jones and Bartlett.

Pharmaceutical Strategies Group (PSG). 2010. Understanding Specialty Pharmacy Management and Cost Control. Available at http://www.psgconsults.com/Understanding_Specialty_Pharmacy_Management_and_Cost_Control_FINAL.pdf; accessed on July 7, 2011.

Phillips DT. 1992. *Lincoln on Leadership.* New York, NY: Warner Books.

Siracuse MV, Clark BE, Garis RI. 2008. Undocumented source of pharmacy benefit manager revenue. *Am J Health Syst Pharm* 65:552–7.

Stern D, Reissman D. 2006. Specialty Pharmacy Cost Management Strategies of Private Health Care Payers. *J Manag Care Pharm* 12(9):736–44.

US Office of Personnel Management. Federal employment statistics: Executive branch civilian employment since 1940. Available at http://www.opm.gov/feddata/HistoricalTables; accessed on May 2, 2011.

Vanscoy GJ. 2000. The emergence of specialty pharmacy. *J Manag Care Pharm* 6(4):280–84.

West-Strum D. 2009. *2009 NCPA Digest Sponsored by Cardinal Health.* Alexandria, VA: National Community Pharmacists Association.

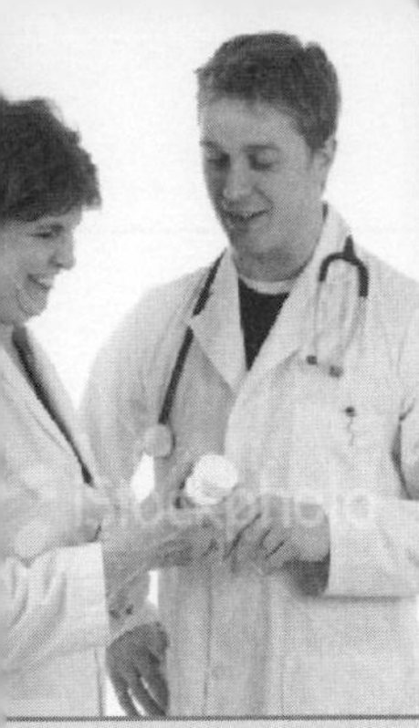

35

APPLICATIONS IN SAFETY NET CLINICS

Steven Chen, Melvin Baron, Laura Feeney, and Stephanie Iniguez

About the Authors: Steven Chen, Pharm.D., is associate professor and the hygeia centennial chair in clinical pharmacy at the University of Southern California (USC) School of Pharmacy. His clinical practice experience is in ambulatory care for government-insured, privately insured, and under-/uninsured patient populations. Dr. Chen's research interests include evaluating the impact of pharmacy services on health outcomes, medication safety, and costs. He is a member of research and practice teams that have been awarded the Best Practices Award from the American Society of Health-System Pharmacists in 2002 and 2008, the American Pharmacists Association Pinnacle Award in 2007, and the American Association of Colleges of Pharmacy Inaugural Community Transformative Award in 2009. Dr. Chen is cochair emeritus of the Health Resources and Services Administration (HRSA) Patient Safety and Clinical Pharmacy Services Collaborative, a government-supported program promoting the spread of clinical pharmacy service integration in medical homes across the nation.

Melvin F. Baron, Pharm.D., M.P.A., is associate professor of clinical pharmacy at the University of Southern California School of Pharmacy. He received his Doctor of Pharmacy degree in 1957 and his Masters degree in Public Administration in 1973, both from University of Southern California (USC). He was in private practice from 1957 to 1987 and developed a unique home health care center providing infusion therapy, durable medical equipment, and respiratory, ostomy, and incontinence care. Dr. Baron joined the USC School of Pharmacy fulltime in 1990. He is director of the Level I Externship program, teaches a pharmacy administration clerkship, and also is director of the Pharm.D./MBA program at USC. His research interests include implementation and expansion of clinical pharmacy services in community clinics and development of educational tools for low-literacy, low-income Latino populations. Dr. Baron was the team leader for the development and production of bilingual fotonovelas for clinic patients. Dr. Baron partnered with The National Institute of Transplantation and was awarded a grant from the UniHealth Foundation to fund a kidney transplant series of videos, in both English and Spanish, to educate patients and their families about the transplant process. Dr. Baron is a recognized leader in providing expanded pharmacy services in safety net clinics. On June 27, 2011, Dr. Baron received the American Pharmacists Association Foundation Pinnacle Award for Individual Career Achievement.

Laura L. Feeney, Pharm.D. is adjunct assistant professor of pharmacy practice at the USC School of Pharmacy, and Clinical Pharmacist at Clinicas Del Camino Real, Inc., a federally qualified health center in Ventura, California. She received her Pharm.D. and completed a PGY1 Residency in ambulatory care at USC. Dr. Feeney provides comprehensive pharmacy services at Clinicas Del Camino Real, including disease state/medication therapy management, and operates an in-house 340B pharmacy.

Stephanie M. Iniguez, Pharm.D., is clinical pharmacist and in-house 340B pharmacy manager at Clinicas Del Camino Real. Dr. Iniguez received her Pharm.D. and completed a PGY1 Residency in ambulatory care at USC. She initiated disease management programs and medication access programs at Clinicas Del Camino Real, Inc. Dr. Iniguez serves as a faculty coach for Health Resources and Services Administration's (HRSA) Patient Safety and Clinical Pharmacy Services Collaborative.

LEARNING OBJECTIVES

After completing this chapter, readers will be able to

1. List key components of a safety net clinic.
2. Describe the 340B Drug Discount Program and list requirements for participation.
3. Identify the legal requirements for dispensary operation.
4. Describe the role of a consultant pharmacist in a safety net dispensary.
5. Discuss the responsibilities of the clinic and the pharmacy entering into a contractual agreement.
6. Describe the general characteristics of patient assistance programs (PAP).
7. List the steps involved in establishing a clinical pharmacy service in a safety net clinic.

SCENARIO

Paul Gant, an administrator at a federally qualified health center called Comprehensive Health Center (CHC), has been meeting regularly with senior leaders from other local safety net clinics to share strategies for providing care to their large number of uninsured and Medicaid patients. As a result of these meetings, Paul is now convinced that CHC's medication budget is much higher than it should be. CHC contracts with a local pharmacy to provide prescriptions for their uninsured patients, which Paul thought would save money by eliminating the need to build a pharmacy or dispensary and pay for personnel to run it. However, Paul noticed that most other local clinics have either built a pharmacy or dispensary, and many have recently hired a clinical pharmacist.

Paul contacts his friend Bethany Kim, CEO of Holy Cross Clinic, and asks if she knows of a consultant that can help him determine whether building a dispensary or pharmacy is financially feasible. Bethany refers Paul to Sarah Pike, a pharmacist working at Fair Oaks Pharmacy with a faculty appointment at a school of pharmacy. Beth states that Sarah has consulted on this matter for several safety net clinics. Paul contacts Sarah and offers to hire her as a consultant. If Sarah accepts the offer, what steps should she take to determine whether a pharmacy or dispensary makes good business sense at CHC? What can Sarah do to help reduce CHC's medication budget? And how can Sarah implement a clinical pharmacy program and produces outcomes of interest to Paul and CHC's stakeholders including potential payers?

CHAPTER QUESTIONS

1. What defines a safety net clinic?
2. How important are patient assistant programs to the clinic dispensary and why?
3. Who can legally operate a clinic dispensary?
4. How can a clinic dispensary be operated without a computer system to generate prescription labels?
5. How can a clinic dispensary become eligible for 340B?
6. Can clinical pharmacy services in safety net clinics be self-sustaining? If so, how?

BACKGROUND

This chapter will discuss pharmacy management applications in a safety net clinic setting. But what is a safety net clinic? How does it differ from other community clinics? Safety net clinics are largely defined by the patient populations they serve (Altman and Lewin, 2000; Saviano and Powers, 2005). These clinics provide health care services to the medically underserved, including the uninsured, underinsured, and Medicaid populations. These groups must make up a substantial portion of the clinic's patient population for the clinic to qualify as a safety net clinic. Safety net clinics may provide primary, specialty, or urgent care services and provide these services regardless of a patient's ability to pay. In many cases, these clinics are mandated to serve the indigent population to receive government funding as well as reimbursement from other public health programs.

The need for safety net clinics has increased over the years for several reasons. The U.S. population continues to gray. According to the California Department of Aging, between the years 1990 and 2020, the elderly age group will experience an increase of about 112 percent (California Department of Aging, 2011). Furthermore, the market environment has seen an augmented emphasis on prevention (US Dept of Health and Human Services, 2010). The current emphasis on prevention has created an overall rise in consumerism as it pertains to the medical field.

Many of the patients requiring health care services are uninsured or underinsured, so they often look to safety net clinics for alternative, more affordable options. The growth of underinsured populations is due in part to recent federal legislation that limits Medicaid and other benefits to legal immigrants (see http://www.cms.gov/MedicaidDrugRebateProgram/). This legislation clearly excludes illegal immigrants from many of the benefits available to other populations. Since illegal immigrants tend to have high rates of chronic illnesses, they benefit from either free or less expensive alternatives, like safety net clinics. As a result of this legislation, the demand for safety net providers has increased. Fortunately, many safety net organizations have demonstrated outstanding quality of care despite high demand and limited resources, serving as examples for others (Keller et al., 2011)

THE 340B PROGRAM

The 340B Drug Discount Program provides highly discounted medications to eligible safety net clinics (see https://www.340pvp.com). The name 340B comes from the section of the law from which the program was created: The Veteran's Health Care Act of 1992 under section 340B of the Public Health Service Act (PHSA). However, the origin of this law dates back to 1990 when Congress created the Omnibus Budget Reconciliation Act (OBRA). This act introduced a Medicaid rebate program that reduced the cost of medications reimbursed by state Medicaid agencies. Under OBRA, drug companies were required to enter into a rebate agreement with the Secretary of the Department of Health and Human Services (HHS) to have their drugs covered under Medicaid. This rebate paid to Medicaid is based on the manufacturer's "best price"[1] on that drug offered to any organization. Thus, if a drug company offered a discounted price to another organization, they would end up having to pay larger reimbursements to state Medicaid agencies. This deterred drug companies from offering large discounts on drugs to non-Medicaid agencies. As a result, drug manufacturers began raising their prices to avoid paying larger rebates to Medicaid. Consequently, government spending actually increased from drug purchases by other government funded non-Medicaid providers, as these costs offset any savings achieved through the rebate program.

To rectify this situation, the 340B program was created in November of 1992. The Veteran's Health Care Act requires manufacturers to provide covered outpatient drugs to certain covered entities (see next section for explanation of covered entities) at a reduced price. The drugs included in the 340B discount program are medications used on an outpatient basis, either administered to the patient onsite, or dispensed to the patient from the pharmacy or dispensary (a dispensary is further defined later; it does not require continuous staffing by a pharmacist). This includes prescription drugs as well as any over-the-counter medications that may be prescribed. Prescription drugs administered in an inpatient setting and vaccines are not included.

To provide the discounts, the 340B program establishes a maximum price that a covered entity would have to pay for a given drug, referred to as a "ceiling price" (von Oehsen, 2003). These prices would be offered to any establishment enrolled in the 340B program, regardless if the drugs are purchased directly from the manufacturer or through a wholesaler. Drugs purchased through this program cannot be subject to a Medicaid rebate. The 340B discounted prices are roughly 25 percent to 50 percent less than the average wholesale price[2] (AWP), thus providing substantial cost savings to the covered entities. In addition, the 340B bill established a "prime vendor" leading to the creation of the Prime Vendor Program (PVP). The prime vendor is the single preferred wholesaler that can serve all entities enrolled in the 340B program. The PVP offers subceiling prices on these covered drugs because they are able to negotiate with the drug manufacturers through their bulk purchases. Covered entities may obtain additional savings by enrolling in and purchasing their medications through the PVP.

The 340B program mandated certain provisions that a covered entity must follow while enrolled in the program. First, 340B participants may not transfer or resell the discounted drugs to anyone other than a patient of that entity. For example, a covered entity reselling its discounted drugs to another pharmacy or hospital would be a violation of the 340B contract. Another restriction, as previously mentioned, is that drugs purchased through the 340B program are not eligible for Medicaid rebates because they are already being purchased at a discounted price. This helps prevent the drug manufacturers from having to give multiple discounts on the same medications. If a covered entity does not comply with these regulations it could become disqualified from participation in the 340B program.

Who Qualifies for the 340B Program?

The 340B program is managed by the Health Resources and Services Administration (HRSA) Office of Pharmacy Affairs (OPA). It establishes the guidelines and eligibility criteria for participation in the 340B drug discount program. Organizations that qualify for the 340B pricing program are referred to as "covered entities" and are specified government-funded facilities. These organizations are those that cater to medically underserved populations. Covered

[1] Best price: The lowest price paid to a manufacturer for a drug, factoring in any rebates, discounts, or other price adjustments.

[2] Average wholesale price (AWP): The national average price that drug manufacturers suggest wholesalers charge pharmacies.

entities include Federally Qualified Health Centers[3] (FQHCs), FQHC look-alikes[4], AIDS, tuberculosis, and black lung clinics, other outpatient clinics funded by the Public Health Services Act (PHSA), and disproportionate share hospitals[5] (DSH) (see Table 35-1 for full list of covered entities or HRSA OPA Web site at http://www.hrsa.gov/opa/). For a hospital to qualify for the 340B program, it must be nonprofit, owned or operated by or under contract with state or local governments, and have a substantial percentage of its patients that are low-income or Medicaid patients, with the exception of critical access hospitals. (For more information, refer to Safety Net Hospitals for Pharmaceutical Access at http://www.safetynetrx.org.)

For an eligible organization to utilize the 340B program, they must complete the appropriate registration form and submit it to HRSA OPA. Registration applications are accepted on a quarterly basis and forms can be found on the HRSA OPA Web site (http://www.hrsa.gov/opa). After registering and being deemed eligible for the 340B program by OPA, the covered entity must inform its wholesaler of enrollment in the program when ordering medications. The wholesaler will then set them up with a 340B account and provide access to all of the 340B prices. The covered entity may then begin purchasing the discounted drugs either through their wholesaler, directly from the drug manufacturer, or through the Prime Vendor Program.

[3]Federally qualified health centers (FQHC's): Health centers that receive federal grants under Section 330 of the Public Health Services Act (PHSA). They must provide primary care services for all ages and preventative health services on site or by arrangement with another provider. Health centers must provide sliding fee scale discounts based on patient family size and income.

[4]FQHC look-alike clinic or health center that meets all eligibility criteria of an organization that received a PHS section 330 grant (an FQHC), but does not actually receive any grant funding. These health centers are eligible to receive many of the same benefits as FQHC's.

[5]Disproportionate share hospitals (DSH): Hospitals that serve a disproportionately large proportion of low-income patients.

How do 340B Programs Support Medication Needs of Health care Organizations?

The 340B program offers a number of ways to support the medication needs of health care organizations. Covered entities are able to reduce the price of covered medications significantly to the patients to whom they are prescribed when dispensing from their pharmacies and dispensaries. This greatly improves access to medications for the medically underserved, who otherwise might be unable to afford these drugs. This could lead to greater adherence among patients who may have chosen not to purchase their medications due to cost.

The large selection of drugs available through the 340B program allows entities to expand their drug formularies to include more therapeutic classes of medications as well as many brand name drugs that otherwise would be much too expensive. In addition, through the cost savings for the entire health center, covered entities can increase the number of patients they serve, and may be able to expand the range services offered. These factors can all lead to greater access to and quality of health care for the indigent and medically underserved populations that safety net clinics serve.

Providing 340B Medications to Patients

Once a 340B-covered entity has begun purchasing drugs at the discounted prices, it may begin dispensing it to their patients. As mentioned previously, the 340B regulations state that the medications may be dispensed only to someone who is a patient of a covered entity. The 340B program defines patients of covered entities as those who

- Have their medical records maintained at that covered entity.
- Receive health care services from a health care professional employed by that entity or under contract with them, such as an outside referral from the covered entity.
- Receive a health service or services for which FQHC funding is provided.

Table 35-1. Organizations Eligible to Apply for the 340B Drug Discount Program

340B-Covered Entities
Federally qualified health centers
• FQHC look-alikes
• Consolidated health centers
• Migrant health centers
• Health care centers for the homeless
• Healthy schools/healthy communities
• Health care centers for residents of public housing
• Office of tribal programs or urban Indian organizations
Family Planning clinics
Sexually transmitted disease clinics
Entities receiving grants for early HIV intervention services under the Ryan White Care Act (RWCA[a])
State-operated AIDS Drug Assistance Program (ADAP)
Black lung clinics
Hemophilia treatment centers
Tuberculosis clinics
Native Hawaiian health centers
Qualified hospitals
• Disproportionate share hospitals
• Children's hospitals
• Cancer hospitals exempt from the Medicare prospective payment system
• Sole community hospitals
• Rural referral centers
• Critical access hospitals

[a]Ryan White Care Act (RWCA) provides federal funding for early intervention and primary care services for people with HIV infection. Clinics funded by RWCA provide HIV counseling and testing, medical evaluation and clinical care, and other essential services.

Dispensaries and In-House Pharmacies

The easiest way for a covered entity to provide its discounted drugs to a patient is directly onsite at their dispensary or in-house pharmacy. In this situation, a covered entity would purchase the medications from its wholesaler or directly from the manufacturer and keep the medications onsite. The patients can then be dispensed the medications as they are prescribed by their providers, abiding all laws regarding the dispensing of any prescription drugs. In addition, the dispensaries and in-house pharmacies must comply with the 340B guidelines of dispensing only to patients of the covered entity and not obtaining any Medicaid rebates on the dispensed medications. The low prices paid through the 340B program often allow the medications to be dispensed to patients at a largely discounted price.

Contracting with Community Pharmacies

Although dispensing 340 medications onsite is the easiest way to provide medications to patients, many covered entities do not possess a dispensary or in-house pharmacy. To enable such entities fully to utilize these drug discounts, the 340B program allows contracting with an outside community pharmacy. Initially, the

340B allowed a covered entity to contract with only a single outside pharmacy; however, that has since been modified, allowing entities to now contract with multiple pharmacies. This arrangement can be established with any community pharmacy willing to enter into such a contract.

In a contract pharmacy arrangement, the covered entity, not the pharmacy, would purchase the medications with their 340B discounted prices. The covered entity then often establishes a "ship to bill" arrangement with its wholesaler or the drug manufacturer, allowing the shipment of 340B medications directly to the contracted pharmacy. The pharmacy keeps the 340B medications stocked separately and maintains records for these medications; alternatively, 340B medications can be mixed with non-340B medications if a virtual inventory is maintained through computer software capable of such management. Records must be kept for all financial statements, status reports of medication collections, and all receiving and dispensing summaries for the 340B drugs. The contracted pharmacy also must develop a tracking system to ensure that the 340B medications are dispensed only to patients of the covered entity, to ensure compliance with the 340B regulations.

PATIENT ASSISTANCE PROGRAMS

Patient assistance programs (PAPs) are available by drug manufacturers to provide indigent patients with free or low-cost medications (Medicine for People in Need, 2003). PAPs are a vital component in providing medication access to a great number of safety net patients. Manufacturers have specific criteria a patient must meet to qualify for a PAP medication. Eligibility criteria for most programs include

- Income and asset guidelines
- Citizenship status
- Veteran's benefit status
- Insurance status

Most programs will not accept patients who are currently receiving prescription drug coverage through private insurance, Medicaid, or Medicare. Patients also must verify their financial status by submitting a variety of income documentation (e.g., Federal tax returns). Each application involves the patient's provider, since a prescription and provider signature is required on most applications. Upon completion of the application and approval by the manufacturer, the medication is either mailed to the clinic or to the patient's home. Although the day supply amount can vary depending on the medication, a qualified patient typically receives a 3-month supply of a medication with 3 refills. Safety net providers often develop a system to help navigate through the PAP process. Although the PAP process is considerably time consuming for a health center, there are many safety net providers across the country providing thousands of PAP medications to indigent patients.

Patient Assistance Programs and Safety Net Organizations

PAPs can be beneficial for both the patient and the 340B safety net organization (Felder et al., 2011). These programs allow providers to prescribe and maintain indigent patients on a variety of brand-name medications that otherwise would be inaccessible. The availability of PAPs provides an avenue to decrease the number of samples utilized by the providers at the health center. Health centers that provide PAP services often run well-organized PAP operations that can decrease the 340B costs accrued by the health center. In addition, safety net organizations that aid patients in completing the entire PAP process may choose to charge patients a fee for processing individual applications, tracking the medication, and dispensing the medication. This fee is known as an administrative fee and typically does not exceed $10. A successful PAP program usually requires at least one full-time staff member who is responsible for overseeing the program, ensuring that paperwork is complete and timelines are met.

Although PAP programs save patients money and give providers additional options to optimize therapy, managing a PAP program can be challenging (Walter, 2004). Review of eligibility information for each individual application is tedious and time consuming. In the safety net population, a noncitizen/resident may present with additional barriers that lead some manufacturers to deem these patients ineligible. Some patients may not be able to provide the detailed financial documentation that is sometimes required by manufacturers. Applications and eligibility requirements are frequently changed without advance notice by the manufacturers; as a result, advocates or clinic staff must spend time on the phone or on various Web sites to find the most updated application information. Once an application is accepted by the manufacturer, it can take up to 4 to 6 weeks for the medication to arrive at the clinic or patient's home. Due to this lag time, most individual PAP medications are more appropriate for chronic therapy as opposed to short-term/acute therapies. All of these challenges and the considerable amount of time and staff required to manage a PAP must be taken into account when a safety net clinic is dispensing both 340B and PAP medications (Carroll, 2007). To maximize a 340B and PAP program, a PAP formulary will help direct providers to efficiently and effectively prescribe medications that are not alternatively provided through the clinic 340B program. A structured program with committed staff is the key to providing a win-win Patient Assistance Program within a safety net clinic (Fig. 35-1). A variety of resources are available to help organizations navigate the plethora of PAP applications.

PAP Resources for Patients and Advocates

Fortunately, most resources for PAP applications are readily available online. There are two ways clinics have chosen to manage PAPs: (1) Manually by utilizing free Web sites or (2) computerized using commercial software. Most health centers launching a PAP will begin the process by downloading individual applications from a variety of free comprehensive Web sites. Once the application is downloaded and completed, these clinics will track the PAP process in a spreadsheet or database program. Large safety net clinic organizations frequently purchase commercial software designed to manage the 340B process by charging a fee per patient per month to process and track active PAP applications. Installation and annual fees might be charged by the software companies. A variety of useful reporting templates and outputs are provided in commercial PAP software programs.

WEB SITES FOR FREE PATIENT ASSISTANCE PROGRAM RESOURCES

www.hrsa.org
www.medpin.org
www.needymeds.org
www.pparx.org
www.rxassist.org
www.rxhope.com

A third option in integrating PAPs into a health center in-house 340B pharmacy is to participate in bulk donation or replacements program by pharmaceutical manufacturers. These programs are commonly known as Institutional Patient Assistance Programs. Institutional PAPs are available from some of the larger pharmaceutical companies, such as Pfizer and AstraZeneca. An agreement between the health center and the manufacturer would allow an in-house 340B pharmacy (and in some cases a 340B dispensary) to obtain bulk quantities of PAP medications to dispense as part of the health center's existing stock. The benefit to institutional PAPs is time saved from completing individual PAP applications. Institutional PAP medications can

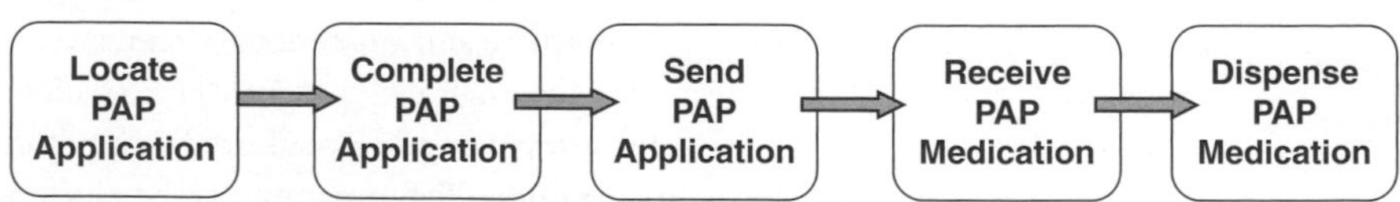
Locate PAP Application
Complete PAP Application
Send PAP Application
Receive PAP Medication
Dispense PAP Medication

Figure 35-1. The Patient Assistance Program (PAP) process.

easily integrate into the pharmacy or dispensary's workflow. Furthermore, there is no longer a wait time of 4 to 6 weeks because the PAP medications would be readily available at the health center. The health center facility can charge a nominal dispensing fee for PAP medications received from institutional programs.

The Pharmacist's Role in PAPs

A clinical pharmacist plays a vital role in implementing and maintaining a successful PAP within a safety net clinic organization. The pharmacy is the key to integrate the 340B medications available for purchase with available PAP medications. Pharmacists can analyze the cost-effectiveness of purchasing a 340B medication at a very low acquisition versus assigning staff to complete and manage individual PAP applications. This is an essential component of the clinical pharmacist's role in comprehensive formulary management for a safety net clinic.

Along with creating a concise and cost-effective PAP formulary, a pharmacist can educate the clinic's providers on newly available PAP medications or changes to various programs that can potentially affect patient outcomes. Clinical pharmacy services can be integrated with medication formulary management to improve patient outcomes. For example, a protocol can be approved by the medical director of the health center to have primary care providers refer all chronic disease patients receiving PAP medications to the clinical pharmacist for medication reconciliation and disease state management.

OPERATING A DISPENSARY VERSUS A PHARMACY IN A SAFETY NET CLINIC

This section summarizes the requirements for a dispensary license and for operating a dispensary in the state of California. The pharmacy laws and regulations discussed in this unit apply to the state of California, but may not necessarily apply to other states. Readers should check with regulations that apply to their own state.

Dispensary versus Pharmacy

Dispensaries and pharmacies have important regulatory differences that must be considered when deciding which is best for a given safety net organization (California Board of Pharmacy, 2011). A licensed pharmacy falls under the series of laws and regulations set forth by each state's Board of Pharmacy. A dispensary in California has a different set of less stringent criteria that allows for personnel flexibility in exchange for some safety assurances. For example, a licensed pharmacy requires having a pharmacist on duty at all times that the pharmacy is open. A clinic dispensary does not require a pharmacist to be on duty when it is open, but a pharmacist consultant review is required quarterly. Dispensaries cannot supply patients with Schedule II controlled substances. It is recommended that no scheduled drugs be part of the dispensary formulary. Dispensaries are not eligible for professional dispensing fees that are authorized under the Medicaid program.

Memorandum of Understanding

With the rising number of safety net providers, clinics often approach pharmacists requesting their services as a consultant for dispensaries. It is important for pharmacists to create a Memorandum of Understanding (MOU) for the consultative services that will be rendered to the safety net clinic or dispensary. In the MOU, the clinic can specify what it wants from the pharmacist, and the pharmacist can articulate what he or she is willing to do.

The MOU usually opens with a formal and simple greeting that can be accomplished in a small paragraph. Following the greetings, a detailed list or explanation of the services to be provided is summarized, often in bullet-point format. The fee for the services rendered should follow the list of services, including a statement of how the invoices will be billed. Agreement cancellation procedures should be specified. The MOU usually closes with a small paragraph that highlights key points in the memorandum, and explains briefly the next steps to forming the collaboration. The last line is polite and appropriate salutation. MOUs are an important tool to specify relationships among any of myriad business entities, including but not limited to health care organizations. (See Appendix A for a Sample Memorandum of Understanding)

Requirements for a Dispensary License

To obtain a dispensary license in the state of California, the Rules and Regulations outlined in 2001 Pharmacy Law 2011 apply (see http://www.pharmacy.ca.gov/forms/clinic_app_pkt.pdf.) In Article 13 of "Business and Professions Code," Section 4181, the requirements to obtain a clinic license, as well as an explanation of who may dispense medications at the clinic is provided. Only a physician, a pharmacist, or a person legally authorized to dispense drugs may dispense medications. In addition, they must comply with the rules and regulations outlined in Pharmacy Law in order to legally dispense the medications.

A key requirement for opening a safety net clinic with a dispensary is to have a consulting pharmacist. According to "Article 13, Section 4182: Duties of Professional Director; Consulting Pharmacist Required":

> The consulting pharmacist shall be required to visit the clinic regularly and at least quarterly. However, nothing in this section shall prohibit the consulting pharmacist from visiting more than quarterly to review the application of policies and procedures based on the agreement of all the parties approving the policies and procedures. The consulting pharmacist shall certify in writing quarterly that the clinic is, or is not, operating in compliance with the requirements of this article (Pharmacy Law 2011, p. 92).

Again, the legal requirements for a dispensary may vary from state to state; however, the preceding description, requirements for, and distinctions between a dispensary and a pharmacy are fairly typical across the United States.

Policies and Procedures Manual

Each clinic must develop a Policies and Procedures Manual. A pharmacist, or a combination of a pharmacist and a director or physician, can create the Manual, but it is the consulting pharmacist's duty to verify and approve the policies and procedures. The Policies and Procedures Manual contains specifications related to the laws and regulations of the State Department of Public Health. For example, Manuals often contain licensing requirements that outline who can dispense medications, whether the clinic has a pharmacy permit, and who is responsible for inspection, training, recordkeeping, and so on.

The Policies and Procedures Manual also contains the licensing requirements and duties of the dispensing physician, hours of operation of the clinic, patient rights, pharmacy services offered, medication handling, labeling, and storage procedures, security procedures and dispensary infection control, and patient consultation that considers the health and well-being of the public. In addition, the Policies and Procedures Manual should include information about drug utilization review. The protocol and policies of drug utilization are clearly outlined in the Manual, along with formulary review and formulary manual protocol.

Lastly, it is recommended that the Policies and Procedures Manual include information on pharmacy purchasing. The regulations and procedures involved in initiating, processing, and receiving a purchase may be included.

Options to Reduce Drug Costs for Patients

One of the advantages of safety net clinics is the amount of options they have to help reduce drug cost. As described previously, safety net clinics usually can take advantage of 340B and Patient Assistant Programs. Integrating these efficiently into a comprehensive formulary system can dramatically reduce medication costs to the clinic, as well as drug samples.

Drug samples may be used at clinic dispensaries, but there are certain conditions for the samples to be valid or permitted at the clinics. The most important of these conditions is that the sample must be received in its original, unopened packaging with its label intact. Once drug samples are received, they must store them under the conditions that will maintain the sample's stability, integrity, and effectiveness. In addition, complete and accurate records of donation, receipt, inspection, inventory, and dispensing (i.e., sample medication control record) must be maintained. Donation records must be kept on file for 3 years from the date of donation. The sample drug donation records must include the following:

- Name, address, and telephone number of the donator
- Manufacturer information
- Brand name and quantity
- Lot or control number of the drug sample donated
- Date of donation

Most importantly, the clinic must conduct an inventory of the drug samples, and all other medications, annually.

Dispensaries without Computer Systems

Dispensaries that do not have a computer system may use a manual labeling system, unit-of-use packaging, or an alternative automated labeling system. Manual labeling systems provide dispensaries with a ready-to-go label. The prescriber must then complete the label by writing the patient's name, date of issue, instructions on how to take the medication, and pertinent prescriber information. After this is done, the prescriber peels the label and affixes it to the prepackaged bottle.

Unit-of-use packaging refers to a sealed, prelabeled prescription drug package. Using currently available pharmacy software, the prescriber has the option of using an automated labeling system. The prescriber can simply write the prescription and generate labels using a printer. This is helpful in maintaining each patient's profile, and tracking spending with periodic reports.

Pros and Cons of an In-House Dispensary, In-House Pharmacy, or Contract with Retail Pharmacy

Perhaps one of the most important decisions made by safety net clinics is whether to create an in-house dispensary or contract with a retail pharmacy to provide 340B medications for their patients. Ultimately, the right decision will depend on the payer mix for the clinic and the prescription volume. If the payer mix and prescription volume are adequate to cover or nearly cover the cost of a pharmacist providing dispensing services, than an in-house pharmacy should be considered. Even if the pharmacy does not generate a profit and only breaks even, having the in-house pharmacy allows all patients (third-party, Medicaid, Medicare, uninsured) to fill prescriptions in the clinic, allowing the clinic pharmacist to ensure optimal medication safety by reviewing every prescription and troubleshoot potential problems for every patient. As discussed previously, the drawbacks of an in-house pharmacy include the need to comply with the stringent laws applicable to pharmacy regulation.

Sometimes, these regulations along with the prescription volume become a barrier to finding time for the pharmacist to develop more comprehensive clinical pharmacy services such as medication therapy or disease state management (please see next section). In this case, and in cases where a pharmacy business model is cost prohibitive, an in-house dispensary can be considered to at least provide 340B medications through the clinic with more flexibility in personnel and management. If other variables work against implementation of an in-house dispensary, such as space or personnel limitations, then contracting with an outside retail pharmacy can be considered. The Health Resource and Services Administration (HRSA) Pharmacy Services Support Center (PSSC) offers excellent tools, resources, and free expert consultations to help 340B program participants optimize the value of the program and provide clinically and cost-effective pharmacy services that improve medication use and advance patient care (see http://pssc.aphanet.org/).

DEVELOPMENT AND IMPLEMENTATION OF CLINICAL PHARMACY SERVICES IN SAFETY NET CLINICS

According to the Institute of Medicine, medication errors are a major source of medical harm that affects more than 1.5 million people annually and is the cause of death for 44,000 to 98,000 Americans each year (the Institute of Medicine, 2000). Medication errors that are deemed "preventable" account for over $3.5 billion in annual hospital expenses alone (the Institute of Medicine, 2007). While it is estimated that 300,000 preventable adverse events occur in America's hospitals each year, it is believed that the number that occurs in outpatient environments is undoubtedly greater but very challenging to quantify (US FDA, 2011).

The pharmacy literature includes numerous examples of clinical pharmacy service integration into medical homes that are associated with improvements in medication safety and health-related outcomes (ACCP, 2007). Although the majority of these reports are not from safety net clinic settings, the principles of initiating and expanding clinical pharmacy services in safety net clinics is similar. Two very helpful resources that provide excellent examples and guidance are the Patient-Centered Primary Care Collaborative (PCPCC) resource guide on Integrating Comprehensive Medication Management to Optimize Patient Outcomes (http://www.pcpcc.net/files/medmanagepub.pdf) and the Health Resources and Services Administration (HRSA) Patient Safety and Clinical Pharmacy Services Collaborative (PSPC) Change Package (healthcarecommunities.org/WorkArea/DownloadAsset.aspx?id=10312). The PCPCC resource guide was produced by a multidisciplinary group of health care professionals, including physicians, nurses and pharmacists, as well as representation from multiple health care stakeholders including health plans, government health leaders, and pharmaceutical manufacturers. The guide is written in terms that allow non–health care professionals to understand the content, yet provides clear explanations and powerful examples of the value of clinical pharmacy services in the outpatient setting.

The HRSA PSPC Change Package provides specific steps that are often needed to implement and/or spread clinical pharmacy services in safety net clinic settings. The HRSA PSPC is the first government-led effort to spread the practice of clinical pharmacy across the nation, beginning with safety net entities (see http://www.hrsa.gov/publichealth/clinical/patientsafety/index.html). The PSPC has demonstrated that integration of clinical pharmacy services into outpatient medical practices is associated with dramatic improvement in the control of common chronic conditions, including diabetes mellitus, hypertension, dyslipidemia, asthma, HIV/AIDS, depression, and anticoagulation therapy.

The safety net clinic setting is clearly an area that can benefit from comprehensive clinical pharmacy services, but implementing a clinical pharmacy practice in this setting is challenging. The majority of safety net clinics are unfamiliar with clinical pharmacy services. Safety net clinics have very limited budgets and are overwhelmed with a continually increasing demand for appointments with primary care providers. Providers are overworked and turnover is high among physicians. Fortunately, when approached methodically, all of these concerns can be appeased through integrated clinical pharmacy services.

Six-Step Process for Establishing and Sustaining Clinical Pharmacy Services in Safety Net Clinics

The following 6-step process includes elements from both the PCPCC resource guide and PSPC Change Package, and is based largely on experience developing or consulting in the development of over a dozen integrated clinical pharmacy services in Southern California as well as in other states. All of these steps are essential for establishing a successful, self-sustaining service.

Step 1 Identify a Physician Champion and Key Collaborators, Initial Start-up

This is without question the first and most important step in the process. Clinical pharmacy services have little chance of successfully meeting program goals and long-term sustenance without the support of a well-respected physician. Usually, this physician champion should be the Chief Medical Officer/Medical Director. However, in some cases, the physician champion can be the physician that the medical staff respects and turns to for leadership and direction; this is typically a senior-level staff physician who understands health care quality, the evolving health care system, and the special needs of the population served. A good physician champion needs to understand the role of integrated clinical pharmacy and embrace the concept of team-based care. The physician should be able to anticipate skepticism and questions from colleagues that will allow the program to address these before they become barriers. Sometimes the initial barrier is start-up funding to generate results that can persuade senior leadership that the clinical pharmacy service is well worth the investment. Partnerships with schools of pharmacy are a natural win-win collaboration: Clinics can benefit from the expertise that pharmacy faculty has in providing comprehensive pharmacy services and can bring pharmacy residents and students to help provide extended care to patients, while pharmacy schools benefit by having a practice site for faculty, teaching, and scholarly activity in the form of practice-based research. Another option that is often linked to pharmacy schools is applying for government or foundation grants to support starting up the clinical pharmacy program.

Step 2 Identify a High-Risk Population

Having pharmacists involved in ensuring the safe and effective use of medications throughout the health system is essential to prevent medication-related harm. However, when developing a focused, individualized MTM or disease management service, it is important to recognize that pharmacists are not an inexpensive investment; therefore, it is important to target patient populations that are at the highest risk for medication-related problems and expensive medical care. These include patients receiving multiple chronic medications, patients with multiple disease states, and patients seeing multiple health care providers within a system that does not facilitate efficient communication of health-related information. Other populations that can be targeted include patients receiving medications that require frequent monitoring or are very expensive, patients with chronic illnesses that are difficult to control, and conditions in which medications critical for reducing morbidity and/or mortality are frequently underutilized. Last but certainly not least, patients who frequently utilize high-cost health care resources (emergency department visits, hospitalizations, and readmissions) should be considered as initial targets for MTM. Improving quality of care for these patients can dramatically reduce the use of these expensive resources and help justify the cost of clinical pharmacists. Resources that may be helpful for identifying a target population include electronic health record queries, disease registries, utilization review and hospitalization reports, quality improvement committee reports, and diagnostic/laboratory test results.

Regardless of the initial target population, it is important to include medication reconciliation as a "baseline" service for every patient. The importance of medication reconciliation is strongly emphasized by several government health care agencies including Agency for Health Care Research and Quality (AHRQ), Institute for Health Care Improvement (IHI), Centers for Disease Control and Prevention (CDC), and HRSA.

When initiating clinical pharmacy services, it is highly recommended that the service be limited to only one or two target populations. Many challenges unique to the safety net clinic setting need to be experienced and resolved (see Step 5), and trying to do so with multiple target populations can be overwhelming.

Step 3 Develop a Proposal for the Clinical Pharmacy Service Role in Managing the High-Risk Population Including Protocols and Assignment of Responsibilities

Upon receiving approval to provide clinical pharmacy services for a targeted high-risk population, the next or concurrent step is to develop a protocol outlining the purpose of the service, individuals involved and their responsibilities (pharmacists, supervising physicians, support staff, pharmacy students, etc.), the process by which targeted patients will be referred and receive clinical pharmacy services, how patient information will be communicated, and how appointments will be managed. A flow diagram can be very helpful for explaining the process to senior leaders and other members of the health care team, and is highly recommended for inclusion in the protocol or for explaining patient flow through the service (see Fig. 35-2).

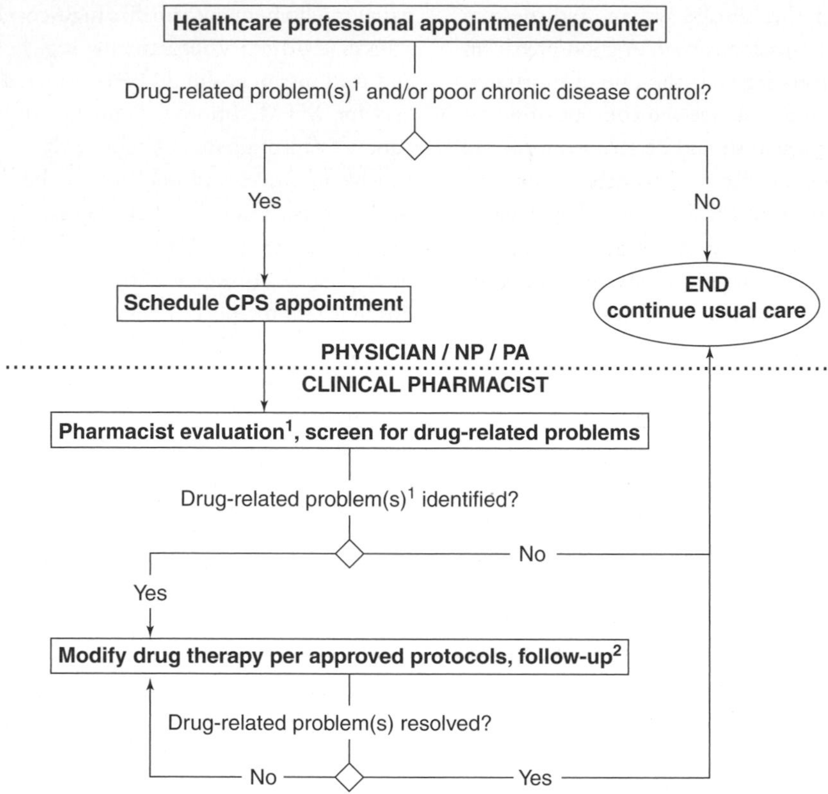

Figure 35-2. University of Southern California Clinical Pharmacy service flow.

Under the pharmacist responsibilities, the scope of the pharmacists' practice must be clarified in accordance with requirements and limitations set forth by the state board of pharmacy. The clinical pharmacy protocol must be signed off by the appropriate oversight group within the organization, typically the chief medical officer. Other resources are available that offer detailed guidance on pharmacy protocol development.

Step 4 Establish Key Measures of Success

Establishing metrics to quantify the value, impact, and quality of clinical pharmacy services is essential for long-term sustenance and to support spread to other high-risk populations. These metrics should be established prior to starting the service in order to integrate the collection of data elements into the service; otherwise, data collection is viewed as an additional burden and never gets done.

The most widely used method of evaluating health quality utilizes three categories of measures: structure, process, and outcomes (Donabedian, 1966) (See Chapter 9). Outcome measures of quality evaluate the end result of health care services from multiple perspectives including clinical, economic, patients satisfaction, and quality of life. Clinical measures include both primary endpoints (e.g., reduction in cardiovascular events among patients with diabetes or coronary artery disease) and surrogate markers that are correlated with primary endpoints (e.g., hemoglobin A1C, blood pressure, lipid levels). Common economic measures are changes in acute care resource utilization or projections in medical cost savings based on changes in surrogate markers of disease control that are correlated with medical costs (e.g., dollars saved per point reduction in A1C). Evaluating patient satisfaction or quality of life requires the use of survey instruments that have been scientifically validated in the target population.

Step 5 Pilot the Service and Collect All Measures Starting Day 1

Even if given permission to launch a clinical pharmacy service organization-wide, it is best to pilot the service with a few or even a single physician, preferably the physician champion. Despite the best planning, a new clinical pharmacy service will experience problems (e.g., confusion with scheduling, patients referred but not showing up for appointments, limited space/rooms, etc.) Resolving these problems can be accomplished much more simply with the support of a physician mentor than with the entire medical staff.

In addition to the daily logistics associated with providing patient care, piloting the service at a small scale is important for helping the clinical pharmacist understand the unique needs and challenges of the underserved. Many patients, particularly the homeless, lack access to a refrigerator. The majority have very low literacy levels, and cultural beliefs/preferences are powerful determinants of whether patients will adhere to instructions. Transportation in many cities can make follow-up care very difficult to provide. Learning to work efficiently with these challenges would be very difficult if clinical pharmacy services were initiated at a large scale.

Collection of measures established for evaluating the service must occur from the first day. The pilot phase is the time to figure out how to integrate collection of measures into the daily workflow. If this integration is not established, the measures will, at best, be extremely difficult and time-consuming to collect retrospectively. Ongoing evaluation of these measures is critical to support the sustainment and spread of clinical pharmacy services.

Step 6 Share Results with All Stakeholders to Sustain Existing and Expand New Services

To sustain a clinical pharmacy service and grow it to additional sites, data reflecting the impact of the service needs to be shared with all health care stakeholders, including payers/plan vendors, physicians, administrators, allied health professionals, patients, legislators and the community, and potential key collaborators. However, it is important to recognize that each of these stakeholders has slightly different priorities:

- Payers, health plans, and administrators are most interested in economic data reflecting cost savings and clinical data reflecting improved quality of care and medication safety. Cost savings reports also should include the impact of the clinical pharmacist on medication costs through optimization of the 340B program, PAPs, and overall medication formulary management; our experience has demonstrated that health systems can save literally millions of dollars annually by having a clinical pharmacist closely managing medication use.
- Physicians and allied health professionals are most interested in clinical data and patient satisfaction.
- Patients, legislators, and the community are most interested in economic data reflecting cost savings to consumers, clinical data, and patient satisfaction.

As a result, the specific data shared and reporting format will differ depending on the stakeholder.

Spreading the news about the clinic's successes through public relations will generate broad awareness among other payers, patients, providers and elected officials of the impact that integrated clinical pharmacy services have on patient health outcomes, medication safety, and cost savings. Some ideas on how to be successful in promoting your program include

- *Develop a public relations strategy.* The strategy employed should emphasize the integration of clinical pharmacy services into the organization, focusing on the complexity of medication regimens today in light of the increased prevalence and incidence of chronic diseases, particularly among the underserved and elderly, and that integrated clinical pharmacy services help improve health care quality while lowering costs in the form of more efficient and cost-effective drug formularies and less use of health care resources.

- *Seek local targets.* Focus promotion of the service on local targets: local newspapers, TV, and radio. Further, getting the story shared through trade groups and associations is a good approach to reaching the target audiences in local markets. For example, reaching out to chambers of commerce and similar groups provides an opportunity to showcase the value of integrated clinical pharmacy services and gives local media a reason to cover the story.
- *Employ effective public relation tactics.* Identify "media stars" on the team (physicians, pharmacists, patients, payers) and develop a media advisory (one pager—who, what, where, why, how). Patient testimonials can be particularly powerful for the general media, particularly those involving a major transformation in health care associated with clinical pharmacy service integration. Make available interviews with the players on the team. Make available clinic photo/video shooting.
- *Offer a Q&A for local print media, radio, and TV with the clinical pharmacy service professionals on a hot topic that is dealt with in the clinic* (getting patients immunized, diabetes management, smoking cessation, childhood obesity, cost savings, etc). Tell the story of the clinic while also providing readers/viewers/listeners with clinical pharmacy service expertise applicable to the needs of the general public, as well.
- *Keep everything in simple terms.* For example, keep in mind:
    - Today's medicines are complex, and the "traditional" role of physicians as solo practitioners has resulted in a rushed and overworked system of health care.
    - Adding clinical pharmacy services to the health care team for medication therapy management in clinics nationwide is improving patient health outcomes, avoiding dangerous medication side effects, and saving money.
    - If asked whether this is a novel, untested program, emphasize that integrating clinical pharmacy services into medical homes is nothing new; it has been done for decades in the Department of Veterans Affairs, Kaiser Permanente, and medical practices across the country in states that have supported an expanded role for pharmacists. The current program is just expanding these past successes to meet today's needs—helping the most vulnerable in clinics across the country but also working shoulder-to-shoulder with physician colleagues in clinics, hospitals, and community pharmacies.

Publishing in peer-reviewed health care journals will increase acceptance and credibility of the clinical pharmacy program within and outside the organization, and is an important method of spreading program successes to a broader audience in a manner that is objective and validated. However, submitting a manuscript can be challenging, particularly for organizations unfamiliar with the publication process. Selecting a journal should be done judiciously, with preference for journals that are not pharmacy-specific; otherwise, the publication ends up being primarily read by a pharmacy audience only.

Revisiting the Scenario

If Sarah accepts Paul's offer to serve as a pharmacist consultant for CHC, she should first establish a Memorandum of Understanding so that her duties are clearly specified. Next, Sarah should find out if CHC has a formulary. What is the clinic's current drug cost? Is the clinic eligible for the 340B program? Does the clinic have a P& T Committee? She should review the CHC medication formulary and determine whether there are untapped opportunities to save medication costs (e.g., 340B or Patient Assistance Program medications that have not been considered). Organizing the formulary to ensure that maximal cost savings is achieved without compromising the selection of medications available should immediately help CHC's medication budget.

Sarah should next inquire about the patient population. This information will give her some idea as to the number of uninsured, Medicaid, or partially insured patients. Based on the payer mix and prescription volume, Sarah can consider whether the clinic is better off running an in-house pharmacy, a dispensary, or contracting with an outside pharmacy to provide 340B medications. She can seek further guidance from the HRSA Pharmacy Services Support Center.

When exploring the possibility of introducing a clinical pharmacy program into a safety net clinic, Sarah should speak with the lead physician at CHC (typically the Chief Medical Officer) to determine the level of interest and support for improving health care quality and medication safety. Sarah's affiliation with a school of pharmacy can be helpful if start-up resources are needed; schools sometimes seek practice sites for faculty, or are interested in submitting grants to fund clinical pharmacy demonstration projects. She will need to identify an initial target population for clinical pharmacy services based on evidence of treatment gaps, known high-risk patient populations, and/or perceived medication-related burdens to physicians. After establishing a practice protocol and nationally aligned metrics for evaluating the quality of clinical pharmacy services, Sarah should pilot the service with a limited group of physicians (even a single physician mentor) to refine the clinical pharmacy program and ensure that it runs smoothly. She should aggregate the outcome data at least quarterly and share the results with all stakeholders to support the service and spread it to other high-risk populations. Over time, fiscal and clinical outcomes from the clinical pharmacy service will confirm that it is self-sustaining and essential.

CONCLUSION

Safety net clinics offer pharmacists the opportunity to provide comprehensive services ranging from acquisition and dispensing of medications to providing all levels of medication therapy management, including medication safety screening/reconciliation and disease management for the most challenging patients. The aging U.S. population and forecasts of continued economic struggles are straining all levels of the health care system, perhaps none more so than those organizations that care for the underserved. As health care reform shifts the U.S. health care system toward one that pays for health care quality instead of quantity, many of these quality measures relate to medication use. With government support from major health care branches including HRSA, CMS, and FDA, pharmacists can step forward and accept the invitation to integrate into health care teams and provide medication-related expertise to settings in the public health arena.

QUESTIONS FOR FURTHER DISCUSSION

1. Check your state regulations that apply to the storage and dispensing of medications from safety net clinics. Are dispensaries allowed? What are the opportunities for pharmacists to be involved?
2. Talk to an administrator at a local safety net clinic about how medications are managed. Is there a formulary? Does the clinic participate in the 340B program or receive drugs though PAP? Does the clinic provide drug samples? How are these accounted for and managed? Are there opportunities for pharmacists to make improvements in cost or efficiency of the processes related to medication acquisition and dispensing?
3. What are the needs that clinical pharmacy programs can fulfill for safety net clinics? What does the profession of pharmacy need to do to take ownership of these opportunities and ensure optimal medication-related health quality and safety?

REFERENCES

Altman S, Lewin ME. 2000. America's Health Care Safety Net: Intact but Endangered. National Academy of Sciences. Washington D.C: National Academy Press.

American College of Clinical Pharmacy (ACCP). 2007. Clinical pharmacy: A healther America through safer, more appropriate medication use. Available at http://www.accp.com/docs/govt/advocacy/ga_overview.pdf; accessed on Sep 2, 2011.

California Board of Pharmacy. 2011. Article 13: Nonprofit or Free Clinics. In: *Pharmacy Law—Rules and Regulations.* California: Lawtech Pub, 2011. 4180–186.

California Department of Aging. 2011. Statistics/demographics—Facts about California's elderly. Available at http://www.aging.ca.gov/stats/fact_about_elderly.asp; accessed on Sep 2, 2011.

Carroll NV. 2007. Pharmaceutical patient assistance programs: Don't look a gift horse in the mouth or there's no such thing as a free lunch. *J Manag Care Pharm* 13:614–6. [PubMed: 17874870]

Donabedian A. 1966. Evaluating the quality of medical care. *Milbank Mem Fund Q* 44:166–206

Felder TM, Palmer NR, Lal LS, Mullen PD. 2011. What is the evidence for pharmaceutical patient assistance programs?: A systematic review. *J Health Care Poor Underserved* 22:24–49.

Keller A, Arch M, Joseph A, et al. 2011. *Promising Practices in Safety-Net Clinic Design: An Overview.* Oakland, CA: California HealthCare Foundation.

Medicine for People in Need. 2003. PAP information management resources for clinics to help uninsured patients. Available at http://www.medpin.org/docs/pap-2003.pdf; accessed on Sept 2, 2011.

Saviano EC, Powers M. 2005. *California's Safety-Net Clinics: A Primer.* Oakland, CA: California HealthCare Foundation.

The Institute of Medicine. 2000. *To Err Is Human: Building a Safer Health System.* The National Academies Press. Available at: http://books.nap.edu/openbook.php?record_d=9728&page=1.

The Institute of Medicine. 2007. *Preventing Medication Errors: Quality Chasm Series.* The National Academies Press. Available at http://books.nap.edu/openbook.php?record_id=11623&page=R1

US Dept of Health and Human Services. 2010. The Affordable Care Act: Preventive Care Services. Available at: http://www.healthcare.gov/law/provisions/preventive/index.html; accessed on Sept 2, 2011.

US Food and Drug Administration (US FDA). 2011. FDA Drug Safety Initiative Fact Sheet. Available at http://www.fda.gov/Drugs/DrugSafety/ucm188760.htm; accessed on Sept 2, 2011.

von Oehsen W, Ashe M, Duke K. 2003. Pharmaceutical discounts under Federal Law: State Program Opportunities. *Am J Health Syst Pharm* 60:551–3.

Walter JM. 2004. *Starting a Pharmaceutical Access Program. A Volunteers in Health Care Guide.* Pawtucket, RI: Volunteers in Health Care.

APPENDIX A: SAMPLE MEMORANDUM OF UNDERSTANDING

SAMPLE MEMORANDUM

Date

Address

Dear __________ :

I am pleased to have the opportunity of working with you and your staff advising you regarding pharmacy services. To ensure complete understanding between us, I am setting forth the terms of my engagement and the nature of the services I will provide. I understand that you will provide me with all of the basic information required and that you are responsible for the accuracy and completeness of that information to the best of your knowledge. I will advise you about appropriate pharmacy law and its application to your facility. I will attend appropriate meetings and be available for consultation.

In addition, I will provide:

-
-
-
-

My __________ fee for these services will be __________ for the clinic, etc. My invoices will be__________ rendered __________ and are payable upon presentation. This agreement is cancelable by either party on a 30-day notice.

I appreciate the opportunity and look forward to be of service to__________ clinic and believe this letter accurately summarizes the significant terms of our engagement. If you have any questions, please let me know. If the foregoing is in accordance with your understanding, please sign the copy of this letter and return to me.

Very truly yours,

John Smith, PharmD.

Approved by: ______________________________

Title: ______________________________

Date: ______________________________

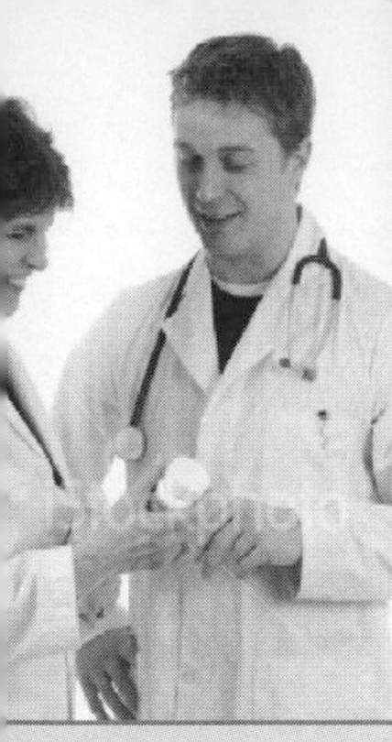

36

APPLICATIONS IN VARIED HEALTH CARE SYSTEMS

Jason Perepelkin

About the Authors: Dr. Perepelkin is assistant professor of social and administrative pharmacy at the University of Saskatchewan's College of Pharmacy and Nutrition, Saskatoon, Saskatchewan, Canada; he is also an associate member of the Department of Management and Marketing, Edwards School of Business. Dr. Perepelkin received his B.A. (social and cultural geography), B.Com. (marketing), M.Sc. (pharmaceutical policy), and Ph.D. (pharmacy management) from the University of Saskatchewan. Dr. Perepelkin collaborates closely with pharmacy regulatory and advocacy bodies and strives to bridge practice and research. Dr. Perepelkin teaches in the areas of pharmacy management, marketing, leadership, communications, health and pharmaceutical policy, organizational behavior, and human resources management. His research interests are in branding and marketing of pharmacists, pharmacy services and pharmacies, pharmacy management curriculum, the interaction between professional and business obligations in community pharmacy, and service quality and trust in community pharmacies.

LEARNING OBJECTIVES

Building on the foundations in pharmacy management outlined in previous chapters, this chapter will explore pharmacy management functions in various health care systems outside the United States, with particular emphasis on Canada. After completing this chapter, readers will be able to

1. Understand the process Canadian-educated pharmacists go through to practice in Canada.
2. Describe alternatives to the United States health care and pharmacy delivery and reimbursement systems.
3. Identify commonalities and differences between pharmacy management within and outside the United States.
4. Apply management theories and concepts in Canada and other countries with alternative health care systems.
5. Discuss implications of systems in some additional countries, such as those of the United Kingdom, New Zealand, and Australia, on pharmacy management.

SCENARIO

As a student in her fourth and final year of pharmacy school, Julia was used to facing billing issues with numerous third-party insurance companies. However, this time was exceptionally frustrating as Julia was having to deal with getting an aerosol chamber covered for a patient through noninsured health benefits (NIHB); NIHB is the insurance program for First Nations and Inuit peoples in Canada, which is a federal program that covers a limited range of health care goods and services that are not insured through the Canada Health Act, so as to help First Nations and Inuit peoples reach overall health comparable to other Canadians. NIHB would cover only one size of aerosol chamber per child per year, and the patient already received one 6 months earlier, yet Julia knew that without coverage the patient would not receive the proper dose of his asthma medication and that his parents could not afford to pay out of pocket for another one. While Julia had been taught in her courses about management situations such as this, she did not think they might be so prevalent in a pharmacist's practice.

CHAPTER QUESTIONS

1. What is the formal education process to become a registered pharmacist in Canada?
2. What pharmacy services are covered under the Canada Health Act?
3. What are some specific responsibilities of pharmacy managers?
4. What are some of the commonalities and differences among pharmacy management in the United States compared to other countries?
5. What are some managerial considerations when implementing new services within a pharmacy?
6. Why might having an appreciation for pharmacy practice outside of one's region be beneficial?

INTRODUCTION

It would be an understatement to say that pharmacy has gone through many changes over the past 50 + years. In the 1960s community pharmacy practice, or as it was referred to back then, "retail pharmacy," operated in small retail business operations, focusing on prescription dispensing, with limited disclosure of medication information to patients. On the other hand, hospital pharmacy practice focused on manufacturing, repackaging, and drug distribution.

Since that time, health care systems and pharmacy care have evolved considerably all around the globe, in some ways minor and in others, major, beginning with the educational process one undertakes to become a registered pharmacist.

Formal Education of Pharmacists in Canada

In Canada, there are currently 10 schools of pharmacy (CPhA, 2011a); see Table 36-1 for an overview of Canadian schools and the degrees offered. While the process is underway in many schools to convert to a Pharm.D. entry-to-practice curriculum, similar to what is standard in the United States (US), most programs currently prescribe to a 1-year prepharmacy, plus 4-year pharmacy model (Austin and Ensom, 2008). In all the schools, interns must complete various structured practical experiences (SPEPs), including community and hospital pharmacy rotations. Once an intern has completed all their formal training, they write the national licensing exam (Pharmacy Examining Board of Canada—PEBC), which includes a 2-day multiple-choice portion, testing on everything from pharmacokinetics to pharmacy management, followed by a half-day of various objective structured clinical examination (OSCE) scenarios; the PEBC is similar to the North American Pharmacist Licensure Examination (NAPLEX) in the United States (APhA, 2011). Some provinces allow pharmacy degree graduates who passed the PEBC to practice as a pharmacist immediately, while other provinces require additional internship hours.

The one exception is for interns educated in Quebec, as that province has a separate system to obtain licensure that involves providing evidence that one has graduated from a pharmacy degree program deemed equivalent to a Quebec pharmacy program; the individual must also be fluent in French, pass a jurisprudence exam, and complete 600 hours of training in

Table 36-1. Colleges/Schools/Faculties of Pharmacy in Canada

College/School/Faculty	Location	Web Site	Degrees Offered
Dalhousie University College of Pharmacy	Halifax, Nova Scotia	http://pharmacy.dal.ca/	Baccalaureate in Pharmacy—BScPharm; Master of Science in Pharmaceutical Sciences—M.Sc.
Memorial University of Newfoundland School of Pharmacy	St. John's, Newfoundland	http://www.mun.ca/pharmacy/about/	Baccalaureate in Pharmacy—B.Sc. (Pharm); Master of Science in Pharmacy—M.Sc.; Doctor of Philosophy in Pharmacy—Ph.D.
Université de Montréal (University of Montreal) Faculté de pharmacie (Faculty of Pharmacy)	Montréal, Québec	http://www.pharm.umontreal.ca/	Bachelor of Science in Biopharmaceuticals (Baccalauréat en sciences biopharmaceutique)—B.Sc.; Doctor of Pharmacy (Doctorat en pharmacie)—Pharm.D. (as the 1st professional degree in pharmacy); Master of Science (Maîtrise ès sciences) in Pharmacy Practice (Pratique pharmaceutique) and Pharmaceutical Sciences (Sciences pharmaceutiques)—M.Sc.; Doctorate of Philosophy (Doctorat de philosophie) in Pharmaceutical Sciences (Sciences pharmaceutiques)—Ph.D.
Université Laval (Laval University) Faculté de pharmacie (Faculty of Pharmacy)	Québec City, Québec	http://www.pha.ulaval.ca/	Doctor of Pharmacy (Doctorat en pharmacie)—Pharm.D. (as the 1st professional degree in pharmacy); Master of Science in Hospital Pharmacy (Maîtrise ès sciences en pharmacie d'hôpital)—M.Sc.
University of Alberta Faculty of Pharmacy & Pharmaceutical Sciences	Edmonton, Alberta	http://www.pharm.ualberta.ca/	Baccalaureate in Pharmacy—B.Sc. (Pharm); Master of Science—M.Sc.; Doctor of Philosophy—Ph.D.

(*continued*)

Table 36-1. Colleges/Schools/Faculties of Pharmacy in Canada

College/School/Faculty	Location	Web Site	Degrees Offered
University of British Columbia Faculty of Pharmaceutical Sciences	Vancouver, British Columbia	http://www.pharmacy.ubc.ca/	Baccalaureate in Pharmacy—B.Sc.Pharm.; Doctor of Pharmacy (post-bacc—Pharm.D.; Master of Science—M.Sc.; Doctor of Philosophy—Ph.D.
University of Manitoba Faculty of Pharmacy	Winnipeg, Manitoba	http://www.umanitoba.ca/faculties/pharmacy/	Baccalaureate in Pharmacy—B.Sc. (Pharm); Master of Science—M.Sc.; Doctor of Philosophy—Ph.D.
University of Saskatchewan College of Pharmacy and Nutrition	Saskatoon, Saskatchewan	http://www.usask.ca/pharmacy-nutrition/	Baccalaureate in Pharmacy—B.S.P.; Master of Science—M.Sc.; Doctor of Philosophy—Ph.D.
University of Toronto Leslie Dan Faculty of Pharmacy	Toronto, Ontario	http://www.pharmacy.utoronto.ca/Page4.aspx	Baccalaureate in Pharmacy— B.Sc.Pharm.; Combined Baccalaureate in Pharmacy—Doctor of Pharmacy—B.Sc.Pharm.-Pharm.D.; Specialist in Pharmaceutical Chemistry—B.Sc.; Doctor of Pharmacy (post-bacc)—Pharm.D.; Master of Science in Pharmaceutical Sciences—M.Sc.; Doctorate of Philosophy in Pharmaceutical Sciences—Ph.D.
University of Waterloo School of Pharmacy	Waterloo, Ontario	http://www.pharmacy.uwaterloo.ca/	Baccalaureate in Pharmacy— B.Sc.Pharm.; Master of Science—M.Sc.;

Note: Web sites are current as of June 15, 2011.

Quebec (OPQ, 2011). Regardless of jurisdiction, all pharmacists must pass a jurisprudence exam to obtain licensure.

According to the Canadian Constitution, education and licensure for all health professions falls within the jurisdiction of each of the ten provinces and three territories. However, for the sake of reciprocating licensure across provinces/territories, agreements were put in place to make this possible by having comparable levels of education. While many organizations existed previously, the Canadian Council for Accreditation of Pharmacy Programs (CCAPP) was granted Letters Patent by the Canadian government on January 5, 1993 (CCAPP, 2011a). CCAPP ensures a standard level of education across Canada; CCAPP is the Canadian equivalent to the Accreditation Council for Pharmacy Education (ACPE) in the United States.

The PEBC was established in 1963, and all provinces and territories, except Quebec, through the National Association of Pharmacy Regulatory Authorities (NAPRA), signed the Mutual Recognition Agreement in 2000, requiring PEBC registration as a prerequisite for licensure in Canada (CCAPP, 2011a). Of note is that the College of Pharmacists of Quebec (L'Ordre des Pharmaciens du Québec) is a member of NAPRA; they just do not follow the PEBC requirement for licensure to practice in Canada.

As can be seen in Table 36-2, there are many parallels between the education of pharmacists in Canada and the United States. While there are some differences that reflect various educational and regulatory variances, the education of pharmacists in both countries continues to increase its focus on cognitive services provided to patients, and away from the historical focus on the product. With a greater focus on cognitive services, the importance of appreciating and having a working knowledge of management concepts plays an increasingly significant role in practice.

Practicing Pharmacy in Canada

As of 2011, there were 33,734 pharmacists practicing in Canada, with 63 percent practicing in community pharmacy settings (NAPRA, 2011). In Canada, each province has a 'college of pharmacists,' similar to state boards/colleges of pharmacists in the United States that serves as the regulatory agency with a mandate to protect the public. NAPRA is the national organization consisting of all regulators across Canada; NAPRA is similar to the National Association of Boards of Pharmacy (NABP) in the United States.

MANAGING THE DISTRIBUTION OF DRUGS AND PHARMACEUTICAL SERVICES

In Canada, the health care system is primarily a publicly funded, privately delivered system of 13 interlocking, but independent, health insurance plans. All the systems share common characteristics, yet each one has unique aspects that reflect the local jurisdiction. While Canada-wide, publicly funded health care (Medicare) came into effect of July 1, 1968, some jurisdictions, most notably the province of Saskatchewan, had some form of publicly funded health care for some time before Medicare. Medicare today involves a complex system of financial transfers from the federal government to provincial/territorial government that has been for the most part in place since the Canada Health Act of 1984. The premise of the Canada Health Act rests on five principles: public administration, comprehensiveness, universality, portability, and accessibility. While the specifics of these principles are beyond the focus of this chapter, one can access more information by accessing the Health Canada Web site (www.hc-sc.gc.ca/hcs-sss/medi-assur/index-eng.php).

What may be surprising to some is that Medicare in Canada does not cover many outpatient procedures, costs, and services, including prescription drugs. As a result, many Canadians have some sort of third-party insurance coverage to help pay for some or all of the costs incurred for prescription drug therapy. Some of the coverage may come from provincial/territorial drug plans, federals plans for certain segments of the population, private insurance provided through an employer, or private insurance paid for by the individual.

Due to the number of drug plans available to Canadians, pharmacists spend a lot of time, and far

Table 36-2. Chronology of Pharmacy Education in Canada and the United States

Date	Canada	Date	The United States
Pre-1930s	Entry to practice via apprenticeships and programs affiliated with provincial universities	1920s–1930s	2- and 3-year programs leading to a Ph.C. (pharmaceutical chemist) or Ph.G. (graduate in pharmacy) designation
1930s–1950s	Introduction of 4-year university B.Sc. programs for entry to pharmacy practice, apprenticeships still exist in some provinces up to the 1940s	1940s	4-year B.Sc. programs become the universal standard for entry to practice
1930s–1970s	Technology school pharmacy diploma programs still in place in some provinces.	1950	The General Report of the Pharmaceutical Survey recommended that the pharmacy curriculum be extended to 6 years, leading to the Pharm.D. degree
1960s	Introduction of 5-year B.Sc. pharmacy programs	1950s	Ohio State University introduces a 5-year B.Sc. program (most other schools remain with the 4-year program)
1960s–1980s	2-year post-B.Sc. Masters of Pharmacy programs available for pharmacists seeking to advance management/clinical academic credentials especially for hospital pharmacy	1950s	USC and UCSF introduce entry-level Pharm.D. programs
Late 1960s–1970s	Hospital pharmacy residency programs introduced	Early 1960s	American Association of Colleges of Pharmacy adopts the 5-year program as the entry-level degree policy
1980s–1990s	Entry to pharmacy practice only via B.Sc. pharmacy degree, all schools now standardized on 5-year program (i.e., 1 + 4 or 2 + 3)	1960s–1980s	Wide spread availability of post-B.Sc. Pharm.D. programs
Early 1990s	First post-B.Sc. Pharm.D. programs start at UBC and Toronto	Mid-1970s	Universities of Nebraska and Michigan introduce entry-level Pharm.D.
1990s	Post-B.Sc. diploma in community pharmacy practice introduced at Laval University	1980s	Slow implementation of more entry-level Pharm.D. programs (B.Sc. still dominates as entry-level professional degree by approximately 2:1 margin)
1990	Community pharmacy residency programs reintroduced at two sites in Canada	1990s	ACPE notice to revise standards to accredit only professional pharmacy programs, awarding the Pharm.D. as the entry-level degree credential greatly accelerates pace conversion for US schools of B.Sc. curricula into Pharm.D. programs

1991	University of British Columbia established Canada's first 2-year postbaccalaureate Pharm.D. program in Canada; University of Toronto introduced a 2-year postbaccalaureate Pharm.D. program in 1992	Late 1990s	Large number of remaining post-B.Sc. Pharm.D. programs likely reflect the last entering classes of traditional B.Sc. programs and implementation of 'nontraditional' Pharm.D. programs geared to midcareer B.Sc. pharmacists wanting to enhance professional academic credentials
2001	PEBC introduced practice-based performance assessment for licensure of pharmacists (Objective Structured Clinical Examination—OSCE)	2000	Only colleges and schools offering Pharm.D. as the first professional degree could apply for accreditation, and graduates of baccalaureate programs would not be from accredited programs after July 1, 2005
2007	Université de Montréal moves to a Pharm.D. entry-level professional degree program, the first in Canada	2007	AACP Center for the Advancement of Pharmaceutical Education (CAPE) releases Social and Administrative Sciences Supplemental Educational Outcomes Based on the CAPE 2004 document focusing on educational objectives and outcomes
2009	Université de Montréal begins offering the Bachelor of Biopharmaceuticals (B.Sc.) degree; focuses on manufacturing and drug development to prepare students to enter the pharmaceutical industry or similar areas, but not to practice pharmacy	2011	124 colleges and schools of pharmacy with accreditation status; all 124 offer Pharm.D. as first professional degree and 27 offer Pharm.D. as a post-BS in pharmacy degree
2011	Ten Colleges and Schools of Pharmacy with accreditation status (8 offer program in English, two offer program in French); nine offer baccalaureate as first professional degree, one offers Pharm.D. as first professional degree, and two offer Pharm.D. as post-BS in pharmacy degree	2011	ACPE releases revised Accreditation Standards and Guidelines for the Professional Program in Pharmacy Leading to the Doctor of Pharmacy Degree
2011	Université Laval becomes the second school in Canada to offer the Pharm.D. as the first professional degree program		
2011	University of Toronto begins to offer a combined Bachelor of Science in Pharmacy–Doctor of Pharmacy Program; the program begins in a student's 4th year of the B.Sc.Phm. program, where students complete the requirements for the B.Sc.Phm. program in the Fall term and simultaneously begin coursework for the Pharm.D. program		

Source: Hill, 1999; AACP, 2007; Blackburn, 2007; Austin and Ensom, 2008; ACPE, 2011a; ACPE, 2011b; AACP, 2011; CCAPP, 2011b.

too much time dealing with the management of drug plan coverage. Thinking back to the scenario that began this chapter, Julia was dealing with one of the federal drug plans (NIHB) with a billing mechanism that is quite different from other drug plans.

In the province of Saskatchewan, the first province in Canada to offer some form of drug coverage for its residents (September 1, 1975), the Drug Plan now captures all prescription medications in a database. This allows the government to assess prescribing and dispensing patterns, and help track potential abuses of the system. As well, in case a patient has third-party coverage by a private insurer, the private insurer may limit reimbursement if coverage was not attempted to be received from the provincial drug plan first. Therefore, pharmacists must continually understand each unique drug plan and recall which organization to put billing through first; otherwise, an audit of drug claim submissions may result in discrepancies that result in the pharmacy repaying money it received for past claims that were not billed properly.

One major issue continuing to affect pharmacy in North America and beyond is that of prescription drug shortages (CPhA, 2011b; Chustecka, 2011). This may appear to be a relatively recent event to some, yet this has been a recurring issue. In an effort to help reduce the negative impact of drug shortages, new legislation is being proposed that would require prescription drug manufacturers to provide early notification to the US Food and Drug Administration (FDA) about potential shortages in supply (Chustecka, 2011). For example, if a manufacturer is having trouble obtaining ingredients for a drug, they would notify the FDA so that a contingency plan can be put in place.

While many view drug shortages as a clinical issue, minimizing their potentially deleterious effects is a management issue. The FDA is seeking to help manage and prevent shortages so that patient care is not impacted negatively. For example, if the FDA predicts a potential future shortage of a drug, it will work directly with the manufacturer(s) to help mitigate any potential negative affects by asking for the manufacturer(s) to increase production if possible (Chustecka, 2011).

It is also the individual pharmacist who plays a role in helping diminish any potential negative impact of drug shortages. For example, if a pharmacist notices a trend with a particular drug being hard to stock, the pharmacist should inform the FDA, Health Canada, or other federal regulators in a country. Not only is patient care potentially negatively impacted by drug shortages, by at the very least having to switch the patient to a different drug therapy, but the patient might have the perception that the pharmacist/pharmacy is at fault for the shortage. This negative impression may cause patients to switch pharmacies to another one; that is, unless the pharmacist does a good job managing the situation through such means as good communication with the patient and prescriber.

While many pharmacists might view drug shortages as a threat due to decreasing access to needed medications and as a result negatively impacting patient care, others may view it as an opportunity to more fully utilize pharmacists' expertise and compound drugs for patients. For example, phenazopyridine, the only approved urinary tract analgesic used to treat urinary tract pain, is no longer available in some jurisdictions. Realizing that many patients found pain relief from the medication, some pharmacists have started to compound phenazopyridine, turning a negative situation into a positive one, specifically for the patient, but also for the benefit of the pharmacy business. Additionally, in advocating for an enhanced scope of practice for pharmacists, the Canadian Pharmacists Association used the May 2011 Canadian federal election as an opportunity to draw attention to the vital role pharmacists can play to help mitigate the negative effects of drug shortages (CPhA, 2011c). For example, the CPhA argued that by increasing the scope of practice for pharmacists that the change would increase the opportunity for pharmacists to advise on alternative therapies when the one prescribed is shorted without the patient needing to revisit their physician (CPhA, 2011c).

Requirements of Pharmacist Managers

Whether one has an official title as 'manager' or not, all pharmacists manage people, places, and processes. "As *managers* pharmacy graduates use management skills in their daily practice to optimize the care of patients, to ensure the safe and effective distribution of medications, and to make efficient use of health resources" (AFPC, 2010). To address the requirement of all pharmacists to be managers in some respect, and draw attention to its importance, the Association of Faculties of Pharmacy of Canada (AFPC) (similar to the American Association of Colleges of Pharmacy) recently highlighted/reinforced the seven main educational outcomes for entry-level pharmacy degree programs (AFPC, 2010).

The seven outcomes focus on the pharmacist as care provider, communicator, collaborator, manager, advocate, scholar, and professional. The outcomes of pharmacist as manager center around five main areas of competence; that is, pharmacists manage their personal practice; manage the safe and efficient distribution of medications, participate in quality assurance and improvement programs, manage the staff under their direct supervision, and manage to maintain the sustainability of the practice.

Once in practice, pharmacy graduates use management skills routinely when seeking to optimize the care of patients, ensuring the safe and effective distribution of medications, and when making efficient use of health resources, including utilizing expertise to its fullest extent. Ultimately, it is up to individual pharmacists, and in particular managers, to take full responsibility for the care provided to patients, which may include no drug therapy at all. As well, in community practice, pharmacists must balance the business and professional realities of practice.

The pharmacist as manager, whether having the title formally or not, is required to (AFPC, 2010):

- *Manage their personal practice*
    - Set priorities and manage their time to balance patient care, workflow, and practice requirements
    - Adapt their practice to fulfill evolving professional roles
- *Manage the safe and efficient distribution of medications*
    - Utilize inventory control concepts to maintain an inventory control system
    - Manage the distribution of medication in a variety of settings
    - Evaluate the factors critical to safe and efficient medication distribution systems including pharmacy layout/design, workflow, technology and automation
    - Anticipate, recognize and manage human, environmental and medication distribution situations that place patients at risk
- *Participate in quality assurance and improvement programs*
    - Evaluate the quality of care and cost effectiveness of services they provide
    - Disclose, manage, and report adverse drug events
    - Disclose, manage, and report errors, incidents, and unsafe practices
    - Participate in formal planning for practice change and implementation of services to meet patient's needs and/or improve the quality of care provided
    - Adapt to change, providing new or emerging services as consistent with management's practice change plans
- *Manage the staff under their direct supervision*
    - Supervise members of the pharmacy team, including pharmacy technicians, to ensure competent performance of functions
    - Ensure that pharmacy technicians and staff are delegated and undertake functions appropriate to their training and legislation
    - Manage workload to prioritize provision of professional services
    - Function as a role model for professional and support staff
    - Participate in staff selection, training, development, and evaluation
- *Manage to maintain the sustainability of the practice*
    - Understand the impact of funding and payment policies on the provision of professional services
    - Create a business plan for the provision of professional services

- Participate in strategic planning for their practice site
- Understand marketing principles in the context of supply and demand for professional services
- Incorporate the use of technology

Province-Specific Example of an Increased Focus on Responsibilities of a Pharmacy Manager

In the province of Saskatchewan, the Saskatchewan College of Pharmacists (SCP), the provincial regulator for the profession, brought an increased focus on the significant role and responsibilities of licensed pharmacists that take on the role of pharmacy manager. On top of the regular role and responsibilities that comes with being a pharmacist, the pharmacy manager, on an operational level, is required to (SCP, 2010)

1. Ensure adherence to the legislation governing pharmacy practice, including, but not limited to, the following:
   a. Food and Drugs Act and Regulations
   b. Controlled Drugs and Substances Act
   c. Narcotic Control Regulations
   d. The Pharmacy Act, 1996, and Bylaws
   e. Saskatchewan College of Pharmacists policies, guidelines, and standards
2. Be responsible for establishing policies and procedures to be followed by pharmacy personnel that are in accordance with pharmacy law, acceptable pharmacy practice, and professional standards
3. Be accountable to SCP for all professional activities within the pharmacy
4. Provide information to the Registrar concerning the operation or conduct of the pharmacy and pharmacists employed, if so required by the College
5. Ensure a system of communication and documentation of information to provide consistency of care that includes
   - Ensure relief pharmacists have all required operational information.
   - Ensure there is a pharmacist–patient interaction with each prescription and that there is documentation of the interaction on the patient's profile.
   - Ensure there is a communication log book in which relevant practice information can be documented and shared with all pharmacy staff.
   - Ensure there is an orientation manual for all staff to be able to reference.
6. Ensure the prescription processes and procedures used by the pharmacy are designed to minimize errors, protect the public, and adhere to the Standards of Practice.
7. Ensure a system is in place for the implementation/maintenance of a medication error follow up and reporting protocol.
8. Ensure an adequate staffing complement for a safe practice.

The roles and responsibilities listed above are common in many jurisdictions, including for example in the United States. In North Carolina, that state's Board of Pharmacy has a document outlining the *Pharmacist-Manager Responsibilities* (NCBP, 2010). While one may not have the intention of becoming a pharmacy manager, especially when first entering practice, this is not always an option, as some employers will appoint new graduates as pharmacy manager out of necessity. Ultimately, it is up to the individual to understand what is required of them as a pharmacy manager, but employers and regulators also have a duty to inform managers of their roles and responsibilities.

MANAGERIAL ISSUES SURROUNDING AN EXPANDED SCOPE OF PRACTICE

Like other countries and jurisdictions around the world, pharmacists in Canada are receiving various levels of prescriptive authority, ability to provide injections, and expanding their scope of practice in various other ways. While the actual services performed rely on an advanced level of therapeutic skills and knowledge, for the services to be provided safely and efficiently, pharmacists must consider the managerial implications of offering these value-added services. For example, if a pharmacy has focused typically on prescription counts, and is now also adding prescribing and providing injections, managerial implications, from the logistics to financial viability, come into play; the managerial implications may be ensuring appropriate staffing levels or that the counseling room is ready for consultations. Otherwise, the services may be hindering the level of patient care as opposed to raising it.

Furthermore, one must consider also the target market in which the pharmacy exists and whether a new service aligns with the needs of the community/market (see Chapters 21–22). For example, a pharmacist may have received certification to conduct lung function testing and be remunerated for providing such services, and therefore want to implement it into the service offering at your pharmacy; however, if there is a negligible prevalence of asthma/COPD in the community (as recognized by a low number of prescriptions for asthma/COPD-related medications), then providing it would likely be a unwise decision.

In all Canadian provinces except one, pharmacists have the ability to provide emergency prescription refills and renew/extend prescription for chronic medications (CPhA, 2011d). Further to this, in most provinces pharmacists can make therapeutic substitution and change the drug dose/formulation, and two provinces (Saskatchewan and Nova Scotia) recently passed legislation authorizing pharmacists to prescribe drugs as part of a minor ailment scheme (CPhA, 2011d).

Of course, with any expansion to the scope of practice of pharmacists comes the need to obtain further training; training focuses mainly on the clinical aspects, including differential diagnosis, but also the managerial and administrative aspects of the expanded scope. For example, Saskatchewan pharmacists recently received training for three minor ailments: cold sores, insect bites, and acne (CPDP, 2011). As part of the training, pharmacists reviewed a decision-making framework and discussed issues around billing.

PROGRAM-SPECIFIC MANAGERIAL CONSIDERATIONS

In the province of Saskatchewan, the advocacy organization for pharmacists in the province is the Pharmacists' Association of Saskatchewan (PAS), and along with the support of the Saskatchewan Ministry of Health (provincial government), a program was created to help individuals wanting to quit using tobacco. PAS started the Partnership to Assist with Cessation of Tobacco (PACT) in 2004; the PACT program was created without any financial support, but in 2008, the Program was awarded funding from Health Canada (federal government). It was in 2010 that the Saskatchewan Ministry of Health aligned with the ongoing work of the program because it fit well into the cessation pillar of the tobacco reduction strategy—*Building a Healthier Saskatchewan* (Saskatchewan Ministry of Health, 2010a). As well, in 2010, the Tobacco Addiction Recovery (TAR) program was developed and implemented targeting a specific demographic—Aboriginal peoples. While both programs utilize pharmacists' expertise in smoking cessation and require pharmacists to obtain additional training, the TAR program targeted Aboriginal peoples, who use tobacco products in traditional ceremonies and as offerings, and therefore have specific needs regarding reducing tobacco use (Saskatchewan Ministry of Health, 2010b).

While there are examples of smoking cessation and other programs in various jurisdictions around the world, like implementing any new service offering into an existing practice setting, managerial and administrative considerations, such as advanced training for pharmacists and adequate staffing levels, can be overlooked; this can cause the uptake of the program to be suboptimal, and in some instances, lead to complete failure of the program of a clinically proven intervention. The PACT program faced many hurdles in implementing the program in Saskatchewan, many of which are not discussed here; one change that was made to better target and meet the needs of high users of tobacco, in particular, Aboriginal peoples who are two to three times more likely to smoke tobacco than non-Aboriginal people, was to develop the TAR program. For example, the TAR program acknowledges the sacred use of tobacco and focuses on the elimination of nonsacred tobacco, while the PACT program focuses on eliminating all tobacco. TAR offers culturally relevant services to Aboriginal peoples, services that were not offered prior to the implementation of the program, and many times were not always appropriate.

Another aspect that has caused some adjustment to the PACT program is in regard to billing. PACT-trained pharmacists are able to bill the Alternative Reimbursement Fund, administered by the Saskatchewan Health Drug Plan, $2.00 per minute to a maximum of $300 per patient, per calendar year (Saskatchewan Ministry of Health, 2009); yet, many PACT-trained pharmacists were not billing at all, while others billed regularly. Moreover, there are some pharmacists who were PACT trained and providing smoking cessation interventions, yet not billing for their services. PACT pharmacists in the province continue to inform the PACT/TAR program coordinator that the billing process is too cumbersome for pharmacists to navigate. For example, there are different levels of PACT services—bronze, bronze plus, silver, and gold, as well as follow-up; with all the different levels of potential services and corresponding levels of billing, and the fact that billing is done through the Drug Plan Web site, and not the pharmacy computer system, a pharmacy that does not have an adequate management strategy in place could lose out on remuneration, not to mention the ability of pharmacists to practice to a higher level clinically. As a result of the insight PACT pharmacists have provided, and with the assistance of the Ministry of Health, the billing system is being revised so that PACT fees can be billed just like a prescription or other prescriptive authority assessment fees, using pseudo-DINs (billing codes).

Overall, the provision of services by pharmacists/pharmacies in Canada is dynamic, resulting in no single, uniform method of delivering services. This is the result of different public drug plans in each province, influence from third-party programs and the willingness to cover pharmacist services beyond basic dispensing fees and markups, and the ability and desire for individuals to pay for services out of pocket, among other factors. Therefore, understanding and appreciating the ways in which to manage a pharmacy, from the procurement of inventory, to conducting a thorough environmental scan, to using the appropriate promotional tools are key to the success of a pharmacy.

These managerial considerations, while primarily focused on community pharmacy examples, do apply to other practice types, in particular hospital practice. While Canada and most other Western countries have a public health care system, all hospitals/health regions work within budgetary constraints. Therefore, if one wants to provide new counseling services on a patient's new drug therapy post-MI, a strategy needs to be formulated, from the clinical benefits, to the financial benefits, to considerations of whether it is a service that should be publicly funded or whether it is an out-of-pocket expense to the patient, and presented to the appropriate administrative personnel. Otherwise, a clinically effective intervention may never be realized within ones institution if it does not consider how it may impact stakeholders, from patients, to other health care practitioners.

As of January 1, 2011, Canada had just under 34,000 licensed pharmacists, with the majority (63 percent) practicing in community pharmacies; furthermore, there were 8,637 community pharmacies and 290 inpatient hospital pharmacies (NAPRA, 2011). While there are no accurate figures on the number of chain versus independent pharmacies, the Canadian Association of Chain Drug Stores (CACDS)–similar to the National Association of Chain Drug Stores (NACDS) in the United States—boasts a membership that operates 6,200 community pharmacies in Canada (71.8 percent) (CACDS, 2011a); however, some independent pharmacy groups are members of CACDS, so the accuracy of this figure may be limited.

Revenues for Canadian community pharmacies have traditionally, like in the United States, been derived from dispensing/professional fees and markups; in other words, from the provision of a product. While this remains as a primary and significant portion of revenues derived directly from the dispensary, alternative mechanisms of revenue generation are being implemented; some of this is forced on the profession by changes in government pharmaceutical policy, while others are proactively looking for alternative revenue sources realizing that the traditional sources of revenue are not sustainable, nor professionally rewarding.

Some governments, that pay for between ~31.8 percent and ~54.5 percent of drug expenditures in Canada (the remainder comes from private third-party plans and out of pocket), have implemented changes to policies regarding reimbursement of prescribed medications (CACDS, 2011b). For example, a recent study examining international generic drug prices discovered that Canadian generic drug prices were, on average, more than double those in the United States and more than five times higher than in New Zealand (PMPRB, 2010). In Canada, the Patented Medicine Prices Review Board (PMPRB) is in place to control the market prices, or the maximum amount a manufacturer can charge in Canada, for patented/brand name medications; specifically, the PMPRB has two mandates—regulatory, to ensure that prices of patented medicines in Canada are not excessive, and reporting, to report on pharmaceutical trends of all medicines, and on the research and development spending of innovative pharmaceutical companies (PMPRB, 2011). Since there is no agency like the PMPRB that regulates the prices for generic prescription medications in Canada, the report stating that prices were higher for generics in Canada was not an entirely new, nor surprising, finding; however, it is one area that provincial governments could focus on to reduce the growing prescription drug budgets.

In 2006, in the province of Ontario, the provincial government changed the price paid by the public Ontario Drug Benefit (ODB) Plan to 50 percent of the branded equivalent reference price; in July 2010, it further reduced the price paid for generics by the ODP to 25 percent, while what manufacturers could charge private payers was set at 50 percent; by April 2012, it will be at 25 percent (Law et al., 2011). Furthermore, the Ontario government eliminated promotional allowances (funding provided to pharmacies for using a specific generic manufacture for its drugs), funding that many pharmacies, particularly independent pharmacies, relied on to help to remain sustainable; the markup paid for ODB prescriptions also was reduced, but the government implemented policies to remunerate professional services provided by pharmacists (Ontario Ministry of Health and Long-Term Care, 2011).

Standing offer contracts (SOCs) are another example of administrative measures managed by pharmacists. These are implemented through policy changes to reduce drug expenditures. An SOC is similar to the professional allowance the Ontario government eliminated, but the funding is provided to the drug plan via savings realized through volume purchasing from a single manufacturer (economies of scale), as opposed to the individual pharmacy. As an example, the Saskatchewan Ministry of Health, for high-volume drugs in select interchangeable categories, seeks to obtain the lowest price possible from a manufacturer by signing an SOC (Saskatchewan Ministry of Health, 2010c). Once the Ministry has accepted and signed a SOC, the successful manufacturer has to guarantee delivery of the given drug to Saskatchewan pharmacies in return for the manufacture's almost exclusive contract to supply the drug for a finite period of time (Saskatchewan Ministry of Health, 2011c). The only time a pharmacy can fill an equivalent to the SOC drug is when the manufacturer fails to supply the drug; as one can imagine, with this comes a requirement to ensure pharmacies are adhering to the Ministry's SOC by conducting audits, and the onus also falls on pharmacists to know which drugs have an SOC.

PHARMACY MANAGEMENT IN ALTERNATIVE SYSTEMS OUTSIDE NORTH AMERICA

Regardless of where one practices, an awareness of the environment, micro and macro, should be gained through an environmental scan. In particular, discussion occurred in chapters on strategic planning (Chapter 4) and marketing applications (Chapter 22) that highlighted the need to conduct environmental scanning on a regular basis. By having an up-to-date appreciation for what is happening in the current market, the pharmacist is able to have a proactive strategy in place and will be less likely to be taken by surprise when changes occur. This also aids the pharmacist to shape the practice environment, as those who do not plan and understand the market in which they practice are taking a reactive approach to practice, and as a result, are continually following practice changes dictated to them by others.

The provision of services around the world differs, sometimes dramatically, as do the resultant managerial implications arising from unique delivery, reimbursement, and financing mechanisms in each country. While this textbook and chapter has focused primarily on practice in North America, there is considerable value to consider alternative health care delivery systems and their financing, as change is inevitable, and understanding the ramifications of systems on management allows pharmacists to be prepared for future shifts in practice.

Australia

Over 30,000 pharmacists currently practice in Australia, with the majority practicing in community pharmacies (PCHR, 2011). There are currently 18 schools/colleges of pharmacy in Australia, offering the Bachelor of Pharmacy (B.Pharm.) or Master of Pharmacy (M.Pharm.) entry-level degree (APC, 2010); the M.Pharm. entry-to-practice degree is a postgraduate degree that one can pursue once they have select Bachelor degrees, such as biology, chemistry, and so on. (Marriott et al., 2008; UC, 2011).

Many changes to practice that are beneficial for pharmacists, and more importantly patients, have occurred in Australia (Roberts et al., 2003; Roberts et al, 2004). Australia continues to be one of the only jurisdictions around that world that provides compensation to pharmacists for providing clinical interventions where they identify, resolve, and document drug-related issues (CPhA, 2011b); this program increases the number of clinical interventions provided and documented, and also improves communication between patient, prescriber, and pharmacist. This program is similar to medication therapy management programs in the United States.

On July 1, 2010 the Fifth Community Pharmacy Agreement (Fifth Agreement) between the Australian Government and the Pharmacy Guild of Australia began; this agreement covers pharmacy services for a 5-year term (Australian Government, 2010). The Pharmacy Guild of Australia is an organization that advocates for the interests of community pharmacy. These agreements allow services to be more or less standardized across Australia, as opposed to having separate state agreements.

The Fifth Agreement "recognises the key role played by community pharmacy in primary health care through the delivery of Pharmaceutical Benefits Scheme (PBS) medicines and related services" (Australian Government, 2010). This agreement focuses on value for money and looks to increase patient-centered approaches and services by better targeting pharmacy services using a quality framework (Australian Government, 2010). Some of the highlights of the Fifth Agreement include (Australian Government, 2010):

- Total funding for the delivery of professional services over the 5-year agreement of $663 million (AUD)
- Timelier and easier access to services in a pharmacy, patient's home, or aged care facility;
- Greater focus on patient services, including a patient service charter to inform patients about services offered, and information and advice patients should receive from their community pharmacy
- A continued focus on Aboriginal, Torres Strait Islander, and Rural Programs to ensure equity of access and to support the rural pharmacy workforce

The continuing relationship between the Australian Government and organized pharmacy (through the Guild) recognizes the expertise of pharmacists and the role pharmacists can and should play in patient care. With these agreements come a lot of administrative and managerial aspects that must be followed in order to receive remuneration, and to ensure that these agreements continue on a go forward basis.

New Zealand

There are currently two schools/colleges of pharmacy in New Zealand, both offering the Bachelor of

Pharmacy (B.Pharm.) as the entry-level degree (PCNZ, 2011). Over 3,000 pharmacists currently practice in New Zealand, with most being community pharmacists (PSNZ, 2011). Organized pharmacy in Australia and New Zealand tend to work rather closely together; part of this may be the fact that New Zealand only has two schools/colleges of pharmacy.

In New Zealand, pharmacists, pharmacy technicians, and pharmacy assistants all have distinct roles, especially in community pharmacy. There are four main professional leadership and advocacy organizations representing pharmacists in New Zealand, and a regulatory council that is responsible for upholding the Health Practitioners Competency Assurance Act (Scahill, 2011). Each leadership/advocacy organization supports a specific sector of pharmacy: Pharmaceutical Society of New Zealand (www.psnz.org.nz) primarily supports community pharmacists; the Pharmacy Guild of New Zealand (www.pgnz.org.nz) supports community pharmacy owners; the New Zealand Hospital Pharmacists' Association (www.nzhpa.org.nz) largely supports hospital pharmacists; and the Clinical Advisory Pharmacists Association (http://capanz.org) whose members are largely primary care pharmacists.

Like pharmacy in North America, pharmacy in New Zealand is seeing a shift in focus to greater collaboration between health care practitioners, a greater focus on enhanced cognitive services, and away from the product-centered approach to pharmacy, and a greater focus on population health (Scahill, 2011). Community pharmacists must embrace new approaches to practice and drive a clearly defined agenda of renewal to meet the needs of health funders, patients, and other primary care providers. There are significant barriers that need to be overcome to change; some of these are financial but many are professional and organizational and require a genuine commitment from the whole primary health care sector (Scahill, 2011).

United Kingdom

More than 49,000 pharmacists practice in the United Kingdom (UK), with approximately 70 percent of pharmacists practicing in community pharmacies (RPSGP, 2011a). There are currently 26 schools/colleges of pharmacy in the United Kingdom, all offering the 4-year Master of Pharmacy (M.Pharm.) entry-to-practice degree (Sosabowski and Gard, 2008; RPSGP, 2011b). In many respects, the United Kingdom has been the leader in pharmacy practice change.

In the United Kingdom, the National Health Service (NHS), the publicly funded (through general taxation) health care system, born in 1948, is "free" at the point of use, but a patient must first register with a family physician to 'enter' the system; it is the first time in the United Kingdom that hospitals, pharmacists, physicians, nurses, opticians and dentists are brought under one administrative organization (NHS, 2009). In 1952, the NHS charged one shilling (5 pence ≈8 cents) for prescriptions; in 1965, prescription charges were eliminated and prescriptions were free until 1968 when charges for prescriptions were reintroduced (NHS, 2009).

The NHS is constantly changing to adapt to the needs of citizens and the economic realities of health care delivery; changes to the economic aspects of the NHS in the United Kingdom in the 1990s coincided with changes in the way services were delivered, including new professional groups such as primary care pharmacists (Silcock et al., 2004). While the NHS is UK wide, decisions about specific aspects are devolved to the administration in each country (Scottish Parliament, National Assembly for Wales, Northern Ireland Executive).

The changes to the funding model in the United Kingdom created Primary Care Trusts (PCTs), which are similar to traditional family physician practices that employ other clinical (many times including pharmacists) and administrative staff. The difference between traditional practices and PCTs is that PCTs are given a global budget for a set "roster" of patients, commonly around 120,000; the amount given to a PCT is based on many indicators, but one is the patient history of the roster (Silcock et al., 2004). For example, a PCT would receive minimal annual funding for a healthy, 6-year-old female whose health care needs are projected to be minimal, whereas a PCT would receive substantially more annual funding for a 85-year-old female with diabetes, requires dialysis, has congestive heart failure, and is on 11 chronic medications.

Pharmacy in the United Kingdom is more similar to practice in North America than to other European countries. The two main streams of practice are community and hospital pharmacy, with primary care pharmacy being a relatively new area of practice. Community pharmacists practice in a similar fashion in the United Kingdom to that in North America, while the primary role of hospital pharmacists is on providing clinical advise, as opposed to supplying medications (Silcock et al., 2004). Primary care pharmacists have emerged as a hybrid of sorts between community and hospital pharmacists. Primary care pharmacists work within PCTs in a clinical and administrative role; many times, they are pharmaceutical care advisors who develop policy and manage budgets, and also work with family physicians regarding drug audits and medication reviews (Silcock et al., 2004).

With the changing roles of pharmacists within the United States come new administrative and managerial roles. Therefore, while the clinical skills and expertise of pharmacists are being better utilized in the changing roles, the challenge is to ensure that the roles continue to evolve through proper management, including evaluation. As well, the role of advocacy, for the profession and for patients, is vital.

As can be seen in the short review of pharmacy management in a select number of countries outside North America, many issues and the way in which they are handled share commonalities. Overall flexibility and the ability to adapt and change one's practice, ideally proactively, will benefit the individual pharmacist, as well as many other stakeholders, most importantly the patient; understanding pharmacy management will allow one to thrive in the dynamic pharmacy practice environment.

REVISITING THE SCENARIO

After sitting on the phone with NIHB and trying to advocate for her patient to get the new aerosol chamber covered, Julia decided to ask the patient's parents if they could afford the device if she could offer it to them at cost. After talking to her manager, Julia was able to sell the aerosol chamber to the patient's parents at cost. Once the patient and his family left the pharmacy, Julia's manager pulled her aside to complement her on the way she handled the situation, and for the fact that she did not just say "no," to the patient's parents; instead she searched for a solution. Her manager was even more impressed considering she was an intern, and her manager said that he has worked with numerous pharmacists over his 20 years of community practice that simply would have said "no, it is not covered". He could tell Julia was going to make an excellent pharmacist and patient advocate.

CONCLUSION

As can be discerned through this brief overview of pharmacy practice and management outside the United States, there are many similarities between the way pharmacy is practiced in the United States in comparison to the countries discussed in this chapter. Where the differences occur are in the more micro details of practice, such as third-party insurance, billing issues, and cognitive services offered and remunerated. Knowledge of practice management in these other systems will allow the pharmacist to appreciate the way pharmacy is practiced in their current system but also be prepared to adapt when the current system changes.

QUESTIONS FOR FURTHER DISCUSSION

1. Are there examples in this chapter that you could see working in a pharmacy environment to which you have been exposed?
2. How might understanding the way pharmacy is practiced outside of the United States improve your own effectiveness as a pharmacist and benefit your career?
3. Regardless of practice setting, why is it important to continually conduct environmental scanning? What is the result of failing to adequately understand one's market?

REFERENCES

Accreditation Council for Pharmacy Education (ACPE). 2011a. *Accreditation Standards and Guidelines for the Professional Program in Pharmacy Leading to the Doctor of Pharmacy Degree.* Chicago, IL: Accreditation Council for Pharmacy Education.

Accreditation Council for Pharmacy Education (ACPE). 2011b. Frequently asked questions: Accreditation statistics. Available at http://www.acpe-accredit.org/deans/faqs.asp; accessed on June 14, 2011.

American Association of Colleges of Pharmacy (AACP). 2007. Social and administrative sciences supplemental educational outcomes based on CAPE 2004. Available at http://www.aacp.org/resources/education/Documents/SocialandAdminDEC06.pdf; accessed on June 24, 2011.

American Association of Colleges of Pharmacy (AACP). 2011. Academic pharmacy's vital statistics. Available at http://www.aacp.org/about/Pages/Vitalstats.aspx; accessed on June 14, 2011.

American Pharmacists Association (APhA). 2011. Getting your license. Available at http://www.pharmacist.com/AM/Template.cfm?Section=Career_Resources&Template=/CM/ContentDisplay.cfm&ContentID=11570; accessed on June 14, 2011.

Association of Faculties of Pharmacy of Canada (AFPC). 2010. *Educational Outcomes for First Professional Degree Programs in Pharmacy (Entry-to-Practice Pharmacy Programs) in Canada.* Vancouver, BC: Association of Faculties of Pharmacy of Canada.

Austin Z, Ensom M. 2008. Education of pharmacists in Canada. *Am J Pharm Educ* 72(6):128.

Australian Government. 2010. *Fifth Community Pharmacy Agreement Between the Australian Government and the Pharmacy Guild of Australia.* Canberra, ACT, Australia: Department of Health and Ageing.

Australian Pharmacy Council (APC). 2010. Accredited pharmacy schools. Available at http://www.pharmacycouncil.org.au/accreditation_accreditatedpharmacyschools.html; accessed on June 21, 2011.

Blackburn J. 2007. Supporting Professional Education. In Gillis C, Rantucci M (eds.) *Canadian Pharmacists Association 1907–2007: 100 Years of Leadership in Pharmacy.* Ottawa, ON: Canadian Pharmacists Association, pp. 105–14.

Canadian Association of Chain Drug Stores (CACDS). 2011a. Home. Available at http://www.cacds.com/en/; accessed on July 28, 2011.

Canadian Association of Chain Drug Stores (CACDS). 2011b. Canadian pharmacy outlook 2011. Available at http://www.cacds.com/pdf/2010_12_06-CDR_Canadian_Pharmacy_Outlook_2011.pdf; accessed on July 28, 2011.

Canadian Council for the Accreditation of Pharmacy Programs (CCAPP). 2011a. History and mission. Available at http://www.ccapp-accredit.ca/the_council/history_and_mission/; accessed on June 3, 2011.

Canadian Council for the Accreditation of Pharmacy Programs (CCAPP). 2011b. University degree programs in pharmacy. Available at http://www.ccapp-accredit.ca/accredited_programs/degree/; accessed on June 14, 2011.

Canadian Pharmacists Association (CPhA). 2011a. Canadian faculties and schools of pharmacy. Available at http://www.pharmacists.ca/content/about_cpha/about_pharmacy_in_can/directory/associations.cfm?main_heading=Canadian$Faculties$and$Schools$of$Pharmacy; accessed on June 21, 2011.

Canadian Pharmacists Association (CPhA). 2011b. *CPhA Stakeholder Update: June 2011.* Ottawa, ON: Canadian Pharmacists Association.

Canadian Pharmacists Association (CPhA). 2011c. Talking points—Drug shortages. Available at http://www.pharmacists.ca/content/about_cpha/whats_happening/government_affairs/pdf/TalkingPoints-DrugShortages_Election2011.pdf; accessed on July 28, 2011.

Canadian Pharmacists Association (CPhA). 2011d. *Pharmacists' Medication Management Services: Environmental Scan of Canadian and International Services.* Ottawa, ON: Canadian Pharmacists Association.

Chong E. 2011. *Cross-Jurisdictional Scan of Legislative and Policy Framework.* Ottawa, ON: Canadian Pharmacists Association.

Chustecka Z. 2011. Early warning system for prescription drug shortages. *Medscape Medical News.* Available at http://www.medscape.com/viewarticle/737038; accessed on June 23, 2011.

College of Pharmacists of Quebec/L'Ordre des pharmaciens du Québec (OPQ). 2011. Admission à la pratique. Available at http://www.opq.org/fr/admission; accessed on June 24, 2011.

Continuing Professional Development for Pharmacists (CPDP). 2011. Sunday Seminar Series: Prescriptive Authority for Pharmacists Minor Ailments Training. Saskatoon, SK. Available at http://www.usask.ca/pharmacy-nutrition/services/Sunday%20Seminar%20Brochure%202011%20final.pdf; accessed on June 1, 2011.

Hill D. 1999. *Association of Faculties of Pharmacy of Canada Background Paper: The "Entry-Level" Doctor of Pharmacy (Pharm.D.) Degree Issue for Schools of Pharmacy in Canada.* Vancouver, BC: Association of Faculties of Pharmacy of Canada.

Law MR, Ytsma A, Morgan SG. 2011. *The Short-term Impact of Ontario's Generic Pricing Reforms.* Vancouver, BC: University of British Columbia Centre for Health Services and Policy Research.

Marriott J, Nation R, Roller L, et al. 2008. Pharmacy education in the context of Australian practice. *Am J Pharm Educ* 72(6):1–12, 131.

National Association of Pharmacy Regulatory Authorities (NAPRA). 2011. National Statistics. Available at http://129.128.180.43/pages/Practice_Resources/National_Statistics.aspx?id=2103; accessed on June 14, 2011.

National Health Service (NHS). 2009. NHS History. Available at http://www.nhs.uk/NHSEngland/thenhs/nhshistory/Pages/NHShistory1948.aspx; accessed on June 24, 2011.

North Carolina Board of Pharmacy (NCBP). 2010. Pharmacist-Manager responsibilities. Available at http://www.ncbop.org/Forms%20and%20Applications%20-%20Pharmacies/Pharmacist-MgrResponsibilities.pdf; accessed on June 8, 2011.

Ontario Ministry of Health and Long-Term Care. 2011. Transparent drug system for patients Act, 2006. Available at http://www.health.gov.on.ca/english/public/legislation/drugs/hu_drugsact.html; accessed on July 27, 2011.

Patented Medicine Prices Review Board (PMPRB). 2010. Generic drugs in Canada: Price trends and international price comparisons, 2007. Available at http://www.pmprb-cepmb.gc.ca/cmfiles/npduis/NPDUIS-GenDrugs-PriceTrends-e.pdf; accessed on July 25, 2011.

Patented Medicine Prices Review Board (PMPRB). 2011. About the PMPRB. Available at http://www.pmprb-cepmb.gc.ca/english/View.asp?x=175&mp=87; accessed on July 28, 2011.

Pharmaceutical Society of New Zealand (PSNZ). 2011. Keeping the profession strong. Available at http://www.psnz.org.nz/public/home/index.aspx; accessed on June 21, 2011.

Pharmacist Coalition for Health Reform (PCHR). 2011. Pharmacists: The best kept secret in health care. Available at http://pharmacistsforhealth.com.au/; accessed on June 21, 2011.

Pharmacy Council of New Zealand (PCNZ). 2011. Universities. Available at http://www.pharmacycouncil.org.nz/links; accessed on June 21, 2011.

Roberts A, Benrimoj SI, Chen T, Williams K, Aslani P. 2003. *An Investigation into Business and Professional Facilitators for Change for the Pharmacy Profession in Light of the Third Guild/ Government Agreement.* Sydney, NSW, Australia: Pharmacy Practice Research Group, University of Sydney.

Roberts A, Benrimoj SI, Chen T, Williams K, Aslani P. 2004. *Quantification of Facilitators to Accelerate Uptake of Cognitive Pharmaceutical Services (CPS) in Community Pharmacy.* Sydney, NSW, Australia: Pharmacy Practice Research Group, University of Sydney.

Royal Pharmaceutical Society of Great Britian (RPSGP). 2011a. What do pharmacists do? Available at http://www.rpharms.com/ipharmacist/what-do-pharmacists-do-.asp; accessed on June 21, 2011.

Royal Pharmaceutical Society of Great Britian (RPSGP). 2011b. Where can I Study? Available at http://www.rpharms.com/what-qualifications-do-i-need-/where-can-i-study-.asp; accessed on June 21, 2011.

Saskatchewan College of Pharmacists (SCP). 2010. Responsibilities of a pharmacy manager. Available at https://scp.in1touch.org/uploaded/58/web/refmanual/Responsibilities%20of%20a%20Pharmacy%20Manager-February%202010.pdf; accessed on June 9, 2011.

Saskatchewan Ministry of Health (SK Health). 2009. *PACT – Partnership to Assist with Cessation of Tobacco, Claims Payment – Cognitive Services.* Regina, SK: Saskatchewan Ministry of Health.

Saskatchewan Ministry of Health (SK Health). 2010a. Building a healthier saskatchewan: A strategy to reduce tobacco use. Available at http://www.health.gov.sk.ca/Default.aspx?DN=9909877e-a9e7-4288-9cb8-49fcc350342e&l=English; accessed on June 9, 2011.

Saskatchewan Ministry of Health (SK Health). 2010b. Partnership to Assist with Cessation of Tobacco (PACT). Available at www.makeapact.ca; accessed on May 19, 2011.

Saskatchewan Ministry of Health (SK Health). 2010c. Cost saving measures. Available at http://www.health.gov.sk.ca/drug-plan-cost-saving; accessed on July 25, 2011.

Scahill S. 2011. Summary of the New Zealand pharmacy scene. Personal communication. School of Pharmacy, The University of Auckland. June 20, 2011.

Silcock J, Raynor DKT, Petty D. 2004. The organisation and development of primary care pharmacy in the United Kingdom. *Health Policy* 67:207–14.

Sosabowski M, Gard P. 2008. Pharmacy Education in the United Kingdom. *Am J Pharm Educ* 72(6):1–7, 130.

United States Food and Drug Administration (FDA). 2011. Drug shortages. Available at http://www.fda.gov/Drugs/DrugSafety/DrugShortages/default.htm; accessed on June 23, 2011.

University of Canberra (UC). 2011. Faculty of Health: Pharmacy. Available at http://www.canberra.edu.au/faculties/health/pharmacy; accessed on June 21, 2011.

INDEX

Page numbers with f and t indicates figure and table.